Diseases in a FLASH!

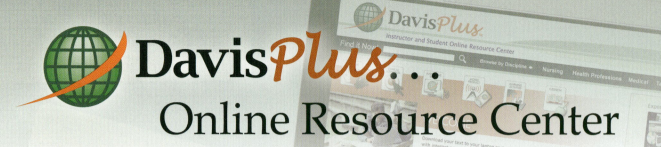
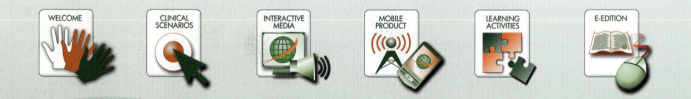
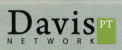
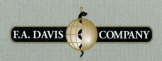

Diseases in a FLASH!

An Interactive, Flash-Card Approach

Sharon Eagle, RN, MSN
Nursing Educator
Wenatchee Valley College Nursing Program
Wenatchee, Washington

 F.A. Davis Company • Philadelphia

F. A. Davis Company
1915 Arch Street
Philadelphia, PA 19103
www.fadavis.com

Printed in the United States of America

Last digit indicates print number: 10 9 8 7 6 5 4 3 2 1

Senior Acquisitions Editor: Andy McPhee
Manager of Content Development: George W. Lang
Developmental Editor: Nancy Hoffmann
Art and Design Manager: Carolyn O'Brien

As new scientific information becomes available through basic and clinical research,
recommended treatments and drug therapies undergo changes. The author(s) and
publisher have done everything possible to make this book accurate, up to date, and in
accord with accepted standards at the time of publication. The author(s), editors, and
publisher are not responsible for errors or omissions or for consequences from
application of the book, and make no warranty, expressed or implied, in regard to the
contents of the book. Any practice described in this book should be applied by the
reader in accordance with professional standards of care used in regard to the unique
circumstances that may apply in each situation. The reader is advised always to check
product information (package inserts) for changes and new information regarding dose
and contraindications before administering any drug. Caution is especially urged when
using new or infrequently ordered drugs.

ISBN: 978-0-8036-1574-8

DEDICATION

To my children, Brad, Brian, and Nicole; my grandsons, Gabe, Seth, Isaac, and Corban; and future grandchildren, whom I've not yet met. You are my greatest gift to this world. I love you more than words can say, now, always, and forever.

PREFACE

Does the world of health care seem mysterious and confusing to you? Have you ever found yourself struggling to understand what your health-care provider was saying? Have you ever wanted to find medical information on your own that is easy to locate and easy to understand? Perhaps you are currently a student in an allied health program—such as medical assisting, radiological technology, or nursing—and you need a reference book that provides basic data about human diseases, but you find pathophysiology books intimidating and overwhelming. Whether your needs are personal or professional, this book is designed for you. You may be required to buy it for a course of study, or you may choose it because of its user-friendly, informative nature.

If you plan to use this as a reference book, then you may approach your information search in a couple of ways. First, identify the body system involved. For example, if you want to learn more about heart disease, the easiest thing is to flip to the chapter on cardiovascular diseases and disorders, scan the headings, and read whatever information appeals to you. On the other hand, you may have a term that you want to learn about but have no idea where to start or which body system is involved. For example, you may have heard that a friend has *ascites,* but you have no idea what it is, much less what caused it or how it is treated. In this case, the best approach is to look in the *glossary* near the back of the book, where *key terms* are listed and defined alphabetically. After reading the definition, you might refer to the *index* at the back of the book, where you will find page numbers listed for each place in the book where ascites is discussed.

If you are reading this book as a part of a course of study, you may be required to commit certain terms and information to memory. This can feel overwhelming and intimidating. There is no question that it does require some work on your part. However, this book comes with some great tools to help you in your journey.

Plan for Success

This text provides some great tools and suggested strategies to make the task of learning and remembering terms and information much easier.

Textbook

This textbook has many features to support your learning:

- **Learning style information** in the first chapter will help you identify and understand your own style and learning needs. This is critically important information, so please don't skip over it. Understanding your style will allow you to devote your valuable, limited study time to activities that are most likely to ensure your success.
- **Learning style tips** are included at the end of each chapter. Be sure to read them and try them out. You may be surprised to find what does and does not work for you. Honing your study strategies in this course as you read this text will pay off big for you in the future, as you go on to take other classes.
- **Chapter exercises** allow you to research information within the chapter (or even in other chapters). This provides repetition and review of key information and, more importantly,

guides you in applying what you have just learned to lifelike situations. This helps you take learning beyond mere memorization and go much deeper into understanding the whys.

- **Full-color illustrations and photos** provide visual information and explanation of a wide variety of topics. Some may illustrate parts of human anatomy. Others may diagram the steps in a certain disease process. Still others provide actual photographs of the physical changes caused by the disease in question. The oft-repeated saying "A picture is worth a thousand words" has never been so true as with this book because the artwork provides accurate, interesting, colorful, powerful, and memorable information.

Flash Cards

Flash cards corresponding to many of the diseases and disorders described in this text may accompany your book. Each card includes a short definition of the disease or disorder, and most contain visual cues as well. They are designed to appeal to the needs of students with various learning styles. Because repetition is the key to memorization, flash cards make repetition easier for you. Read and try the strategies described here to find what works best for you.

Solitary learners: Use the cards when you are alone and away from the distractions of others.
- Select cards for terms you've just read about. Hold them in your hands with the terms and visual cues facing you; challenge yourself to remember any related information for the top card. Then flip the card over to read the definition. Read it aloud two or three times. Then flip the card back over and recite the definition while looking at the term and visual cue. Do this with the rest of the cards in your hand.
- Use the system just described, only now reverse it: Hold the cards in your hands with the definitions facing you. Challenge yourself to recall and recite the name of the disease or disorder on the top card. Also describe (without looking at it) the visual cue included.
- Use the flash cards in these ways during quiet study times. Also try placing a few cards in your purse or pocket, and pull them out for a quick review during otherwise "wasted" moments during the day (waiting in line at the store, sitting in a waiting room, etc.). By using this method, you can memorize eight terms a day—or 56 new terms each week—without using your "official" study time. Over 10 weeks, that adds up to 560 new terms!

Social learners: Using the flash cards on your own is helpful, but using them with a partner or in a group is even better. Take turns running through the cards with your partner in a manner similar to that described previously.
- Make sure that the person being quizzed verbally recites all information. Other individuals may verbally repeat the information, but only afterward. Discussion may follow, but only if you all promise to stay on track and only talk about the subject of study, not your plans for the weekend.
- If you lack a classmate to study with, just hand your flash cards to another person (friend, family member, etc.), and let that person quiz you by showing you one side of the card and challenging you to remember and recite the information on the opposite side. Then use the opportunity to "teach" them about the disorder by sharing any information you can recall about the disease, cause, symptoms, treatment, and so on. Verbalizing the information to another person appeals to your need for social interaction; because you are also very likely a verbal and auditory learner, it meets those needs as well. Your partner doesn't need to know the subject matter but may find it an interesting bonus to learn some things along with you.
- Liven things up by playing games. One example is speed. You need two players and at least two sets of flash cards (more is better). Each player selects the designated cards from their sets and shuffles their newly created deck. When ready, begin laying down cards near to each other (each in a separate pile) at the same time. When you happen to lay down identical cards, the first of you to correctly say the name of the disease or disorder and correctly define it wins the matching cards from both piles; put them aside. Matches will be infrequent at the beginning but will occur more and more frequently as cards are eliminated from play. The game continues until all cards are out of play. The winner is the one who collects the most pairs.

Additional Activities on DavisPlus

There are also interactive exercises for each chapter available at http://davisplus.fadavis.com in the following four formats:

- electronic flash cards
- fill in the blank
- drag-and-drop matching
- quiz show

These activities allow you to review content from the book in a third way, reinforcing further the information you have just read.

CONTRIBUTORS

Cindi Brassington, MS, CMA (AAMA)
Professor of Allied Health
Quinebaug Valley Community College
Danielson, Connecticut

Bennita Vaughans, MSN, RN
Formerly Nursing Instructor and Medical Assisting Program Coordinator
H. Council Trenholm State Technical College
Montgomery, Alabama

REVIEWERS

CAROLE BERUBE, MA, MSN, BSN, RN
Professor Emerita
Bristol Community College
Health Sciences Department
Fall River, Massachusetts

SUSAN A. BOULDEN, BSN, CMA (AAMA)
Instructor
Mt. Hood Community College
Allied Health Department, Medical
  Assistant Program
Gresham, Oregon

VICTOR G. BUCKINGHAM, NHA, RMA
Instructor
Stevens-Henager College, Boise Campus
School of Medical and Health Sciences
Boise, Idaho

CARMEN CARPENTER, RN, MS, CMA
  (AAMA)
Chair
South University
Department of Allied Health Science and
  Medical Assisting
West Palm Beach, Florida

CAROLYN SUE COLEMAN, LPN, AS
Director of Healthcare Education
National College
Medical Department
Lynchburg, Virginia

MARTHA COSTELLO, RMA, BS, DC
Assistant Professor and Program Director
Clayton State University
Health Care Management Department
Morrow, Georgia

DEBRA CRAFT, RN, BSN, MED
Allied Health Coordinator
Moultrie Technical College
Academic Affairs Department
Moultrie, Georgia

BARBARA M. DAHL, CMA (AAMA), CPC
Coordinator and Chair
Whatcom Community College
Medical Assisting Program
Bellingham, Washington

CANDACE S. DAILEY, RN, MSN, CMA
  (AAMA)
Instructor and Director
Nicolet Area Technical College
Medical Assistant Program
Rhinelander, Wisconsin

ROSANA DARANG, MD
Program Chair
Bay State College
Health Studies and Medical Assisting
  Program
Boston, Massachusetts

ANNE DAVIS-JOHNSON, CMA (AAMA)
Instructor
Central Carolina Community College
Health Occupations Department, Medical
  Assisting Program
Lillington, North Carolina

CYNTHIA DESTAFANO, BS, RRT, CCS
Coordinator
Consolidated School of Business
Medical Department
Lancaster, Pennsylvania

TAMMY T. GANT, CMA (AAMA), CPC,
  RHIT, AHI
Director
Surry Community College
Business Technologies Department,
  Medical Assisting Program
Dobson, North Carolina

PAIGE GEBHARDT, BA, RMT
Instructor and Program Coordinator
Sussex County Community College
Health Sciences Department
Newton, New Jersey

REBECCA GIBSONLEE, MSTE, CMA
(AAMA), ASPT
Professor and Director
University of Akron
Department of Allied Health Technology,
  Medical Assisting Program
Akron, Ohio

BRENDA K. HARTSON, MSM, BSM, CMA
(AAMA)
Manager
Colorado Technical University
Medical Assisting Program
Sioux Falls, South Dakota

JOANNA L. HOLLY, MSHSA, RN, CMA
(AAMA)
Director, Allied Health
Midstate College
Peoria, Illinois

KRIS LINDAHL, CMA (AAMA)
Director
Lake Area Technical Institute
Health Division, Medical Assisting
  Program
Watertown, South Dakota

MARTHA LOGAN-BIELER, RHIT, RMA
Faculty
Raritan Valley Community College
Health Science Education Department,
  Medical Assistant Program
Branchburg, New Jersey

BARBARA MARCHELLETTA, AS, BS, MBA
Program Director/Advisor
Allied Health, Medical Assisting, Medical
  Coding, Health Information Technology
  and Medical Transcription
Beal College
Bangor, Maine

TAMMY MARTIN-GRIFFIN, CMA (AAMA)
Faculty
Springfield Technical Community College
Medical Assisting Department
Springfield, Massachusetts

CHERIE MATTSON, CMA (AAMA), LPN
Instructor
Ridgewater College
Medical Assistant Program
Willmar, Minnesota

SUZANNE MOE, RN
Instructor
Northland Community and Technical
  College
Health Division
East Grand Forks, Minnesota

LISA NAGLE, CMA (AAMA), BSEd
Director
Augusta Technical College
Health Department, Medical Assisting
  Program
Augusta, Georgia

ELIZABETH PEACE, RN
Instructor, Medical Assisting
Moultrie Technical College
Allied Health Department
Moultrie, Georgia

KAROLYN K. RYAN, RN, BSN
Faculty, Clinical Instructor
Springfield Technical Community College
Medical Assistant Department
Springfield, Massachusetts

AMY SAGER, RN, BSN, MS
Instructor
Seward County Community College/Area
  Technical School
Allied Health Division, Medical Assistant
  Program
Liberal, Kansas

TAMMY SAVAGE, RN
Coordinator, Medical Programs
Douglas Education Center
Medical Department
Monessen, Pennsylvania

ACKNOWLEDGMENTS

Thank you to the people at F. A. Davis who helped turn this manuscript into a book. A special thanks to Andy McPhee, Senior Acquisitions Editor, for your unwavering support, your guidance, and your good humor. Thank you also to George Lang, Manager of Content Development; Elizabeth Stepchin, Developmental Associate and Project Editor; Stephanie Rukowicz, Associate Developmental Editor; Amanda Frederick, Production Editor at Graphic World, Inc.; and Nancy Hoffmann, Freelance Developmental Editor. All of you had a hand in moving this book forward.

A special thank you goes to Cindi Brassington for all of your contributions—from providing up-to-date codes to being a second set of eyes on the chapters and a valued friend. I appreciate your support. Thank you as well to Bennita Vaughans for your contributions to Chapter 4.

Finally, thank you to the reviewers who provided valuable feedback on the chapters and helped shape them into a great book.

CONTENTS IN BRIEF

CONTENTS

LEARNING STYLES

1

Overview

Learning style theory suggests that individuals learn information in different ways according to their unique abilities and traits. Therefore, while all humans are similar, the ways in which you perceive, understand, and remember information may be somewhat different from other people's.

In truth, all people possess a combination of styles. You may be especially strong in one style and less so in others. You may be strong in two or three areas or may be equally strong in all areas. No style is inherently good or bad; styles simply indicate how you most effectively perceive and process new information. As you learn about the styles described in this chapter and come to identify your own, you will then be able to modify your study activities accordingly. This will aid you in making the very most of your valuable study time, will enhance your learning, and will support you in doing your very best in this and any future classes.

Sensory Learning Styles

Experts have identified a number of learning styles and given them a variety of names. Some are described in an abstract and complex manner, while others are relatively simple and easy to grasp. For ease of understanding this book uses the simpler learning styles. This is done so you can quickly come to understand the basic elements of learning style theory and, more importantly, identify and understand your own style.

When learning, there are several ways to perceive and grasp new information. You may use your senses to see it and hear it. You may use touch and manipulation or your sense of taste or smell. You might find it useful to think aloud as you discuss the new information with someone else. Because the senses are so often involved in the acquisition of new information, many learning styles are named accordingly: visual, auditory, kinesthetic (hands-on or tactile), and so on.

Visual Learners

Most people are strongly visual learners. To most accurately and quickly grasp new information, these people need to see it represented visually. The more complex the data, the more this is true. Visual learners especially like data that is colorful and visually striking. Visual information can be presented in many ways. Examples include:

- Written words
- Diagrams
- Shapes
- Patterns
- Colors
- Symbols

- Illustrations
- Graphs
- Photos
- Tables
- Flowcharts
- Time lines
- Maps
- Handouts
- Posters
- Flash cards
- PowerPoint presentations
- Internet data
- Videos
- Live demonstrations

If you are a visual learner you may have already noticed that you are drawn to visual information. Unless you are also an auditory learner, you may have some difficulty remembering information that is shared only verbally. Consequently you may ask others to repeat themselves, or better yet, to write it down. When looking through books, magazines, or instruction manuals, you are especially drawn to photos and any visual illustrations because they help you to more accurately see what is being discussed. Within the classroom, you prefer instructors who use written outlines and lots of visual aids.

Visualization is a powerful tool for you. In your health-care program you will very likely learn specific skills and procedures. Examples may include giving injections, drawing blood, and recording a patient's electrocardiogram. The first time you do this with a real patient you will likely feel nervous. You can use visualization to help you prepare. Find a quiet place such as a break room or even a supply closet. Close your eyes. Take a deep breath and exhale slowly to relax. Now visualize approaching the patient and performing the procedure. Picture each step exactly as you will perform it; be sure to visualize yourself using any necessary equipment. Not only will this process help you mentally rehearse the procedure, but it will also allow you to make a supply list as you note each of the needed items. This form of mental rehearsal is nearly as good as the real thing and will allow you to enter the patient's room feeling calmer, more clearheaded, and more prepared to competently perform the procedure.

As a visual learner, you find writing notes helpful, and you often like to study alone where you can occasionally close your eyes and see in your mind's eye the situation or circumstances being studied. When learning tasks or procedures, you like to have written instructions. You are also able to close your eyes and mentally rehearse through the process of visualization because you can picture everything clearly. During exams you recall information by seeing it in your mind's eye, whether it is an actual picture or diagram or a fragment of written text. During conversations or discussions you tend to use visual words such as "see," "look," and "picture." Examples include:

- Let me see if I understand.
- Let's look at this.
- See what you think of this.
- I see what you mean.
- I'm trying to picture it.

You generally have a good sense of direction, rarely get lost, and can easily interpret and use maps. Your office and home may be littered with lists and notes that you've written to organize yourself and to remember things. You love self-adhesive note pads. You find listening to a lecture without stimulating visuals to be boring and tedious. You need to take notes, draw, or doodle to keep from falling asleep. In fact, you may appear to other people as if you are distracted or daydreaming when doodling on paper. However, you know that it actually helps you listen better. Your work and hobbies include activities that make use of color, shapes, and design or visual art. Just a few examples are drawing, painting, quilting, photography, and scrapbooking.

Study Strategies for Visual Learners

If you are a visual learner, try using any study or memory technique that aids you in visually seeing and recalling information. You may find **mnemonics** (memory aids) especially helpful for remembering lists or sequenced pieces of information. Generally speaking, the more creative, whimsical, funny, or absurd they are, the better you will remember them. There are many different types of mnemonics. Some examples are:

- Children use the well-known alphabet song, a musical mnemonic, to learn their ABCs.
- Students in anatomy classes use one of several mnemonic variations to remember the 12 cranial nerves (olfactory, optic, oculomotor, trochlear, trigeminal, abducens, facial, acoustic, glossopharyngeal, vagus, spinal accessory, and hypoglossal). One example is "On old Olympus' tower tops, a Finn and German viewed some hops." Note that the first letter of each word is the same as the first letter of the name of one of the cranial nerves.
- Most people use this spelling mnemonic to remember where to place the I and E: "I before E, except after C."

Another form of commonly used mnemonic is the **acronym.** An acronym is an abbreviation created by using the first letters or word parts in names or phrases. Examples of acronyms include:

LASER — **L**ight **a**mplification by **s**timulated **e**mission of **r**adiation
INTERPOL — **Inter**national Criminal **Pol**ice Organization
FAQ — **F**requently **a**sked **q**uestions
CD-ROM — **C**ompact **d**isc **r**ead-**o**nly **m**emory
PIN — **P**ersonal **i**dentification **n**umber
OLD CART — **O**nset, **l**ocation, **d**uration, **c**haracter, **a**ggravating factors, **r**elieving factors, **t**reatments
VS — **V**ital **s**igns

The seven warning signs of cancer can be remembered in the acronym CAUTION:

Change in bowel or bladder habits
A sore throat that does not heal
Unusual bleeding or discharge
Thickening or a lump in the breast or other area
Indigestion or difficulty swallowing
Obvious change in a mole or wart
Nagging cough or hoarseness

And finally, the warning signs of malignant melanoma are shown by the acronym ABCD:

Asymmetry — One half of the mole does not match the other half.
Border — The edges of the mole are irregular or blurred.
Color — The color varies throughout, with shades including tan, brown, black, blue, red, or white.
Diameter — The mole is larger than 6 millimeters.

Auditory Learners

Many people are auditory (or *aural*) learners. To most accurately and quickly grasp new information, these people need to hear it spoken. The more complex the data, the more this is true. The most common example of auditory information sharing is during a classroom lecture; however, there are other ways to hear information. Examples include audio recordings, computer tutorials (with audio), and oral discussions.

If you are an auditory learner, you may have already noticed that you are drawn to information presented aloud. Unless you are also a visual learner, you may have some difficulty remembering written information without some verbal discussion or review. You may often ask others to elaborate on details orally or to repeat themselves so you can hear it again. When recalling events, you can sometimes hear how someone else spoke. You notice subtle inflections that convey meaning. Chances are you enjoy music and have a good sense of rhythm. You may play an instrument or sing. At the very least, you are an avid appreciator of music and may prefer a radio, stereo, or mp3 player over the television at least part of the time. Music evokes emotion in you. For example, you notice that you feel energized, joyous, or melancholy in response to certain music. You may also notice that songs or jingles pop into your head and stay there for hours. Your work and your hobbies often involve sound. Examples include playing musical instruments, attending concerts, composing music, or working as a sound engineer or even a band or orchestra conductor. During conversations or discussions you tend to use auditory words such as "sound" and "hear." Examples include:

- That sounds like...
- Music to my ears.
- This rings a bell.
- I hear what you're saying.
- You are coming through loud and clear.
- I'm tuned in.

Study Strategies for Auditory Learners

If you are an auditory learner, try using any study or memory techniques that allow you to hear information aloud, whether it is the spoken word or data set to music or any other auditory format. Auditory learners are also usually verbal learners as well. If this is true for you, then you learn best when you have the chance for a verbal exchange. This allows you to speak to and listen to others. For this reason you are probably a social learner and often prefer studying with a partner or in a study group. You find mnemonics helpful, especially if they include rhymes or are catchy and fun to say out loud. A common example is the following mnemonic used to help people remember the number of days in each month:

Thirty days hath September,
April, June, and November;
All the rest have thirty-one
Excepting February alone:
Which has twenty-eight, that's fine,
Till leap year gives it twenty-nine.

Another example of a mnemonic that relates to health care is the acronym MONA. This is often used by nurses and other health-care workers when providing emergency care for patients experiencing possible myocardial infarction (heart attack):

Morphine
Oxygen
Nitrates
Aspirin

Verbal Learners

It is sometimes said that some people must think (first) in order to speak. For verbal learners the reverse may be true: They feel compelled to speak in order to think. What this means is that speaking aloud helps them to process information and think things through. This is especially true when the information is complex or the situation feels stressful. These people often talk to themselves. Such individuals may state that doing so helps to slow their brain down and help them to focus and think more clearly.

Many people are verbal learners. This includes use of the spoken and the written word. If you are a verbal learner, you may seek out a trusted friend to act as a sounding board. You do not expect this person to solve your problem; rather, you need them to listen as you think aloud and bounce things off of them. They may offer no advice at all, yet you usually find these sessions enormously helpful. You very likely love to read and enjoy some type of writing. This could take a professional form such as becoming an author or personal forms such as writing poetry for your own enjoyment or simply writing in a private journal. You enjoy learning new words and incorporating them into your vocabulary. You find rhymes and tongue twisters entertaining. You may enjoy reading poetry aloud because speaking it is more enjoyable than silently reading it. Your occupation or hobbies may include public speaking, writing, or politics. You enjoy a lively discussion or even a debate, as well as interactive social activities such as playing games or simply visiting, because this includes verbal exchange. During conversations you tend to use verbal words such as "talk," "spell," and "word." Examples include:

- Let talk about this.
- I will spell it out.
- In other words.
- The best word to describe...

Study Strategies for Verbal Learners

If you are a verbal learner, try using any study or memory techniques that allow you to speak aloud in order to recite data or explain concepts. Like auditory learners, you find mnemonics helpful, especially if they are fun to say or include rhyming. You may also find writing to be very helpful. Writing down important data such as outlines, summaries, and vocabulary helps you remember the content. You are very likely also a social learner who benefits from studying with a partner or in a study group. This provides ample opportunity for discussion. You especially benefit from explaining challenging concepts or "teaching" your study partners about a given topic. For example, the members of your study group may decide to teach one another about the four major joint types in the body: hinge, ball-and-socket, pivot, and gliding. Each person describes the appearance and function of a type of joint and gives an example. One person may compare a hinge joint like those found in the knee and elbow to a door hinge, and describe how it moves back and forth like a door that swings open and shut. The next person may compare a pivot joint, such as the one in the neck, to a chair that turns back and forth in a 180-degree half circle. Other students go on to teach about their assigned joints and give examples. To maximize the value of this exercise for verbal learners, you can add a requirement that all members of the group must verbally repeat key information or phrases after the "teacher."

Kinesthetic Learners

Most people have some kinesthetic (tactile) aspects to their learning style even though it may not be their most dominant style. People who are strong kinesthetic learners need to use their bodies as they learn. They like to touch and manipulate objects. This is especially important when learning physical skills. When assembling things, they may forgo reading the instructions and just assemble the product based on feel and instinct. They are usually successful, but if not, they may check the instructions, which will now make much more sense to them since they have become physically acquainted with the parts. Examples of physical learning include:

- Demonstrations
- Simulations
- Practicing a skill

If you are a kinesthetic learner, you may have already noticed that you are eager to get your hands on objects and do things yourself. When the information being learned is theoretical, you are still eager to move your body somehow, even if it is to draw a diagram or fidget in your chair. Sitting through lengthy lectures feels tedious and almost painful to you. You like to touch things, and very likely have hobbies that include manipulating objects or making things with your hands, such as woodworking, gardening, baking, assembling puzzles, putting models together, sewing, acting, and sculpting. You notice textures and like how they feel. Your most productive thinking time occurs when you are on the move in activities such as biking, hiking, walking, or even running on a treadmill. You get restless if you sit around too long, and feel eager to do something. You are very physical when communicating and may use big hand and arm gestures. You may enjoy dancing, sports, and other physical activities. During conversations or discussions you tend to use physical action or sensation words like "feel" and "touch." Examples include:

- This doesn't feel right.
- I follow you.
- Get a grip.
- Keep in touch.
- This just doesn't sit right.
- I feel it in my gut.
- I need to get a handle on this.
- I'm trying to get a feel for...

Study Strategies for Kinesthetic Learners

If you are a kinesthetic learner, try using any study or memory techniques that allow you to move your body or touch objects. When learning skills or procedures, your best strategy is to actually get your hands on the needed supplies and practice the procedure. For example, consider again the study group in which you and your friends are each describing major types of body joints. In addition to verbally describing the joints and giving examples, add a requirement that each person must somehow act out or physically mimic the joint movement—something like a charades game with talking allowed. The person describing the hinge joint now must physically get up and find a door to open and shut while describing its function. Better yet, the person might play the part of the door and move back and forth. The next person compares a pivot joint, such as the one in the neck, to a chair that turns back and forth in a 180-degree half circle. While describing this, the person literally turns his or her head back and forth and then turns the chair back and forth in a 180-degree half circle. After each person performs a physical demonstration, other members of the group must perform the same movement. This gives everyone full kinesthetic value from the activity.

When actual physical practice of a skill is not possible, visualization is a great alternative. It gives you the chance to "practice" skills in your mind and even move your body, arms, and hands as you would when performing the actual skill. When the content is theoretical, you still benefit from physical movement. Play learning games, use flash cards, complete activities included in your textbook, use the student activity disc that accompanies many textbooks (including this one), and interact with a study partner or group.

Social Preferences

In addition to your sensory learning style, you also have a social preference for learning. If you notice that interacting with others helps you to grasp and understand information, you are most likely a social learner. On the other hand, if you do your best when working alone without the distraction of others, you are very likely a solitary learner.

Social Learners

Many people are social learners. They learn most effectively when they are able to interact with other people. They enjoy group **synergy** (the enhanced action of two or more agents working together cooperatively) and are able to think things through with the verbal exchange that occurs during a lively discussion. Examples of social learning include:

- Discussions about specific topics
- Question-and-answer sessions
- Group projects
- Group games

If you are a social learner, you may have already noticed that you are drawn to social situations and don't like to study alone. You communicate and interact well with others. You enjoy listening to and helping others. You may also be a verbal-auditory learner and may enjoy discussions and bouncing your ideas off other people. You are drawn to social situations and may stay after class to talk with others. If you are athletic, you may prefer group sports to solo activities. You also enjoy social activities such as dancing and board games. You like working through problems with a partner or a group. Work activities may include teaching, coaching, or working in a people-oriented setting such as a restaurant or retail store. During conversations or discussions, you tend to use social wording, which includes "we" and "let's." Examples include:

- If we work cooperatively...
- Let's work it out.
- Let's explore this.
- We should get together and...

Study Strategies for Social Learners

If you are a social learner, you may find that you feel restless and have difficulty staying focused when you try to study alone. You need to seek out opportunities to study with one or more other people. If there isn't a study group available, consider starting one. Group activities can include discussion, learning games, role-playing, and creating mnemonics together. Your study group will be most effective if you set and adhere to some ground rules that provide structure. It's your group, so the rules are up to you; but here are some suggestions:

- Identify a group leader—preferably someone with some knowledge or experience in the subject being studied.
- Have the group complete specified readings or assignments prior to each meeting.
- Have the group members agree to stay on task so the group doesn't deteriorate into a social group or complaint session.
- Set and follow time limits.
- Encourage all members to contribute.

Solitary Learners

Many people are solitary learners. They learn most effectively when they are able to study alone without distraction from others. They are often somewhat private, and enjoy time alone to ponder and reflect. They are strongly independent and know what works for them; trying to conform to the group can be a source of frustration.

There are many ways that solitary learners study. The important thing is that they do it alone. They may read, review notes, and listen to recorded lectures (if they are also auditory), or they may incorporate any number of other strategies. During conversations or discussions, they tend to use solitary "me" or "I" language. Examples include:

- I need to think this over.
- Let me ponder it.
- I'll get back to you.
- I'll let you know what I decide.

Study Strategies for Solitary Learners

If you are a solitary learner, you may feel frustrated trying to study with a partner or a group. You may feel like they are wasting your time and believe you would do better by yourself. You focus and concentrate best when alone. You are somewhat analytical and goal oriented. You are also a self-starter and don't need anyone else to prompt you or provide structure. You have learned to enjoy your own company and enjoy solitude. Many people, especially your social friends, may find this difficult to understand, since they may not like being alone. You may be known to travel alone, dine out alone, and go to movies or concerts alone. You don't feel that you are missing out when you do this; in fact, you may prefer it because you don't have to negotiate with anyone else about what to do or where to eat. You may enjoy solitary hobbies and may work for yourself or dream of working for yourself one day. You are self-reflective and interested in personal improvement. Strong solitary learners often end up in jobs where they work independently. Examples include writing, farming, forestry, and other outdoor occupations.

Global Versus Analytical Preferences

In addition to the styles described above, most people tend to initially grasp information either as a whole, looking at the "big picture," or in a more sequential fashion in which the individual parts are studied first to comprehend the whole. If you are in the first group, you are a global learner; if you are in the second group, you are an analytical learner.

Global Learners

Global learners, sometimes called *holistic* learners, generally see the big picture first and later pay more attention to details. For example, when studying the human body, global learners first see it as a whole, complete organism. With that picture in mind, they are then able to begin studying the parts. This is true even when studying individual body systems, such as the cardiovascular system. Global learners first grasp the big picture of the entire system as it circulates blood throughout the body. With further study and thought, they appreciate how the system delivers oxygen and nutrients and eliminates waste through a complex network of vessels including veins, arteries, and capillaries.

If you are a global learner, your primary learning style may be a mix of visual and auditory. You are also probably a social learner. If you are a global learner, you often respond based on intuition or emotion and are able to grasp symbolism. You may be able to accept rules, such as a math equation, without necessarily understanding how the steps work. You may be more interested in general themes than little details and are good at paraphrasing ideas and concepts. Along the same lines, you are good at recognizing relationships and reading between the lines. You are flexible and do well with multitasking. When studying new concepts, you usually compare them with concepts you already understand. For example, when first learning about the lymphatic system, you may think, "This is very similar to what I know about the cardiovascular system. They both have a complex network of vessels that convey fluid through the body." As you study the lymphatic system in detail, you then begin to distinguish the important differences.

All learning styles provide benefits as well as potential challenges. If you are a global learner, you may experience periods of frustration relieved by moments of insight when the "light comes on" and you suddenly "get it." When reading, you desire to know the main point or bottom line. When you encounter a term or concept you don't understand, you may skim over it, hoping that it will make sense as you continue on. This strategy sometimes works for you, but you risk missing important details. You may not like being asked to explain details to others or to write out how you achieved your final answer. You may resist accepting critical feedback and may often be late to class or work. You usually feel a need to know the whys before you commit your enthusiasm and energy to a project.

Study Strategies for Global Learners

If you are a global learner, you are probably also a visual-auditory learner. Therefore, be sure to try the study and memory techniques previously described for those styles. If you find studying details to be tedious and boring, try to find other, more creative and fun ways to learn the same material. For example you may prefer drawing your own colorful diagrams or may enjoy using audiovisual tutorials or other activities that are often on the student discs that accompany textbooks or are available online.

Use your strengths. You are flexible. You are a multitasker. Don't be afraid to mix it up a bit to make your study efforts more lively and enjoyable. You are good at seeing the big picture and recognizing relationships; therefore, begin each study session by identifying the relationship between what you are currently studying and your future career ambitions.

Here is a study activity that might help you connect current studies with future career goals. Meet with a group of fellow students or with a study partner. In addition to verbalizing or explaining terms and concepts, add an additional requirement: Give a hypothetical example of a time in your future career when knowing this information will be necessary. For example, imagine that today your group is studying the structure and function of the neurological system, in particular the structure of the basic neuron. As a global learner, you are more interested in whether the human body works as it should, and you may be less attuned to details. Furthermore, you wish to get on with learning about your role as a future medical assistant, nurse, or whatever occupation you are pursuing.

As you study the structure of the neuron today, you are challenged with seeing the value of such detailed trivia in your future role and career. Consider then the important function of that little neuron in transmitting signals, and the way each of its structural parts supports it in that function. Then ask yourself what might happen if some of the protective coating (myelin sheath) began to erode. How might that affect the function of the body? And how might that lead the person to show up in the clinic or hospital you will be working in? How might your understanding of that little neuron help you to understand your patient, her symptoms, her diagnosis, and her needs? One day you may be responsible for providing care to a patient with multiple sclerosis or another degenerative neuromuscular disorder. Keep this in mind as you study the neurological system today. Then challenge yourself to get the maximum value from your investment of time and energy.

Beware your tendency to overlook details. You can compensate with strategies that help you identify and remember details of significance. While reading, make note of terms, concepts, or sections that you skipped over or did not understand. You can do this by highlighting these areas in a specific color or by writing notes in the margins. Once you've completed your initial read-through, force yourself to return to each of these areas and investigate them further. When deciding how much time and energy to devote to each one, ask yourself the following questions:

- Is there a learning objective in the syllabus that pertains to this content?
- Might this content impact my understanding of the whole?
- How likely is the instructor to include a test question on this content?
- How relevant is this content to the remainder of this class, to future classes, or to my future career?

Analytical Learners

Analytical learners, sometimes called *logical, linear, sequential,* or *mathematical* learners, generally need to see the parts before fully comprehending the whole. For example, when studying the human body, analytical learners prefer to study in a methodical fashion beginning with the smallest parts and working up to the whole. Such people will prefer to take classes such as chemistry and cellular biology before taking classes like anatomy and physiology. As they continue learning about each of the body systems, they begin to appreciate how each relates to the others and constitutes the whole organism.

Analytical learners readily identify patterns and like to group data into categories for further study. They love to create and follow agendas, make lists with items ranked by priority, and approach problem-solving in a logical, methodical manner. They like to create and follow procedures and may grow impatient with others who do not. They are often linear and orderly in their thinking and seek to quantify things whenever possible. They often pursue careers in accounting, sciences, computer technology, engineering, law enforcement, and mathematics.

If you are an analytical learner, your primary learning style may be verbal. If this is true, then you process information verbally, which means you sometimes talk to yourself and think aloud. You may also have a visual dimension to your style since this lends itself so well to grouping information into categories and drawing connections. However, you could be a mix of any of the styles previously described. Because you are so methodical, you may also be a solitary learner and prefer a quiet environment. Working with others who are not analytical may frustrate you. You tend to respond to problems logically rather than emotionally. This serves you well in some cases but may cause you to be labeled by others as cold and unfeeling. On the other hand, you have an eye for detail and are organized and forward-thinking. Most work teams need at least one person with your skills to ensure accuracy and quality. Your logical mind makes you especially good at noting errors or flaws in other people's reasoning; however, those people may not always appreciate this. You are especially good at mathematics or any pursuit that requires logic and strategy. You may enjoy brainteasers such as sudoku or games of strategy like chess and certain computer games. However, your less analytical friends may grow weary of playing games with you, since you nearly always win.

Some of the same qualities that are your strengths can, at times, become a source of frustration. For example you may get stuck in "analysis paralysis" as you study details. This can stall forward movement and impair decision-making. Some may accuse you of being stubborn, rigid, or inflexible. You may also struggle in fast-paced, stressful environments where quick decisions are required. You may feel frustrated when other people issue personal opinions as facts. To you, facts are only facts when they are indisputably accurate and supported by reliable data. In turn, other people may become frustrated by your need to gather more data and process information in detail (often verbally). In most cases they really don't want to hear all of your logic and rationale, and instead wish you would just get to the point.

Study Strategies for Analytical Learners

If you are an analytical learner, use your style to maximize learning, but take care not to get stuck in analysis paralysis or sidetracked with insignificant detail. Try the study and memory techniques previously described that are relevant to your basic style. Put your organizational talent to work to make your study efforts productive: Make an agenda or create a list of topics to be studied. Prioritize topics to ensure that you address the most important things first. This is your "Must Know" list. Set and follow time limits but don't overanalyze your plan. It is most important to get busy studying. Rather than getting sidetracked with interesting (but low-priority) items, make another list of topics as you go along titled "It Would Be Nice to Know." Come back to this list later if—and only if—time permits. Use your gift for identifying patterns by noting patterns within the material you are studying. This can be useful when you prepare for exams, because test questions often focus on features that are similar and those that are different. For example, a myocardial infarction (MI) and angina both cause chest pain. In both cases, the pain is caused by inadequate blood supply to the heart. These are two important and similar features when comparing these disorders—chest pain and lack of oxygen. On the other hand, an MI causes actual death of heart muscle tissue, while angina does not. This is an important difference.

As an analytical learner, you may not be able to hear new information while you are focusing on and processing other information. Consequently, you may often feel like the instructor moves too quickly during lecture. However, you must remember that if she speaks slowly enough for you to hear, write, and process the data, your global-learner classmates class will grow uninterested and restless. They may perceive the class as boring and may believe the instructor moves too slowly. Therefore, your best bet is to use multiple strategies that allow you to get good class notes, identify important details, and delay much of your detailed information-processing until a later time. This might mean that you focus on writing during class and record the lecture (with your instructor's permission) so you can hear it later. Such a plan keeps you from missing significant details. This should lower your stress and allow you to enjoy class more. Another option is to get notes at a later time from a classmate, so you can devote your in-class energy to listening. If you do this, be sure to select someone who is a very thorough and accurate note taker.

To make the most of some study strategies, you must give yourself permission to be illogical or even silly. If a technically "inaccurate" mnemonic or silly song will help you remember something, then why not use it? Your global-learner classmates can help you with this if you will let them.

You are a good reflective thinker and are able to evaluate your own performance. However, this can also become a flaw since you are probably a perfectionist and may be too hard on yourself. You must learn to let the small stuff go, not let other people bug you, and give yourself permission to be less than perfect. If other students distract or annoy you with their behaviors or chosen study tactics, try to ignore them. You may need to physically separate yourself from them to do so. You need to do your "analytical thing" and allow them to do their "global thing." You will both achieve the same goals in different ways. The exception is when you must work with others as part of a group assignment. This can be challenging for students of different styles, but this mirrors real life. In fact, this is the main reason instructors assign group work: It gives you the opportunity to practice communication and teamwork skills. In this case it will help if everyone on the team begins by sharing information about their individual styles, including strengths, flaws, and needs. Group roles and tasks can be divided according to each person's style and strengths.

As an analytical learner, you may sometimes feel overwhelmed by unstructured environments and unexpected events. For this reason, you must think carefully about your career choice. The same abilities that serve you very well in some settings could hold you back in others. Since you are reading this book, you may be embarking on a career in health care. Fortunately, there are many paths within this arena. Be sure to select one that allows you to use your talents to their fullest. It is for you to decide what this might be. However, someone with your ability to methodically process and analyze data, ensure accuracy, and work independently might do especially well in certain settings, such as medical coding, research, laboratory technology, quality control, or utilization review. On the other hand, you generally do not like unpredictability or group work. Therefore, trying to work in a fast-paced, unpredictable environment might prove frustrating for you and your team. Examples might include roles in which you must provide patient care in an emergency department, urgent care center, or other medical units with very ill patients.

Identifying Your Style

How do you identify your learning style? In reading through this chapter you may have recognized yourself in one or more of the styles described. Remember that nobody has one style exclusively. Your style may have a combination of some or all of these but may be especially strong in one or two areas. Identifying the dominant aspects of your learning style will help you understand yourself better. It will also help you to identify study strategies that will be most effective for you. This allows you to make the most of your valuable and limited study time. It will help you to be more successful in this course than you might have otherwise been. It will also help you to be more successful in any future classes that you take. Therefore, taking a few minutes now to clearly identify your style will pay off in the long run.

Learning Styles and Learning About Human Diseases

Most medical courses require students to learn and remember a huge amount of information. This one is no exception. As you learn about various diseases and disorders, you must find a way to commit key points to memory. In other words, you must *memorize* a lot of data. There is no way around it; you are learning a foreign language, and to become fluent in this language you must develop a large, accurate vocabulary and must know how to use it.

So how does learning style theory apply to learning about human disease? By having a clear understanding of your style, you will be able to use your strengths and abilities to their fullest. Knowing what *not* to do becomes as important as knowing what to *do*. Because learning and remembering memorized data are key to this course, understanding how memory works will help you to accomplish this.

Memory

Human memory is the process by which people store, retain, and retrieve information. Perceiving, processing, and storing information are complex processes that involve many parts of your brain. It is beyond the scope of this book to describe the process in detail. However, a few key points are worth mentioning.

Sensory memory involves the first brief impression during which your brain registers patterns, sounds, smells, or other sensory data. You then almost immediately forget it, although you do store some data for later retrieval (see Fig. 1-1).

Perception and storage of information requires a complex combination of electrical and chemical functions within the nervous tissue of your brain, usually in your **short-term memory.** This allows you to retrieve it for a very short span of time, usually several seconds to several minutes. In general, most people are able to retrieve four to seven items of information from short-term memory. This capability is increased if the data is clustered into groups; this is known as *chunking.* For example, you may have noticed that it is easier to remember a string of numbers, such as a telephone number, if you chunk the numbers, such as in 233 467 901 rather than 233467901.

Memorization is a method that allows you to recall data through a process known as rote learning. It can be an effective strategy for you if you use it in the right way. It has been shown that most people's ability to retain memorized information is enhanced if they rehearse the data intermittently over an extended period of time rather than using the last-minute cram-and-forget method. In other words, cramming may or may not get you through the next exam, but it certainly will not support your long-term success in future classes or your career. To get important memorized data into your **long-term memory** you must do more than cram. Long-term memory is capable of storing an infinite amount of data for an indefinite period of time, perhaps for a lifetime. However, getting the information you wish to remember into your long-term memory is sometimes challenging. A number of factors are required, among them healthy functioning of several parts of the brain and sufficient quantity and quality of sleep. Others include:

- Attention (the extent to which you consciously attend to and focus on the data)
- Repetition (rehearsal of the data over and over)
- Information-processing method (strategies used to analyze and remember data; examples include chunking or other means of organization and using creative tricks such as mnemonics and acronyms)
- Study effort (the degree of mental and physical energy combined with the amount of time you devote to learning)
- Emotional relationship (relating the information being studied to strong emotional feelings or significant events)
- Connection (relating new information to a prior experience or previously learned information)

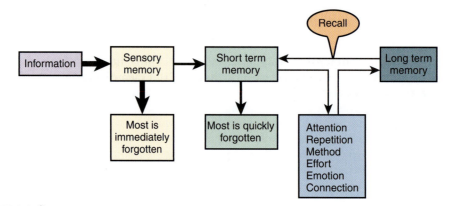

FIGURE 1-1 Sensory memory.

Some activities hamper your ability to store and recall information in both your short-term and long-term memory banks. Examples include:

- Interference (stimuli that hamper your ability to attend to information as you learn)
- Cramming (extensive memorization of a large amount of data over a short period of time; results in very poor recall and may displace other data in short-term memory)

Some general measures can help you in this process. General self-care activities that enhance memory include healthy nutrition, stress-reduction activities, regular exercise, socialization activities, and regular, good-quality sleep.

Plan for Success

To ensure your success in this course, you must take a bit of time now to do a self-assessment. It won't take long, and the information you gather will pay off big-time. Completing the chapter activities will guide you in this process. Once you've identified your own style, you can then proceed through this book.

Student Resources

http://www.studygs.net/memory/
http://www.academictips.org
http://vark-learn.com/english/index.asp
http://www.edutopia.org/multiple-intelligences-learning-styles-quiz

Note: The self-assessment tool at vark-learn.com is user-friendly. Students can complete it online or print a hard copy.

Chapter Activities

1. **Visit the websites listed below and take their free self-assessment tests.**
   - http://vark-learn.com/english/index.asp
   - http://www.edutopia.org/multiple-intelligences-learning-styles-quiz

   Describe your results.

2. **Now that you know what your dominant style is, read again the sections of this chapter about your style. Briefly describe the type of study strategies most likely to be effective for you.**

3. **Describe the plan that you believe will help you to be most effective in this course. Include approximate study times and techniques and whether they will be solitary or social.**

4. **Describe the activities you plan to employ to transfer as much human-disease data as possible into your long-term memory.**

Practice Exercises

Answers to Practice Exercises can be found in Appendix D.

True or False

1. True   False   Many learning styles are named according to the special senses.

2. True   False   Few people are strongly visual learners.

3. True   False   Visual learners prefer data to be presented simply in black and white.

4. True   False   *Auditory* and *aural* have similar meanings.

5. True   False   Kinesthetic learners like to touch and manipulate objects.

Multiple Choice

1. Diagrams, shapes, and patterns are examples of which type of data?
    a. Kinesthetic
    b. Visual
    c. Solitary
    d. Verbal

2. Posters, flash cards, and PowerPoint presentations all appeal to:
    a. Kinesthetic learners
    b. Visual learners
    c. Auditory learners
    d. Social learners

3. Which of the following statements is true regarding visual learners?

    a. They can recall information by seeing it in their mind's eye.

    b. During conversations they use visual words such as "touch" and "feel."

    c. They like to bounce things off of their friends.

    d. None of these.

4. All of the following techniques are helpful to visual learners **except:**

    a. Mnemonics

    b. Acronyms

    c. Flow charts

    d. Rhymes

5. Oral discussions appeal to students with which learning style?

    a. Verbal

    b. Auditory

    c. Social

    d. All of these

6. Which of the following statements is true regarding global learners?

    a. They are sometimes called sequential learners.

    b. They like to analyze details.

    c. Their learning styles are probably a mix of visual and auditory.

    d. They approach problem-solving in a very logical manner.

7. All of the following words of advice are specifically appropriate for global learners **except:**

    a. You are a multitasker, so don't be afraid to mix it up a bit and make your study efforts more lively and enjoyable.

    b. Begin each study session by identifying the relationship between what you are currently studying and your future career ambitions.

    c. Beware your tendency to get stuck in analysis paralysis.

    d. While reading, make note of terms or concepts that you skipped over and later take time to look them up.

8. All of the following statements are true regarding analytical learners **except:**

    a. They approach problem-solving in a logical, methodical manner.

    b. They dislike following official procedures.

    c. They seek to quantify things whenever possible.

    d. They often pursue careers in accounting, sciences, and engineering.

9. Which of the following words of advice are specifically appropriate for analytical learners?

    a. Prioritize items of importance for studying.

    b. Consider seeking work in an area that allows you to process and analyze data.

    c. Consider recording lectures.

    d. All of these.

10. Which of the following statements about memory is true?

    a. Most data moves easily from short-term to long-term memory.

    b. Emotional feelings affect whether some information is stored in long-term memory.

    c. Cramming is an effective method of transmitting data into long-term memory.

    d. All of these.

INFECTION AND DISEASE

2

Learning Outcomes

Upon completion of this chapter, the student will be able to:

- Define and spell the key terms
- List and describe five risk factors for disease
- Describe the medical response to disease, including diagnosis, prognosis, treatment, and evaluation
- Identify disease-producing microorganisms
- List common infectious diseases
- Identify the links in the chain of infection
- List and describe the three types of infection
- Differentiate between the stages of disease

KEY TERMS	
aerobe	microorganism that needs oxygen to grow
anaerobe	microorganism that grows without oxygen
asymptomatic	free of symptoms
bacterium	one-celled organism; some bacteria are capable of producing disease
disease	any condition characterized by subjective complaints, a specific history, clinical signs, symptoms, and laboratory or radiographic findings
etiology	cause
fomite	any object that adheres to and transmits infectious material (e.g., comb, countertop, drinking glass)
fungus	organism such as yeast, mold, or mushroom; most are not pathogenic
homeostasis	state of dynamic equilibrium in the body
idiopathic	having an unknown or uncertain cause
incubation	interval between exposure to infection and the appearance of the first symptoms
infectious disease	any disease transmitted directly or indirectly between individuals; also called *communicable disease*
microorganism	living organism too small to be seen by the naked eye
normal flora	organisms commonly found on and in the body that do not cause disease
nosocomial	acquired within the hospital
palliative care	medical care aimed at alleviating disease symptoms and enhancing quality of life
parasite	pathogen requiring another living organism in order to live
pathogen	disease-producing microorganism

Continued

KEY TERMS—cont'd	
pathologist	one who is devoted to the study of human tissues, cells, and body fluids for evidence of disease
prodromal	occurring between earliest symptoms and the appearance of a rash or fever
protozoan	organism; most protozoans live in soil, and some are capable of producing disease
symptomatic	having symptoms, such as fever, sore throat, nausea, or vomiting
vector	carrier, usually an insect, that transmits a disease from an infected person to a noninfected person
virus	pathogen which grows and reproduces after infecting a host cell

Disease

A *disease* is defined as a condition characterized by subjective (not perceptible to an observer) complaints, a specific history, clinical signs, symptoms, and laboratory or radiographic findings. A disorder is defined as a pathologic (diseased) condition of the mind or body. Because the terms are similar, both are used throughout this text to refer to abnormal conditions of body systems.

All diseases and disorders of the human body involve the disruption of *homeostasis,* which is the state of dynamic equilibrium (balance or stability) of the internal environment of the body. To some extent, all medical persons are *pathologists* (those who study disease). Yet the term is usually used in reference to medical professionals who devote their careers to the study of human tissues, cells, and body fluids for evidence of disease. Individuals within this field may specialize in research, teaching, postmortem examinations (autopsies), and other areas.

Understanding the *etiology* (cause) of diseases and disorders is generally considered the first important step toward finding a cure or effective treatment. When the cause is unknown, the disease may be referred to as *idiopathic* in nature. Some conditions are iatrogenic, meaning they developed as a complication to the medical or surgical treatment of another disorder. An example is the individual who suffers severe immune suppression secondary to chemotherapy (a type of cancer treatment). A *nosocomial* condition is one that was acquired within the hospital, such as the staphylococcal infection a patient develops in the incision while recovering from surgery.

Flashpoint

When the etiology is unknown, the disease is idiopathic.

Risk Factors for Disease

Risk factors, also called predisposing factors, are factors known to increase the likelihood of certain diseases and disorders. They are not the direct causes of disease, but they do increase the chances that an individual will develop disease. Some of these factors are beyond the individual's control, but others can be eliminated or modified to varying degrees.

Age
Premature and newborn infants have immature immune systems and immature kidneys. This makes them vulnerable to some types of infection and dehydration. Advanced age is also considered a risk factor for many diseases and disorders, since the immune system, as well as most other body systems, weakens with advancing age. For example, the elderly are vulnerable to conditions such as cardiovascular disease, cancer, osteoporosis, arthritis, and various forms of dementia.

Heredity
Certain hereditary traits—such as a family history of breast cancer or of cardiovascular disease—are known risk factors for disease. In some cases hereditary disorders are passed from

parent to child via identified genes. Examples are Huntington disease (a degenerative and ulti-mately fatal neuromuscular disease) and hemophilia (a disease that impairs the blood's ability to form clots).

Lifestyle

Many lifestyle practices have a positive or negative impact on health, leading to increased or decreased resistance to disease. Factors known to promote health and boost disease resistance include regular exercise and a healthy diet. Factors that lead to vulnerability to disease include sedentary lifestyle, poorly managed stress, poor nutrition, and abuse of alcohol, drugs, and tobacco.

Gender

Gender is considered a risk factor for some disorders; for example, osteoporosis, breast cancer, and autoimmune disorders such as multiple sclerosis are more prevalent (more common) in women, while others like Parkinson disease and lung cancer are more common in men.

Environment

In some cases, environment is known to contribute to disease. For example, individuals who suffer exposure to chemicals, radiation, or air pollution are known to have higher risk for certain types of cancer and respiratory disorders. Those who live in crowded conditions with poor sanitation, low income, and inadequate access to quality education and health care are known to suffer a higher incidence of nutritional deficiencies and communicable (contagious) diseases.

Combination of Factors

Some disorders are thought to be triggered by a combination of the factors discussed previously. In some cases, a triggering event is also thought to play a role. For example, the onset of multi-ple sclerosis is thought to be from a combination of genetics, a possible triggering event such as pregnancy, and a dysfunctional response of the immune system.

The Medical Response to Disease

Health-care providers are trained to provide medical care in a thoughtful and methodical manner, which helps to ensure a thorough, efficient response. This care includes several predictable features, including diagnosis, prognosis, treatment, and evaluation.

Diagnosis

Patients usually present to the provider with complaints about various signs and symptoms. Before determining the diagnosis, the provider must collect certain data (information). This is done by performing a physical examination and questioning the patient to gather information about medical history, family history, medication use, current health practices, allergies, and risk factors. In some cases the diagnosis is arrived at easily; in others it may not be readily apparent. To keep from overlooking important clues, the provider begins with a list of dif-ferential diagnoses, which are all of the possible diagnoses that may apply. The provider may next elect to perform diagnostic tests or procedures such as blood tests or radiological studies (see Box 2-1). As data is collected, the provider is able to cross diagnoses off the list of potentials and eventually narrow the list down to one diagnosis.

Flashpoint

Some diagnoses are easy to make, while others are more elusive.

Prognosis

The prognosis is the anticipated outcome of the disease. In many cases it is quite predictable; for example, the common cold typically lasts 7 to 10 days, and individuals generally recover fully unless they are in a weakened state from some other disease or disorder.

Treatment

Once the diagnosis has been determined, the provider and patient discuss treatment options. Ideally, this should be a collaborative process in which the patient makes a decision after being informed about the potential risks and benefits of all treatment choices. Treatment plans vary widely by patient situation and disease. Features often include medication, surgery, education, physical therapy or other forms of therapy, exercise, nutritional counseling, and complementary therapies such as biofeedback, acupuncture, chiropractic, and massage. Forms of treatment which completely resolve or eliminate the problem are considered curative. An example is the use of antibiotics to eliminate infection. Forms of treatment aimed at reducing the likelihood of disease, such as implementation of regular exercise and a low-fat diet to reduce the risk of heart disease, are considered preventive. Some forms of treatment are considered *palliative.* These types of treatment do not cure a disease, but are aimed at preventing or relieving associated pain and suffering. An example is the use of morphine and other medications to ease the pain and suffering of cancer patients.

Evaluation

The evaluation process may be so simple as to seem invisible. In cases of uncomplicated conditions, the responsibility falls on the patient to contact the physician after treatment if improvement does not occur. A provider who hears nothing further from the patient assumes that the patient has recovered completely, as in the case of a patient who is prescribed antibiotics for a simple bacterial infection and then does not return for further care. In other cases, when the condition is more complex or chronic, the patient will be asked to return for one or more follow-up appointments so the provider can evaluate the response to treatment. This allows for further examination, testing, education, and modification of the treatment plan as needed. An example of this situation is the continued care an individual with severe hypertension requires to ensure that blood pressure is being managed adequately.

Abbreviations

There are many lengthy terms in the world of health care. To make verbal and written communications easier, these terms are often abbreviated (see Table 2-1). It is important, though, that providers use only approved abbreviations, to avoid miscommunication.

TABLE 2-1			
ABBREVIATIONS			
Abbreviation	**Meaning**	**Abbreviation**	**Meaning**
DD, DDx, ddx	differential diagnosis	Sx	symptom
Dx	diagnosis	Tx	treatment
Rx	prescription		

Infectious Disease

The health-care environment is intended to be a place where people can find help and healing. However, because it brings many individuals together who have infectious diseases or weakened immune systems, it sets the stage for the very real possibility of disease transmission between patients and even health-care staff. To prevent such transmission, health-care workers must have an understanding of how disease is transmitted and how to take every reasonable precaution to reduce disease transmission in the medical office. *Infectious diseases,* also called *communicable diseases,* are those that may be transmitted directly or indirectly between individuals (see Box 2-2).

Microorganisms and Pathogens

Microorganisms are living organisms too small to be seen with the naked eye. Many different types of microorganisms exist in the environment; however, not all are connected to disease. Those that normally live on and in the human body are generally harmless and are known as *normal flora.* They are present in and on areas such as the skin, nasopharynx, gastrointestinal tract, and vagina. A healthy balance of these microorganisms normally exists, and rather than causing disease, they usually provide protection from organisms that are not part of the body's normal flora. However, when this balance is disturbed or when bacteria are spread to another site, infection can occur. For example, *Escherichia coli* is a bacterium that normally resides within the gastrointestinal tract. If it is transmitted into the urinary tract, a urinary tract infection may develop.

Box 2-2 Wellness Promotion

PREVENTING DISEASE TRANSMISSION
Microorganisms are introduced into the health-care environment on a daily basis by ill patients who speak, cough, sneeze, and touch things with contaminated hands. By doing so, they spread pathogens throughout the reception area and examination rooms. To help break the chain of infection, health-care workers must team up in their efforts to keep the environment as clean as possible. Administrative medical assistants or receptionists may be responsible for cleaning countertops, windows, and other surfaces in the reception area. Clinical medical assistants or nurses may be responsible for cleaning surfaces and equipment in the clinical areas between patient visits. Preventing disease transmission is everyone's job, so all members of the team should work together in a cooperative fashion. In addition, they can make sure hand sanitizers and tissues are available to patients in all areas and teach patients the importance of hand washing.

Flashpoint
Normal flora often help to keep you healthy.

Pathogens are microorganisms that are capable of producing disease. To grow and thrive, most pathogens require nutrients, moisture, warmth, and a suitable-pH (usually neutral) environment. Thus, some parts of the human body tend to provide a more hospitable environment for pathogenic growth than others. Some pathogens, called ***aerobes***, require oxygen; those that must have an oxygen-free environment are called ***anaerobes***. The main types of pathogens are bacteria, viruses, fungi, protozoans, and parasitic worms.

Flashpoint
Most pathogens thrive in a warm, moist, pH-neutral environment.

Bacteria

Bacteria are one-celled organisms that cause such diseases as staphylococcus infection, streptococcus infection, gonorrhea, and Lyme disease. Bacteria are classified according to their shape (see Fig. 2-1):

Flashpoint
Bacteria are classified by their shape.

* Cocci: round or spherical in shape; grouped in pairs (diplococci), double pairs with a square appearance (tetrads), chains (streptococci), and clusters (staphylococci)
* Bacilli: rod-shaped; arranged as single, separate rods (single bacilli), pairs (diplobacilli), chains (streptobacilli), and rods with rounded ends (coccobacilli)
* Spiral: curved rods (spirilla) and helical or corkscrew-shaped (spirochetes)

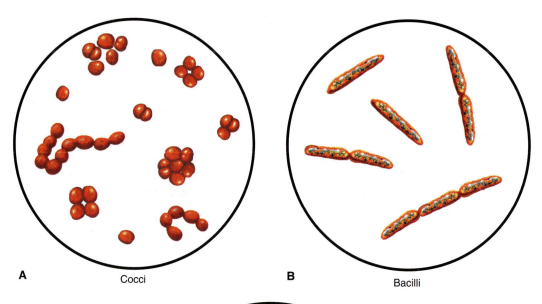

A   Cocci   B   Bacilli

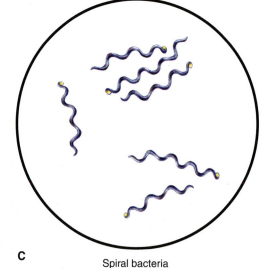

C   Spiral bacteria

FIGURE 2-1 Classification of bacteria based on shape (From Eagle, S, et al. *The Professional Medical Assistant: An Integrative Teamwork-Based Approach.* 2009. Philadelphia: F.A. Davis Company, with permission.)

Viruses

A **virus** is a pathogen that grows and reproduces after infecting a host cell. There are more than 400 types of viruses in many shapes and sizes. They are classified by their shape and size and whether they contain DNA or RNA (see Fig. 2-2). They are generally named after the illness they cause or the family in which they are classified. They cause diseases such as the common cold, hepatitis, chicken pox, and AIDS.

Viruses usually act in a parasitic fashion by invading and dominating the host individual's healthy cells. They then use the host cell's nutrients to multiply. The cells subsequently burst and spill more virus into the body. Viruses are the smallest of pathogens and can only be seen with an electron microscope. They contain RNA or DNA and are difficult to treat because the protein in their outer cell membrane prevents antibiotics from affecting them.

Fungi

A **fungus** may be a simple, single-celled organism such as yeast or a multicellular colony such as mold or a mushroom (see Fig. 2-3). Most fungi do not cause disease and are present in the body's normal flora; however, some do cause diseases in humans, including:

- Yeasts, such as *Candida albicans* (a cause of local infections such as vulvovaginal infection and thrush) and *Cryptococcus neoformans* (a cause of serious systemic infections, such as meningitis, particularly in those with weakened immune systems)
- Molds, such as the black mold *Aspergillus niger* (a cause of lung and ear infections)

Protozoans

Protozoans are single-celled microscopic organisms that live mainly in soil and water (see Fig. 2-4). Most do not cause infection, but a few can cause serious illness that can be difficult to diagnose, because the protozoans have a dormant stage in which they exist in cyst form. During this stage they are resistant to environmental factors that might otherwise kill them. Once a cyst is ingested by a human, the protozoan's life cycle begins and human infection occurs. Protozoans commonly infect persons with low immunity. They are spread through the fecal-oral route, when individuals ingest contaminated food or water, or by contact with mosquitoes or other infected insects. Protozoans that cause illness include *Plasmodium* species, *Pneumocystis carinii*, *Giardia lamblia*, and *Cryptosproridium* species.

> **Flashpoint**
> People with weakened immune systems are most vulnerable to protozoal infections.

Parasitic Worms

Parasitic worms are present in soil and water and require other living organisms to survive. Infection occurs when individuals unknowingly ingest the tiny worm eggs, which then hatch within the intestinal tract. Less commonly, worms or eggs may migrate to other organs, such as the liver or lungs. Common offenders are *Enterobius vermicularis* (pinworms) and *Ascaris lumbricoides* (roundworms).

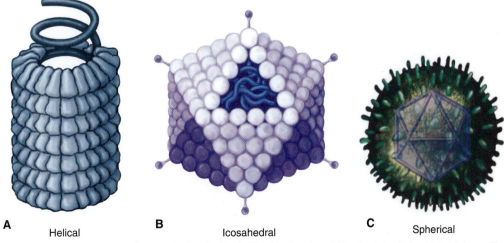

A	B	C
Helical	Icosahedral	Spherical

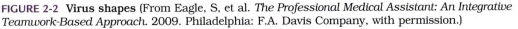

FIGURE 2-2 Virus shapes (From Eagle, S, et al. *The Professional Medical Assistant: An Integrative Teamwork-Based Approach.* 2009. Philadelphia: F.A. Davis Company, with permission.)

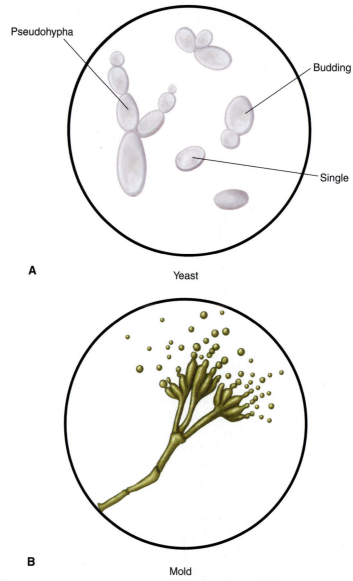

A   Yeast

B   Mold

FIGURE 2-3 **Fungi** (From Eagle, S, et al. *The Professional Medical Assistant: An Integrative Teamwork-Based Approach.* 2009. Philadelphia: F.A. Davis Company, with permission.)

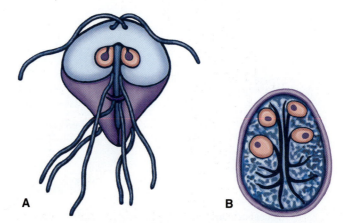

A   **B**

FIGURE 2-4 *Giardia lamblia:* **(A) Trophozoite (active) stage; (B) Cyst stage** (From Eagle, S, et al. *The Professional Medical Assistant: An Integrative Teamwork-Based Approach.* 2009. Philadelphia: F.A. Davis Company, with permission.)

The Chain of Infection

The chain of infection describes a series of steps that must occur for disease to spread. Learning about the chain of infection helps health-care workers understand how microorganisms are transmitted and how people become infected. This understanding helps workers more effectively protect themselves and their patients. Infectious diseases can only spread if all of the links in the chain of infection are active. Therefore, health-care workers can stop the spread of disease by breaking any link in the chain. The chain consists of the pathogen, reservoir host, means of exit, mode of transmission, means of entry, and susceptible host (see Fig. 2-5).

Pathogen

Pathogens are the first link in the chain of infection. Those that are present in the blood and can be transmitted through blood or body fluids are called bloodborne pathogens. Examples of common bloodborne pathogens are HIV, hepatitis B, and hepatitis C. Organisms that are usually harmless but become pathogenic under specific circumstances, such as exposure to an immunocompromised host, are called opportunistic pathogens.

Reservoir Host

A reservoir host is an organism from which pathogens such as bacteria and viruses obtain their nourishment. It provides a hospitable environment in which the pathogens can grow. Living infected hosts may be *symptomatic* (having noticeable signs of disease) or *asymptomatic* (free of symptoms). The reservoir host is considered contagious and can spread the disease to others.

Flashpoint
Pathogens thrive in warm, moist places.

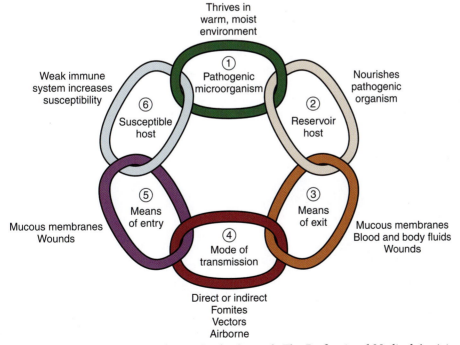

FIGURE 2-5 The chain of infection (From Eagle, S, et al. *The Professional Medical Assistant: An Integrative Teamwork-Based Approach.* 2009. Philadelphia: F.A. Davis Company, with permission.)

Means of Exit

A common way for pathogens to leave a reservoir host's body is via the mucous membranes. Therefore, any opening of the body that is lined with mucous membranes becomes a potential exit site, including the eyes, nose, mouth, throat, vagina, and rectum. Another type of exit site might be an interruption in the normal protective structures of the body, such as injury or surgical incision into the skin and underlying tissues. Pathogens can also exit the body via blood and such body fluids as semen, vaginal secretions, urine, and feces.

Mode of Transmission

A pathogen can be transmitted to another person by direct or indirect contact. Examples of direct contact include skin-to-skin contact, such as shaking hands or kissing, and the exchange of body fluids, such as needle-sharing or sexual contact. Pathogens may also be transmitted via indirect contact with inanimate objects called *fomites.* Virtually any object can be a fomite. Common examples are countertops, hairbrushes, combs, doorknobs, drink containers, handles of shopping carts, and pencils. Another type of transmission occurs via *vectors,* which are usually insects (or other arthropods, such as lice, ticks, and vermin) that carry pathogens from infected to noninfected individuals.

Airborne transmission, a form of indirect transmission, occurs when an infected individual sprays pathogens into the air by coughing or sneezing. Another individual then inhales the pathogens from the air and becomes infected. Tuberculosis is one disease that is spread by airborne transmission.

Means of Entry

Pathogens gain entry to the body in much the same way as they exit the reservoir host's body, usually via contact with mucous membranes or a break in the skin. Therefore, potential entry sites include the eyes, nose, mouth, throat, vagina, and rectum, as well as any wounds to the skin.

Susceptible Host

If a host is susceptible, pathogens will grow and multiply, eventually reaching an infectious level. A number of conditions increase host susceptibility; most contribute to a weakened immune system. Common examples include poor hygiene, poor nutrition, stress, other underlying diseases or disorders, some medications, age (extreme youth or senescence), and self-destructive behaviors such as tobacco use, excessive alcohol intake, and use of illicit drugs (see Box 2-3).

Types of Infection

Infections can be categorized according to their general duration and whether they occur only once or recur repeatedly. There are three types of infection:

- *Acute* infections typically have a quick onset and short duration. There may or may not be a clear prodromal phase, which is when early symptoms are nonspecific. The duration is usually one to three weeks. An example is the common cold.
- *Chronic* infections last for a long time, sometimes for years or even a lifetime. The patient may be asymptomatic or symptoms may fluctuate. Individuals with some types of chronic disease may experience periods of exacerbation (worsening of symptoms) and remission (improvement or disappearance of symptoms). Examples of chronic infection include hepatitis C and AIDS.

Box 2-3 Wellness Promotion

BREAKING THE CHAIN
The following common-sense strategies will help protect you from pathogens.

- Wash your hands:
  Frequently throughout the day, especially during cold and flu season
  After using the toilet
  After blowing your nose
  Before eating
- Teach children how to wash or sanitize their hands
- Avoid crowds during cold and flu season, if possible
- Avoid others who are ill
- Avoid going to work when you are ill
- Keep ill children home from school
- Cover coughs and sneezes with your arm rather than your hand
- Avoid sharing drink containers and eating utensils
- Use hand sanitizer when warm water and soap are not available
- Avoid unprotected sexual encounters
- Avoid touching your eyes, nose, and mouth
- Use hand sanitizers if available in medical offices and grocery stores

- *Latent* infections are those in which patients experience alternating periods of being symptomatic (relapse) with periods of being asymptomatic (remission). The infecting organism, usually a virus, never leaves the body, but lies dormant between relapses. A common example is the herpes viruses, which can cause intermittent outbreaks of oral or genital lesions and shingles.

> **Flashpoint**
> Infections can be acute, chronic, or latent.

Stages of Disease

There are several stages in the disease process (see Fig. 2-6). The first begins when pathogens first come in contact with and gain access to the body, and the last ends when patients are no longer ill and have fully recovered. The duration and severity of the entire process is highly variable; in some cases it lasts a few short days, and in other cases for weeks or even months. Some diseases are so disabling that infected individuals are bedridden, yet others are so mild that infected individuals experience few symptoms and continue to carry out their normal daily activities. The stages of disease are:

- Incubation
- Prodromal
- Acute
- Declining
- Convalescent

> **Flashpoint**
> Disease stages are variable in length but usually predictable in order.

Incubation Stage

The **incubation** stage, sometimes called the *latent* period, is the beginning stage of an infectious disease, starting at first contact with the pathogen. It is the interval between exposure and the appearance of the first symptoms. During this stage, patients may be asymptomatic but are commonly considered contagious. Incubation time varies from days to weeks or months, depending on the disease.

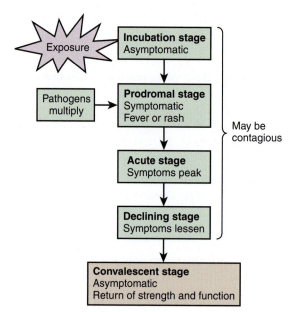

FIGURE 2-6 **The stages of disease** (From Eagle, S, et al. *The Professional Medical Assistant: An Integrative Teamwork-Based Approach.* 2009. Philadelphia: F.A. Davis Company, with permission.)

Prodromal Stage

The ***prodromal*** stage marks the interval between the earliest symptoms and the appearance of a rash or elevated temperature. Patients who are febrile (with a fever) also commonly complain of such generalized symptoms as malaise (a feeling of discomfort), fatigue, weakness, and generally feeling unwell.

Acute Stage

The acute stage is when symptoms peak and the patient feels the worst. Patients in this stage continue to be contagious and should avoid others, to keep from spreading the disease. They should heed medical advice, which often includes taking prescribed medications, resting, and drinking nonalcoholic and noncaffeinated beverages.

Declining Stage

The declining stage begins with the end of the acute stage. It is characterized by a continuation of the disease but a lessening of the symptoms. Patients notice that they are beginning to feel better and may wish to begin resuming normal activities.

Convalescent Stage

The convalescent stage of disease is the recovery period. It begins when disease symptoms disappear and continues until the patient has regained full strength and returned to a normal state of health. During the declining and convalescent stages, patients must be cautioned to avoid overexerting themselves or prematurely discontinuing their medication or other therapies. Either one could, in some cases, cause a relapse (see Box 2-4).

 STOP HERE.
Select the flash cards for this chapter and review them at least three times before moving on to the next chapter.

Box 2-4 Wellness Promotion

FINISH YOUR MEDICATION

Patients sometimes fail to take or complete their medication as prescribed and as a result may be labeled "noncompliant" by their health-care providers. However, many patients may not understand *why* the medication should be taken a certain way. If health-care providers explain to patients why it is important to take medications as prescribed, patients will be more likely to comply with the treatment plan. Here are some common scenarios in which patients do not take medications as prescribed:

- **Feeling better.** Some patients think they no longer need the medication when they begin feeling better. However, the effectiveness of medications such as antibiotics depends on completion of the full course of treatment. Discontinuing early could cause a relapse and worsening of the illness. Furthermore, discontinuing medication early exposes the pathogens to the medication without fully destroying them. This brief but inadequate exposure is a major contributor to the rise in antibiotic-resistant organisms so prevalent today.
- **Saving some for later.** Some patients discontinue medication early so they will have some left for future use. This practice is dangerous, because the current medication may not be the best choice for whatever future illness arises. Furthermore, having only a small amount of medication like antibiotics may be worse than having none at all, leading to relapse or drug resistance.
- **Fitting the schedule.** Some patients change dosing times or frequencies to better fit with their daily schedule. Sometimes this is OK, but patients should be encouraged to check with their physician before making any changes.
- **Increasing the dose.** Some patients take more than the prescribed dose, hoping for an increased effect or a faster response. Doing so puts them at risk for drug toxicity but does not increase the healing benefit.
- **Reducing the effects or cost.** Some patients take less than the prescribed dose, hoping to reduce unpleasant adverse effects, save money, or make the medication last longer. Doing so results in decreased effectiveness of the medication and provides no benefits to the patient. In these situations, patients should consult with their physician regarding possible solutions.

Student Resources

Centers for Disease Control and Prevention: http://www.cdc.gov
Mayo Clinic Infectious Disease Center: http://www.mayoclinic.com/
Occupational Safety and Health Administration: http://www.osha.gov
World Health Organization: http://www.who.int/en/

Chapter Activities

Learning Style Study Strategies

Try any or all of the following strategies as you study the content of this chapter:

Visual learners: Look closely at the photos, illustrations, and other visual material. You will very likely be able to see them later in your mind's eye, which will help you recall details.

Kinesthetic learners: Use the flash cards; also make and use your own additional flash cards as needed.

Auditory learners: Read sections from the book aloud to yourself; consider recording challenging sections to replay repeatedly until you fully comprehend the material.

Verbal learners: Explain or "teach" specific topics, such as the chain of infection, to a study partner or friend.

Practice Exercises

Answers to Practice Exercises can be found in Appendix D.

Case Studies

CASE STUDY 1

While working in a medical clinic, you are assigned to help provide care for a patient suspected of having influenza.

1. Describe the precautions you will take to keep from catching the flu from your patient.

2. Describe the education you will provide to your patient so that she can reduce the risk of transmitting her illness to others.

CASE STUDY 2

You observe a coworker placing patients into examination rooms and taking their vital signs without washing her hands in between patients. When you comment on this, she states that she just doesn't have time. How will you respond?

CASE STUDY 3

You have been asked to speak to your child's second-grade class about germs and how to keep from getting sick. Describe how you will do this.

Multiple Choice

1. Which of the following terms is matched with the correct definition?

   a. Fungus: Microorganism that needs oxygen to grow

   b. Parasite: Organism found on and in our bodies that does not cause disease

   c. Protozoan: A genus of bacteria that are intracellular parasites

   d. Idiopathic: Having an unknown cause

2. Which of the following terms is matched with the correct definition?

   a. Prodromal: Interval between earliest symptoms and the appearance of a rash or fever

   b. Incubation: Ability of a pathogen to produce disease

   c. Symptomatic: Interval between exposure to infection and the appearance of the first symptoms

   d. Virulence: Forming or containing pus

3. Which of the following is **not** one of the links in the chain of infection?

   a. Antibody

   b. Reservoir host

   c. Means of exit

   d. Susceptible host

4. Which of the following is **not** a type of infection?

   a. Latent

   b. Acute

   c. Chronic

   d. Intermittent

5. Which of the following is **not** one of the stages of the disease process?

   a. Incubation stage

   b. Prostration stage

   c. Prodromal state

   d. Acute stage

Short Answer

1. **Describe some simple measures that can be taken to help prevent transmission of pathogens in the waiting room of a medical office.**

2. **Describe the following three types of infection:**

   a. Acute

   b. Chronic

   c. Latent

3. **List at least three reasons why individuals should take all of their medications as prescribed.**

3 DISEASE PREVENTION

Learning Outcomes

Upon completion of this chapter, the student will be able to:

- Define and spell the key terms
- Describe the body's defense mechanisms
- Explain the steps in the inflammatory response process
- List and describe four different types of immunity
- Explain standard precautions
- List common types of personal protective equipment
- Describe three types of biohazardous waste and list precautions that must be followed for disposal
- Discuss the employer's role in providing vaccinations to employees
- Describe strategies to increase health and safety in the workplace
- Describe the appropriate response when a worker is exposed to a blood-borne pathogen
- Describe the appropriate response when a biohazard spill occurs in the health-care workplace
- Differentiate between medical asepsis and surgical asepsis
- Describe symptoms of burnout
- Discuss factors that contribute to burnout
- Design and describe a self-care plan that will prevent burnout

KEY TERMS	
antibody	substance produced by white blood cells in response to a specific antigen that then acts to destroy the disease-causing organism
antigen	marker that identifies a cell as being part of the body (self) or not part of the body (nonself)
burnout	syndrome of feeling physical, emotional, or mental exhaustion caused by ongoing intensive demands without sufficient physical or emotional rest
histamine	chemical which causes the dilation of blood vessels and other activities in the inflammatory response
interferon	chemical produced by white blood cells in response to pathogen invasion that inhibits virus production within infected cells
kinins	chemicals that increase blood flow and increase the permeability of small blood capillaries as a part of the inflammatory response
leukocytes	white blood cells that act against infection and tissue damage
lysozyme	enzyme present in tears, saliva, and other secretions which protects against pathogens
medical asepsis	destruction of pathogenic organisms after they leave the body
phagocytosis	process in which specialized white blood cells engulf and destroy microorganisms, foreign antigens, and cell debris

KEY TERMS—cont'd	
prostaglandins	hormones that stimulate receptors and produce localized vasodilation, vascular permeability, and platelet aggregation
self-care	any activity which supports and nurtures one's physical, mental, spiritual, or emotional health and well-being
standard precautions	guidelines for the handling of any blood or body fluids (except sweat) that might contain blood or infectious organisms
surgical asepsis	destruction of pathogenic organisms before they enter the body

Abbreviations

There are many lengthy terms in the world of health care. Table 3-1 lists some of those most common to disease prevention.

The Body's Defense Mechanisms

The body's natural protective mechanisms normally work amazingly well to protect human beings from pathogens. There are three main types of defense mechanism:

- mechanical
- chemical
- cellular

Mechanical Defenses

Mechanical defenses include certain structures and functions of the body. For example, the skin is a structure that protects a person from the external environment. Tiny hairs within the nasal cavity help filter the air by removing debris. The lower airways are lined with special membranes that have cilia (threadlike projections) that move in a wavelike fashion to propel debris upward

TABLE 3-1
ABBREVIATIONS

Abbreviation	Meaning	Abbreviation	Meaning
Ab	antibody	MMR	measles-mumps-rubella (vaccine)
Ag	antigen	PPD	purified protein derivative (Tuberculosis test)
ANA	antinuclear antibody	WBC	white blood cell
DPT	diphtheria-pertussis-tetanus (vaccine)		

so that it can be coughed out or swallowed. Protective reflexes, such as coughing and sneezing, are triggered by the presence of foreign debris in the respiratory tract. A cough is a forceful expiratory effort that is difficult, if not impossible, to suppress and can literally be lifesaving. When an individual sneezes, air is expelled forcefully though the nose and mouth by a spasmodic contraction of muscles that normally facilitate respiration. This action helps clear irritating debris and microorganisms from the nasal passages.

Flashpoint

The body's mechanical defenses keep pathogens from entering the body and help expel them from the body.

Other mechanical protective mechanisms in the body include the flushing action of certain body fluids. For example, the tear glands of the eyes produce a fluid that continually bathes and cleanses the eyes. Because the eyes are extremely sensitive, when foreign particles enter them the tear glands respond by increasing production of tears to flush the debris away. Flushing action also occurs in the urinary tract, where urine is produced in the kidneys and follows a one-way path through the ureters (long narrow tubes) to the bladder and out of the body via the urethra. This one-way flow of fluid helps prevent pathogens from moving upward through the urethra into the urinary tract, where they might cause infection.

Chemical Defenses

The body has some chemical barriers that help protect it from pathogens. For example, the skin contains sebaceous glands nearly everywhere except the palms of the hands and soles of the feet. These glands secrete an oily substance that not only helps keep skin supple and healthy but actually kills some types of pathogens. The fluids in the stomach are normally very acidic, which effectively kills most swallowed pathogens. The fluids in tears and the urinary tract are also somewhat acidic, which is generally not conducive to bacterial growth.

In addition, the body produces a group of glycoproteins (compounds of carbohydrates and proteins) called *interferons* that have antiviral activity. Some are produced by *leukocytes* (white blood cells) in response to invasion by pathogens, especially viruses. They help mark the invading pathogens for destruction. They also inhibit virus production within infected cells. Various types of interferons are used to treat diseases such as hepatitis B and C, Kaposi sarcoma, and multiple sclerosis.

Also, some enzymes produced by the body protect against pathogens. A great example is *lysozyme.* This enzyme, which is present in tears, saliva, and other bodily secretions, acts to inhibit the growth of bacteria by damaging their cell walls.

Cellular Defenses

Various cells also act to protect the body from pathogens. Their defenses include:

- inflammatory response
- immunity

Inflammatory Response

The inflammatory response is the body's immediate immunological defense against injury, infection, or allergy (see Fig. 3-1). This response protects the body from invasion by foreign pathogens and sets in motion a series of events that repair tissue damage. In the inflammatory response, tissue trauma sets off the release of several chemicals that cause inflammation:

- *Histamine* is a chemical that causes a variety of responses, depending on the site of injury. In soft tissue it causes the dilation of blood vessels, which helps improve circulation to the injured area and speeds the arrival of white blood cells to the scene.
- *Prostaglandins* are hormones that are formed rapidly and act in the immediate area of the injury. They stimulate receptors and produce local vasodilation, vascular permeability, and platelet aggregation.
- *Kinins* are chemicals that increase blood flow and increase the permeability of small blood capillaries.

As a result, localized inflammation occurs, indicated by redness, swelling, heat, pain, and decreased function. Some of these changes indicate that the body is at work healing itself; for

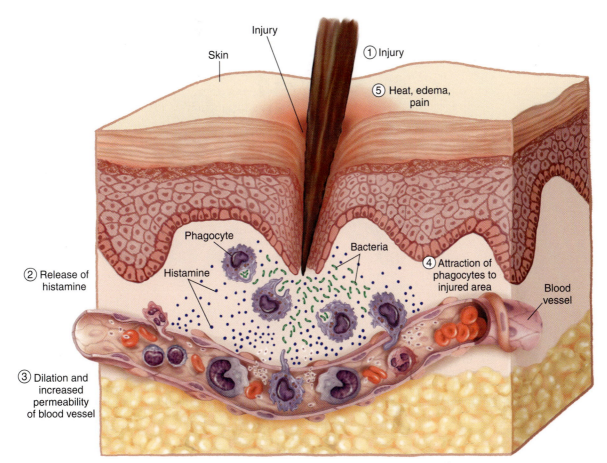

FIGURE 3-1 **Inflammatory response** (From Eagle, S, et al. *The Professional Medical Assistant: An Integrative Teamwork-Based Approach.* 2009. Philadelphia: F.A. Davis Company, with permission.)

example, the increase in circulation and vessel permeability allows white blood cells to enter the injured area and begin engulfing bacteria and cellular debris in a process known as **phagocytosis** (see Fig. 3-2). Increased circulation also brings oxygen and nutrients to the area so that repair can occur. However, edema (swelling) can contribute to the patient's discomfort. In addition, the chemicals that set the whole process in motion also cause increased pain perception.

When the body's natural defenses are unsuccessful in eliminating invading organisms, infection may occur. However, inflammation and infection are not the same. Symptoms of localized infection are similar to those of inflammation but may become more pronounced. In infection, such signs of inflammation as redness, swelling, heat, and pain may be present along with fever and generalized malaise. Localized sites of injury may produce purulent (pus-containing) drainage, which is rich in necrotic (dead) WBCs, bacteria, and cellular debris.

Immunity

Immunity is defined as protection from infectious disease. It is categorized as active or passive, with active and passive immunity further categorized as naturally or artificially acquired (see Fig. 3-3).

Active Natural Immunity

Active natural immunity develops when the body is exposed to a pathogenic microorganism. All microorganisms contain **antigens,** which are markers that identify cells as being part of the body (self) or not part of the body (nonself). Antigens on the body's own cells are called *autoantigens;* all others are *foreign antigens.* Antigens are capable of triggering an immune response or binding with an antibody to neutralize or destroy pathogens. During the initial exposure to the

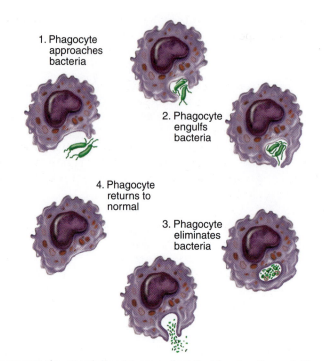

1. Phagocyte approaches bacteria

2. Phagocyte engulfs bacteria

4. Phagocyte returns to normal

3. Phagocyte eliminates bacteria

FIGURE 3-2 **In phagocytosis, specialized types of white blood cells engulf and eliminate pathogens and cellular debris.** (From Eagle, S, et al. *The Professional Medical Assistant: An Integrative Teamwork-Based Approach.* 2009. Philadelphia: F.A. Davis Company, with permission.)

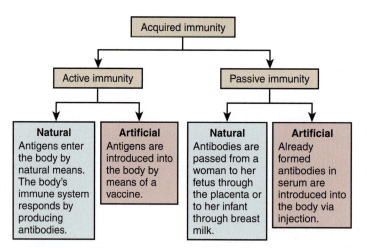

FIGURE 3-3 **Types of immunity** (From Eagle, S, et al. *The Professional Medical Assistant: An Integrative Teamwork-Based Approach.* 2009. Philadelphia: F.A. Davis Company, with permission.)

pathogen, a person usually develops symptoms of disease. This initial exposure also stimulates white blood cells to develop *__antibodies,__* which are immunoglobulins (a diverse group of plasma proteins) specifically tailored to that pathogen's antigen. Those antibodies later combine with that antigen when it presents itself again (during a second exposure) to mark the microorganism for destruction by macrophages, another type of white blood cell.

Active Artificial Immunity

Active artificial immunity develops when an antigen is purposely introduced into a person's body in the form of a vaccine. Examples of vaccines include measles, mumps, and rubella (MMR) and oral poliomyelitis vaccine. Vaccines generally contain a live, altered (weakened) microorganism or all or part of a dead microorganism. The antigen in the vaccine has been altered in some way so that it will stimulate antibody formation without causing disease. When an individual's immunity status or exposure to disease is in question, an antibody titer check may be done (see Box 3-1).

Passive Natural Immunity

Passive natural immunity develops when already formed antibodies are passed from mother to fetus across the placenta during pregnancy. A pregnant woman has, through the course of her life, been exposed to a variety of pathogenic organisms and developed antibodies against many of them. Some of these antibodies cross the placenta to the fetus. After the infant is born, the antibodies continue to provide protection against disease for several months. If the woman breast-feeds the infant, additional antibodies are passed to the infant through breast milk. In both cases, the preformed antibodies temporarily help to protect the infant until the infant's body begins developing its own antibodies.

Passive Artificial Immunity

Passive artificial immunity develops when preformed antibodies are developed in an animal or in another human and are then injected into an individual who has experienced a known exposure. This introduction of antiserum provides the individual with temporary passive immunity. Situations in which such an injection might be given include known exposures to rabies, botulism, venomous snakes or spiders, hepatitis, and diphtheria.

Flashpoint
Infants are given temporary immunity by antibodies received through the placenta before birth and through breast milk after birth.

Standard Precautions

Safety in the medical office is of utmost importance—including the safety of staff and patients from injury and disease transmission. Two organizations that play an important role in safety guidelines and regulation in medical offices are the Centers for Disease Control and Prevention (CDC) and the Occupational Safety and Health Administration (OSHA).

In the 1980s the CDC created a set of guidelines called *universal precautions* to instruct health-care providers on how to minimize the risk of disease transmission when providing care. The CDC later revised the guidelines and renamed them **standard precautions.** The revision expanded the guidelines to cover more body fluids and routes of exposure. In general, standard precautions advise health-care providers about the handling of any blood or body fluids (except sweat) that might contain blood or infectious organisms. Such body fluids include semen, vaginal secretions, cerebrospinal fluid, synovial joint fluid, pleural fluid (from the lining of the lungs), peritoneal fluid (from the abdominal cavity), pericardial fluid (from between the heart and its lining), amniotic fluid, and any other body fluid or substance that contains visible blood.

OSHA is regulated by the U.S. Department of Labor to ensure safe, healthy working conditions for Americans. OSHA guidelines for bloodborne pathogens were developed to decrease the transmission of diseases in the workplace. Upon being hired, health-care workers learn about OSHA guidelines relevant to medical-office safety and must review them on a regular basis,

Box 3-1 Diagnostic Spotlight

ANTIBODY TITER

An antibody titer is a test that identifies the presence and amount of antibodies in the blood. To perform the test, blood is drawn from a vein (or in some cases obtained by puncturing the skin on the patient's fingertip). The test is useful in determining whether exposure has occurred. It is also sometimes used to determine whether a patient has sufficient immunity to certain diseases and whether a booster dose of the vaccine should be administered.

usually annually. OSHA guidelines dictate that employers provide workers with personal protective equipment (PPE), supplies, and equipment required for the safe disposal of contaminated or dangerous items. Regulations also include mandatory vaccinations against communicable diseases and protocols to follow in the event of an exposure.

Personal Protective Equipment

Flashpoint

Personal protective equipment is worn by health-care workers to protect them from pathogenic organisms.

The practice of standard precautions requires health-care providers to wear PPE that is appropriate to each situation, depending on the degree of risk. In the medical office, common PPE includes gloves, masks, eye protection, shoe covers, and gowns to wear during minor office surgeries and procedures when there is a risk of contact with blood or body fluids (see Fig. 3-4). Health-care workers should wear PPE that fits adequately and should replace it if it becomes contaminated or damaged. They should appropriately discard gloves that have become contaminated, punctured, or torn and replace them immediately. Appropriate eye protection includes a face shield or safety glasses that prevent splashing into the eyes.

Disposal of Biohazardous Waste

Health-care workers must develop careful habits when handling materials that are considered "sharps," such as needles, scalpel blades, capillary tubes, microscope slides, cover slips, and broken glass. They must dispose of such items in puncture-resistant containers. They should never recap an uncapped contaminated (used) needle, and they should only recap sterile needles

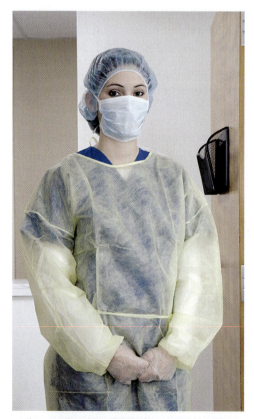

FIGURE 3-4 **Personal protective equipment (PPE)** (From Eagle, S, et al. *The Professional Medical Assistant: An Integrative Teamwork-Based Approach.* 2009. Philadelphia: F.A. Davis Company, with permission.)

when absolutely necessary, using the one-handed scoop technique. Furthermore, they should carefully examine trays and work areas for needles or any sharp objects after procedures are completed. This can be done safely by sorting through instruments and supplies with a pair of forceps, rather than by hand. Workers can then use the forceps to pick up and discard items as needed.

Health-care workers must also be in the habit of properly closing, removing, and replacing sharps and biohazard containers before they are full. This reduces the risk of injury from trying to place items in a too-full container. Furthermore, workers must know the policy and procedure for disposal of biohazardous waste at the facilities where they work (see Box 3-2).

In 2000 the U.S. Congress passed the Needlestick Safety and Prevention Act in an effort to reduce occupational exposure to sharps injuries. This act was a modification of OSHA's Bloodborne Pathogens Standard and provided more specific directives to employers to identify, evaluate, and implement safer medical devices and to maintain a sharps-injury log.

Vaccinations

In most cases, a health-care worker must provide documentation of all necessary vaccinations prior to employment. Examples include the hepatitis B vaccination and testing for tuberculosis exposure. If a worker has not completed certain vaccinations, the CDC requires the employer to provide them at no cost to the employee within 10 days of employment. The hepatitis B vaccine is administered in a series of three injections; the second injection is administered 1 month to 6 weeks after the first, and the third injection is administered 6 months later. An employee can decline to receive the immunization by completing and signing the proper paperwork, which the employer keeps on file. If the employee later requests the immunization, the CDC requires the employer to make it available.

Flashpoint

Employers are required to provide certain immunizations to employees at no cost.

Exposure Control

In the event of exposure to a pathogen, health-care workers must follow facility policy, which is dictated by several guidelines and requirements set by government agencies. Most exposure-control guidelines address exposure to a bloodborne pathogen and a biohazard spill.

Box 3-2 Wellness Promotion

PROTECTING ONE ANOTHER IN THE WORKPLACE

Sadly, there are too many true stories about health-care workers exposed to contaminated substances due to sloppy habits of their coworkers. Consider the following true events:

- A hospital housekeeper is stuck by a contaminated needle left in a bundle of soiled linens.
- A medical assistant cleaning up after a procedure is stuck in the finger by a suture needle left on the tray.
- As a nursing assistant reaches for an overflowing biohazard container placed on an upper shelf in a dirty utility room, it opens and spills its contents over his face.
- A nurse sits on a contaminated needle left on a chair in a patient's room.
- A kitchen worker in a local hospital is poked by a contaminated needle left on a meal tray.

All of these events might have been avoided, had the individuals involved used better work habits. Everyone's safety matters, and everyone needs to look out for one another.

Bloodborne Pathogen Exposure

If health-care workers are exposed to a bloodborne pathogen, they must first wash or flush the exposed area and then report the incident to the employer right away. OSHA guidelines require employers to develop exposure-control plans and make these plans known to employees. Workers must document the event by completing an incident report. Employers are required to follow up on the exposure incident by documenting the exposure and related circumstances and identifying the source individual and the status of the source individual, if that individual consents to testing for HIV or hepatitis B virus (HBV). Employers must offer employees the option of having their blood tested for HIV and HBV, as well as postexposure treatment in accordance with current recommendations from the U.S. Public Health Service. Furthermore, employers must provide counseling to the employees regarding precautions they must take and possible illness signs or symptoms to report.

Biohazard Spill

Health-care workers must be familiar with office protocol and CDC recommendations for responding to a biohazard spill. The first priority is to self-protect by applying gloves and other PPE. Next, workers should contain the spill with paper towels and then cover the entire spill with 10% bleach solution and let it stand for at least 20 minutes. When cleaning up the spill, they must use a mechanical device rather than their hands. They should then place all items in a biohazard container and repeat the bleach application, waiting another 20 minutes. They must document the incident according to office policy.

Asepsis

Important to the discussion of disease prevention are the practices of medical and surgical asepsis. All health-care workers must learn and practice the principles of medical asepsis; depending upon their duties, many must also learn and implement the principles of surgical asepsis (see Box 3-3).

Medical Asepsis

Medical asepsis refers to the destruction of pathogenic organisms after they leave the body. More specifically, medically aseptic technique refers to a method of performing procedures and providing patient care so that pathogenic organisms are not transmitted from the ill patient to other

---

Box 3-3 Wellness Promotion

MEDICAL VERSUS SURGICAL ASEPSIS

In general, medically aseptic technique is used to protect health-care providers and others from patients' pathogenic microorganisms. Surgically aseptic technique is used to protect patients from any pathogenic organisms external to their bodies. Here are some examples of procedures that require medical and surgical asepsis:

Medical Asepsis
- Taking a patient's temperature
- Removing an old dressing from a patient's wound
- Scrubbing and disinfecting used surgical instruments
- Emptying an emesis basin

Surgical Asepsis
- Inserting a urinary catheter
- Administering an intramuscular injection
- Applying a new dressing to a patient's wound
- Opening a sterile package
- Setting up a tray for the physician to perform suturing

patients or anyone else. The simplest way to apply medical asepsis is to follow standard precautions consistently. Health-care workers should always consider collected specimens to be contaminated, whether labeled or not. Body fluids that are not considered contaminated are tears, sweat, and saliva; but workers should always be cautious and wear examination gloves when there is any possibility of contamination.

Surgical Asepsis

Surgical asepsis is the practice of destroying pathogenic organisms before they enter the body. More specifically, surgically aseptic technique refers to a method of performing invasive procedures so that patients are protected from pathogenic microorganisms. When performing invasive procedures, health-care workers must use surgically aseptic technique. Invasive procedures are those in which the patient's normal protective barriers are punctured or disrupted in some manner, including injections, urinary catheterization, wound care, and such surgical procedures as tissue biopsy or repair and suturing of lacerations.

Flashpoint
Surgical asepsis protects patients from infection.

Self-Care

Most people are drawn to the health-care professions because of a combined interest in medicine and desire to help others and make a difference in the world. This desire will serve them well in their careers but can also be their undoing, because caregivers sometimes have a tendency to take good care of everyone but themselves. Ignoring their needs can eventually put them at great risk of *burnout,* a syndrome in which an individual feels physical, emotional, or mental exhaustion caused by ongoing intensive demands without sufficient physical or emotional rest (see Box 3-4). New health-care workers are usually so enthusiastic about their careers that they find it difficult to imagine themselves ever feeling burned out. However, no one is immune. Furthermore, burnout rarely occurs suddenly; rather, it usually develops slowly over a period of time and may become profound before an individual is fully aware of it. Therefore, all new health-care workers should develop a plan now to avoid burnout later.

Many factors contribute to burnout, but a key factor is the neglect of *self-care.* Self-care is any activity that supports and nurtures an individual's physical, mental, spiritual, or emotional health and well-being. Providing effective self-care entails taking full responsibility for nurturing and keeping oneself physically, emotionally, and mentally healthy. Some people have a hard time doing this and feel guilty when they spend time on themselves. Yet they may find themselves feeling needy and resentful when their needs go unmet and may even begin to feel neglected by others for failing to meet their needs. This has a negative impact on their relationships. Such individuals are at high risk for eventual burnout. To avoid this risk, they must learn to grant themselves permission to provide self-care, understanding that caring for themselves is a critical

Box 3-4 Wellness Promotion

SYMPTOMS OF BURNOUT
Health-care workers should watch out for these common symptoms of burnout:

- fatigue
- depression
- loss of interest in or enthusiasm for the job
- insomnia
- excessive need for sleep
- loss of empathy for clients
- feelings of anger or frustration

first step in being able to effectively care for others. A key principle in self-care is finding ways to create balance between work, play, rest, family obligations, and self-care needs. Health-care workers who develop and consistently use a plan of self-care find that their effectiveness in their professional and personal lives is enhanced (see Box 3-5).

For most busy professionals, finding time for self-care activities is challenging. Yet when one weighs the many benefits of self-care against the risks of burnout or injury, the choice becomes easier. For most individuals, it is helpful to view the time spent in self-care activities as an investment in their career and relationships that will reap benefits for years to come.

Flashpoint

Practicing good self-care is an important first step in being able to provide care for others.

STOP HERE.
Select the flash cards for this chapter and run through them at least three times before moving on to the next chapter.

Box 3-5 Self-Care Strategies to Avoid Burnout

BURNOUT FACTORS AND SELF-CARE STRATEGIES
This table lists some of the most common factors that contribute to burnout, as well as self-care strategies that can help avoid them.

Burnout Factor	Self-Care Strategy
stressful work environment	utilize stress-reduction strategies (meditation, exercise, relaxation, etc.)
feeling unsupported by boss or manager	set and adhere to healthy, effective boundaries in work and personal relationships
conflict among coworkers	create positive, nurturing relationships; participate in meaningful spiritual activities
long work hours; inability or unwillingness to take time off	make time for fun and recreational activities
insufficient or poor-quality sleep	get an adequate amount of quality sleep each night (7 to 8 hours for most adults) by developing good sleep habits; • go to bed and get up at the same time each day • avoid caffeinated beverages late in the day • avoid large meals before bed • seek treatment for sleep apnea and other sleep disorders • use a good-quality mattress and pillow • use earplugs or a fan to create white noise
substance abuse (self or family members); dysfunctional or stressful relationships; pent-up anger or frustration over unresolved issues	seek professional counseling for major unresolved issues or dysfunctional relationships
poor nutrition	follow a common-sense balanced nutritional plan (avoid fad diets)
lack of quality physical exercise	participate in regular physical exercise (minimum of 3 days per week)
medical illness	practice good body mechanics; achieve and maintain optimal body weight
financial stress	develop and follow a budget; get advice from a credit counselor if necessary

Student Resources

EngenderHealth infection-prevention course: http://www.engenderhealth.org/IP/index.html
Helpguide: http://www.helpguide.org (enter "burnout" in search box)
National Institutes of Health Office of Disease Prevention: http://prevention.nih.gov

Chapter Activities

Learning Style Study Strategies

Try any or all of the following strategies as you study the content of this chapter:

Visual learners: As a visual learner, you are especially aware of colors and will better remember key data later if you color-code it. So buy a variety of brightly colored markers and highlighters to code your notes and key data within the text.

Kinesthetic learners: Physical movement is key for you. It helps you keep focused on the topic at hand and greatly increases the odds that you will later remember what you study now. Therefore, try using your finger to trace the illustrations and tables in this text as you study them.

Auditory learners: Hearing information verbalized aloud helps you to process and remember it. Therefore, you may benefit from joining a study group or studying with a partner. Just make sure that you stay on task; don't let yourselves get sidetracked with socializing.

Verbal learners: Speaking aloud helps you think things through, process information, and achieve better understanding. Try reading aloud when you come across sections of text that you find complex or difficult to grasp. You may need to read certain passages more than once.

Practice Exercises

Answers to Practice Exercises can be found in Appendix D.

Case Studies

CASE STUDY 1

Mary is a medical assistant who works in an urgent-care clinic. One day, after drawing blood for testing, she accidentally dropped the Vacutainer on the floor. It broke, splattering blood over a 3-foot area. She wasn't sure, but thought she felt something moist hit her right eye at the moment of the splatter. She is concerned that she might have gotten a tiny drop of the patient's blood in her eye. What measures should she take?

CASE STUDY 2

Veronica is a nurse who has worked in a family medical clinic for the past 5 years. She confides in you one day that she is feeling unhappy and just isn't enjoying her work like she used to. She notices that she feels impatient with her clients and sometimes even resents them. She finds herself feeling overwhelmed and exhausted most of the time, even though she says she sleeps 8 to 10 hours most nights. She states that she would like to quit work for a while, but being a single mother of two teenagers, she cannot afford to do this. You suspect that she may be experiencing burnout.

1. What potential symptoms of burnout is Veronica exhibiting?

2. What questions might you ask her to further determine whether she is experiencing burnout?

3. Since she cannot afford to quit working, what advice might you offer to help her experience greater job satisfaction?

Multiple Choice

1. Which of the following is an example of a mechanical defense?
   a. Sebaceous glands
   b. Stomach acid
   c. Cilia
   d. All of these

2. Which of the following is an example of a chemical defense?
   a. Skin
   b. Mucous membranes
   c. Nasal hair
   d. Enzymes

3. Which of the following statements is true of antigens?
   a. They are markers that identify cells as self or nonself.
   b. They engulf bacteria and cellular debris in a process known as phagocytosis.
   c. They are enzymes produced by the body which guard against pathogens.
   d. They are responsible for artificial passive immunity.

4. Which of the following statements is **not** true of the inflammatory response?
   a. It is the body's immediate immunological defense against injury, infection, or allergy.
   b. It causes blood vessels to constrict to reduce blood loss.
   c. It is responsible for the release of histamine.
   d. It protects from invasion by foreign pathogens and sets in motion a series of events which serve to repair tissue damage.

5. Which of the following is **not** considered a part of personal protective equipment?

a. Gloves

b. Mask

c. Hand sanitizer

d. Shoe covers

Short Answer

1. **Describe the process for getting immunized against hepatitis B.**

2. **List at least three items that are considered sharps and describe their correct disposal.**

3. **Describe activities that you enjoy in your nonwork time that reduce your feelings of stress and help you feel nurtured, rested, or energized.**

4. **List at least two different activities that you will do a least once a week to contribute to your physical, emotional, psychological, or spiritual well-being.**

4 CHILDHOOD DISEASES AND DISORDERS

Learning Outcomes

Upon completion of this chapter, the student will be able to:

- Define and spell key terms
- Describe structures and functions unique to the infant and child
- Discuss characteristics of each of the disorders in this chapter, including:
  - description
  - incidence
  - etiology
  - signs and symptoms
  - diagnosis
  - treatment
  - prognosis

KEY TERMS

abscess	localized collection of pus
afebrile	without fever
anorexia	loss of appetite
communicable	contagious, capable of being passed between individuals
cyanosis	bluish color due to lack of oxygen
dysphagia	pain or difficulty with swallowing
dyspnea	difficulty breathing
exudate	substance that drains out
febrile	having a fever
lesions	skin wounds or sores
malaise	discomfort, weakness, fatigue
neonatal	newborn
orthopnea	difficulty breathing that is eased by sitting, rather than lying down
pathogenic	disease-causing
pharyngitis	sore throat
pruritus	itching
stridor	high-pitched breathing sound
tachycardia	rapid heartbeat
tachypnea	rapid breathing

Abbreviations

There are many lengthy terms in the world of health care. Table 4-1 lists some of the most common abbreviations related to infants and children.

Anatomy in Children

It has often been said that children should not be treated as if they are merely small adults. This is especially true in the medical profession. Before studying diseases and disorders that are common to children, a systematic review of the anatomical differences of children from adults is in order.

Flashpoint
Children should not be treated as if they are just small adults.

Sensory System

Sense organs begin to develop well before birth—during embryonic life—and continue to mature until approximately the ninth year of life. Infants are able to hear, taste, smell, and see from the time of birth. The eustachian tubes, which connect the middle ear to the nasopharynx, are smaller and straighter than an adult's, making it easier for bacteria to enter from the nose and throat. This makes children more vulnerable to middle-ear infections (see otitis media, Chapter 15).

Respiratory System

Infants born prematurely may be lacking sufficient amounts of surfactant, a substance which increases the surface tension of the fluid that lines the inside of the alveoli (tiny air sacs within the lungs). Lack of surfactant makes the alveoli more likely to collapse and impairs oxygen–carbon dioxide exchange.

Compared to adults, children have larger heads, shorter necks, and larger tongues. This makes them more vulnerable to airway obstructions. They also breathe mainly through the nose, rather than the mouth, yet their nasal passages are smaller than adults'. Children have larger adenoids, tissues similar to tonsils located at the back of the nose and upper throat, than adults do. When adenoids swell they can block the eustachian tubes, increasing the risk of middle-ear infection. Children also have smaller-diameter lower airways, which increases their risk of respiratory compromise.

TABLE 4-1			
ABBREVIATIONS			
Abbreviation	Meaning	Abbreviation	Meaning
AGA	appropriate for gestational age	PKU	Phenylketonuria
APGAR	activity, pulse, grimace, appearance, respiration	RSV	respiratory syncytial virus
FTT	failure to thrive	SIDS	sudden infant death syndrome
Peds	Pediatrics		

Cardiovascular System

The cardiovascular system begins to develop within the first 8 weeks of gestation (pregnancy). The cardiovascular system of infants and children is smaller than that of adults. Heart rate is higher in infants—approximately 130 beats per minute, compared with the adult average of 75— and systolic (top-number) blood pressure in infants is lower—approximately 65, compared with the normal adult value of 120.

Muscle tissue in the newborn heart is stiffer than in older individuals, which may result in decreased blood output with each heartbeat. The foramen ovale, an opening between the atria (two upper chambers of the heart), does not fully close until the infant reaches 3 to 12 months of age. Hemoglobin (an oxygen-carrying protein in red blood cells that contains iron) in infants 3 months and younger does not deliver oxygen as efficiently as in adults. To compensate for this, infants have a higher hemoglobin concentration (around 17 grams per deciliter) than adults (around 14 grams per deciliter).

Gastrointestinal System

Development and maturation of the child's digestive system continues throughout the first year. During the first few months of life, infants most readily digest and absorb maternal breast milk; when breast milk is not a viable option, good-quality infant formula is an adequate replacement. Infants younger than 9 months should not be given cow's milk, because their immature gastrointestinal system will have difficulty digesting the milk protein and absorbing the fat.

Nervous System

The nervous system grows from approximately 6 weeks after conception until well after birth. The sympathetic nervous system in infants is still immature. One of the roles of this system is to prepare the body to respond during times of stress (the fight-or-flight response).

Renal System

The kidneys begin excreting small amounts of urine approximately 3 months after conception. However, newborn kidneys are not fully mature, and as a result they have less ability to filter fluids and electrolytes and to concentrate urine than adult kidneys. They do not achieve full maturity until approximately 12 months of age. Therefore, infants cannot handle large volumes of water and cannot excrete electrolytes as readily as adults. Infants and small children also lack the fat pads in the flank around the kidneys that adults have. This makes their kidneys more vulnerable to traumatic injury. Because of fecal incontinence, infants are sometimes more susceptible to urinary tract infections.

Immune System

Flashpoint

Kidneys are not fully mature until infants are a year old.

A child's immune system is immature, which increases the child's susceptibility to infectious disease. The thymus, located within the chest, is proportionately larger in infants than in adults. It plays an active role in the maturation of white blood cells, which are important players in the body's immune response.

Skeletal System

Infants are born with a greater amount of cartilage than adults have. They also are born with a greater number of bones, some of which later fuse together. The infant's bones are softer and more flexible than the adult's but slowly harden as mineral content increases. Bone growth occurs in places called growth plates. Thus, injury to growth plates during childhood can impair normal bone growth.

Muscular System

Muscle development progresses from before birth into adulthood. In infants, the muscles of the head, neck, and trunk develop more quickly than those of the arms and legs. This allows infants to hold their heads up and sit up before developing fully coordinated movements of their extremities.

Endocrine System

Structures of the endocrine system develop within the first 3 months after conception. Maternal hormones cross the placenta during pregnancy, resulting in the swollen appearance of the breasts and genitalia of both male and female newborns.

Reproductive System

Infants are born with immature reproductive systems. Development and maturation does not occur until puberty, when the pituitary gland in the brain signals the release of sex hormones.

Temperature Regulation

Infants are not able to regulate body temperature as efficiently as adults; they lose body heat more readily, especially from their heads. Infants younger than 3 months are unable to shiver to generate body heat.

Flashpoint
Infants cannot regulate body heat as efficiently as adults.

Infectious Diseases and Disorders

Infectious diseases are those caused by the growth of **pathogenic** (disease-causing) microorganisms in the body. Children are more susceptible to infectious diseases and disorders because they are less likely to use precautions such as proper hand washing. They are also more prone to putting objects in their mouths. Many infectious diseases are also **communicable,** meaning they are contagious and can be passed between people.

A number of infectious diseases can now be prevented through immunization (see Box 4-1). These include chickenpox, measles, mumps, rubella, tetanus, diphtheria, pertussis, and the human papillomavirus (HPV), which is discussed in Chapter 8.

Chickenpox

ICD-9-CM: 052.9   [ICD-10: B10.9 (without complication)]
Chickenpox is a highly contagious viral fever and rash.

Incidence
Prior to the vaccine, developed in 1995, approximately four million Americans (mostly children) contracted chickenpox each year. Widespread administration of the vaccine has reduced the number of cases and hospitalizations.

Box 4-1 Wellness Promotion

GET IMMUNIZED

Routine childhood immunizations are state mandated for children who attend public schools. The Centers for Disease Control and Prevention (CDC) gives specific guidelines about the ages at which a child should receive vaccines, as well as how many times the child should receive the vaccines. Although the CDC strongly recommends that parents and caregivers follow these guidelines, parents may elect to delay a vaccine for any reason, including illness or allergy. Many pediatricians also routinely delay administration of a vaccine if the child is ill.

The complete immunization schedule includes ranges for catch-up immunizations for children who were incompletely immunized, as well as recommendations for high-risk populations. This table gives the general immunization schedule. Many immunizations are administered in several doses over a period of time; the dose number is indicated in the table by a number in parentheses.

Age	Immunization
birth	hepatitis (hep) B (1)
1 to 2 months	hep B (2)
2 months	rotavirus (rota) (1) diphtheria and tetanus toxoids and acellular pertussis protein (DTaP) (1) *Haemophilus influenzae* type B conjugate (Hib) (1) pneumococcal conjugate vaccine (PCV) (1) inactivated poliovirus (IPV) (1)
4 months	rota (2) DTaP (2) Hib (2) PCV (2) IPV (2)
6 months	rota (3) DTaP (3) Hib (3) PCV (3)
6 to 18 months	hep B (3) IPV (3)
12 to 15 months	Hib (4) PCV (4) measles, mumps, rubella (MMR) (1) varicella (1)
15 to 18 months	DTaP (4)
12 to 23 months	hep A (1 and 2*)
6 months to 5 years	influenza (yearly)
4 to 6 years	DTaP (5) IPV (4) MMR (2) varicella (2) influenza (yearly)

Box 4-1 Wellness Promotion—cont'd

Age	Immunization
11 to 12 years	tetanus and diphtheria toxoids and acellular pertussis (Tdap) human papillomavirus (HPV) (1, 2, and 3**) MCV4 influenza (yearly)

*Separated by at least 6 months
**Administered to females only, with 2 months separating the first and second doses
  and 6 months separating the second and third doses

Etiology

Chickenpox is highly contagious for those who have not previously had it or the vaccine. It is caused by the varicella-zoster virus, which is part of a group of viruses called herpesviruses. The virus spreads easily from person to person through direct contact with the rash or through droplets dispersed into the air by coughing or sneezing.

Signs and Symptoms

The primary sign of chickenpox is the classic red, itchy rash on the face, scalp, chest, and back. The rash can spread to the entire body, including the throat, eyes, and vagina. The chickenpox rash usually appears less than 2 weeks after exposure to the virus and begins as superficial (surface) spots. These spots quickly turn into vesicles (small, fluid-filled blisters) that break open and crust over (see Fig. 4-1). New spots continue to appear for several days and may number in the hundreds. Itching may range from mild to intense. The rash may be preceded or accompanied by fever, abdominal pain, *anorexia* (loss of appetite), headache, *malaise* (discomfort, weakness, fatigue), lethargy, and irritability. Individuals may have a mild cough and runny nose for the first 2 days of illness before the rash appears. A person who has chickenpox can transmit the virus for up to 48 hours before symptoms appear and remains contagious until all spots crust over.

The health-care provider should instruct the parent or caregiver to call the office if any of the more severe effects occur. These include a marked increase in warmth, tenderness, or redness of the rash (which may indicate a secondary bacterial skin infection), spreading of the rash to one or both eyes, dizziness or disorientation, *tachycardia* (rapid heartbeat), *dyspnea* (difficult breathing), tremors or loss of coordination, stiff neck, worsening cough, vomiting, or fever above 103°F.

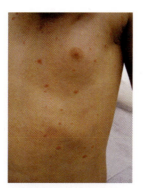

FIGURE 4-1 **The vesicular rash of chickenpox** (From Barankin, B, and Freiman, A. *Derm Notes: Clinical Dermatology Pocket Guide.* 2006. Philadelphia: F.A. Davis Company, with permission.)

Treatment

Treatment for chickenpox involves acetaminophen for pain and fever, and rest at home. Aspirin should be avoided because of the risk of Reye syndrome. Children with chickenpox should avoid going to school until all **lesions** (skin wounds or sores) have crusted over.

Prognosis

Chickenpox usually lasts about 2 weeks and rarely causes complications. Although the disease is generally mild in healthy children, it can be serious for anyone; thus, most states have made the chickenpox vaccine a requirement for attendance in public school. For most patients, the vaccine is a safe, effective way to prevent chickenpox. In the small number of cases where the vaccine does not stop chickenpox completely, the resulting infection is much milder than it would have been without it. Many people who experience chickenpox as a child later develop shingles, a painful reemergence of the varicella-zoster virus that usually occurs in older adults.

Flashpoint

People who have had chickenpox are at risk for developing shingles.

Measles

ICD-9-CM: 055.9   [ICD-10: B05.9 (without complication)]

Measles, also known as *rubeola,* is an uncommon, highly contagious viral infection.

Incidence

In the early 1970s there were approximately 35 measles deaths each year, most commonly in those under 12 months of age. Fortunately, measles is now fairly rare in the United States, due to immunization: Incidence has dropped from thousands of cases in 1950 to just 66 cases in 2005. While measles is no longer considered native to the United States, vaccinations are important because it is still a common disease worldwide. This is illustrated by the fact that there were nearly a quarter of a million measles deaths globally in 2006. Most of the U.S. cases that do arise are due to importation (infected individuals traveling here) or Americans becoming infected when traveling abroad.

Flashpoint

Measles is very contagious.

Etiology

Measles is caused by a virus. It is very contagious and is spread via respiratory droplets when individuals cough, sneeze, or share eating utensils or drink containers.

Signs and Symptoms

Measles causes flu-like symptoms that include a fever, cough, runny nose, and rash. The child's eyes become red, teary, and sensitive to light. The rash is characterized by red-brown blotches that first appear on the face and then spread down the body (see Fig. 4-2).

Diagnosis

Diagnosis of measles is based upon the child's presenting signs and symptoms. Further testing is rarely needed.

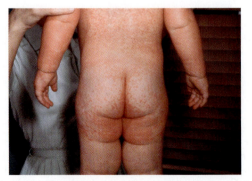

FIGURE 4-2 Measles rash (Courtesy of the Centers for Disease Control and Prevention.)

Treatment

Treatment is aimed at relieving symptoms. Parents should encourage children to drink fluids and get plenty of rest. Acetaminophen may be given to relieve fever and discomfort. Children should be kept home from school or day care and away from anyone who has not been immunized until symptoms have resolved. A cool-mist vaporizer can relieve coughing and soothe irritated mucous membranes.

Prognosis

The prognosis for individuals with measles is very good. Symptoms usually resolve on their own after the virus has run its course, which takes about 2 weeks. Occasionally other problems may develop, such as *croup* (a severe respiratory illness), *bronchitis* (inflammation of the bronchial airways), *pneumonia* (viral or bacterial infection), *bronchiolitis* (inflammation of the small lung airways), *conjunctivitis* (eye inflammation), *myocarditis* (heart inflammation), *otitis media* (middle-ear infection), or *encephalitis* (brain inflammation).

Mumps

ICD-9-CM: 072.9   [ICD-10: B26.9 (without complication)]

Mumps, technically known as *epidemic parotitis,* is a contagious viral disease known for causing severe swelling of the parotid (salivary) gland on one or both sides of the face.

Incidence

Before vaccination, mumps was a common childhood disease. More than 150,000 cases were reported in 1967. But by 1993 the reported number had dropped to 1,692. However, it is still common in countries where vaccination is not readily available.

Etiology

Mumps is caused by a virus which is quite contagious. It is spread through oral secretions when an infected person coughs, sneezes, or shares utensils or drink containers with others.

Signs and Symptoms

Individuals with mumps develop painful, swollen salivary glands, fever, malaise, anorexia, and headache (see Fig. 4-3). Males may also develop swollen, painful testicles.

Flashpoint
Mumps can affect one or both sides of the face.

Diagnosis

Diagnosis is usually based upon physical examination and the patient's symptoms. Laboratory testing is not usually needed, but it can be done on saliva or blood to confirm diagnosis.

Treatment

Treatment is aimed at relieving symptoms. Children should be kept home from school or day care to prevent infecting others. Application of cold compresses to the neck may soothe discomfort. Analgesics such as acetaminophen or ibuprofen may help relieve pain. Aspirin should be avoided, due to the risk of Reye syndrome. Rest and fluid intake are encouraged. Gargling with warm salt water may help to soothe the throat.

Prognosis

Most individuals recover fully. Impaired fertility in males is an unlikely but potential complication. Other uncommon complications include meningitis (inflammation of the lining of the brain), encephalitis, hearing loss, **pancreatitis** (inflammation of the pancreas), and **oophoritis** (inflammation of the ovaries) in girls.

Rubella

ICD-9-CM: 056.9   [ICD-10: B06.9 (without complication)]

Rubella, also known as *German measles* or *3-day measles,* is a viral infection that affects the skin and lymph nodes. It is not the same illness as measles (rubeola).

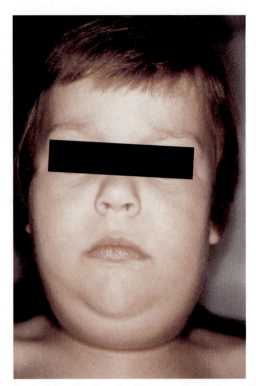

FIGURE 4-3 **Mumps** (Courtesy of the Centers for Disease Control and Prevention, Patricia Smith, and Barbara Rice.)

Incidence

Prior to the advent of the rubella vaccine in 1969, epidemics occurred every 6 to 9 years, primarily affecting children between the ages of 5 and 9. It is currently listed as a rare disease by the National Institutes of Health's Office of Rare Diseases Research. Most current cases affect young adults who have not been immunized. This is of concern, since approximately 10% of young adults are estimated to be susceptible, which could pose a risk for any children they may have.

Etiology

Rubella is contagious and is spread via respiratory droplets from the nose or throat of infected people. Individuals are most contagious from 1 week before the rash appears to 1 week after. Rubella can also spread from an infected pregnant woman to her fetus, causing congenital rubella syndrome. Infants with the syndrome can shed the virus in urine and fluid from the throat or nose for a year or more.

Flashpoint

If a pregnant woman catches rubella, her baby could suffer serious birth defects.

Signs and Symptoms

Infection usually begins with a day or two of mild fever and enlarged, tender lymph nodes in the neck or behind the ears. Next, a rash of pink or light-red spots appears on the face and spreads down the body. As the rash resolves, the skin may shed in fine flakes. Other symptoms include headache; anorexia; conjunctivitis; a runny or stuffy nose; enlarged, tender lymph nodes in other parts of the body; and painful joints. Some individuals may be relatively asymptomatic.

Diagnosis

Diagnosis may be based upon the patient's presenting signs and symptoms, but blood tests or identification of the virus through immunofluorescence (microscopic detection of antibodies using fluorescent proteins) is needed to confirm the infection.

Treatment

Treatment is aimed at relieving symptoms. Ill children should be kept at home so as not to infect others. Parents can give them acetaminophen or ibuprofen for fever and discomfort; aspirin should be avoided. The physician should be called if the child runs a fever higher than 102°F or an infant younger than 6 months runs a fever above 100.4°F. Any pregnant woman who becomes exposed to the illness should contact her physician right away.

Prognosis

If a pregnant woman contracts rubella, it may cause congenital rubella syndrome in the fetus. This syndrome can result in growth deficits, mental deficits, abnormalities of the heart and eyes, deafness, and problems with the liver, spleen, and bone marrow. Risk is greatest during the first 20 weeks of pregnancy.

Tetanus

ICD-9-CM: 771.3   [ICD-10: A33 (no mention of complication)]

Tetanus, also known as *lockjaw*, is a noncontagious illness marked by severe, prolonged spasms of skeletal muscle fibers.

Incidence

Incidence of tetanus has decreased radically in the United States since the vaccine was developed and offered as a part of routine childhood immunizations in the 1940s. Currently, approximately 100 individuals become infected each year, and five of them die. Tetanus is still a widespread global health concern, though, with approximately one million cases annually and as many as a half a million deaths. Therefore, getting the tetanus vaccination and booster every 10 years is very important (see Box 4-2). Tetanus occurs most commonly in hot, humid climates with soil that is richly organic, especially manure-treated soils.

Etiology

Tetanus is caused by a neurotoxin called tetanospasmin, which is produced by the bacterium *Clostridium tetani*. Infection usually occurs through a contaminated wound such as a cut or puncture.

Signs and Symptoms

Tetanus causes muscle spasms which first affect the jaw. This is what gives it the common name of lockjaw. As the illness progresses, the individual experiences difficulty swallowing as well as muscle stiffness and spasms in other parts of the body.

Flashpoint

Tetanus is most common in areas with hot, humid climates and rich, organic soil.

Diagnosis

Diagnosis is made using the "spatula test," in which the posterior pharyngeal wall (back of the throat) is touched with a sterile, soft-tipped instrument. Involuntary biting of the spatula caused by contraction of the jaw muscles confirms the diagnosis. The normal response would be a gag reflex.

Treatment

The wound is cleaned and debrided (stripped of dead tissue). The medication metronidazole is given to decrease the number of bacteria, although it has no effect on the toxin. Tetanus

---

Box 4-2 Wellness Promotion

GET YOUR BOOSTER

Don't make the mistake of assuming that you are protected for life once you've completed your initial immunizations. Tetanus immunity is only good for about 10 years; so if your last tetanus vaccination was given at age 12, you should get a booster by age 22 and again every 10 years thereafter. Additionally, if you happen to suffer a contaminated wound or a deep puncture wound, your health-care provider will give you a booster if your last one was more than 5 years ago. This ensures that your immunity is strong so you don't become ill with tetanus.

immunization or a booster must be given. Diazepam (Valium) is given for muscle spasms. In extreme cases the patient may need to be placed on mechanical ventilation and given medication to cause temporary paralysis. A high-calorie, high-protein diet is needed to meet the individual's energy needs related to increased muscle activity.

Prognosis

The mortality rate for tetanus varies between 5% and 30% and is highest in the very young and the very old. The highest mortality rates are also associated with delay in treatment, early onset of convulsions, contaminated lesions of the head and face, and *neonatal* (newborn) tetanus.

Diphtheria

ICD-9-CM: 032.9   [ICD-10: A36.9 (without complication)]
Diphtheria is a serious, contagious bacterial upper respiratory infection.

Incidence

Prior to the common use of a vaccine in the 1930s, diphtheria was much more common than it is today. Since that time, incidence has dropped significantly. Currently there are fewer than five cases reported each year in the United States. However, because vaccinations are not readily available in all countries, diphtheria is still a threat. Those at risk for diphtheria are nonimmunized people who live in crowded areas with poor sanitation and hygiene.

Etiology

Diphtheria is a contagious disease caused by the *Corynebacterium diphtheriae* bacterium. It is spread by direct contact with droplets when infected individuals cough or sneeze or share eating utensils or drink containers. It can also be spread via objects or foods that have been contaminated.

Signs and Symptoms

The onset of diphtheria is gradual. Occasionally it first affects the skin, causing bluish color and lesions. It usually causes sore throat; fatigue; fever; bloody, watery nasal drainage; difficulty swallowing; and the development of a membrane on the tonsils, nasopharynx and oropharynx (back of the nose and upper throat) that can block airways (see Fig. 4-4). Because of this, individuals may exhibit a crouplike barking cough, difficulty breathing, *stridor* (high-pitched

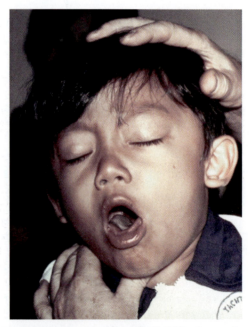

FIGURE 4-4 **The pseudomembrane associated with diphtheria can become large enough to obstruct the airway.** (Courtesy of the Centers for Disease Control and Prevention.)

breathing sound), drooling, and hoarseness. Other signs and symptoms include chills, high fever, nausea and vomiting, and tachycardia. With severe cases, individuals may develop hypotension (low blood pressure) and neck swelling.

Diagnosis

Diagnosis is confirmed by the presence of a membrane in the patient's throat and a throat culture positive for *C. diphtheriae.*

Treatment

Treatment for diphtheria includes administration of an antitoxin (antibody capable of neutralizing a specific biological toxin) and antibiotics. Individuals will be hospitalized, given fluids and oxygen, and put on bedrest. If necessary they may be placed on mechanical ventilation. Anyone exposed to an infected person should be immunized or given a booster.

Prognosis

Individuals who exhibit hypotension and neck swelling have the highest mortality rate. Recovery is slow and long-term deficits caused by the diphtheria toxin may include peripheral neuropathy (nerve pain or paralysis), kidney damage, and cardiomyopathy (diseased heart muscle). The overall mortality rate is 10%.

> **Flashpoint**
> Diphtheria causes a fibrous membrane to develop in the upper throat that can block airways.

> **Flashpoint**
> Diphtheria is treated with an antitoxin and antibiotics.

Pertussis

ICD-9-CM: 033.9 [ICD-10: A37.9 (without complication)]

Pertussis, also known as *whooping cough,* is a highly contagious bacterial respiratory disease. The name is taken from the severe cough, which is followed by breathing in that creates a "whoop" sound, most typical in children.

Incidence

After the development of the vaccine, the incidence of pertussis dropped to a low in the United States of 1,010 cases in 1976. However, since then it has risen to a disturbing 29,000 cases per year.

> **Flashpoint**
> Pertussis is sometimes called whooping cough.

Ninety percent of all cases occur in underdeveloped countries. Globally, there are between 30 million and 50 million cases each year, causing 300,000 deaths, making it a leading global cause of death from vaccine-preventable illness. Most vulnerable are infants younger than 6 months and children between 11 and 18 whose immunity is fading.

Etiology

Pertussis is caused by the bacterium *Bordetella pertussis.* It is spread by respiratory secretions when infected individuals cough, sneeze, or share eating utensils or drink containers.

Signs and Symptoms

Infants and children with pertussis initially display mild symptoms such as coughing, runny nose, sneezing, and low-grade fever. At 1 to 2 weeks the cough becomes more severe and frequent, with a characteristic inspiratory barking sound. Coughing may be so severe as to cause the individual to turn red or purple, or cause vomiting. This may lead to problems with nutrition and hydration.

Diagnosis

Diagnosis is based upon the patient's presenting signs and symptoms and the positive results of a throat culture for *B. pertussis.*

Treatment

Administration of antibiotics does not stop the disease but does decrease the severity of symptoms and the length of infection time. Individuals who have come in close contact with the ill person should also be treated.

During the recovery period, children should be kept home to rest. A cool-mist vaporizer will help sooth an irritated throat and lungs and loosen secretions. The home should be kept free of irritants that might trigger coughing spells, such as tobacco smoke, wood-fire smoke, and aerosol sprays. Because the child may have difficulty eating and drinking enough, frequent small snacks and fluids should be offered. If signs of dehydration occur (thirst, lethargy, tearless crying, fewer diaper changes or trips to the bathroom), the parent should contact the health-care provider.

Prognosis

Episodes of coughing slowly resolve over 1 or 2 months during the convalescent stage. Potential complications include secondary bacterial infection, pneumonia, encephalitis, and pulmonary hypertension (elevated blood pressure in the arteries of the lungs). Mortality is highest among unvaccinated or incompletely vaccinated infants.

Respiratory System Diseases and Disorders

Respiratory illnesses are among the most common illnesses, because they are spread so easily. In most cases they are spread via respiratory droplets that are released into the air when individuals cough, sneeze, or even laugh. They may also be transmitted by kissing, or sharing eating utensils or drink containers. Children are especially prone to sharing their illness because they are more apt to put things into their mouths and often play very close together at home, day care, or school. The first and best strategy in helping them to stay healthy is teaching about simple measures such as proper hand washing (see Box 4-3).

Influenza

ICD-9-CM: 487.0–487.9   [ICD-10: J09–J11 (specify organism)]

Influenza is a respiratory viral infection that attacks the nose, throat, bronchi, and lungs. Young children are especially vulnerable, including those who have weakened immune systems. It is easily spread through the air in droplets when someone with the infection coughs, sneezes, or talks near objects such as toys that children play with. See Chapter 11 for a detailed description of influenza.

Upper Respiratory Infection

ICD-9-CM: 465.9   [ICD-10: J00–J06]

Upper respiratory infection (URI), often called the *common cold*, is a group of symptoms that may be caused by several viruses. Young children are especially susceptible to common colds because

---

Box 4-3 Wellness Promotion

STOP THE GERMS

Respiratory illnesses, including the common cold, are highly contagious and are readily spread between young children. You can help children stay healthy by teaching them and their parents the following measures to reduce the number of respiratory illnesses that everyone catches:

- Wash your hands frequently using warm water and soap—singing "Happy Birthday" twice will ensure adequate scrub time.
- Cover your mouth with your arm (not your hand) when you cough or sneeze.
- Avoid sharing drink containers, eating utensils, face cloths, or towels with others.
- Keep your hands and other objects away from your face, especially during cold and flu season.
- Stay home from school or day care when you are ill.

their immature immune systems have not yet developed resistance to most of the viruses that cause them. Children, especially preschoolers, can have a cold eight to 10 times per year, compared to the average adult, who has a cold two to four times per year. See Chapter 11 for a detailed description of URI.

Epiglottitis

ICD-9-CM: 464.30   [ICD-10: J05.1]
Epiglottitis is an uncommon but serious condition in which the epiglottis (a flap of tissue above the larynx or voice box) becomes swollen due to inflammation or infection.

Incidence
Epiglottitis most often affects children between the ages of two and seven.

Etiology
In the past, the most common cause of epiglottitis was the bacterium *Haemophilus influenzae.* However, since the development of the influenza vaccine, the most common causative organisms are *Staphylococcus aureus* and *Streptococcus pneumoniae.* There have also been reported cases of epiglottitis caused by respiratory syncytial virus (RSV) and *Candida albicans.*

Signs and Symptoms
The child with epiglottitis may initially appear to have croup, a condition that is usually not life threatening. Signs and symptoms include sore throat, chills, fever, **dysphagia** (difficulty swallowing) with subsequent drooling, and stridor and a muffled voice. The child will prefer to sit upright with the neck hyperextended to ease breathing.

Diagnosis
The child's physical presentation should alert the health-care provider to the possible presence of epiglottis. No attempt should be made to look at or swab the throat by anyone other than a trained health-care provider who is prepared to deal with an airway-obstruction emergency; doing so may trigger spasms that could completely obstruct the airway. A lateral x-ray view will show the swollen epiglottis. Once the child's airway is stabilized, a throat culture and blood specimens may be obtained to identify the causative organism.

> **Flashpoint**
> The child with epiglottitis could develop trouble breathing.

Treatment
Epiglottitis is a medical emergency that usually requires hospitalization. Tracheal intubation (the insertion of a breathing tube) may be done and humidified oxygen administered to improve the child's respiratory status. Intravenous antibiotic therapy is also initiated. Health-care providers should be aware that this is a very frightening situation for the parents and the child. Parents should be given emotional support and kept informed about the child's status. The organisms that cause epiglottitis are communicable; therefore, people who have been in contact with the child should be evaluated and treated if necessary.

Prognosis
Epiglottitis is a serious and potentially life-threatening illness. Early recognition and treatment usually results in a favorable outcome.

Bronchiolitis

ICD-9-CM: 466.1   [ICD-10: J21.0–J21.9]
Bronchiolitis is an inflammation of the smallest airways in the lungs.

Incidence
Bronchiolitis is most commonly seen in children under 2 years of age, with a peak incidence around 6 months of age, and occurs more often in the winter and spring months. Children who attend day care and who are exposed to cigarette smoke are at a greater risk for developing this condition.

Etiology

Bronchiolitis can be caused by an adenovirus, influenza virus, and parainfluenza virus, but the most common culprit is the respiratory syncytial virus (RSV). Bronchiolitis is a more serious condition for children than for adults because of the small diameter of the child's airways.

Signs and Symptoms

The child with bronchiolitis initially displays cold symptoms (clear nasal drainage and low-grade fever). Within a couple of days, breathing becomes more difficult and the child experiences **tachypnea** (rapid breathing), nasal flaring, retraction of respiratory muscles, wheezing, and tachycardia. **Cyanosis** (bluish color due to lack of oxygen) develops as the child's condition worsens. In severe cases, overinflation of the alveoli (tiny air sacs of the lungs) can be seen on the chest x-ray.

Diagnosis

Diagnosis is based upon physical examination, the child's signs and symptoms, and risk factors. A swab of the nasal passage for RSV will also be obtained. A chest x-ray may be ordered to screen for overinflation of the alveoli and to rule out other respiratory disorders.

Treatment

Mild cases of bronchiolitis can be treated at home with rest, humidified air, saline nose drops, and increased fluid intake. Hospitalization is recommended if the child demonstrates signs of severe respiratory distress—retractions, nasal flaring, tachypnea, and lethargy—or is at serious risk of dehydration. Humidified oxygen and intravenous fluids are usually initiated for children requiring hospitalization. Children can breathe with greater ease if placed in the semi-Fowler position (semireclining). An infant seat can be used for this purpose. If RSV is the causative organism, precautions should be taken to prevent spreading it to others. In more serious cases the child may require artificial ventilation and ribavirin therapy. Ribavirin is administered via oxygen hood, tent, or mask; it is potentially **teratogenic** (causing cancer in a fetus), therefore pregnant health-care providers should avoid exposure to the child receiving this type of therapy.

> **Flashpoint**
>
> Nasal flaring, tachypnea, and retractions are signs of respiratory distress.

Bronchodilators are not effective in the treatment of bronchiolitis because small children do not have adequately developed smooth muscles in their airways to respond well.

Patient education covers avoiding exposure to anyone with the viruses during peak cold and flu seasons, hand washing, covering the mouth when coughing, and avoiding exposure to cigarette smoke. Two preventive medications, RSV-IGIV (RespiGam) and palivizumab (Synagis), can be given to high-risk children. Palivizumab is the preferred medication because it is easier to administer.

Prognosis

Children with mild cases of bronchiolitis usually recover without complication. There is a tendency, however, for those children who experience repeat episodes of this disease to develop asthma.

Croup

ICD-9-CM: 464.4   [ICD-10: J05.0]

Croup is a severe viral respiratory illness that involves edema of the upper respiratory passages due to inflammation or spasms.

Incidence

Croup is most often seen in children between the ages of 6 months and 5 years, and it occurs most often during the winter and early spring months.

Etiology

Croup may be caused by several viruses, most commonly the parainfluenza virus or, less commonly, respiratory syncytial virus (RSV), the measles virus, or other viruses. On rare occasions it is caused by bacterial infection. Allergies, psychological stressors, and gastroesophageal reflux (spilling of stomach fluid into the esophagus) are other infrequent causes. Additionally, young children have small airways that can quickly accumulate mucus and lead to airway obstruction and severe respiratory distress.

Signs and Symptoms

There are two types of croup: spasmodic and viral. Both are characterized by the classic "barky cough," similar to the noise of a barking seal, that usually first appears in the middle of the night. The child experiencing spasmodic croup is usually *afebrile* (without fever), and the onset is sudden and without warning. The child with viral croup may have a fever, runny nose, and other cold symptoms for several days prior to the onset of croup symptoms. In both types of croup, stridor may be present.

Flashpoint

Croup causes the child to have a cough that sounds like a seal's bark.

Diagnosis

Diagnosis of croup is usually made on the basis of the parent's description of the child's symptoms and on the findings of the physical examination. Consideration is also given to historical data such as prematurity and recent foreign-body aspiration (inhalation of anything other than air). Occasionally, x-ray, CT scan, and visualization of the airway may be necessary. A classic finding on the x-ray of a child with croup is the "steeple sign," a critical area of airway narrowing in the upper centimeter of the trachea.

Treatment

Most cases of croup can be treated at home with humidified air (see Box 4-4). Placing a humidifier in the child's room at night helps moisten the air and prevent the nighttime episodes of coughing and distress. Acetaminophen is given to manage fever. A health-care provider should be contacted if the child does not respond to treatment. Parents should also be instructed to call their local emergency response number (usually 911) if the child has bluish skin color, is drooling, or has persistent stridor at rest. Children who are brought to the emergency room with signs and symptoms of croup may be treated with a corticosteroid (a potent anti-inflammatory medication). Corticosteroids provide quick relief of symptoms and diminish the need for hospitalization. Severe cases of croup require hospitalization, oxygen, nebulized adrenaline, and possible tracheal intubation. Regardless of the treatment setting, the child should be allowed to remain as close as possible to parents (who should be kept informed of the child's condition and plan of care). This will minimize the child's anxiety and assist with controlling respiratory distress.

Flashpoint

Using a humidifier can help relieve coughing and dyspnea.

Prognosis

Children usually respond well to treatment and recover completely within a week. While croup is usually self limiting, it occasionally results in death from complete obstruction of the airway.

Box 4-4 Wellness Promotion

TREATING CROUP AT HOME

The following guidelines are useful for the parent providing home care for the child with croup:

- Administer moist air using a humidifier or turn on a hot shower and sit in the bathroom with the child.
- Encourage fluid intake and rest.
- Remain calm to help the child relax and avoid panic.

Go to the emergency room if the child:

- makes noisy, high-pitched breathing sounds when inhaling (stridor)
- has difficulty swallowing or begins to drool
- is extremely irritable or agitated
- has difficulty breathing
- develops blue or grayish skin around the nose, mouth, or fingernails

Respiratory Syncytial Virus

ICD-9-CM: 079.6   [ICD-10: B97.4]

Respiratory syncytial virus (RSV) is a virus that causes infections of the respiratory tract and the lungs. It is the leading cause of serious respiratory infection in infants and children.

Incidence

RSV is so common that most children have been infected with the virus by the time they reach age two. Approximately 100,000 people are hospitalized each year with the virus and approximately 11,000 die. Most of the deaths are in the elderly population.

Etiology

RSV is caused by exposure to the virus and is spread by the respiratory secretions of infected people. Signs and symptoms of severe RSV in young children include a fever of 103°F or higher, severe cough, wheezing, tachypnea, retractions, dyspnea, **orthopnea** (difficulty breathing that is eased by sitting, rather than lying down), cyanosis, and poor appetite. Children at higher risk of RSV include those with weakened immune systems or congenital heart or lung disease, those born prematurely or with a low birth weight, and those attending child care or with siblings attending child care. Infants who are exposed to cigarette smoke or high levels of air pollution are also at increased risk of developing RSV.

Signs and Symptoms

In severe and mild cases, signs and symptoms typically appear about 4 to 6 days after exposure to the virus. In older healthy children and adults, the symptoms of RSV are the same as those of the common cold, including runny nose or congestion, dry cough, sore throat, fever, mild headache, lethargy, and malaise.

Diagnosis

Diagnosis of RSV is made by analysis of a sputum (mucus) sample obtained from the patient's nasopharyngeal passage. A positive result reveals the presence of the virus, viral antigens, or viral RNA (see Box 4-5).

Treatment

Treatment for severe RSV includes acetaminophen for discomfort and fever and possible hospitalization to administer intravenous fluids, electrolytes, oxygen therapy, and sometimes mechanical ventilation. Ribavirin aerosol may be used to treat some patients with severe RSV. Treatment for less severe RSV includes fluids and acetaminophen.

Box 4-5 Diagnostic Spotlight

THE RAPID RSV TEST

The rapid RSV test identifies the presence of respiratory syncytial virus in nasopharyngeal secretions. For greatest accuracy, it must be done within the first few days of infection; this is when the largest amount of virus is being shed. Careful collection of the specimen is critical for test-result accuracy. One technique involves the insertion of a nasopharyngeal swab into the back of the patient's nostrils. It is gently rotated back and forth and then withdrawn. A more accurate technique involves instillation (insertion of a liquid) of a small amount of sterile saline into the patient's nose followed by gentle aspiration (withdrawing) of it back out. This is sometimes called a *wash* because it literally washes the specimen (bacteria, cells, etc.) from the patient's nasal passages.

The advantage of this rapid test is the speed with which it provides results; however, in some cases a traditional culture of the specimen is necessary, which generally takes 2 to 3 days.

Prognosis

Most children completely recover from RSV in 8 to 15 days. Death from RSV infection is relatively rare; however, it can occur in high-risk infants under 6 months old. RSV in infancy may increase a child's risk of developing asthma and allergies later. RSV in children ages three and under can lead to a lower respiratory tract illness, such as pneumonia or bronchiolitis; RSV is the most common cause of these disorders.

Tonsillitis and Adenoiditis

ICD-9-CM: 463.0   [ICD-10: J35.0]

Tonsillitis is an inflammation of the palatine tonsils and adenoiditis is an inflammation of the adenoids.

Incidence

Approximately 30 million people develop tonsillitis each year in the United States; approximately one in 10 children see their doctor for this problem.

Etiology

Tonsillar tissue is frequently exposed to microorganisms entering the body through the mouth, nose, and upper airway. Scientists believe that the tonsils provide protection to children during a time when they are at a greater risk of contracting upper respiratory infections. This theory is further supported by the fact that the tonsillar tissue shrinks considerably after childhood.

> **Flashpoint**
> One in 10 children see their doctor each year because of tonsillitis.

Signs and Symptoms

Key manifestations of tonsillitis are sore throat, drooling secondary to painful swallowing, fever, and tonsils that are red and enlarged with white patches (see Fig. 4-5). Adenoiditis may cause snoring, mouth-breathing, and bad breath.

Diagnosis

Correct diagnosis is essential for appropriate treatment of tonsillitis and adenoiditis. Diagnosis of tonsillitis is based on the presenting symptoms and results of lab tests such as the rapid strep test, throat culture, and Monospot test. Additional tests may be needed to rule out more serious disorders such as epiglottitis and peritonsillar *abscess* (localized collection of pus).

Treatment

Treatment for viral tonsillitis and adenoiditis is symptomatic. Rest and fluids are encouraged. A soft diet can be offered if the child demonstrates an interest in eating. Saline gargles, acetaminophen, and ibuprofen should be used to control fever and pain. Aspirin should not be used to treat viral infections in children, because of its association with Reye syndrome.

Tonsillectomy or adenoidectomy may be necessary for chronic tonsillitis or adenoiditis that is unresponsive to antibiotic and symptomatic treatment.

> **Flashpoint**
> Tonsillectomy may be necessary for children with chronic tonsillitis.

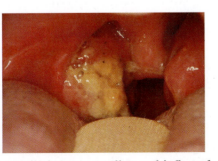

FIGURE 4-5 In tonsillitis the tonsils become swollen and inflamed, with pockets of pus on them. (From Dillon, PM. *Nursing Health Assessment: A Critical Thinking, Case Studies Approach, 2nd edition.* 2007. Philadelphia: F.A. Davis Company, with permission.)

Prognosis

Most children respond well to antibiotic treatment. There is a risk of respiratory arrest if the tonsils swell enough to block the airway. Those children not responding to medical treatment usually respond well to surgical interventions. Some children may experience regrowth of the adenoids or may experience enlargement of one or more of the tonsils; if so, they may continue to experience presurgical symptoms.

Strep Throat

ICD-9-CM: 034.0   [ICD-10: J02.0]

Strep throat is a common bacterial infection that causes *pharyngitis* (sore throat).

Incidence

Strep throat can occur at any age; however, it is rarely seen in children younger than age three.

Etiology

Flashpoint

Some people are carriers of streptococcus bacteria but may be asymptomatic.

Strep throat is caused by infection with group A streptococci. Family members who carry the streptococcus bacteria may be asymptomatic. These family members can pass the infection to children, who then experience repeated infection. Some people, called carriers, harbor the bacteria in their throats but never experience symptoms.

Signs and Symptoms

Common signs and symptoms of strep throat include throat soreness, inflammation and tenderness of cervical lymph nodes, and fever. Infants and small children may exhibit sleeplessness, irritability, fever, refusal to breastfeed or drink from a bottle or cup, and occasionally a fine red rash on the torso, arms, and legs.

Diagnosis

Diagnosis is based upon the patient's complaints and examination findings. A rapid strep test may be done to confirm a positive diagnosis (see Box 4-6); however, a throat culture may still be needed to confirm negative results.

Treatment

Treatment of strep throat involves administration of antibiotics, acetaminophen, fluids, and rest. Health-care providers should encourage the parent or caregiver to administer the entire prescription of antibiotics to avoid superinfection (see Box 4-7).

Prognosis

Most cases of strep throat resolve with treatment. Recurrence is common, though, in part because the disease is so easily spread to other family members and friends. The recurrence of

---

Box 4-6 Diagnostic Spotlight

THE RAPID STREP TEST

The rapid strep test is used to identify whether group A streptococcus bacteria are present in the patient's throat. Although it is less accurate than the traditional throat culture, it has two distinct advantages: it is less expensive and the results are obtained very quickly. If the results are positive, this allows the initiation of immediate antibiotic therapy. On the other hand, a negative result is less conclusive. It indicates that strep bacteria are *probably* not present, but a traditional strep test may still be necessary to confirm the results.

To perform the test, the health-care provider rubs a cotton-tipped swab over the patient's tonsils or back of the throat to obtain a mucus sample. The specimen is tested for the presence of a protein associated with the strep bacteria. Most rapid strep tests take only hours or even minutes to provide results. By comparison, the traditional throat culture takes 2 or 3 days.

Box 4-7 Wellness Promotion

ANTIBIOTICS AND SUPERINFECTION

Make sure that parents understand the importance of having their child complete the entire prescription of antibiotics. This helps avoid superinfection, which can occur when the patient takes some of the antibiotic but stops taking it when he or she starts feeling better. When this happens, the antibiotic kills only the weakest bacteria, leaving the stronger to survive and reinfect the patient. Then the patient experiences a relapse, which may be much worse than the initial infection.

In addition, the remaining bacteria may acquire resistance to the antibiotic, forcing the physician to select a different antibiotic to treat the patient. As the process continues it may eventually become difficult for the physician to find any antibiotic that will kill the infection.

strep throat is likely not a sign of an underlying problem with the child's immune system. Complications of strep throat include rheumatic fever, which produces skin rash, joint inflammation, and possibly damage to heart valves and kidneys.

Asthma

ICD-9-CM: 493.9   [ICD-10: J45.9 (unspecified)]

Asthma is a disorder characterized by inflammation and spasms of the bronchi, increased mucous secretions in the bronchi, and narrowing of the airways (see Fig. 4-6).

Incidence

Asthma affects about 15% of all children in the United States, making it the most common chronic disease in children and the most common disorder seen in the pediatric office. It is increasing in prevalence among children and affects minority and inner-city children more than others.

Flashpoint

Asthma is the most common chronic disease in children.

Etiology

Specific causes of asthma vary; triggers can include cigarette smoke and other inhaled irritants, respiratory infections, weather extremes, emotional distress, exercise (called *exercise-induced asthma*), and environmental allergens. The tendency to have asthma sometimes runs in families. Allergens are the most common type of trigger and include house dust, pet dander, mold, pollen, and less often foods such as milk and eggs.

Signs and Symptoms

Signs and symptoms of asthma include frequent respiratory infections, dyspnea, wheezing, chest tightness, difficulty speaking, and anxiety. Coughing may also be present, especially after the

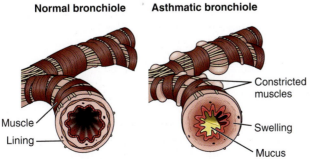

Normal bronchiole   **Asthmatic bronchiole**

Constricted muscles

Muscle

Swelling

Lining

Mucus

FIGURE 4-6 **Asthma causes the bronchioles to constrict, swell, and produce mucus.**

child has been running or crying. Mild wheezing may not be noticeable until the child is 18 to 24 months of age and may go unrecognized by the child and parents. Some children are asymptomatic or have very mild symptoms ("hidden asthma").

Diagnosis

Asthma is difficult to diagnose in children younger than 5 years and in those with "hidden asthma." History and physical examination, along with results from pulmonary function tests (PFTs, also called *spirometry*) and chest x-rays, help confirm the diagnosis. PFTs measure lung capacity; because many patients with chronic asthma exhibit normal spirometry results, they may also be asked to measure peak expiratory flow twice daily for 2 weeks. Although peak flow varies normally, variability of greater than 20% confirms a diagnosis of asthma. Because PFTs are not always possible on small children, diagnosis may be confirmed by a positive response to treatment. A diagnosis of mild intermittent asthma, mild persistent asthma, moderate persistent asthma, or severe persistent asthma is made depending on the presenting symptoms. The classification will determine the treatment approach selected for the child.

Flashpoint
PFTs are performed to measure lung capacity.

Treatment

Effective management of asthma depends on (1) control of triggers, (2) medication therapy, (3) therapy-effectiveness monitoring, and (4) active involvement of the parent and child in the plan of care. Triggers are identified through self-reporting and allergy testing. Once identified, the triggers should be avoided. Enrollment in a desensitization program may be beneficial.

Treatments for asthma include bronchodilator medication delivered via an inhaler or nebulizer, anti-inflammatory medications, and avoidance of common triggers. Administration of an oral corticosteroid within 45 minutes of the onset of an acute attack may prevent hospitalization. Patients who experience more than two asthma attacks per week should be referred to a respiratory specialist.

Prognosis

Asthma is a potentially life-threatening disease. Most children who have well-controlled asthma can participate in usual childhood activities except during periods of acute illness. Prognosis for childhood asthma is generally good, with more than 50% of patients outgrowing asthma after 10 years. With proper treatment, the extent of permanent lung damage is minimal.

Gastrointestinal System Diseases and Disorders

Many diseases and disorders affect the gastrointestinal tract, either directly or indirectly. Most are addressed in Chapter 12; however, because diarrhea, constipation, and parasitic worm infestations are so common in children, they are instead addressed in this chapter.

Diarrhea

ICD-9-CM: 787.91   [ICD-10: A09.0 (infectious origin)]

Diarrhea is the passage of large amounts of watery stool and mucus from the gastrointestinal tract. It is not a disease or disorder per se, but it is a symptom of many health problems, especially gastrointestinal infections, which can pose a serious threat to the infant or child.

Incidence

Diarrhea is common across all populations, regardless of age, sex, race, or socioeconomic status. Outbreaks of diarrhea may occur within a family or at a day-care center, where widespread transmission of the offending pathogen causes the condition in many people.

Etiology

The most common causes of diarrhea in children are bacterial, viral, and parasitic infections. Less commonly, diarrhea is caused by a food allergy or adverse reactions to medication. Because the body attempts to rid itself of the offending organism, the digested food, called chyme, moves too quickly through the digestive tract to provide sufficient time for the intestines to absorb water. The irritated, inflamed lining of the digestive tract secretes mucus to protect the surface of the intestines from the irritant. The result is watery stool with strings of mucus.

Signs and Symptoms

The key symptom of diarrhea is frequent passage of loose or watery stools. It is often accompanied by abdominal pain and cramping.

Diagnosis

Diagnosis is based on the parent or caregiver's report that the child has had two or more loose or watery stools within a 24-hour period. If bloody stool is present, the pediatrician will order collection of a stool sample to identify the causative agent.

Treatment

Treatment of diarrhea aims to replenish fluids and resolve the underlying cause. If stool cultures are positive for bacteria, the pediatrician will prescribe an antibiotic.

In addition to replenishing fluids, an infant or a child recovering from diarrhea must eat. Withholding food can damage the intestines. The parent should continue to offer the infant breast milk or formula. The toddler and older child should be offered a mild, high-carbohydrate diet and lots of fluids (see Box 4-8). Water and electrolyte-replacement drinks for children, such as Pedialyte, are the best choices. If necessary, the electrolyte drink can be diluted with water so that the child tolerates it better.

Prognosis

Most cases of diarrhea resolve with dietary changes. If diarrhea is left untreated, it can lead to increased pulse rate, hypotension, diminished urine output, kidney failure, confusion, acidosis (increased acidity of the blood), and possibly death.

> **Flashpoint**
> Diarrhea is commonly caused by bacterial, viral, or parasitic infection.

> **Flashpoint**
> Infants and children should be given lots of fluids to prevent dehydration.

> **Flashpoint**
> Most cases of diarrhea resolve with time and TLC.

Constipation

ICD-9-CM: 564.00   [ICD-10: K59.0]

Constipation is a condition in which a person has hard stools that are difficult to expel or defecation that is painful and infrequent.

Incidence

Constipation occurs in approximately 2% of the general population but is most prevalent in children. Women and elderly people suffer more bouts of constipation than young men.

Etiology

The primary causes of constipation in most children are lack of dietary fiber and fluids and sedentary lifestyle. Medication may also be a cause in some cases.

> **Flashpoint**
> The most common cause of constipation is lack of fiber and fluid.

Signs and Symptoms

Signs and symptoms of constipation include hard, dry stools that are difficult to pass, infrequent urge to defecate, and stomach discomfort. Because babies and young children are not able to communicate sensations of pain or difficulty passing stool, the parent or caregiver may notice the child straining and turning red when trying to defecate. The parent may also note the child holding his or her abdomen or complaining of a bellyache. Stools that the child is able to pass may be small lumps that look like nuts.

Diagnosis

Diagnosis is usually easily made based upon the child and parents' description of recent bowel-elimination patterns and physical examination. Occasionally, radiological testing is done to confirm the presence of retained stool in the bowel.

Treatment

Health-care providers can encourage the constipated child and the parents to make dietary changes (see Box 4-9). If dietary changes are inadequate, the physician may prescribe a stool softener. However, parents should be cautioned to avoid giving the child too much stool softener, because it could cause diarrhea and dehydration.

Box 4-8 Wellness Promotion

THE DIARRHEA DIET

When a child has diarrhea, temporary dietary modification can help. The child should avoid foods that stimulate peristalsis (movement of food through the digestive tract).

Foods to Avoid

Fruits such as prunes, peaches, and pears and dairy products such as milk, cheese, and yogurt.

Foods to Eat

When a toddler or older child is recovering from diarrhea, the caregiver should provide foods that are high in carbohydrates, to help enhance fluid and sodium absorption, and mild, to avoid irritating the intestines. For this reason, most pediatricians recommend the BRAT diet, which consists of:

- **B**ananas
- **R**ice
- **A**pplesauce
- **T**oast

Watch for Dehydration

Prolonged diarrhea will cause dehydration, electrolyte imbalance, and diaper rash in infants. Parents should be educated to look for the signs of dehydration that accompany diarrhea, including:

- lack of tears when crying
- lethargy
- fewer wet diapers than normal
- dry mouth and lips
- weight loss
- irritability

Rehydrate

The pediatrician may recommend the use of oral rehydration products, such as Pedialyte or Infalyte. Caregivers should give small amounts of these products, approximately three tablespoons every 15 minutes.

When to Come to the Office

Parents or caregivers should bring a young child who has diarrhea for more than 2 days to see the physician to determine the cause and appropriate treatment.

Prognosis

Flashpoint

Most cases of constipation get better with dietary changes.

Most children respond favorably to dietary changes, and normal bowel function returns. In some cases, constipation can lead to hemorrhoids or anal fissures (tears of the skin around the anus). Rectal bleeding may occur from hemorrhoids and anal fissures. The parent or caregiver should be instructed to bring the child to the pediatrician if there is blood in the child's diaper or underwear. In severe cases, constipation can lead to a bowel obstruction.

Parasitic Worms

ICD-9-CM: 129.0 (unspecified organism)   [ICD-10: B65-B83 (code by organism)]

Parasitic worms, also called *helminths,* are present in soil and water and require other living organisms to survive. Infection occurs when individuals unknowingly ingest the tiny worm eggs, which hatch within the intestinal tract. Less commonly, they may migrate to other organs, such

Box 4-9 Wellness Promotion

THE CONSTIPATION DIET
The health-care provider should teach the pediatric patient and parents or caregivers about foods that cause constipation and others that help alleviate it.

Foods to Encourage
- Fruit and fruit juices, including apples, oranges, plums, and prunes
- High-fiber cereals
- High-fiber, whole-grain bread
- Water

Foods to Avoid
- Bananas
- Pudding
- Cheese
- Rice
- White bread

as the liver or lungs. Common offenders are *Enterobius vermicularis* (pinworms) and *Ascaris lumbricoides* (roundworms).

Incidence
Pinworms are the most common form of parasitic worm, with an estimated 42 million people infected in the United States, and widespread infection worldwide. Infections are most common in preschool-aged and school-aged children, institutionalized individuals, and those who come into contact with these individuals. Consequently, infection generally occurs in multiple members of the household and among those in child-care centers.

An estimated 4 million people in the United States are infected with roundworms, mainly in rural areas of the Southeast. An estimated one billion individuals are infected worldwide. Roundworm infection is most common in tropical areas where individuals live with poor sanitation and hygiene.

Flashpoint
Pinworm infestation is very common in children.

Etiology
Infection with pinworms and roundworms occurs though the fecal-oral route, by accidental ingestion of mature eggs. Any object (food, drink, hands, etc.) that has been contaminated with feces and then put into the mouth promotes infection. Pinworms exit the intestine through the anus while individuals sleep, and lay their eggs on the surrounding skin (see Fig. 4-7).

Signs and Symptoms
Common symptoms of pinworm infection include perianal **pruritus** (itching), especially at night.

Diagnosis
Diagnosis is based on the patient's complaints of perianal itching, identification of the worms from cellophane tape pressed over the anal opening, and identification of the worms in stool and blood samples.

Flashpoint
The most common symptom of pinworm infestation is perianal itching, especially at night.

Treatment
Treatment includes the prescription of antiparasitic medication such as albendazole, mebendazole, ivermectin, and others. Education about sanitation and hand washing will help patients break the reinfection cycle.

Prognosis
Prognosis is good for those with light to moderate infections. Occasionally the parasite may migrate to other sites and cause complications such as ulcerative lesions in the intestines, appendicitis, and chronic salpingitis (inflammation of the fallopian tubes).

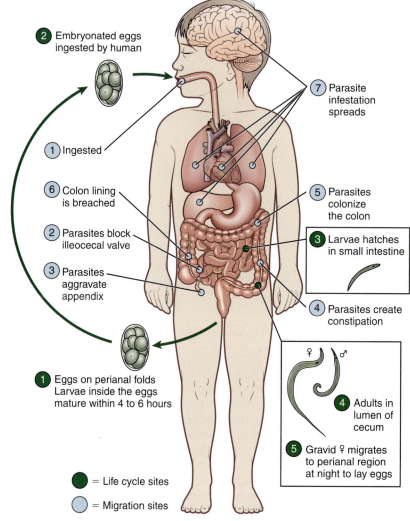

② Embryonated eggs
ingested by human

⑦ Parasite
infestation
spreads

① Ingested

⑥ Colon lining
is breached

② Parasites block
illeocecal valve

③ Parasites
aggravate
appendix

⑤ Parasites
colonize
the colon

③ Larvae hatches
in small intestine

④ Parasites create
constipation

① Eggs on perianal folds
Larvae inside the eggs
mature within 4 to 6 hours

♀   ♂

④ Adults in
lumen of
cecum

⑤ Gravid ♀ migrates
to perianal region
at night to lay eggs

● = Life cycle sites

○ = Migration sites

FIGURE 4-7 Lifecycle of the pinworm.

Sensory System Diseases and Disorders

Children are vulnerable to many of the same sensory diseases and disorders as older individuals. However, they are especially prone to developing conjunctivitis and otitis media.

Conjunctivitis

ICD-9-CM: 372.00 (unspecified acute or chronic)   [ICD-10: H10.9]

Conjunctivitis, commonly called *pinkeye*, is a bacterial or viral inflammation or infection of the conjunctiva, which is the transparent membrane that lines the eyelid and part of the eyeball. A recent study estimated that 4% of schoolchildren and 6% of high schoolers see a physician for conjunctivitis each year.

Neonates are sometimes born with incompletely opened tear ducts, making them more prone to infection. They are also susceptible to bacteria normally present in the mother's birth canal. In rare cases, these bacteria can cause infants to develop a serious form of conjunctivitis known as *ophthalmia neonatorum,* which requires immediate treatment to preserve sight. To prevent this serious complication, most hospital policies require administration of a preventive antibiotic application, such as erythromycin ointment, to the eyes of every neonate. For a detailed description of conjunctivitis, see Chapter 15.

Otitis Media

ICD-9-CM: 381.00   [ICD-10: H65.0 (acute serous)]

Otitis media (OM) is an infection of the middle ear that occurs commonly in babies and children between ages 4 months and 5 years. It accounts for an estimated 16 million pediatric visits each year in the United States. About 17% to 20% of American children have had at least one case of otitis media by age two. Because infants are not able to verbally communicate, OM can be difficult to recognize in them; however, they may have a fever and cough and may pull at their ears and be fussier than normal. For a detailed description of otitis media, see Chapter 15.

Integumentary System Diseases and Disorders

Children are vulnerable to many of the same integumentary system diseases and disorders as older individuals. However, they are especially prone to developing oral candidiasis, impetigo, and warts.

Oral Candidiasis

ICD-9-CM: 112.0 (neonate: 771.7)   [ICD-10: B37.0]

Oral candidiasis, commonly called *oral thrush* and sometimes *oral yeast infection*, is a fungal infection of the mouth. Although it can affect anyone, it occurs most commonly in infants under age 6 months and older individuals who are taking antibiotics or whose immune system is weakened. Oral thrush is caused by *Candida albicans*. A healthy neonate with oral thrush usually develops symptoms during the first few weeks of life. In addition to the distinctive white lesions in the mouth, the parent or caregiver may notice that the infant is irritable and fussy and may not want to eat. During breastfeeding, the neonate can pass the infection to the mother. Occasionally, oral thrush may spread to the roof of the mouth, gums, tonsils, or back of the throat.

Oral thrush is a minor problem for healthy children, but for those with weakened immune systems, symptoms of oral thrush may be more severe, widespread, and difficult to control. Uncontrolled thrush may lead to diaper rash and vaginal yeast infections. Severe complications that spread to the esophagus, brain, heart, and joints are rare but may occur in immunocompromised infants, such as those with HIV. For a more detailed description of oral candidiasis, see Chapter 5.

Impetigo

ICD-9-CM: 684.0   [ICD-10: L01.0]

Impetigo is a common, highly contagious skin infection that accounts for 10% of all skin problems seen in the pediatric office. It is most common in preschoolers and easily spreads through day-care centers and preschools. It first appears as small, fluid-filled vesicles around the mouth or nose. The vesicles quickly enlarge and rupture, excreting a yellow ***exudate*** (drainage). The lesions then crust over, and the crusty area is inflamed and moist. For a more detailed description of impetigo, see Chapter 5.

Warts

ICD-9-CM: 078.1 [ICD-10: B07]

Common warts are noncancerous skin growths. Approximately 4% of 9- to 14-year-olds in the United States develop common warts, which are caused by HPV. Warts appear as small, fleshy, grainy bumps that are rough to the touch and usually painless. They may occur singly or in multiple clusters. They commonly contain one or more tiny black dots, which are small, clotted blood vessels. They usually occur on the hands or fingers or near the fingernails. Nail biting can also cause warts to spread onto the fingertips and around the nails. For a more detailed description of warts, see Chapter 5.

Miscellaneous Diseases and Disorders

There are many childhood disorders that do not easily fit into a specific category. Yet some are important enough to address in this text: Kawasaki disease, failure to thrive, lead poisoning, Reye syndrome, phenylketonuria, sudden infant death syndrome, infantile colic, and child abuse.

Kawasaki Disease

ICD-9-CM: 446.1 [ICD-10: M30.3]

Kawasaki disease, also known as mucocutaneous *lymph node syndrome* and *Kawasaki syndrome,* is a self-limiting vasculitis (inflammation of vessels) that affects various structures including the mouth, skin and lymph nodes, blood vessels, and the heart in children.

Incidence

Kawasaki disease affects 1,000 to 2,000 children in the United States per year, 80% of them younger than 5 years—boys more than girls. It is most common among those of Japanese or Korean descent and is the leading cause of acquired heart disease in children.

Etiology

The cause of Kawasaki disease is unknown.

Signs and Symptoms

The hallmark sign of Kawasaki disease is a high fever (102°F to 104°F) that lasts for at least 5 days and is not responsive to antibiotics. Other principal symptoms include red-purple palms and soles; swollen hands and feet; peeling skin around the fingers and toes; a diffuse red skin rash over the trunk and extremities; severe eye redness without exudate; red, cracked lips; reddened, swollen tongue; sore throat; and swollen cervical lymph nodes. Additionally, the child may be irritable and complain of joint pain and gastrointestinal symptoms.

> **Flashpoint**
>
> Kawasaki disease causes high fever and purple, swollen hands and feet.

Diagnosis

Diagnostic criteria for Kawasaki disease include a fever of at least 5 days accompanied by four or more of the principal symptoms already described. Alternately, a patient meeting the temperature criterion who has fewer than four of the principal symptoms but also has coronary disease may be diagnosed. There is no specific diagnostic test for Kawasaki disease; however, blood studies may reveal anemia and thrombocytosis (high platelet count), increased erythrocyte sedimentation rate, and elevated C-reactive protein. Liver function tests may indicate hepatic (liver) inflammation.

Treatment

Treatment includes high-dose intravenous gamma globulin, which may be repeated if fever does not improve. It is most useful if given within 1 week of fever onset. Salicylate therapy in the form of high-dose aspirin is initiated and then continued in smaller doses for 2 months. Aspirin use is usually discouraged in children due to risk of Reye syndrome, but it is given for this disorder because it helps to control the fever, reduce inflammation, and prevent blood-clot formation.

Prognosis

Most children respond well to treatment and recover in several days, although relapses may occur. If treatment is not initiated early, the child may develop vasculitis damage to the muscles, lining, and valves of the heart. Abnormal heart rhythm and even heart attack can occur. The mortality rate is 2%.

Flashpoint

Normally aspirin should not be given to children, but a child with Kawasaki disease is an exception to this rule.

Failure to Thrive

ICD-9-CM: 783.41   [ICD-10: R62.8]

Failure to thrive (FTT) is a condition of insufficient weight gain according to standardized growth charts. Children experience irregular growth patterns, gaining height and weight at irregular intervals commonly called *growth spurts*. As long as toddlers are growing and developing, there is little cause for concern. However, infants who do not gain sufficient weight will not develop normally.

Incidence

Although the exact incidence of FTT is not known, approximately 10% of children under age two who have parents with psychological problems and low socioeconomic status exhibit FTT. The FTT category includes infants whose weight is below the third percentile.

Etiology

The most common cause of FTT is inadequate nutrition. Colic, mothers who used alcohol or had poor nutrition during pregnancy, and new mothers who experience fatigue and postpartum depression can all contribute to FTT. Causes can also include cleft palate, which affects the infant's ability to suck, and malabsorption syndrome, which compromises the body's ability to absorb formula or breast milk. Social and economic factors that can promote FTT include poverty, drug and alcohol abuse, depression, abuse, and immature parents.

Flashpoint

Infants and children whose weight is under the third percentile may have FTT.

Signs and Symptoms

Children with FTT demonstrate insufficient growth and weight gain according to standardized growth charts.

Diagnosis

Diagnosis is based upon documentation of the child's failure to grow, gain weight, and develop according to expected norms. If the rate of growth is normal, the child may simply be small for his or her age; the size of the child's biological parents must also be considered. The health-care provider may question the parent about feeding, bowel habits, financial resources, and social and emotional factors that might affect access to food. Diagnostic testing may be done to identify nutritional disorders or other underlying diseases.

Treatment

Social services may be consulted to obtain financial assistance for the family to buy food and to address issues of abuse, neglect, or drug abuse. Most states have programs for food stamps or nutritional assistance.

Prognosis

Prognosis for the child with FTT depends on the cause. Infants who have a malabsorption syndrome treated with diet modification, or a cleft palate that is surgically corrected, have good outcomes. FTT due to abuse and neglect can lead to permanent lack of growth and possible long-term developmental delay; the duration of the abuse or neglect affects the long-term outcome.

Lead Poisoning

ICD-9-CM: 984.9   [ICD-10: T56.0]

Lead poisoning, or *plumbism,* is a chronic disorder caused by ingestion or inhalation of lead-contaminated paint, soil, or dust.

Incidence

According to the Centers for Disease Control and Prevention (CDC), approximately 2% of children between ages one and five contract lead poisoning. Children of lower socioeconomic status are at greater risk.

Etiology

In the body, lead interferes with minerals such as iron, calcium, and zinc. It replaces these minerals and disrupts their normal function. In the bloodstream, lead replaces iron in the hemoglobin of red blood cells, making them unable to carry oxygen to tissues. In bone, lead interferes with the absorption of calcium needed to make bone cells. Decreased zinc absorption causes immune suppression.

Malnourished children are at greater risk of lead poisoning because they will absorb more lead than children with healthy diets. This is because lead competes for absorption with many vitamins and minerals, including vitamins C and D; when lesser amounts of these vitamins and minerals are present, more lead is absorbed. In addition, the empty stomach of a hungry child will absorb more lead if lead is consumed.

> **Flashpoint**
>
> Lead interferes with the body's ability to absorb important minerals like iron and calcium.

Signs and Symptoms

Signs and symptoms of lead poisoning include recurrent episodes of diarrhea, irritability, and fatigue. Because these symptoms are similar to those of iron-deficiency anemia, the two are commonly confused. In fact, iron-deficiency anemia and lead poisoning are often diagnosed together in children of low socioeconomic backgrounds.

Diagnosis

Diagnosis is based on blood-sample analysis for lead. Lead levels greater than 60 to 70 micrograms per deciliter of whole blood indicate poisoning.

Treatment

> **Flashpoint**
>
> The child's environment must be evaluated for possible sources of lead.

Treatment includes chelation therapy, which involves injection of a chelating agent that binds to lead, making it water soluble so the child can excrete it in urine. Because children with lead poisoning usually have an iron deficiency, iron supplementation typically accompanies chelation therapy. In addition, the identified sources of lead in the child's environment should be removed to prevent further poisoning.

Prognosis

Prognosis is based on the child's lead levels and how long the child ingested lead before diagnosis and treatment. Outcomes vary from mild (complete recovery that takes months to years) to severe (brain damage and permanent reduction in IQ). In addition, lead poisoning suppresses the child's immune system, leaving little protection from infectious diseases.

Reye Syndrome

ICD-9-CM: 331.81   [ICD-10: G93.7]

Reye syndrome is a serious disease associated with aspirin use by children with viral illnesses. It can result in permanent brain damage or even death.

Incidence

Reye syndrome develops predominantly in children between the ages of four and 14. Over 500 cases were reported in 1980. However, since that time physicians and parents have been cautioned to avoid aspirin use in children, and the incidence has declined to about two cases per year (see Box 4-10).

Etiology

The exact cause of Reye syndrome is not understood; however, the syndrome has been linked to the use of aspirin in children who have *febrile* (fever-producing) viral illness.

> **Flashpoint**
>
> Reye syndrome has been linked to aspirin use in children.

Signs and Symptoms

The child with Reye syndrome has nearly always had a viral illness such as a cold, influenza, diarrhea, or chickenpox within the preceding 2 weeks. Some cases are mild and may go unnoticed.

Box 4-10 Wellness Promotion

ASPIRIN FOR CHILDREN?
With very rare exceptions, aspirin should not be given to children, because of the risks associated with Reye syndrome. Other options are available to help relieve fever and discomfort associated with illnesses, including acetaminophen and ibuprofen. When in doubt about what to do, parents should contact their child's health-care provider for guidance. This is especially important for children under the age of two.

Five stages of symptom progression have been identified. In the first stage, children demonstrate persistent vomiting, mental confusion, and lethargy, and complain of nightmares. During the second stage, they display tachypnea and become severely lethargic, yet have hyperactive reflexes. Liver biopsy at this stage reveals fatty liver. During stage three, mental status further deteriorates to a coma. During stage four, the coma deepens. During the fifth and final stage, the child has very high blood ammonia levels, displays deep coma and muscle flaccidity yet may also experience seizures, and may die.

Diagnosis
Diagnosis is based on the child's history of a recent viral illness and aspirin use (these factors correlate 90% to 95% of the time), along with presenting signs and symptoms. Laboratory testing may be done to rule out other disorders and confirm diagnosis. A variety of tests may be done, but the most conclusive are liver function tests, which reveal elevated ammonia levels and other abnormalities during the first three stages of Reye syndrome.

Treatment
There is no cure for Reye syndrome. Children are usually hospitalized and given fluids, electrolytes, and nutritional support. Mechanical ventilation may be indicated. Neurological status is monitored very closely. Brain swelling may be treated with corticosteroids and diuretics.

Prognosis
Mild to severe permanent brain damage may develop. The mortality rate is 20% to 30%. Chances of recovery are greatest if diagnosis and treatment occur early.

Flashpoint
Reye syndrome can cause permanent brain damage.

Phenylketonuria

ICD-9-CM: 270.1   [ICD-10: E70.0]
Phenylketonuria (PKU) is a genetic disorder in which infants are born with a lack of the enzyme phenylalanine hydroxylase. As a result, they are unable to properly utilize protein, specifically the amino acid called *phenylalanine*.

Incidence
It is estimated that one in every 70 people is a carrier for PKU and that the disorder affects one in every 15,000 to 20,000 infants born in the United States.

Etiology
Normally, when a person eats protein the body breaks it down into separate amino acids. In an infant with PKU, one of the enzymes that changes phenylalanine into another amino acid, tyrosine, is missing. As a result, phenylalanine accumulates in the blood and prevents the infant's brain from growing and developing normally.

Signs and Symptoms
In addition to increased levels of phenylalanine, other symptoms of PKU include skin rash, irritable behavior, and a musty body odor.

Diagnosis
A PKU test, mandated by most states, is typically performed before the baby leaves the hospital but may be done after discharge or at the first health-care visit if the newborn was delivered at home. A simple blood test diagnoses the disorder (see Box 4-11).

Box 4-11 Diagnostic Spotlight

THE PKU TEST

The PKU test is done to identify whether a newborn infant has the enzyme necessary to utilize phenylalanine. If the enzyme is not present, the level of phenylalanine builds up in the blood, causing brain damage. All infants in the United States are tested within several days of birth and again at around 7 to 10 days. The test involves obtaining a blood specimen by heel stick and applying it to a card that is sent to the laboratory. Infants should be taking in formula or breast milk for 24 to 48 hours before the blood sample is collected. For infants older than 6 weeks, a urine PKU test is done.

Treatment

Early diagnosis of the disorder allows parents to put the child on a special diet that is very low in phenylalanine. The diet includes phenylalanine-free formula and eliminates foods high in protein, such as dairy products, beans, nuts, meat, eggs, and fish. It also requires monitoring intake of fruits, vegetables, cereals, breads, and pastas. In addition, PKU patients should avoid the artificial sweetener aspartame, which breaks down into two amino acids, one of them phenylalanine.

Prognosis

Flashpoint

Keeping the child on a special PKU diet will prevent brain damage.

The extent of brain damage and disability is directly proportional to the length of time that phenylalanine levels remain high. Thus, untreated PKU will cause progressive mental disability. However, because most cases are identified with neonatal screening, the more serious complications of PKU are rarely seen.

Sudden Infant Death Syndrome

ICD-9-CM: 798.0   [ICD-10: R95]

Sudden infant death syndrome (SIDS) is a diagnosis of exclusion that is made when there is a sudden unexplained death of an infant less than 1 year old.

Incidence

SIDS is the major cause of death in infants between 1 and 12 months of age, with the majority of deaths occurring between 2 and 4 months of age. African American and Native American infants are affected two to three times more than white infants. Boys are affected more than girls.

Etiology

Flashpoint

The exact cause of SIDS is still a mystery.

The cause of SIDS is unknown. Autopsy findings suggest that a nervous system defect is a contributing factor. Maternal risk factors include late or poor prenatal care; tobacco, alcohol, or drug abuse during pregnancy; and a maternal age of less than 20 years. Infants born prematurely or with a low birth weight are at risk. Other identified risk factors include exposure to tobacco smoke after birth, overheating, sleeping in the prone position, sleeping on soft surfaces, and bed-sharing.

Signs and Symptoms

As the name suggests, this disorder is sudden and without any signs or symptoms to warn of its impending occurrence. An otherwise healthy infant is discovered by parents or other caregivers to be lifeless, usually during a sleep period. The infant appears to have experienced no suffering prior to death.

Diagnosis

Diagnosis of SIDS can only be made after death when all other possible causes, such as cardiac disorders, metabolic disorders, accidental death, and abuse, have been ruled out. A diagnosis of

SIDS is made after autopsy, examination of the death scene, and review of the infant's and family's medical history. The very nature of the diagnostic process may lead parents to feel as if they are under suspicion. Professionals involved in this fact-finding process should be trained to avoid stigmatizing the parents, other family members, or caregivers.

Treatment

Incidence of SIDS can be minimized by teaching parents and caregivers how to control risk factors. One of the biggest factors associated with SIDS is the sleep position of the infant. Parents and caregivers should be instructed to place the child in the supine position (lying on the back) for sleep. Additional suggestions include providing a smoke-free environment; breast-feeding; using an approved crib with a firm, snug-fitting mattress; refraining from placing the infant on a soft surface for sleep; removing all soft bedding and toys from the crib; making sure not to overheat the infant; and avoiding bed-sharing.

Prognosis

Since the initiation of the national "Back to Sleep" campaign, SIDS rates have declined significantly. Despite this improvement, SIDS continues to be the number one cause of death during the postneonatal period, and African Americans and Native American babies are still two to three times more likely to die of SIDS than white babies are. Education is the key to further reduction of the prevalence of SIDS.

> **Flashpoint**
> The "Back to Sleep" campaign has helped significantly reduce the number of SIDS cases.

Infantile Colic

ICD-9-CM: 789.0   [ICD-10: R10.4]

Colic is described as crying in an infant less than 3 months of age that lasts more than 3 hours of the day and occurs at least 3 days per week (the "rule of three").

Incidence

Colic usually occurs in otherwise healthy babies.

Etiology

There is no known cause of colic. It is not caused by gas, as once believed; instead, the colicky infant is more likely to have gas from swallowing air while crying.

> **Flashpoint**
> The exact cause of colic is still a mystery.

Signs and Symptoms

The "rule of three" summarizes the main manifestations of colic. Colic can occur at any time of the day, but most often occurs during the evening hours. Additionally, the infant may alternately flex and extend the arms and legs.

Diagnosis

Diagnosis of colic is by exclusion. If the "rule of three" criteria are met and all other causes of crying have been excluded, it is likely that the infant has colic.

Treatment

There is a wide range of suggestions for dealing with colic, but no treatment is consistently effective for all infants. Cuddling, swaddling, using a pacifier, gently rocking the infant, and eliminating potentially irritating foods from the breastfeeding mother's diet may be beneficial. A formula change or the use of simethicone drops are options sometimes suggested by physicians, but there is no conclusive evidence that either of these interventions works consistently. Other treatments, such as herbal tea, crib vibrators, and infant massage, are available but should be used with caution and only after consulting with a pediatrician, because of possible harmful effects. Dealing with a colicky infant can be frustrating; parents should ask a family member or friend for assistance when a break is needed.

> **Flashpoint**
> Colic eventually resolves with time, patience, and TLC.

Prognosis

Colic is a temporary condition that usually disappears by the time the infant is 3 months of age. It is important to rule out other, more serious causes of crying, such as meningitis, otitis media, and abuse. Doing so will minimize the likelihood of unfavorable outcomes.

Child Abuse

ICD-9-CM: 995.54   [ICD-10: T74.1]

Child abuse is generally defined as any act that results in physical, emotional, or sexual harm to a child. In the United States there are nearly one million reported cases of child abuse and 1,500 reported deaths resulting from child abuse annually. There are four forms of child abuse: physical abuse, emotional abuse, sexual abuse, and neglect. Intentional acts that result in bodily injury to the child characterize physical abuse. Sexual abuse includes any sexual act between a child and adult or older child—the act may or may not involve physical contact. Emotional abuse sends the message that the child is worthless, unwanted, and unloved. Neglect is a failure to provide for the child's basic physical, educational, emotional, and medical needs.

Shaken-baby syndrome (SBS) and Munchausen syndrome by proxy are two special types of child abuse. Shaken-baby syndrome occurs when a child, usually under 1 year of age, is shaken vigorously by a frustrated parent or caretaker in an effort to stop the child's crying. Almost 50% of infants who experience SBS die. Those that survive often experience irreversible brain damage that leads to blindness, seizures, and learning difficulties. Munchausen by proxy syndrome is a form of child abuse in which a caretaker or parent, usually the mother, fabricates or deliberately causes illness in the child in order to receive the sympathy and attention of health-care providers. The child undergoes unnecessary testing and may be given medications, hospitalized, and even operated on to determine the cause of the illness. Health-care providers may not be suspicious because the parent appears to be very concerned, attentive, and cooperative.

Flashpoint

Shaken-baby syndrome has a very high mortality rate.

Incidence

Many of the victims of abuse are less than 4 years of age. Children who have physical and mental disabilities are also at great risk.

Etiology

There is no universal motivation for child abuse, but there are numerous associated risk factors, including poverty, domestic violence, substance abuse, unplanned pregnancy, single parenthood, lack of education, and parents who were themselves victims of child abuse.

Signs and Symptoms

The signs of child abuse are variable and often hidden. Recognizing child abuse requires alertness to typical injury patterns and explanations that do not fit with the child's injuries. Injury patterns include bruises in odd places in various stages of healing, handprints, belt marks, human bite marks, cigarette burn marks, rope burns, bald patches from hair being pulled out, greenstick fractures, and burn marks from being dunked in scalding water. Signs that suggest SBS include retinal hemorrhages, skull fractures, and subdural hematomas (bleeding beneath the dura layer in the skull). Unfortunately, a child presenting with SBS may be misdiagnosed, because presenting signs such as lethargy, fussiness, and feeding problems may be attributed to other causes.

Flashpoint

Injury patterns may alert the health-care provider to the possibility of child abuse.

Signs of sexual abuse are more subtle and include difficulty sitting or walking, hesitance to remove clothing for examination, sleep disturbance, bedwetting, inappropriate sexual knowledge for the child's age, bruising or injuries to the genitalia, and the presence of sexually transmitted disease. Emotional abuse may be manifested by extremes in behavior, including excessive cooperation or passivity, extreme aggression, depression, emotional detachment, or attempted suicide.

Signs of neglect include inappropriate clothing for the weather, poor hygiene, malnutrition, lethargy, failure to seek health care, frequent school absenteeism, failure to thrive, and behavioral problems at school, including begging or stealing from classmates.

Diagnosis

Recognizing signs of child abuse can be difficult. The very nature of childhood adds to this difficulty, because injuries such as bumps, scrapes, bruising, and even broken bones can result from normal activities of childhood. Additionally, the consequences of neglect, sexual abuse, and emotional abuse are not always obvious at first glance. Diagnosis is based on presenting signs and symptoms and historical data. Health-care providers must be alert to physical signs of abuse, especially in instances where the injury does not fit the reported cause. Laboratory and radiological testing may provide additional evidence of abuse; for example, x-rays may reveal numerous untreated fractures. The child's demeanor and the parent's or caretaker's behavior should be monitored.

Treatment

Providing care to the child, including ensuring safety, should take priority. Findings should be carefully and objectively documented. Suspected abuse should be reported as soon as possible. Health-care providers, teachers, day-care workers, and law-enforcement officials are required to report suspected cases of child abuse. Failure to do so may result in legal penalties. Emotional support should also be provided to the child and parent. Long-term treatment requires a multidisciplinary approach including family therapy.

Prevention of child abuse is complex and involves addressing societal, family, and individual issues. A key component is education aimed at teaching parents appropriate parenting skills and stress management, and teaching children how to recognize and respond to abusive behaviors.

Prognosis

The consequences of child abuse are far-reaching. Recovery from physical injury is dependent upon the extent of the injury and the timing of treatment. Emotional and psychological consequences may extend into adulthood. There is an increased risk for smoking, substance abuse, eating disorders, depression, and suicide among victims of child abuse. Also significant is the fact that these victims often perpetuate the cycle and become abusers themselves unless they get help.

Flashpoint

Signs of abuse and neglect may be subtle and difficult to identify.

Flashpoint

Professionals like health-care providers, teachers, day-care workers, and law-enforcement officials must report suspected abuse.

STOP HERE.
Select the flash cards for this chapter and run through them at least three times before moving on to the next chapter.

Student Resources

About.com Health Videos (video clips about immunization, chickenpox, mumps, and other topics): http://video.about.com/health.htm
CDC recommendations for immunization: http://www.immunize.org/catg.d/p2010.pdf
Child Abuse Prevention Association: http://www.childabuseprevention.org
CJ Foundation for SIDS: http://www.cjsids.com
Common Cold: http://www.commoncold.org
Immunization Action Coalition Vaccine Information for the Public and Health Professionals: http://www.vaccineinformation.org
MedlinePlus asthma tutorial: http://www.nlm.nih.gov/medlineplus/tutorials/asthma/htm/index.htm
National Institute of Environmental Health Sciences page on lead poisoning: http://www.niehs.nih.gov/kids/lead.htm
National Reye's Syndrome Foundation: http://www.reyessyndrome.org

Chapter Activities

Learning Style Study Strategies

Try any or all of the following strategies as you study the content of this chapter.

Visual learners: Be sure to use the flash cards that come with this book. They were created especially for visual learners. Take a few with you each day and run through them several times throughout the day. By the time you get home in the evening, you will be familiar with those diseases.

Kinesthetic learners: Be creative, have fun, and learn all at the same time. Buy some inexpensive watercolor paints or colored markers. After reading each section about a disease, create a colorful painting or drawing that includes key points that you remember. Read the section again and add more details. The physical motion combined with the visual images will help you remember what you have studied.

Auditory learners: Locate audio tapes or CDs at your college library or at a bookstore that describe and discuss some of the diseases and disorders you are studying. For this chapter it would be especially useful to locate some that pertain to the pediatric population.

Verbal learners: Assign friends or family members specific diseases or disorders to ask you about when they see you or speak with you. This will force you to recite what you know, which will reinforce the information in
your mind.

Practice Exercises

Answers to Practice Exercises can be found in Appendix D.

Case Studies

CASE STUDY 1

A 2-year-old child of Korean descent has been running a temperature of 102°F to 104°F for the past 5 days. The child has been unresponsive to antibiotic therapy. Additionally, the child has a diffuse red skin rash over the trunk and extremities, red eyes without any drainage, swollen hands and feet with peeling around the fingers and toes, and swollen cervical lymph nodes. A diagnosis of Kawasaki disease is suspected.

1. Which of the above-identified findings is most significant to the diagnosis of Kawasaki disease?

2. What are the guidelines for diagnosing Kawasaki disease?

3. What medications are prescribed for treatment of Kawasaki disease?

4. What complications may develop in the child who has Kawasaki disease?

CASE STUDY 2

The mother of a 1-month-old baby boy asks if it is really necessary to have him immunized, since "nobody in our country ever gets sick with any of those diseases anymore." Respond to her, making sure to address the following:

1. Which of "those diseases" are immunizations currently available for?

2. Why might her infant still be at risk for contracting those diseases?

3. If her baby becomes infected with any of these diseases, what complications might he experience?

CASE STUDY 3

A new medical assistant has been hired at the family medicine clinic where you work. The assistant notices a child in the waiting room with bruises on his legs and asks you how to tell if the child is suffering from abuse.

1. What signs of physical abuse will you describe to the assistant?

2. What signs of emotional abuse will you describe?

3. What signs of sexual abuse will you describe?

4. What signs of neglect will you describe?

Multiple Choice

1. All of the following diseases can be prevented by vaccination **except:**

   a. Measles

   b. Rubella

   c. Pertussis

   d. Bronchiolitis

2. Which of the following disorders is matched with the correct description?

   a. Croup: severe viral respiratory illness that involves swelling and edema of the upper respiratory passages due to inflammation or spasms

   b. Phenylketonuria: a common bacterial infection that causes pharyngitis

   c. Kawasaki disease: a potentially fatal disease associated with aspirin use by children with viral illnesses, which can result in permanent brain damage

   d. Reye syndrome: a disorder characterized by inflammation and spasms of the bronchi, increased mucous secretions in the bronchi, and narrowing of the airways

3. Treatment for chickenpox includes:

   a. Acetaminophen

   b. Antibiotics

   c. Antitoxin

   d. Aspirin

4. Which of the following statements is true of respiratory syncytial virus?

   a. It is most common in teenage boys of Asian descent.

   b. A risk factor is exposure to cigarette smoke or high levels of air pollution.

   c. Affected individuals are usually afebrile.

   d. The mortality rate is 50%.

5. Which of the following is the preferred sleeping position for infants?

    a. Prone

    b. On the left side

    c. On the right side

    d. Supine

Short Answer

1. **Describe shaken-baby syndrome.**

2. **Describe Munchausen by proxy syndrome.**

3. **Describe the "rule of three" with regard to infantile colic.**

INTEGUMENTARY SYSTEM DISEASES AND DISORDERS

5

Learning Outcomes

Upon completion of this chapter, the student will be able to:

- Define and spell terms related to dermatology
- Identify key structures of the integumentary system
- Discuss the roles of protection and temperature regulation played by the integumentary system

- Distinguish skin lesions
- Identify characteristics of common skin diseases and disorders, including:
  - description
  - incidence
  - etiology
  - signs and symptoms
  - diagnosis
  - treatment
  - prognosis

KEY TERMS	
abrasion	area where skin or mucous membranes are scraped away
comedones	small skin lesions of acne that include whiteheads and blackheads
debridement	removal of dead or damaged tissue
dermabrasion	process in which outermost layer of skin is scraped away with a wire brush or burr impregnated with diamond particles
dermatome	area of skin associated with a pair of spinal nerves
diaphoresis	profuse sweating
edema	swelling
erythema	redness
febrile	having a fever
friction	rubbing of skin against bedding, linens, a brace, a cast, etc.
hyperkeratosis	thickening of the skin
hyperplasia	increased cell growth
keratinized	hardened
laceration	cut or tear in the flesh
necrosis	tissue death
rhinophyma	large, irregularly shaped, dark-red nose
shearing	sliding downward of deeper structures due to gravity while the skin remains in place

Continued

KEY TERMS—cont'd	
sutures	stitches used to hold tissue together
syncope	fainting
telangiectasia	appearance of dilated vessels on the skin of cheeks and nose

Abbreviations

Table 5-1 lists some of the most common abbreviations related to the integumentary system.

Structures and Functions of the Integumentary System

The integumentary system is made up of skin and related structures, such as hair follicles, tiny blood vessels, fatty tissue, and specialized nerves for detecting heat, cold, pain, and pressure. The integumentary system protects vital organs and helps carry out many essential body functions.

Structures of the Skin

The skin is made up of three layers: the epidermis, the dermis, and the subcutaneous layer (see Fig. 5-1). The top layer is the epidermis, which is a thin outer layer mostly constructed of nonliving, *keratinized* (hardened) cells. It is waterproof and provides protection for the deeper layers. The epidermis is thickest on the palms of the hands and soles of the feet. The base of this layer, aptly named the *basement membrane,* is where new skin cells are produced. These cells are pushed upward as even newer cells form beneath them. Eventually, they rise near enough to the top that they die and slough off, leaving dry, keratinized tissue that becomes a part of the epidermal layer.

The dermis lies just beneath the epidermis and is much thicker. It contains the hair follicles, nerves, blood vessels, and some glands.

TABLE 5-1

ABBREVIATIONS

Abbreviation	Meaning	Abbreviation	Meaning
Bx, bx	Biopsy	MRSA	methicillin-resistant *Staphylococcus aureus*
C&S	culture and sensitivity	OTC	over-the-counter
Decub	decubitus ulcer	PSUs	pilosebaceous units
derm	dermatology	SLE	systemic lupus erythematosus
HPV	human papillomavirus	Sub-Q	Subcutaneous
I&D	incision and drainage	ung	Ointment
ID	intradermal (injection)		

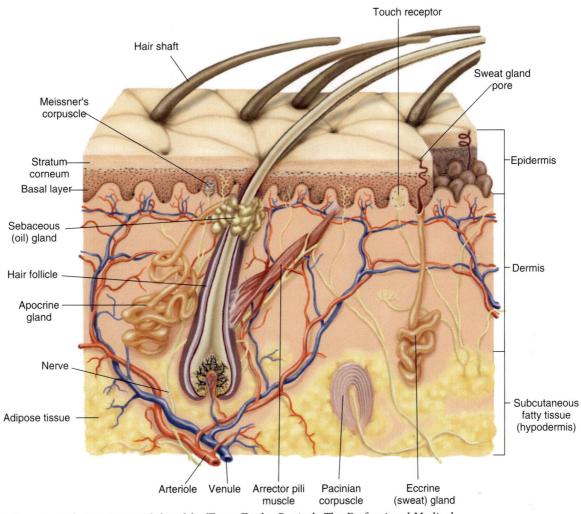

Touch receptor

Hair shaft

Meissner's corpuscle

Sweat gland pore

Stratum corneum

Basal layer

Epidermis

Sebaceous (oil) gland

Hair follicle

Apocrine gland

Dermis

Nerve

Adipose tissue

Subcutaneous fatty tissue (hypodermis)

Arteriole   Venule   Arrector pili muscle   Pacinian corpuscle   Eccrine (sweat) gland

FIGURE 5-1 Layers and structures of the skin (From Eagle, S, et al. *The Professional Medical Assistant: An Integrative Teamwork-Based Approach.* 2009. Philadelphia: F.A. Davis Company, with permission.)

Beneath the dermis is the subcutaneous layer, which contains fatty tissue as well as the deeper blood vessels, nerves, and hair follicles. It also contains elastin, for elasticity, and collagen, for strength. The subcutaneous layer provides insulation for deeper structures.

Accessory structures of the skin include the sudoriferous (sweat) glands, sebaceous (oil) glands, hair, and nails. Sebaceous glands are found at the base of hair follicles all over the body and secrete an oily substance called *sebum*. Sudoriferous glands are located throughout the body but are more concentrated in some areas, such as the soles of the feet and palms of the hands.

Functions of the Skin

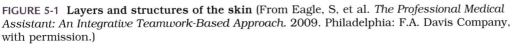

The skin and accessory structures serve important functions in the body, primarily protection and temperature regulation.

Protection

Skin protects the body from bacteria and other microorganisms, the damaging ultraviolet rays of the sun, and extreme temperatures. Because the outer layer of the skin is waterproof, it prevents organisms from entering even when it gets wet, unless there is a break in the skin. Sebaceous glands secrete an oily substance that inhibits bacterial growth and lubricates the skin to keep it soft and supple. If microorganisms gain entry through breaks in the skin, such as **lacerations** (cuts or tears in the flesh) or **abrasions** (areas where skin or mucous membranes are scraped away), an infection may occur. However, as the tissue becomes irritated, a natural inflammatory response occurs. This response triggers increased circulation in the injured area, which is responsible for the appearance of such signs as **edema** (swelling) and **erythema** (redness) that may indicate inflammation or injury. Additional leukocytes (white blood cells) arrive to fight off the invaders and act to engulf the bacteria. The increased circulation also helps speed the process of healing, as debris is cleared away and healthy new cells along with scar tissue fill in the injured area.

The skin also contains melanocytes, which are melanin-forming skin cells. In response to ultraviolet light from the sun, melanocytes secrete melanin, a brown pigment that helps filter ultraviolet light and protect the skin from further damage. These cells are responsible for browning of the skin known as a *suntan*. The amount of melanin in the skin varies depending on the individual's heredity and ethnicity.

Because skin contains a number of specialized nerves and sensory receptors, it plays a vital role in the ability to perceive cold, heat, pressure, and pain. The messages these nerves and receptors send signal the individual to take measures to increase physical comfort, such as putting on a coat for warmth. In addition, they provide an important protective function; if a person accidentally touches a hot surface, the heat and pain receptors immediately send a message to the central nervous system, and the person responds by pulling her hand away. Such a response is a protective reflex, which happens quickly and without conscious thought.

Two accessory structures of the integumentary system play a role in protecting the body. The hair of the head, eyebrows, eyelashes, nose, and ears protects the body by filtering out dust and debris from the air; and nails help protect the ends of the fingers and toes.

Temperature Regulation

The integumentary system also plays an important role in body-temperature regulation. It helps to insulate and maintain warmth when the external environment is too cold. As the environment becomes colder, the hands and fingers become pale in color because the blood vessels near the skin's surface constrict in order to give off less heat and conserve it for deeper organs. When the environment is too hot, these same blood vessels dilate (expand) in order to give off more heat. This response causes a flushed appearance. In addition, the sweat glands secrete sweat, which evaporates on the skin's surface and provides even more cooling.

Flashpoint
The skin provides insulation to keep us warm.

Common Integumentary System Diseases and Disorders

Some of the most common diseases and disorders of the integumentary system include bacterial infections; viral infections; fungal diseases; those caused by vectors, ticks, and parasites; hypersensitivity and inflammatory reactions; pigmentation disorders; and disorders associated with aging. Many disorders are identified by the type of lesion they produce on the skin (see Box 5-1).

Bacterial Skin Infections

A number of common skin disorders are caused by bacterial infection. These include impetigo, cellulitis, folliculitis, furuncles, carbuncles, and paronychia.

Impetigo
ICD-9-CM: 68   [ICD-10: L01.0 (any organism, any site)]
Impetigo is a highly contagious bacterial skin infection caused by group A streptococci or *Staphylococcus aureus*.

Incidence

Impetigo is most common in young children and accounts for 10% of all medical-clinic cases of children with skin problems. Males and females are affected equally. Impetigo is most prevalent in warm, humid environments and is rarely seen in northern states during the winter months.

Etiology

Impetigo is caused by group A streptococci or *S. aureus* on areas of skin with minor injuries such as scrapes and scratches. It is spread by direct contact with secretions from the lesions or items with secretions on them. It is quite contagious and commonly spreads through day-care centers and preschools, where children come into close contact with one another and share toys (see Box 5-2).

Flashpoint

Impetigo is one of the most common skin infections in children.

Box 5-1 Diagnostic Spotlight

COMMON SKIN LESIONS

This table lists some of the most common types of skin lesions, along with a pronunciation guide, definition, and an illustration for each.

Lesion	Definition	Example
Bulla BŬL-lă	large blister or vesicle filled with fluid	From Eagle, S, et al. *The Professional Medical Assistant: An Integrative Teamwork-Based Approach.* 2009. Philadelphia: F.A. Davis Company, with permission.
Fissure FĬSH-ūr	small, cracklike break in the skin	From Eagle, S, et al. *The Professional Medical Assistant: An Integrative Teamwork-Based Approach.* 2009. Philadelphia: F.A. Davis Company, with permission.

Continued

Box 5-1 Diagnostic Spotlight—cont'd

Lesion	Definition	Example
macule MĂK-ūl	flat, discolored spot on the skin, such as a freckle	
Nodule NŎD-ūl	small node	
Scales Skālz	areas of skin that are excessively dry and flaky	

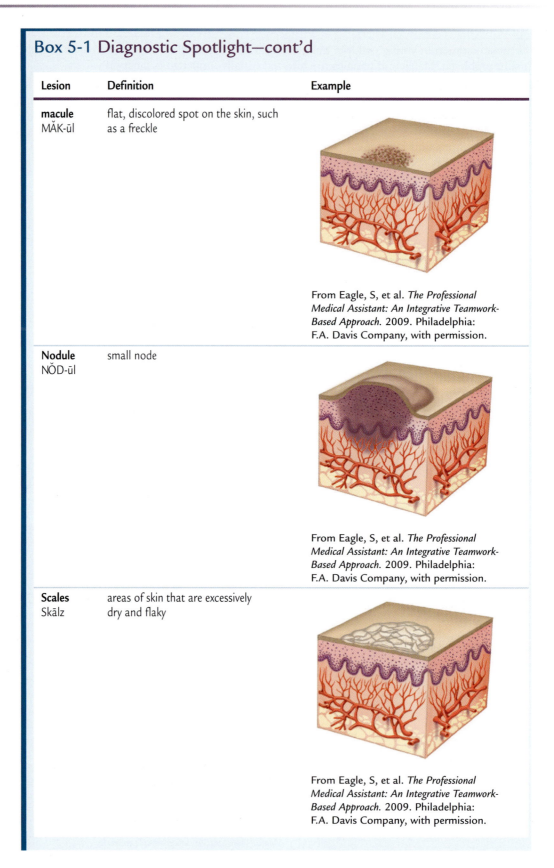

From Eagle, S, et al. *The Professional Medical Assistant: An Integrative Teamwork-Based Approach.* 2009. Philadelphia: F.A. Davis Company, with permission.

From Eagle, S, et al. *The Professional Medical Assistant: An Integrative Teamwork-Based Approach.* 2009. Philadelphia: F.A. Davis Company, with permission.

From Eagle, S, et al. *The Professional Medical Assistant: An Integrative Teamwork-Based Approach.* 2009. Philadelphia: F.A. Davis Company, with permission.

Box 5-1 Diagnostic Spotlight—cont'd

Lesion	Definition	Example
Papule PĂP-ūl	small raised spot or bump on the skin, such as a mole	 From Eagle, S, et al. *The Professional Medical Assistant: An Integrative Teamwork-Based Approach.* 2009. Philadelphia: F.A. Davis Company, with permission.
Pustule PŬS-tūl	small, pus-filled blister	 From Eagle, S, et al. *The Professional Medical Assistant: An Integrative Teamwork-Based Approach.* 2009. Philadelphia: F.A. Davis Company, with permission.
Ulcer ŬL-sĕr	lesion of the skin or mucous membranes marked by inflammation, necrosis, and sloughing of damaged tissues	 From Eagle, S, et al. *The Professional Medical Assistant: An Integrative Teamwork-Based Approach.* 2009. Philadelphia: F.A. Davis Company, with permission.

Continued

Box 5-1 Diagnostic Spotlight—cont'd

Lesion	Definition	Example
Vesicle VĚS-ĭ-kl	clear, fluid-filled blister	 From Eagle, S, et al. *The Professional Medical Assistant: An Integrative Teamwork-Based Approach.* 2009. Philadelphia: F.A. Davis Company, with permission.
Wheal Hwēl	rounded, temporary elevation in the skin that is white in the center with a red-pink periphery; accompanied by itching	 From Eagle, S, et al. *The Professional Medical Assistant: An Integrative Teamwork-Based Approach.* 2009. Philadelphia: F.A. Davis Company, with permission.

Box 5-2 Wellness Promotion

STOP THE SPREAD

Good hygiene is vital to preventing the spread of infection. Lesions that drain should be cleaned frequently. Wash your hands thoroughly after touching any skin lesion. Do not reuse or share washcloths or towels. Wash clothing, washcloths, towels, and sheets or other items that come in contact with infected areas in very hot (preferably boiling) water. Change dressings frequently and discard them in a manner that contains the drainage, such as placing them in a bag that can be closed tightly before discarding.

Signs and Symptoms

Impetigo appears as small, fluid-filled vesicles, usually around the mouth or nose. The vesicles quickly enlarge and rupture, excreting a yellow exudate, then crust over (see Fig. 5-2). Lesions are inflamed and moist, and they may itch.

Diagnosis

Diagnosis is usually based on medical history and physical-examination findings. Occasionally, culture and sensitivity testing may be done to identify the causative organism and determine the most appropriate antimicrobial medication (see Box 5-3).

Treatment

Topical antibiotic ointment is prescribed for small areas, and oral antibiotics are prescribed for widespread infection. To prevent spreading infection, patients and parents are instructed to wash hands frequently, avoid touching the lesions, and refrain from sharing drinking glasses, towels, or facecloths. Skin with lesions should be gently scrubbed daily with an antiseptic soap and covered lightly with a dressing. To help prevent the spread of impetigo, patients' fingernails should be short and clean.

Flashpoint
Impetigo is very contagious.

The health-care provider should be called if the lesions do not begin to heal within 3 days of treatment, if the skin around the rash becomes red, warm, and tender, or if fever develops.

Prognosis

Most cases of impetigo completely resolve with treatment. As the lesions heal, they appear red; however, permanent scarring is rare. Rarely, cellulitis and lymphadenitis (inflammation of local

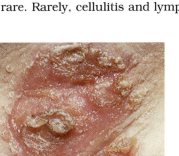

FIGURE 5-2 **Impetigo** (From Eagle, S, et al. *The Professional Medical Assistant: An Integrative Teamwork-Based Approach.* 2009. Philadelphia: F.A. Davis Company, with permission.)

Box 5-3 Diagnostic Spotlight

CULTURE AND SENSITIVITY TEST

The culture and sensitivity test has two parts. *Culturing* involves obtaining a specimen from the site of the suspected infection and propagating microorganisms in a special medium (broth, blood, gelatin, etc.) conducive to their growth. This step usually takes about 24 hours. Once grown, the microorganisms can be examined and identified. During *sensitivity* testing, the susceptibility of the microorganisms is determined by exposing them to various antimicrobial drugs. This step takes another 24 hours and identifies which antibiotics will most effectively kill the microorganisms. The information is then shared with the health-care provider so that the most effective antibiotic can be prescribed for the patient.

lymph nodes) occur, prolonging treatment. Acute poststreptococcal glomerulonephritis, a type of kidney infection, is a rare but serious complication.

Cellulitis

ICD-9-CM: 682.9   [ICD-10: L03.9 (unspecified site)]

Cellulitis is a potentially serious bacterial infection of the dermis and subcutaneous tissues.

Incidence

Cellulitis is a common type of skin infection occurring among all races. Facial cellulitis is more common among adults over age 50 and children ages 6 months to 3 years. Perianal (around the anus) cellulitis is more common among children.

Etiology

Cellulitis is usually caused when pathogenic microorganisms invade the skin through a local injury, such as a scrape or cut. The most commonly involved organisms are group A streptococci and *S. aureus*. Individuals at increased risk include those with weakened immune systems, diabetes, other systemic illness, or impaired peripheral circulation, and those using corticosteroid medication. A more serious type of cellulitis caused by resistant organisms such as methicillin-resistant *S. aureus* (MRSA) is becoming more common.

Flashpoint

MRSA infections are becoming all too common.

Signs and Symptoms

Symptoms of cellulitis include localized pain, erythema, edema, warmth, and fever (see Fig. 5-3). Red streaks may indicate spreading infection. The skin of the lower legs is commonly affected, although cellulitis can develop anywhere on the body.

Diagnosis

Diagnosis is usually based on physical-examination findings. In more complex cases, wound and blood cultures may be ordered to clearly identify the causative organism.

Treatment

Treatment includes administration of antibiotics and, for severe cases, surgery. The affected body part may be elevated to reduce edema. Analgesics may relieve discomfort.

Flashpoint

Untreated cellulitis can lead to septicemia.

Prognosis

Complications can include loss of localized tissue and septicemia (infection in the blood); however, with early diagnosis and appropriate treatment, most people recover fully.

Folliculitis

ICD-9-CM: 704.8   [ICD-10: L73.9]

Folliculitis is the inflammation of hair follicles, which can occur anywhere on the skin.

Incidence

The exact incidence of folliculitis is not known. However, it is very common.

Etiology

Folliculitis develops secondary to irritation caused by the friction of clothing rubbing on the skin or shaving, as well as from the blockage of follicles. Infection with *S. aureus* may follow. Chronic cases are sometimes associated with iron-deficiency anemia.

Flashpoint

Folliculitis commonly develops on the neck, axillae, and groin.

Signs and Symptoms

Folliculitis can occur anywhere on the skin but is especially common on the neck, axillae, and groin. Signs and symptoms vary with the specific type but generally include a rash with small red bumps, pustules, tenderness, and itching (see Fig. 5-4).

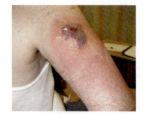

FIGURE 5-3 Cellulitis (From Barankin, B, and Freiman, A. *Derm Notes: Clinical Dermatology Pocket Guide.* 2006. Philadelphia: F.A. Davis Company, with permission.)

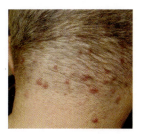

FIGURE 5-4 Folliculitis (From Barankin, B, and Freiman, A. *Derm Notes: Clinical Dermatology Pocket Guide.* 2006. Philadelphia: F.A. Davis Company, with permission.)

Diagnosis

Diagnosis is based on physical-examination findings and symptoms. Occasionally, a culture may be done to identify the infecting organism.

Treatment

Folliculitis can be prevented or minimized by reducing friction from clothing, avoiding shaving if possible, and keeping the skin clean and dry. Treatment includes the application of warm, moist compresses; topical or oral antibiotics; and antifungal medications.

Prognosis

Folliculitis generally responds well to treatment but has a tendency to recur. A potential complication is the spread of infection.

Furuncles and Carbuncles

ICD-9-CM: 680.0 (face), 680.1 (neck), 680.2 (trunk), 680.3 (upper arm and forearm), 680.4 (hand), 680.5 (buttock), 680.6 (leg), 680.7 (foot), 680.8 (other specified site), 680.9 (unspecified site)   **[ICD-10: L02.0 (face), L02.1 (neck), L02.2 (trunk), L02.3 (buttock), L02.4 (limb), L02.8 (other), L02.9 (unspecified)]**

A furuncle, sometimes called a *boil,* is an infection of a hair follicle and nearby tissue. It is more invasive than folliculitis because it involves the sebaceous gland. A carbuncle is a very large furuncle or a cluster of connected furuncles and is more invasive than a single furuncle.

Flashpoint
A carbuncle is a very large furuncle or a cluster of furuncles.

Incidence

The exact incidence of furuncles is unknown. However, they are thought to be quite common, since most people are troubled by them at least once during their lifetime. Carbuncles are rarer than furuncles. Both types of lesions may affect healthy young people, but they are much more common in the obese, the immunocompromised, and the elderly.

Etiology

Furuncles and carbuncles are usually caused by *S. aureus* or *Staphylococcus epidermidis,* which are commonly found on skin surfaces. However, they may also be caused by other bacteria or fungi. Minor injury to the skin or hair follicles, such as in bathing or shaving, permits these pathogens entry into deeper skin tissues. Those at greatest risk for furuncles and carbuncles are people with acne, poor hygiene, obesity, malnutrition, or diabetes. Also at risk are those living in hot, humid climates and patients who have weakened immune systems or are taking corticosteroid medications.

Flashpoint
Minor injury to the skin or hair follicles permits pathogens to enter and cause infection.

Signs and Symptoms

Furuncles begin as inflamed hair follicles that become infected. Localized itching is sometimes an early sign. The areas develop into red, warm, tender, pea-sized nodules filled with pus that may rupture and spontaneously drain foul-smelling fluid. They can develop anywhere on the body but are most common on the face, neck, axillae, back, stomach, shoulders, thighs, and buttocks. They are especially painful when located in the nose or ear canal.

Carbuncles are larger than furuncles, sometimes as large as a golf ball. They become reddened, tender, fluid-filled lumps just beneath the skin's surface and may develop white or yellow centers (see Fig. 5-5). They are commonly located on the neck, back, and thighs. They rarely resolve on their own and should be treated. When multiple furuncles form (sometimes referred to as *chronic furunculosis*), or carbuncles develop, the individual may become **febrile** (having a fever) and develop enlarged, tender lymph nodes nearby. The individual may also experience malaise and fatigue.

Diagnosis

Diagnosis of furuncles and carbuncles is based upon visual examination of the characteristic lesions. In some cases, fluid from the lesion is collected for culture and sensitivity testing.

Treatment

Furuncles are typically treated by the application of warm, moist compresses several times a day. This helps reduce pain and speeds the course of the lesion so that it will eventually rupture and drain. When this occurs, the area should be washed with warm water and soap and then bandaged. Magnesium sulfate paste may also be applied to the lesion to inhibit bacterial growth and dry the lesion. Carbuncles usually require surgical incision and drainage (I&D) for healing to occur. Individuals with severe or chronic conditions may be prescribed topical or oral antibiotics. If antibiotic-resistant pathogens are the cause, other agents may be necessary. Furuncles often recur and may be prevented by that application of topical solutions containing 2% to 3% chloroxylenol or chlorhexidine gluconate with isopropyl alcohol, or by a maintenance dose of antibiotics over 1 or 2 months.

Flashpoint

Furuncles are commonly treated with warm, moist compresses.

Prognosis

Prognosis is generally very good for individuals afflicted with furuncles or carbuncles if the lesions are treated appropriately. Furuncles often recur. Complications include permanent scar formation and the spread of infection to other parts of the body, such as the bones, heart, kidneys, brain, or blood. Meticulous hygiene can help reduce the risk of spread.

Paronychia

ICD-9-CM: 681.02 (finger), 681.11 (toe)   [ICD-10: L03.0 (finger or toe)]

Paronychia is an infection that occurs at the base or side of a finger or toenail.

Incidence

Paronychia is the most common type of hand infection, accounting for 35% of the total. It affects individuals of all ages, women three times as often than men. It occurs most commonly among individuals whose jobs require repetitive or prolonged immersion of their hands in water, including bartenders, bakers, and florists. Also at risk are those with weakened immune systems.

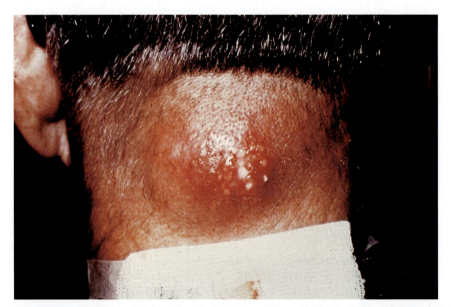

FIGURE 5-5 Carbuncle (From Goldsmith, LA, Lazarus, GS, and Tharp, MD. *Adult and Pediatric Dermatology: A Color Guide to Diagnosis and Treatment.* 1997. Philadelphia: F.A. Davis Company, with permission.)

Etiology

Paronychia develops when pathogens enter through an injury near the cuticle. Risk factors include nail-biting, overly aggressive manicuring, and participating in occupations that require frequently putting the hands in water (see Box 5-4).

Signs and Symptoms

The onset of paronychia may be gradual or sudden. Typical signs and symptoms include warmth, erythema, edema along one of the nail folds, accumulation of pus, and throbbing pain or tenderness (see Fig. 5-6). The nail becomes discolored and thickened.

Diagnosis

Diagnosis is usually based upon physical examination and history, but the health-care provider may test drainage from the site to identify the causative organism, especially in chronic cases.

Treatment

Acute infection is treated with warm-water soaks three or four times per day and antibiotic cream or oral antibiotics. Chronic forms may be caused by a fungal infection, for which antifungal medication is prescribed. The individual is encouraged to keep the nail clean and dry (other than during prescribed warm soaks) and to avoid manicures and any other activities that may further traumatize the nail. In either case, I&D may be done to drain abscesses so the site can heal properly.

Prognosis

With appropriate treatment, acute paronychia usually resolves within 10 days. A rare complication is osteomyelitis (serious infection in the bone and bone marrow). With proper treatment, chronic paronychia should heal within several weeks; however, it may recur unless the individual changes the activities that predisposed him or her to the condition in the first place. Potential complications include felon (infection of tissue within the fingertip) and septic tenosynovitis (infection of tendons and synovial tissues).

Flashpoint
People who bite their nails are at increased risk of paronychia.

Flashpoint
The patient with paronychia should avoid manicures and any other activity that traumatizes the nail.

Box 5-4 Wellness Promotion

BE KIND TO YOUR HANDS

Paronychia is usually associated with minor trauma to the hands, especially the fingernails. Here are some ways to avoid this disorder:

- Keep your hands clean and dry.
- Take care of your nails but avoid overly aggressive or frequent manicuring.
- Do not bite or chew your nails or the skin around them.
- Do not suck on your fingers.
- Wear gloves for prolonged or frequent contact with water or other liquids.
- Think twice about getting acrylic (fake) nails, especially if you are in health care. They may harbor infectious pathogens, increasing your risk of infection, and as a result, could put your patients at risk.

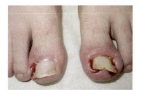

FIGURE 5-6 Paronychia (From Barankin, B, and Freiman, A. *Derm Notes: Clinical Dermatology Pocket Guide.* 2006. Philadelphia: F.A. Davis Company, with permission.)

Viral Skin Infections

Some skin conditions are caused by viruses. Among the most common are those caused by wart viruses and various herpes viruses.

Warts

ICD-9-CM: 078.10 (unspecified), 078.19 (genital)   [ICD-10: B07 (unspecified), A63.0 (anogenital)]

Warts are small, benign skin tumors caused by various strains of the human papillomavirus (HPV). There are many variations of warts, including verruca vulgaris (common warts—see Fig. 5-7), commonly found on the hands; venereal (genital) warts, which are sexually transmitted; and verruca plantaris (plantar warts), on the soles of the feet.

Incidence

Children and young adults most commonly get warts. People with weakened immune systems are especially vulnerable, such as those with AIDS or cancer or those taking chemotherapy or other immunosuppressive medications. Experts estimate that genital HPV infection is the most common type of sexually transmitted disease, with 5.5 million new cases reported yearly and at least 20 million people already infected.

Etiology

Warts are caused by more than 100 different strains of HPV and are contagious via direct contact.

Signs and Symptoms

The physical appearance of warts varies depending on the specific type of virus and the location involved. Warts may be tiny to medium-sized bumps or may have a cauliflower-type appearance. Genital warts may be obvious and extensive or subtle and only perceptible using a Papanicolaou (Pap) test, also called a *Pap smear.*

Diagnosis

Diagnosis is based on physical-examination findings or, in some cases of genital warts, the results of a Pap test.

Treatment

Treatment options include over-the-counter (OTC) topical medications such as salicylic acid and others. For greatest effect, warts should first be softened by soaking in warm water and

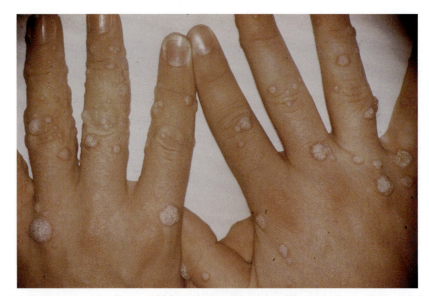

FIGURE 5-7 **Common warts** (From Goldsmith, LA, Lazarus, GS, and Tharp, MD. *Adult and Pediatric Dermatology: A Color Guide to Diagnosis and Treatment.* 1997. Philadelphia: F.A. Davis Company, with permission.)

then reduced by abrasion with a pumice stone, small scrub brush, or emery board. Before applying salicylic acid, the patient can protect the skin around the wart by applying petroleum jelly. Medication is absorbed better if warts are covered with an adhesive bandage or piece of tape after application. Treatment should be repeated daily for best results. If home treatment does not produce satisfactory results, patients may seek treatment from their health-care provider. A common treatment choice is cryotherapy (the use of cold to treat a medical condition), which involves the application of liquid nitrogen to freeze the wart and kill it (see Fig. 5-8). Repeated treatments may be needed. Other forms of treatment include the application of lactic acid or trichloroacetic acid.

Prognosis

Warts usually resolve spontaneously, but it may take weeks, months, or even years. Genital warts in women have been found to cause tissue changes that may result in the development of cervical cancer. This likely accounts for the growing incidence of cervical cancer among young women. Therefore, precautions to prevent transmission, such as use of condoms, should be stressed. Furthermore, women who are sexually active should be encouraged to have regular examinations and Pap tests.

Flashpoint

Genital warts in women can lead to cervical cancer.

Herpes Zoster
ICD-9-CM: 053.9   [ICD-10: B02.9] (without complications for both codes)

Outbreaks of herpes zoster, also called *shingles,* are caused by a reactivation of the varicella-zoster virus. After an initial outbreak of varicella (chickenpox), the varicella-zoster virus incorporates itself into nerve cells and lies dormant until it is reactivated years later.

Incidence

Between 600,000 and one million people develop shingles each year. About 50% of people who live to age 80 will have an outbreak at some time in their life. People at increased risk are those taking immunosuppressive medications and those with weakened immune systems, including elderly patients and those with AIDS, Hodgkin disease, or diabetes.

Flashpoint

Shingles are caused by a reactivation of the varicella-zoster virus.

Etiology

The active virus is present in the fluid from herpetic chickenpox and shingles lesions and may be spread to others through direct contact.

Signs and Symptoms

Symptoms of herpes zoster include unilateral (one-sided) distribution of herpetic vesicles along the affected **dermatome** (region of skin supplied by a single sensory nerve) (see Fig. 5-9). These vesicles usually develop on the trunk or, sometimes, the face or head. Lesions are described as acutely painful; they may burn or itch. Other symptoms may include fever, chills, headache, and malaise, depending on the dermatomes involved.

Diagnosis

Diagnosis is based upon the characteristic appearance and may be confirmed by culture of secretions. It may also be made based on the presence of antibodies in the blood.

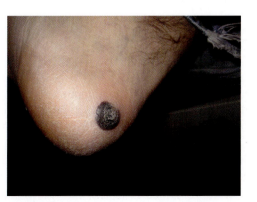

FIGURE 5-8 Black skin from blistering related to liquid-nitrogen treatment for warts (Courtesy of Dr. Benjamin Barankin.)

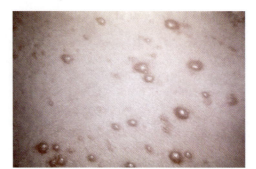

FIGURE 5-9 **Herpes zoster** (Photo courtesy of the Centers for Disease Control and Prevention and Dr. KL Hermann.)

Treatment
Treatment includes antiviral drugs, which reduce viral shedding as well as the severity and duration of the outbreak, if administered within 3 days of onset. Other medications may include corticosteroids, analgesics, and antipruritics.

Flashpoint

Postherpetic neuralgia is a potential complication of shingles.

Prognosis
Outbreaks can last from 10 days to 5 weeks. One potential complication is postherpetic neuralgia, which is continued nerve pain that persists for months after the lesions disappear. Fortunately, repeated outbreaks of shingles are uncommon.

Fungal Skin Disorders

Fungal skin disorders are a common complaint. Two of the most common types are the family of tinea infections, which are named for the various parts of the body affected, and candidiasis.

Tinea

ICD-9-CM: 110.0 (tinea capitis; tinea barbae), 110.1 (tinea unguium), 110.2 (manuum) (hand), 110.3 (tinea cruris), 110.4 (tinea pedis), 110.5 (tinea corporis), 110.9 (unspecified site)

[ICD-10: B35.0 (tinea capitis; tinea barbae), B35.1 (tinea unguium), B35.2 (manuum) (hand), B35.3 (tinea pedis), B35.4 (tinea corporis), B35.6 (tinea cruris), B35.9 (unspecified site)]

Tinea, also called *dermatophytosis* or *ringworm*, is a fungal skin infection on the body. Various forms include tinea capitis (scalp), tinea corporis (trunk), tinea cruris (genital area, also called *jock itch*), tinea barbae (mustache and beard), tinea pedis (feet, also called *athlete's foot*), and tinea unguium (nails).

Incidence
These types of infections are common. Tinea cruris is most common in adult men, and tinea corporis is especially common in children.

Etiology
Tinea is caused by a fungus and is, therefore, contagious. It is transmitted by direct contact or by touching infected items, such as shoes, combs, clothing, or shower or pool surfaces. It may also be contracted from pets; cats are common carriers. Tinea fungi thrive in warm, moist areas, and skin with a minor injury (such as a scratch or scrape) is more vulnerable.

Signs and Symptoms
Symptoms of tinea vary depending on the type and location. Most forms include red, raised, scaly, pruritic (itchy) lesions (see Figs. 5-10, 5-11, and 5-12). Patchy hair loss may be evident on the head or, in men, the face. The rash of tinea corporis has circular lesions. Tinea pedis causes the skin of the feet, especially between the toes, to crack, peel, flake, and redden. Patients may complain of itching, burning, and stinging. There may be blisters that break, ooze, and become

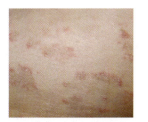

FIGURE 5-10 Tinea corporis (From Barankin, B, and Freiman, A. *Derm Notes: Clinical Dermatology Pocket Guide.* 2006. Philadelphia: F.A. Davis Company, with permission.)

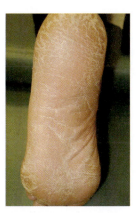

FIGURE 5-11 Tinea pedis (From Barankin, B, and Freiman, A. *Derm Notes: Clinical Dermatology Pocket Guide.* 2006. Philadelphia: F.A. Davis Company, with permission.)

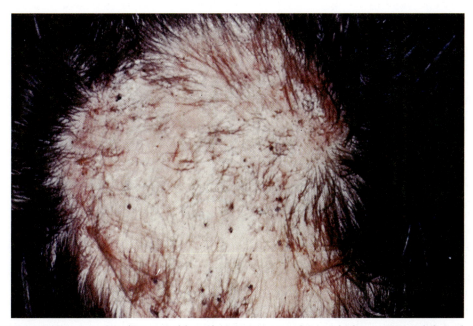

FIGURE 5-12 Tinea capitis (From Goldsmith, LA, Lazarus, GS, and Tharp, MD. *Adult and Pediatric Dermatology: A Color Guide to Diagnosis and Treatment.* 1997. Philadelphia: F.A. Davis Company, with permission.)

crusty. Nails affected with tinea unguium become discolored, thickened, and softened, and they sometimes crumble.

Diagnosis

Diagnosis is based on the appearance of lesions and the patient's description of symptoms. It is confirmed by a skin culture or **biopsy,** a procedure in which a representative sample of tissue is obtained for microscopic examination via surgery, syringe and needle, endoscopy, punch technique, or other means. Examination of the scraping under a blue light (Wood's lamp) in a dark room can also confirm the diagnosis (see Box 5-5).

Treatment

Treatment usually includes OTC or prescription antifungal creams or powders. Patients should be instructed to continue use for 2 weeks after symptoms have resolved, to keep infection from recurring. They should also be instructed to keep the affected skin clean and dry, wear clean cotton socks (for tinea pedis), and wash sheets and pajamas daily. Additionally, they should seek treatment for infected pets.

Prognosis

Tinea infections usually respond well to treatment within 3 to 5 weeks, although recurrence is possible. If the infection does not respond, evaluation by a health-care provider is recommended. There is a risk of a secondary bacterial infection, such as cellulitis, developing because of skin breakdown from scratching.

Candidiasis

| ICD-9-CM: 112.0 (oral thrush), 112.1 (vaginal yeast), 112.3 (skin and nails) | [ICD-10: B37.0 (oral trush), B37.2 (skin and nails), B37.3 (vaginal yeast)] |

Candidiasis, commonly called *yeast infection,* is an infection of the mucous membranes or skin caused by *Candida albicans,* which is part of the body's normal flora. It causes an infection when an overgrowth of the organism develops in warm, moist areas such as the mouth, vagina, nails, or skin folds.

Incidence

The exact incidence of candidiasis is unknown, but candidal infections of various types are known to be extremely common.

Etiology

Candidiasis develops when the composition of the body's normal flora is disrupted, usually due to antibiotic therapy, or when the normal immune defenses are weakened by corticosteroid therapy, chemotherapy, or an immune-disorder such as AIDS. Risk factors for candidiasis include diabetes mellitus and pregnancy.

Signs and Symptoms

Symptoms vary depending on the location of the infection. Oral candidiasis, commonly called *thrush,* causes raised, white patches on the oral mucous membranes and tongue, with an underlying inflammation (see Fig. 5-13). Candidiasis within skin folds causes a reddened, pruritic rash (see Fig. 5-14). Vaginal infections cause a thick, cheesy discharge and pruritis.

Box 5-5 Diagnostic Spotlight

WOOD'S LAMP EXAMINATION

A Wood's lamp or Wood's light is a device that uses blue rays to detect fluorescent materials in the skin and hair. These materials are present in certain disease states and will often appear pink under the light. During the examination, the patient is seated in a chair or positioned on an examination table in a dark room. The health-care provider turns on the lamp and holds it approximately 4 inches from the patient while examining the area of skin in question. This test is useful for identifying certain types of fungal and bacterial infection.

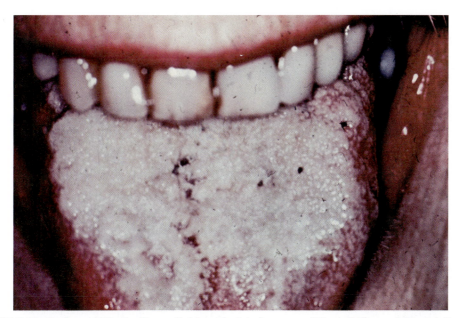

FIGURE 5-13 Oral candidiasis (From Goldsmith, LA, Lazarus, GS, and Tharp, MD. *Adult and Pediatric Dermatology: A Color Guide to Diagnosis and Treatment.* 1997. Philadelphia: F.A. Davis Company, with permission.)

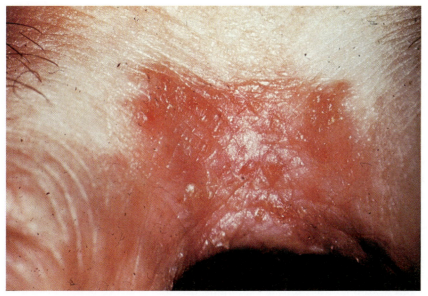

FIGURE 5-14 Candidiasis infection on the skin (From Goldsmith, LA, Lazarus, GS, and Tharp, MD. *Adult and Pediatric Dermatology: A Color Guide to Diagnosis and Treatment.* 1997. Philadelphia: F.A. Davis Company, with permission.)

Diagnosis

Diagnosis is based upon physical examination, the patient's description of symptoms, and occasionally microscopic examination of skin scrapings or vaginal discharge.

Treatment

Most forms of candidiasis respond to systemic antifungal medication. Oral infections may also be treated with antifungal throat lozenges or an oral solution that is swished in the mouth and then swallowed. Antifungal creams or ointments are sometimes applied topically to affected skin folds, and vaginal suppositories may be used for vaginal infections.

Prognosis

Prognosis for most forms of candidiasis is good. Immunocompromised individuals who develop systemic fungal infections may be vulnerable to septicemia, which can be life threatening if septic shock develops.

Skin Diseases and Disorders Caused by Vectors, Ticks, and Parasites

A number of diseases are caused by vectors, ticks, and parasites. A vector is an organism such as a mosquito that transmits infection from one host to another. Parasites are organisms that must live off a host in order to thrive. Some, such as intestinal parasites, must live inside the host; others, like mites and lice, live on or just beneath the host's surface. Some confusion exists between disorders caused by mite and lice, but both cause infestation, are very contagious, and cause itching.

Pediculosis

> ICD-9-CM: 132.0 (Pediculus humanus capitis), 132.1 (P. humanus corporis), 132.2 (*Phthirus pubis*), 132.9 (Infestation unspecified)
>
> [ICD-10: B85.0 (Pediculus humanus capitis, B85.1 (P. humanus corporis), B85.2 (Infestation unspecified), B85.3 (*Phthirus pubis*)]

Pediculosis is the term used to refer to infestation with a species of louse. There are three species: the head louse, body louse, and pubic louse. Head lice and body lice are very similar in appearance and differ primarily in habitat. Nits (eggs) are tiny, yellow-white, and oval in shape. Head and pubic lice attach the nits firmly to the side of the hair shaft near the skin; the nits cannot be transmitted to others. It takes 7 to 10 days for eggs to hatch and then another 7 to 10 days for the new females to mature and begin laying their own eggs. Adult lice—reddish-brown, wingless crawling insects that cannot jump or fly—are about the size of a sesame seed. They are rarely found on pets. They feed on human blood and usually live for about 30 days, but can only live for 1 to 2 days away from the host. Head lice are common and primarily affect the scalp and, infrequently, the eyebrows and eyelashes. Body lice are found on the body and attach their eggs to the inside of clothing, usually along seam lines. Pubic lice are found primarily in the pubic and perianal areas.

Incidence

Head lice are currently considered the most common human parasitic infestation in children in the United States and Europe. Preschool and elementary-school children are mostly commonly affected, girls more commonly than boys. Pubic lice, also called crab lice, are a common infestation transmitted by sexual contact. Body lice are much less common than the other types.

Flashpoint

Head lice are the most common parasitic infestation in American children.

Etiology

Head lice are transmitted via direct contact with the infested person's head or with personal items such as scarves, hats, coats, brushes, combs, and towels (see Box 5-6). Personal hygiene and cleanliness in the home are not factors. Pubic lice are transmitted through sexual contact and occasionally through sharing personal items like undergarments.

Signs and Symptoms

Signs of all types of pediculosis include the appearance of lice on the body and their eggs (nits) attached to hair shafts (see Fig. 5-15). Symptoms include itching and sores on the scalp from scratching, as well as the sensation of something crawling on the skin.

Diagnosis

Diagnosis is made by careful examination of the hair and scalp for nits or lice.

Treatment

Treatment includes manually ridding the body of parasites, controlling itching, and disinfecting the home environment. Medication and treatment recommendations are modified frequently; the latest can be found at http://www.headlice.org.

Box 5-6 Wellness Promotion

DON'T SHARE LICE

Lice can be easily spread from one person to another in situations where people are in close contact or are sharing personal items. To stop the spread, follow these steps:

- Do not assume that only a certain type of person gets head or body lice. Anyone can get them and can spread them to others.
- Do not share combs or brushes.
- Do not share hats, scarves, safety helmets, or other articles of clothing.
- Examine your children's heads regularly, especially if they attend day care or school.
- Immediately treat everyone in the household when anyone in the household has lice.

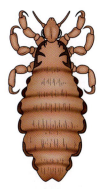 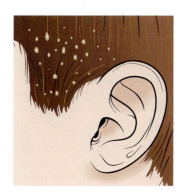

Head louse   **Louse eggs (nits) in hair**

FIGURE 5-15 *Pediculus humanus capitis* (head louse)

Prognosis

Prognosis is good with adequate treatment, although reinfestation is possible.

Scabies

ICD-9-CM: 133.0 (scabies),   **[ICD-10: B86 (scabies)]**
133.9 (acariasis, unspecified)

Scabies is a common, contagious condition in which the skin is infested with microscopic mites. It is one of the most common types of human parasitic-insect infestations.

Incidence

Scabies is common worldwide and crosses all social classes and races.

Etiology

Scabies is caused by the human itch mite, *Sarcoptes scabiei*, which is a wingless parasitic insect. Scabies is very contagious and spreads quickly in crowded conditions where people have close contact. It is spread through direct contact with an infected person or through sharing personal items such as clothing or bed linens. The mites live on human skin, survive on human blood, and lay their nits on human hair.

Flashpoint
Scabies spreads quickly in crowded conditions.

Signs and Symptoms

The rash caused by scabies is intensely pruritic and is made up of scaly papules, insect burrows, and secondary infected lesions (see Fig. 5-16). It is most prevalent in skin folds at the wrists and elbows, between the fingers, under the arms, in the groin, and under the beltline. The scalp, palms of the hands, and soles of the feet may also be affected. Itching is usually worse at night.

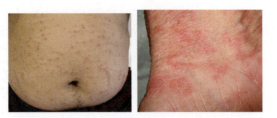

FIGURE 5-16 **Scabies** (From Barankin, B, and Freiman, A. *Derm Notes: Clinical Dermatology Pocket Guide.* 2006. Philadelphia: F.A. Davis Company, with permission.)

Diagnosis

Scabies must be differentiated from other skin conditions such as folliculitis, dermatitis, and impetigo. It may be identified by the characteristic rash. The most common diagnostic test involves scraping the lesion and examining the tissue microscopically for the presence of mites or eggs. An ink test may also be used, in which blue or black ink is applied and then cleaned off. Some of the ink absorbs into the mite burrows, thus revealing them.

Treatment

Traditional treatment of scabies involved the application of products containing lindane; however, its use is no longer advised, due to potentially serious adverse effects. A safer alternative is a topical 5% permethrin cream. Application should be repeated in 7 to 10 days when the nits hatch. Other individuals who live in the same household should be treated as well. The home environment should be disinfected as extensively as possible by washing or vacuuming surfaces and washing linens, towels, and clothing in hot water. Pesticide sprays should not be used.

Prognosis

Flashpoint

Scabies reinfestation may occur if the home and personal belongings are not adequately cleaned.

Prognosis is good with adequate treatment. Itching may persist for several weeks after treatment. Reinfestation is possible if the home and personal belongings are not cleaned adequately.

Lyme Disease
ICD-9-CM: 088.81   [ICD-10: A69.2]

Lyme disease is a bacterial infection transmitted by ticks.

Incidence

Lyme disease makes up 90% of infections in the United States transmitted by vectors: between 1980 and 2005, nearly 270,000 cases were reported in the United States. However, the actual incidence is estimated to be much higher.

Etiology

Lyme disease is caused by the bacterium *Borrelia burgdorferi.* It is carried by ticks (most commonly deer ticks) that attach to a host such as a deer, bird, mouse, dog, cat, horse, or human to feed on its blood. When this occurs, the tick may transmit the infection to the host.

Signs and Symptoms

The majority of individuals with Lyme disease develop the erythema migrans rash within 30 days of being bitten. It is usually a circular rash that slowly enlarges (see Fig. 5-17). The center of the rash tends to clear as the rash enlarges, emphasizing the circular appearance. The rash may subsequently appear on other parts of the body. On dark-skinned individuals the rash may resemble a bruise. Other signs and symptoms include headache, stiff neck, fever, fatigue, chills, swollen lymph nodes, and muscle aches.

If the disease is not treated early, it may disseminate (spread widely) and affect nearly every body system. General symptoms include severe fatigue and muscle pain. Neurological symptoms may include weakness, paralysis, tingling, memory deficits, confusion, severe headache, visual deficits, stroke, meningitis, and numerous others. Emotional and psychiatric symptoms may include agitation, paranoia, hallucinations, and others. Impact on the cardiovascular system may result in irregular heart rhythm, inflammation of heart muscle, and chest pain. Musculoskeletal symptoms include pain, muscle cramps, and loss of muscle tone. The effect on the lungs may be dyspnea (difficulty breathing) and pneumonia. Gastrointestinal symptoms may include anorexia, nausea, vomiting, and diarrhea. Pregnant women may experience premature delivery, miscarriage, or stillbirth.

Flashpoint

Lyme disease can have a profound impact on multiple body systems.

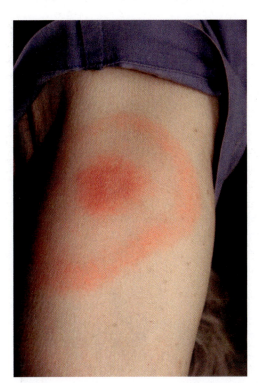

FIGURE 5-17 Lyme disease (Courtesy of the Centers for Disease Control and Prevention and James Gathany.)

Diagnosis

There is no definitive test to diagnose Lyme disease. Therefore, diagnosis is based upon history, physical-examination findings, and presenting signs and symptoms. Testing is done in an attempt to rule out other disorders and to identify Lyme Disease antibodies.

Treatment

Treatment of early disease includes oral antibiotics; disease that has progressed must be treated with intravenous antibiotics. Medication may be given to relieve fever, inflammation, and discomfort. Bedrest may be necessary until the more severe symptoms have resolved.

Prognosis

Prognosis is very good with early identification and treatment. More advanced disease may result in arthritis and chronic neurological symptoms that last for months or even years.

Hypersensitivity and Inflammatory Reactions

Hypersensitivity skin disorders are common, especially in people who suffer from other forms of allergies. Among the most common are eczema and psoriasis.

Urticaria

ICD-9-CM: 708 (general), 708.0 (allergic urticaria), 708.1 (idiopathic urticaria), 708.2 (urticaria due to cold and heat), 708.3 (dermatographic urticaria), 708.4 (vibratory urticaria), 708.5 (cholinergic urticaria), 708.8 (other specified urticaria), 708.9 (unspecified) [ICD-10: L50 (general), L50.0 (allergic urticaria), L50.1 (idiopathic urticaria), L50.2 (urticaria due to cold and heat), L50.3 (dermatographic urticaria), L50.4 (vibratory urticaria), L50.5 (cholinergic urticaria), L50.8 (other specified urticaria), L50.9 (unspecified)]

Urticaria is a skin reaction that includes erythema and extremely pruritic wheals (multiple swollen, raised areas, also called *hives*). It is not actually a disorder in itself, but rather a symptom caused by a severe allergic reaction.

Eczema

ICD-9-CM: 690 (general code for seborrheic dermatitis), 691 (general code for atopic dermatitis), 692 (general code for contact dermatitis); refer to diagnosis for specific code

[ICD-10: L21 (general code for seborrheic dermatitis), L21 (general code for atopic dermatitis), L23 (general code for contact dermatitis); refer to diagnosis for specific code]

Eczema, also known as *dermatitis*, is a general term for a group of conditions that affect people of all ages. The most common type is atopic eczema, which comes from a genetic predisposition; it is associated with asthma and hay fever, and it runs in families.

Flashpoint

Eczema is associated with asthma and hay fever.

Incidence

Eczema is fairly common, affecting 10% to 20% of the general population. It is more common among infants and children and may be acute or chronic.

Etiology

Causes of eczema include allergies, chemicals, scratching the skin, emotional stress, illness, and sun exposure. It is not contagious.

Signs and Symptoms

The appearance and symptoms of the rash vary with the severity and type of eczema and the causative agent. The skin may be hot, dry, and pruritic. In more severe forms it may be red, swollen, cracked, weeping, scaly, and pruritic, and it may even bleed (see Fig. 5-18).

Diagnosis

There is no specific diagnostic test for eczema. Diagnosis is based on medical history, patient symptoms, and physical-examination findings.

Treatment

At present, there is no cure for eczema; however, many children will be free of symptoms by the time they are in their teens. There are a number of treatment options, including the application of aluminum acetate astringent (Burow's solution), which is used in dermatology as a drying agent for weeping skin lesions. Other medications include corticosteroids, emollients, antihistamines, and injections. Known allergens—any substance that causes a hypersensitivity reaction or abnormal immune response—should be avoided. Clothing made from soft-textured cotton is recommended and should be laundered in mild detergent. Keeping room temperatures below 72°F and using room humidifiers may help.

Prognosis

Sensitivity to specific allergens may never disappear entirely, but flare-ups can be minimized and symptoms controlled.

Rosacea

ICD-9-CM: 695.3   [ICD-10: L71.9] (unspecified for both codes)

Rosacea is a chronic skin condition that causes flushing and redness on the face, neck, and chest. It is often mistaken for acne, skin allergies, or eczema.

Incidence

Rosacea is estimated to affect more than 14 million Americans. It affects individuals between the ages of 30 and 60, three-fourths of them female. Individuals with lighter complexions have a higher incidence.

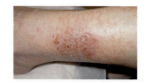

FIGURE 5-18 Eczema (From Barankin, B, and Freiman, A. *Derm Notes: Clinical Dermatology Pocket Guide.* 2006. Philadelphia: F.A. Davis Company, with permission.)

Etiology

The exact cause of rosacea is not fully understood. It is not infectious; rather, it is thought to be due to a combination of heredity and environmental factors. Alcohol use does not cause it but may worsen it. Other factors that may worsen symptoms include hot or spicy foods and beverages, medications that dilate blood vessels, corticosteroids, sunlight, hot baths or saunas, vigorous exercise, and emotions such as anger or embarrassment.

Signs and Symptoms

Four subtypes of rosacea have been identified. Substype 1 is erythematotelangiectatic rosacea, which begins with the tendency to blush noticeably progressing to persistent facial redness, especially on the nose. Subtype 2 is papulopustular rosacea, in which signs and symptoms worsen. *Telangiectasia* develops, which is the appearance of dilated vessels on the skin of the cheeks and nose (see Fig. 5-19). Bumps and pimples may come and go. Subtype 3 is phymatous, in which sebaceous glands slowly enlarge, causing **rhinophyma** (large, irregularly shaped, dark-red nose). This is most common in men. Subtype 4 is ocular rosacea, which causes conjunctivitis, an uncomfortable inflammation of the eyes resulting in a dry, gritty, burning sensation as well as itching.

Diagnosis

Rosacea is sometimes misidentified as other disorders, such as acne. However, it does not cause the typical whiteheads or blackheads associated with acne. The physician will identify rosacea through physical examination and a careful history, noting which factors improve and especially which factors worsen it. In particular, identification of the associated rosacea eye symptoms (ocular rosacea) will help to confirm diagnosis.

Flashpoint
Rosacea sometimes causes rhinophyma, a large, irregularly shaped, dark-red nose.

Treatment

There is no cure for rosacea. Unfortunately, it is often mistaken for acne, causing individuals to waste time using OTC acne remedies which may actually worsen their condition. However, appropriate treatment can help to relieve signs and symptoms and improve appearance. The physician may recommend specific types of skin-care products, including sunscreens, moisturizers, and cleansers. Medications may include topical or oral antibiotics as well as medication to reduce inflammation. In severe cases, isotretinoin may be prescribed to reduce oil production by sebaceous glands. Treatments to reduce the appearance of rhinophyma include electrosurgery and laser surgery.

Prognosis

Rosacea worsens over time if left untreated, although symptoms tend to be cyclic, with periods of worsening and improvement. Because it affects appearance, it tends to have a negative impact on the individual's self esteem. With treatment, individuals generally notice improvement within 2 months; since rosacea is a chronic disorder, treatment may need to be ongoing. Those who use isotretinoin must be monitored by a dermatologist because of the potential for serious side effects, including severe birth defects in children if used by pregnant women. It may also increase levels of cholesterol, triglycerides, and liver enzymes.

Acne Vulgaris

ICD-9-CM: 706.1   [ICD-10: L70.0]

Acne is the term used to describe a disease of the pilosebaceous units (PSUs) in the skin. PSUs include sebaceous (oil) glands and hair follicles.

Incidence

Acne is most common among teenagers of all races and ethnicities but may affect adults as well. It develops most commonly where large numbers of sebaceous glands are located, such as on the face, back, and chest.

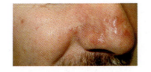

FIGURE 5-19 Telangiectasia associated with rosacea (From Barankin, B, and Freiman, A. *Derm Notes: Clinical Dermatology Pocket Guide*. 2006. Philadelphia: F.A. Davis Company, with permission.)

Etiology

The exact cause of acne is unclear; however, the PSUs apparently become plugged and develop into *comedones,* which are small skin lesions of acne such as whiteheads and blackheads. Contributing factors include hormonal influences, genetics, and the use of some medications or oily cosmetics. Exacerbations may be related to hormonal factors, exposure to oily environments, pollution, humidity, and stress. As infection sets in, the comedones become pustules that can further develop into nodules and cysts.

Signs and Symptoms

Acne manifests as plugged pores, pimples, cysts, and nodules on the face, neck, chest, back, and other areas (see Fig. 5-20).

Diagnosis

Diagnosis is based upon clinical presentation and symptoms.

Treatment

Most young people can adequately manage their skin problems with OTC topical preparations such as benzoyl peroxide, resorcinol, salicylic acid, and sulfur. However, over 40% of acne sufferers develop skin problems severe enough to seek medical care. Prescription medication may be needed for severe cases, including antibiotics, vitamin A derivatives, and others. Some medications, such as isotretinoin, are known teratogens (substances which cause defects in the fetus); use by pregnant women should be avoided. Oral contraceptives or low-dose corticosteroids may be useful for women in whom the cause is excess androgens (male hormones).

Patients must be encouraged to have realistic expectations of treatment, as people respond differently. It commonly takes 6 to 8 weeks for a full response. Acne scars may be removed or minimized by *dermabrasion,* a process in which a plastic surgeon or dermatologist scrapes away the outermost layer of skin using a wire brush or burr impregnated with diamond particles.

Flashpoint

Acne scars can be removed or minimized by dermabrasion.

Prognosis

Acne is not life-threatening, but it may cause disfigurement and permanent scarring that could embarrass the individual. Procedures such as dermabrasion can significantly improve appearance.

Psoriasis

ICD-9-CM: 696   **[ICD-10: L40] (general code for both codes; refer to diagnosis for specific code)**

Psoriasis is a chronic inflammatory skin disorder characterized by the development of red, scaly plaques.

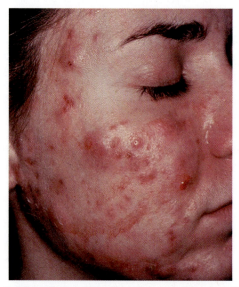

FIGURE 5-20 Acne (From Goldsmith, LA, Lazarus, GS, and Tharp, MD. *Adult and Pediatric Dermatology: A Color Guide to Diagnosis and Treatment.* 1997. Philadelphia: F.A. Davis Company, with permission.)

Incidence

Psoriasis affects 1% to 3% of the world's population and approximately 4.5 million people in the United States. It affects men and women equally and is more common in whites. Age of onset is usually between 15 and 35 years, although it can develop at any age.

Etiology

The specific cause of psoriasis is unknown, although it is thought to be autoimmune (due to a failure of the body to recognize its own tissues as self) in nature. Contributing factors include stress, family history, skin trauma, cold weather, infections, and some medications. It is not contagious.

Signs and Symptoms

The appearance of psoriasis varies with the specific type. The typical presentation of psoriasis includes silvery-white, scaly plaques or patches with reddened skin beneath and sharply defined borders (see Fig. 5-21). Lesions may crack and bleed. They are commonly found on the knees, shins, elbows, buttocks, lower back, ears, and along the hairline; however, the total body surface may be involved in some cases. There is a pattern of exacerbations and remissions, but flare-ups can last for years. Many patients report that psoriasis has a significant impact on their quality of life, affecting clothing choice (to cover lesions), quality of sleep, and self-esteem. Symptoms include itching and pain.

Diagnosis

Diagnosis of psoriasis is based on history, physical-examination findings, and the patient's description of symptoms. Biopsy may be done when typical lesions and scales are not obvious.

Flashpoint

Psoriasis usually causes silvery-white, scaly patches over reddened skin.

Treatment

Treatments for psoriasis include topical corticosteroids, vitamin D, coal-tar derivatives, retinoids, and ultraviolet-light exposure. Relatively new drugs on the market, known as *biologics,* have been approved for the treatment of psoriasis. The term *biologics* refers to a variety of medicinal products derived from natural sources or produced by biotechnology. In addition to using prescribed medications, patients are encouraged to maintain self-care, which includes preventing skin trauma and avoiding known triggers. There is no cure for psoriasis. However, the disorder can be managed by avoiding triggers and using approved treatments and medications.

Prognosis

Approximately 10% to 30% of individuals with psoriasis develop a related form of arthritis known as psoriatic arthritis.

Pigmentation Disorders

Pigmentation disorders usually do not have a serious physical effect on the individual. However, they do affect physical appearance and may therefore impact self-esteem and self confidence. Common pigmentation disorders include melasma, vitiligo, seborrheic keratosis, and actinic keratosis.

Melasma

ICD-9-CM: 709.09   [ICD-10: L81.1]

Melasma, also called *chloasma* or the *mask of pregnancy,* is the development of patches of dark skin on the face.

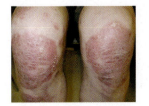

FIGURE 5-21 Psoriasis (From Barankin, B., and Freiman, A. *Derm Notes: Clinical Dermatology Pocket Guide.* 2006. Philadelphia: F.A. Davis Company, with permission.)

Incidence

Melasma is common and can occur in anyone, but it is most common in women who are pregnant or taking hormones. It is also common on the forearms of those of Native American descent and on the face of those of German or Russian Jewish descent. Individuals who live in tropical areas with intense sun exposure are most susceptible.

Etiology

Melasma develops when melanocytes (skin-pigment cells) are stimulated by the female hormones estrogen and progesterone. Less commonly, it can also be caused by thyroid disease, liver disease, or allergic reactions to cosmetics or medication.

Flashpoint

Melasma is most common in women who are pregnant or taking hormones.

Signs and Symptoms

Individuals with melasma gradually develop irregular areas of darker-pigmented skin on the forehead, nose, cheeks, and upper lip (see Fig. 5-22). Distribution is usually symmetrical. There are no other signs or symptoms.

Diagnosis

Melasma is diagnosed based upon the appearance of the skin. Occasionally the skin may be examined with a Wood's lamp, which reveals excess melanin in the epidermis as opposed to the dermis.

Treatment

When hormones are the causative factor, the skin discoloration generally resolves within several months after hormones are discontinued. If pregnancy is the cause, the skin changes resolve within several months of delivery. Depigmenting agents, facial peels, and laser treatment may be used to hasten the process. Cosmetics can also be used to lessen the appearance of melasma and even out skin color.

Prognosis

Melasma causes no physical deficits but can impact self-image and self-esteem. It often fades with time and does not require treatment unless the individual's appearance is a cause of distress.

Vitiligo
ICD-9-CM: 709.01   [ICD-10: L80]

Vitiligo is a chronic skin disease that results in patchy loss of skin pigment.

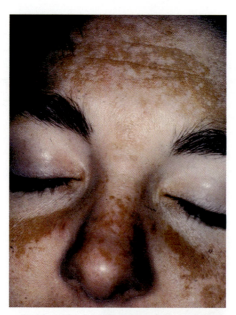

FIGURE 5-22 Melasma (From Goldsmith, LA, Lazarus, GS, and Tharp, MD. *Adult and Pediatric Dermatology: A Color Guide to Diagnosis and Treatment.* 1997. Philadelphia: F.A. Davis Company, with permission.)

Incidence

The global incidence of vitiligo is estimated at 1% to 2%. Approximately one to two million Americans have the disorder. It affects individuals of all races, men and women equally.

Etiology

Vitiligo develops when melanocytes die or become inactive. Why this happens is not fully understood; a combination of genetic, environmental, and autoimmune factors is suspected. Vitiligo has also been associated in some cases with Addison disease (chronic adrenal insufficiency) and autoimmune thyroid disease (thyroid dysfunction caused by an autoimmune response).

Signs and Symptoms

Individuals with vitiligo typically develop symmetrical areas of depigmented, pale skin on the extremities, face, and neck (see Fig. 5-23). Onset is usually in young adulthood, before the age of 20. The condition progresses gradually and may affect hair color, causing white patches or streaks. Additionally, individuals may develop brown or purple patches around the eyes or on mucous membranes. Because of the lack of pigmentation, individuals with vitiligo are especially sensitive to the sun.

Flashpoint
People with vitiligo are very sensitive to the sun.

Diagnosis

Diagnosis of vitiligo is based upon the characteristic appearance of the light, pigment-free patches of skin.

Treatment

Many individuals choose to do nothing about their vitiligo. Those who are troubled by their appearance can avoid the sun to minimize tanning, which accentuates the pale patches, or they can use cosmetics to hide the light areas. Those looking for a longer-term solution may be interested in trying immunomodulating creams, which may stimulate repigmentation of the skin when combined with UVB light therapy. Others may opt for chemical depigmentation of their darker skin, which is irreversible.

Prognosis

Prognosis for vitiligo is quite good, since the condition has little impact on physical health other than making individuals more vulnerable to sunburn and possibly skin cancer. However, some individuals find their appearance to be cause for embarrassment, which decreases self-esteem and contributes to depression.

Skin Disorders Associated With Aging

Skin changes create some of the most visible signs of aging. These changes are accelerated by environmental exposure to pollution and the sun's ultraviolet rays. Skin cells reproduce more slowly, causing the skin to thin and become more vulnerable to tearing and other types of injury. Once injured, the elderly person's skin is slower to heal, especially if the individual also suffers circulatory or immune-system impairment. The skin loses moisture, elasticity, and strength due to changes in elastin fibers, which provide elasticity, and collagen fibers, which provide strength. Lesions

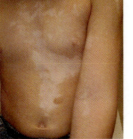

FIGURE 5-23 **Vitiligo** (From Barankin, B, and Freiman, A. *Derm Notes: Clinical Dermatology Pocket Guide.* 2006. Philadelphia: F.A. Davis Company, with permission.)

commonly called "age spots" develop due to changes in pigmentation. A variety of other changes may develop as well; among the most common are seborrheic keratosis and actinic keratosis.

Seborrheic Keratosis

ICD-9-CM: 702.1   [ICD-10: L82]

Seborrheic keratosis causes benign (noncancerous) skin growths of various shapes and sizes.

Incidence

Seborrheic keratosis is extremely common and is present in most people over the age of 65. Additionally, up to 25% of adults below the age of 65 are affected.

Etiology

The cause of seborrheic keratosis is not known. The condition most commonly develops after the age of 40. Lesions originate in the epidermis.

Signs and Symptoms

Seborrheic keratosis lesions are often described as having a "stuck-on" appearance and loose edges. Their surfaces are often flat yet irregular, with an oval shape and somewhat warty, waxy appearance; they may alternatively be smooth with tiny bumps (see Fig. 5-24). They come in a variety of colors, including black, brown, and yellow. They tend to appear in large numbers, often on the chest, face, back, and shoulders, as well as other areas of the body. The lesions often itch and may create a cosmetic appearance that is unacceptable to the individual.

Diagnosis

Diagnosis is made based upon the appearance of the lesions. A biopsy may be used to confirm diagnosis, especially if malignant melanoma is a concern.

Treatment

Unless the lesions are troubling to the individual, no treatment is needed, since this condition is benign and is not related to the wart viruses. However, if the lesions itch or the individual finds their appearance distressing, they may be removed: the health-care provider may apply liquid

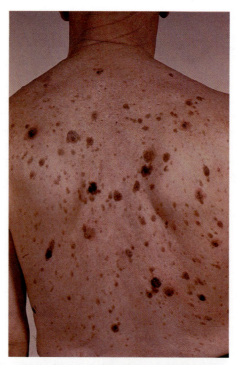

FIGURE 5-24 **Seborrheic keratosis** (From Goldsmith, LA, Lazarus, GS, and Tharp, MD. *Adult and Pediatric Dermatology: A Color Guide to Diagnosis and Treatment.* 1997. Philadelphia: F.A. Davis Company, with permission.)

nitrogen or may "shave" them off and then treat the underlying tissue with silver nitrate or aluminum chloride to stop bleeding.

Prognosis

Prognosis is excellent with or without treatment, since the lesions are not cancerous. Early lesions may sometimes be difficult to distinguish from melanoma, a dangerous form of skin cancer; therefore, individuals should see their health-care provider if they have any concerning lesions. Once removed, growths do not return; however, they may appear in other areas.

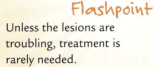

Flashpoint

Unless the lesions are troubling, treatment is rarely needed.

Actinic Keratosis

ICD-9-CM: 702.0   [ICD-10: L57.0]

Actinic keratosis, also known as *solar keratosis,* is a condition in which rough, scaly patches of skin develop, most commonly on sun-exposed areas of skin. These lesions may be precancerous.

Incidence

Actinic keratosis occurs most frequently in light-skinned people who have frequent sun exposure. It follows then that incidence increases with age, living near the equator, and participating in activities or jobs that take place outdoors. Actinic keratosis is more common in men than women, and in those who eat a high-fat diet. Estimated incidence in the United States is as high as 26%. Australia has the highest rate, estimated at 50% among those over the age of 40.

Etiology

Actinic keratosis is caused by exposure to ultraviolet light from the sun. Risk factors include pale skin that burns easily and tans poorly; blond or red hair; and blue, green, or hazel eyes. Those with frequent sun exposure or weakened immune systems are most vulnerable.

Flashpoint

Actinic keratosis is caused by ultraviolet sunlight.

Signs and Symptoms

Actinic keratosis lesions appear as slightly raised, flat patches that are scaly and flesh-colored, pink, or reddish-brown (see Fig. 5-25). Some lesions eventually take on a wartier appearance. They may be as small as several millimeters across or as large as several centimeters (an inch or more). They are most common on sun-exposed areas such as the scalp, neck,

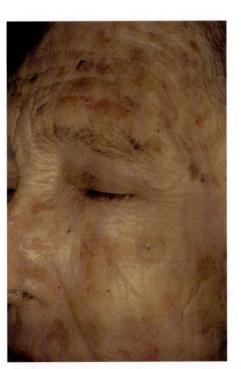

FIGURE 5-25 Actinic keratosis (From Goldsmith, LA, Lazarus, GS, and Tharp, MD. *Adult and Pediatric Dermatology: A Color Guide to Diagnosis and Treatment.* 1997. Philadelphia: F.A. Davis Company, with permission.)

face, ears, lips, hands, and forearms. Occasionally, due to **hyperkeratosis** (thickening of the skin), they may develop a hornlike growth above the surface of the skin.

Diagnosis

Diagnosis of actinic keratosis is based upon the appearance of the lesions. Blood tests are not necessary, but a skin biopsy may be necessary in some cases to rule out squamous cell carcinoma.

Treatment

Several treatment options are available, including cryotherapy, the application of topical medication, chemical peels, curettage (surgical scraping), laser therapy, photodynamic therapy combined with topical application of an approved agent, medication called retinoids, and possibly cosmetic resurfacing procedures. Individuals should consult with their health-care provider to select the one that is most appropriate for their specific circumstances. They are also counseled to protect their skin from further sun exposure.

Prognosis

Prognosis for actinic keratosis is very good as long as lesions are monitored and treated appropriately. They can usually be prevented from evolving into cancer via sun-protection strategies and recommended therapies. Most lesions will remain unchanged and some may even resolve spontaneously. Up to 5% of lesions, though, will develop into squamous cell carcinoma, a serious form of skin cancer which can spread into facial structures and become deadly. The more lesions an individual has, the greater the chance that some will become cancerous.

Flashpoint

Up to 5% of lesions will become cancerous.

Sebaceous Cysts and Epidermoid Cysts

ICD-9-CM: 706.2   [ICD-10: L72.1]

Sebaceous cysts and epidermoid cysts are similar and are often confused for one another. Epidermoid cysts are the more common of the two. Both are small sacs or pouches which slowly develop below the skin surface. They are filled with a thick fluid or semisolid oily substance, produced by sebaceous glands, called sebum.

Incidence

Both types of cysts are quite common. Sebaceous cysts are most common among men in their 30s or 40s and those with a history of acne.

Etiology

Causes of sebaceous cysts include swollen hair follicles, blocked sebaceous glands, and excessive testosterone levels. Common sites include the scalp, face, ears, upper arms, and back. In men, other common areas are the chest and scrotum.

Flashpoint

Sebaceous cysts usually develop on the scalp, face, ears, upper arms, and back.

Epidermoid cysts develop when surface skin cells move deeper into the skin and multiply. This usually happens at hair follicles and larger sebaceous glands. The most common locations are the face, neck, back, and groin. Factors that contribute to the formation of epidermoid cysts include damaged hair follicles, ruptured sebaceous glands (usually caused by inflammatory conditions such as acne), developmental defects that occur during the embryonic stage, and heredity.

Signs and Symptoms

Signs and symptoms of a sebaceous cyst depend somewhat on whether it is inflamed or infected. It may present as a rounded area in the skin that is soft and somewhat movable, meaning that it can be pushed slightly to the side upon examination.

Epidermoid cysts are usually round and freely movable, and they vary in diameter from several millimeters to 5 centimeters. They usually appear pale white or yellow but can be darker on individuals with darker skin. Occasionally they have an opening in the center, through which the sebum might be expressed; it is thick and cheeselike and may have a foul odor, particularly if the cyst is infected.

Either type of cyst can become infected. In this case, they will take on many of the characteristics associated with inflammation: erythema, edema, heat, and tenderness.

Diagnosis

The health-care provider diagnoses both types of cysts based upon appearance and location. Occasionally the patient may be referred to a dermatologist for diagnosis and treatment.

Treatment

In general, cysts of either type do not require treatment or removal unless they become infected or the individual finds them unsightly. Treatment options include corticosteroid injections to reduce inflammation, incision and drainage, excision of the entire cyst, laser treatment to vaporize small epidermoid cysts on sensitive areas, antibiotics (if infection is present), and heat compresses (effective for sebaceous cysts only).

Prognosis

Infected cysts, especially those located on the neck or other sensitive areas, should be evaluated and treated by a physician. A cyst may grow back, depending upon its type and the form of treatment.

Flashpoint
Cysts of either type do not require treatment unless they become infected or are unsightly.

Alopecia

ICD-9-CM: 704.00   [ICD-10: L65.9] (unspecified for both codes)

Alopecia areata is an autoimmune disease that results in patchy hair loss from the scalp. In alopecia capitis totalis the hair loss spreads to the entire scalp. In alopecia universalis, hair loss spreads to the entire body. Both of the latter two forms are rare.

Incidence

Various forms of alopecia affect approximately 5 million American men and women. Onset may occur at any age but is most common during childhood, the late teens, and young adulthood.

Etiology

Alopecia areata is an autoimmune disorder in which the immune system attacks the hair follicles, causing hair growth to cease. Genetics are thought to play a role, as are emotional stress and pathogenic organisms. It may also be caused by vitamin B5 deficiency or Prilosec, a medication for heartburn.

Signs and Symptoms

Alopecia areata often starts with small, round, smooth patches of hair loss on the scalp or beard (see Fig. 5-26). They develop quickly and are usually not symmetrical. These areas may be slightly tender and may tingle. In some individuals the fingernails take on an irregular appearance, with ridges and multiple tiny dents or pits. This is called trachyonychia.

Diagnosis

Diagnosis is made based upon presenting signs and symptoms, primarily the characteristic patchy hair loss. The health-care provider may also test the hair to see if it pulls out more easily than normal by gently tugging a handful of hair along the edge of a bare patch.

Flashpoint
People with alopecia sometimes also develop fingernail changes.

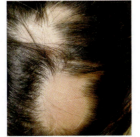

FIGURE 5-26 Alopecia (From Barankin, B, and Freiman, A. *Derm Notes: Clinical Dermatology Pocket Guide.* 2006. Philadelphia: F.A. Davis Company, with permission.)

Treatment

There is no FDA-approved treatment for alopecia areata. However, it may be treated with oral corticosteroids or topical immunotherapy. The latter involves intentionally inducing an allergic reaction on the scalp. Approximately 40% of patients treated in this manner will experience scalp-hair regrowth in about 6 months.

Prognosis

Flashpoint

Ninety percent of the time, hair eventually grows back.

In approximately half of all patients, hair regrows within 1 year without any treatment. In approximately 90%, the hair eventually grows back. For the other 10%, some degree of hair loss is permanent. Until hair growth resumes, individuals must take measures such as wearing hats and applying sunscreen to protect their skin from sunlight.

Decubitus Ulcers

ICD-9-CM: 707.0   [ICD-10: L89]

Decubitus ulcers, sometimes called *pressure ulcers* or *bedsores*, are areas of injury and **necrosis** (tissue death) caused by a variety of factors, especially unrelieved pressure that impedes circulation in the skin and underlying tissues. Decubitus ulcers are categorized into four stages according to degree of severity.

Flashpoint

Decubitus ulcers are also called pressure ulcers and bedsores.

Incidence

As many as 3 million Americans are estimated to have decubitus ulcers. Incidence is highest among the frail elderly and those with decreased mobility.

Etiology

The most common cause of decubitus ulcers is pressure on tissue, which impairs perfusion (delivery of oxygen and nutrients via the blood) and leads to necrosis. Formation is most likely to occur where soft tissue becomes compressed between bony prominences and external forces. Consequently, decubitus ulcers are frequently found on the elbows, heels, sacrum, hips, and anywhere that may be subject to pressure. Major contributors to tissue injury in the immobile individual are the forces of *friction* (rubbing of skin against bedding or linens) and *shearing* (sliding down of deeper structures due to gravity while the skin remains in place). Other risk factors include advanced age, immobility, impaired circulation, impaired sensory or perceptual function, poor nutrition, and moisture from incontinence or perspiration. Most vulnerable are individuals with cognitive impairment, an inability to communicate, or an inability to move spontaneously and change position.

Signs and Symptoms

Signs and symptoms of decubitus ulcers range from mild to extreme. On the mild end, the individual may simply notice mild redness and the dull ache that comes from remaining in the same position for too long. On the extreme end, individuals may lose all soft tissue in the area, including skin, fat, and even muscle, with subsequent bone exposure. A stage system has been created that helps with identification and monitoring of decubitus ulcers (see Fig. 5-27):

- Stage 1 ulcers exhibit temperature changes (warmer or cooler than surrounding skin), color changes—including redness in light-skinned people and blue or purple coloring in dark-skinned people—that do not blanch (become more pale) with briefly applied pressure or resolve after pressure is relieved, discomfort (itching or tenderness), and change in consistency (firmer or softer).
- Stage 2 ulcers exhibit erosion of the epidermis or dermis without subcutaneous exposure; they may appear as abrasions, blisters, or shallow wounds.
- Stage 3 ulcers exhibit erosion or necrosis of all layers of skin down to underlying fascia and appear as deep wounds which may or may not extend beneath the surrounding skin. For this reason they are often much larger than they appear (the "iceberg effect").
- Stage 4 ulcers exhibit erosion and tissue necrosis through all layers of skin and subcutaneous tissue, with damage to supporting structures such as muscle, tendons, and bones.

Flashpoint

Ulcers have the best chance of healing if they are caught at stage 1.

Some individuals deny pain or tenderness even with the most severe decubitus ulcers. This may be due to sensory or perceptual deficits or to localized impairment of circulation and nerve function. Other individuals describe their ulcers as extremely painful.

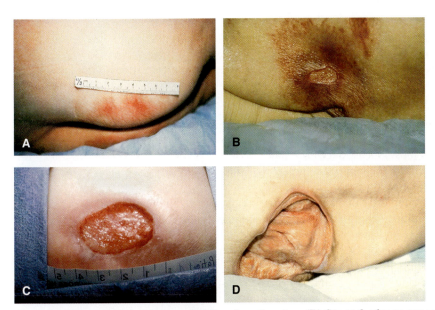

FIGURE 5-27 (A) During stage 1, ulcers exhibit color changes. (B) Stage 2 ulcers are superficial and may appear as abrasions, blisters, or shallow craters. (C) A stage 3 ulcer appears as a deep wound that may undermine adjacent tissues. (D) Stage 4 ulcers involve damage to muscle, tendons, and/or bones. (From Dillon, PM. *Nursing Health Assessment: A Critical Thinking, Case Studies Approach,* 2nd edition. 2007. Philadelphia: F.A. Davis Company, with permission.)

Diagnosis

Decubitus ulcers are generally easy to identify and diagnose based upon appearance; however, the extent and depth of an ulcer may be unclear. Osteomyelitis (infection in the bone) may be diagnosed with radionuclide bone scanning or gadolinium-enhanced MRI. Bone biopsy and culture may be necessary to determine the causative organism.

Treatment

Decubitus ulcers are more easily prevented than treated (see Box 5-7). Once present, ulcers heal most successfully with a multidimensional approach to treatment, including **debridement** (removal of dead or damaged tissue) of necrotic tissue, antimicrobial medication for infection, nutritional support (such as adequate protein intake and the use of vitamins and nutritional supplements), pressure relief through frequent turns, special mattresses and cushions, education of caregivers, consultation with wound and skin-care specialists, and thorough hygiene measures.

Prognosis

When decubitus ulcers are identified early, the prognosis for patients is very good. Approximately 75% of stage 2 ulcers resolve within 8 weeks. However, 38% of stage 4 ulcers never heal. Delays in treatment can result in life-threatening infection, amputation, and even death.

Flashpoint
Some stage 4 ulcers never heal.

Calluses and Corns

ICD-9-CM: 700   [ICD-10: L84]

A callus is a thickened, hardened, toughened area of skin. A corn is a type of small callus that usually develops on smooth, hairless skin surfaces, such as the backs of fingers or tops of toes, in response to pressure and friction. Hard corns are the most common type. They develop on flat, dry skin surfaces such as the sides of feet and tops of toes. Soft corns remain moist with a firm center. They usually develop between toes.

Box 5-7 Wellness Promotion

PREVENTION IS KEY

Pressure ulcers develop quickly in vulnerable people and are often difficult to eliminate. Therefore, these aggressive measures should be taken to keep them from developing in the first place:

- Inspect the person's skin, especially bony prominences like the heels, elbows, sacrum, and hips, at least once each day.
- Turn or reposition the individual frequently—at least every 2 hours—using a written schedule if necessary.
- Teach chairbound individuals to shift their weight every 15 minutes.
- Place soft padding between bony body parts (such as knees) to keep them from pressing on one another.
- Provide heel protection, such as placing a soft pillow or cushion under the calf to keep heels from pressing into the bed.
- Keep the individual's skin clean and dry, but moisturize if it becomes too dry and flaky.
- Provide careful hygiene and skin protection for individuals who are incontinent.
- Provide cushioned or padded surfaces for sitting.
- Consider providing special mattresses for those who are bedbound.
- Turn and reposition the individual carefully to avoid friction and shearing trauma—use turn sheets or mechanical lifting devices if necessary.
- Provide good nutrition and hydration to promote skin health.
- Treat areas of skin breakdown early and aggressively.

Incidence

Calluses and corns are quite common. It is estimated that nearly 7 million people in the United States have calluses and corns at any given time. They are especially common in the working population, since these people tend to spend long hours on their feet. They are more common in women than men.

> **Flashpoint**
>
> The development of calluses and corns is a natural protective skin response.

Etiology

The development of calluses and corns is a natural protective response of the skin; when it is subjected to frequent or chronic pressure or friction, it responds with increased cell growth, known as *hyperplasia.* This frequently occurs on areas of the feet and toes that press against the inside wall of the shoe. Because many individuals have toes that curl downward rather than lying flat, they are prone to corn development at toe joints and on the tips of toes. This is especially true when an individual has a condition called hammertoe, in which the toe is curled in a clawlike shape rather than lying flat. Another common cause of callus formation is a bunion, an inflammation caused by hallux valgus, which is a structural deformity in which the bone forming the base of the great toe is angulated inward. Soft corns commonly develop between the fourth and fifth toes, where they are widest and press against one another. Both types of corns (hard and soft) are worsened by poorly fitting shoes. Shoes with narrow or pointed toes compress the toes. High heels create downward pressure against the toes. Shoes that are too loose allow the foot to rub and slide. A poorly placed seam or other structural defect creates excessive pressure. Absence of socks, or socks with seams or wrinkles, also contributes to the problem. Defects in the foot, such as bone spurs, may also exacerbate the problem.

> **Flashpoint**
>
> A common cause of corns is poorly fitting shoes.

Calluses and corns also commonly develop on the hands due to friction and pressure. Typical causes include the use of hand tools, especially when gloves are not worn to protect the skin. Occasionally the development of a callus is desirable and even intentional: for example, individuals who play the guitar develop calluses on the tips of their fingers from repeatedly compressing the guitar wires. To a certain extent, this increases the ability of the person to play without experiencing undue pain and tenderness in the fingertips.

Signs and Symptoms

Calluses are areas of thickened, hardened skin, as described previously. They are usually not tender and may be dry and flaky. They are most commonly located on the hands and feet. Corns sometimes have areas of inflammation surrounding the hardened center; therefore, they can be painful or tender to the touch and may ache.

Diagnosis

Diagnosis of calluses and corns is easily made based on physical examination. In some cases, the health-care provider may order x-rays to determine whether a structural abnormality is the underlying cause.

Treatment

Calluses and corns do not require treatment unless they are causing discomfort or their appearance is unacceptable to the individual. In most cases, identifying and eliminating the cause of friction or pressure (such as poorly fitting shoes) will allow the condition to resolve (see Box 5-8). Occasionally the insertion of friction-reducing material, such as a special insole, into the shoe will resolve the issue or at least increase foot comfort. An orthotic device—a shoe insert designed by a specialist to address the specific needs of the person's foot—may also be prescribed. Other options for treatment include surgery to correct structural defects such as hammertoe and bunions. A podiatrist may also reduce a hard callus by shaving it down or applying salicylic acid.

Prognosis

While calluses and corns tend to be chronic, they are rarely serious and generally improve with appropriate intervention. Individuals with diabetes must take care to regularly examine the skin on their hands and especially their feet, which are vulnerable to ulceration and infection and may experience delayed healing.

Skin Disorders Caused by Autoimmune Disease

A number of skin disorders are considered autoimmune in nature. In such cases, the underlying cause involves a malfunction of the body's immune response. Common autoimmune skin disorders include scleroderma and systemic lupus erythematosus (SLE).

Scleroderma
ICD-9-CM: 710.1   [ICD-10: L94.0]

Scleroderma is a group of uncommon chronic autoimmune diseases. The name comes from the Greek words *skleros* (hard) and *derma* (skin), and refers to the skin changes caused by the condition. It has also been known as *progressive systemic sclerosis*, but this name has fallen out of

---

Box 5-8 Wellness Promotion

BE KIND TO YOUR FEET

The development of calluses and corns is always related to pressure and friction, and it is preventable. You can avoid these painful problems by being kind to your feet. Here are some suggestions:

- Inspect your feet regularly for areas of redness or tenderness.
- Identify possible hammertoes or bunions early and discuss them with your health-care provider.
- Carefully select new shoes that are comfortable—do not sacrifice your feet for fashion!
- Stop wearing shoes that hurt your feet or toes.
- Avoid wearing heels more than 2 inches high (or avoid wearing heels at all).
- Avoid wearing pointy-toed shoes.
- Wear socks, but avoid those with seams that press against your toes.

favor as it became clear that the disease is not always progressive in nature. See Chapter 9 for a detailed description of scleroderma.

Systemic Lupus Erythematosus
ICD-9-CM: 710.0   [ICD-10: L93]

Systemic lupus erythematosus (SLE) is a chronic autoimmune disorder that causes inflammation and degeneration of various connective tissues in the body, including the skin and the joints. Lupus that affects only the skin is called discoid lupus erythematosus (DLE). One of the most prominent features of both discoid lupus and SLE is the skin rash that may develop anywhere on the body but is most obvious on the face and scalp. It is generally red and flat (but may have raised borders), is painless, and doesn't itch. See Chapter 9 for a detailed description of SLE.

Skin Injuries Caused by Environmental Factors

Injury to the skin occurs as the result of a variety of external forces. Common sources of trauma include burns from fire, electricity, and other sources of heat, as well as chemicals. Frostbite may result from exposure to extreme cold. Lacerations may occur from a wide variety of sources. Injury may also be inflicted by humans, animals, and insects.

Burns
ICD-9-CM: 940.00–949.59; fourth digit indicates degree and fifth digit indicates percentage of body surface involved   [ICD-10: T20–T31 (code by body site and degree)]

Burns are a type of thermal injury to the skin caused by a variety of heat sources. They are classified according to severity as first-degree burns, also called *superficial burns;* second-degree burns, also called *partial-thickness burns;* and third-degree burns, also called *full-thickness burns.*

Flashpoint
Burns are classified as first-, second-, or third-degree.

Incidence
Approximately 4,000 Americans die each year in fires or from burn injuries; 75% of those deaths occur at the scene. A total of 500,000 individuals are treated each year for burn injuries and 40,000 of them are hospitalized, with 25,000 requiring specialized care that is provided in burn centers. Of those admitted to burn centers, 70% are male and 62% are white. The largest percentage of burn injuries occurs in the home (43%); the rest occur in a variety of places, including the workplace and motor vehicles.

Etiology
First-degree burns are usually caused by exposure to heat or, more commonly, the ultraviolet rays of the sun. Second- and third-degree burns usually result from exposure to or direct contact with very hot objects, scalding liquids, flames, chemicals, or electricity.

Signs and Symptoms
First-degree burns involve only the epidermis and are generally considered minor injuries. The skin is red, blanches with pressure, is moderately painful to the touch, and is dry with no blisters. Permanent tissue damage is rare and may consist of minor changes in skin color (see Fig. 5-28). Second-degree burns involve the epidermis and part of the dermis. The skin appears red, edematous, and wet, shiny, or blistered, and it is intensely painful. Third-degree burns destroy the epidermis, dermis, and subcutaneous layers of the skin. Fatty tissue, muscles, bones, and tendons may be involved as well, although some experts further classify such burns as fourth-degree burns. These burns may appear black and charred, brown, yellow, or even white. They are also dry and leathery. The patient feels no pain from third-degree burns because nerves are destroyed. However, superficial and partial-thickness burns in the surrounding area may be very painful.

Flashpoint
Third-degree burns are the worst.

Diagnosis
Diagnosis of burns is based upon a description of the mechanism of injury and examination of the injured tissue.

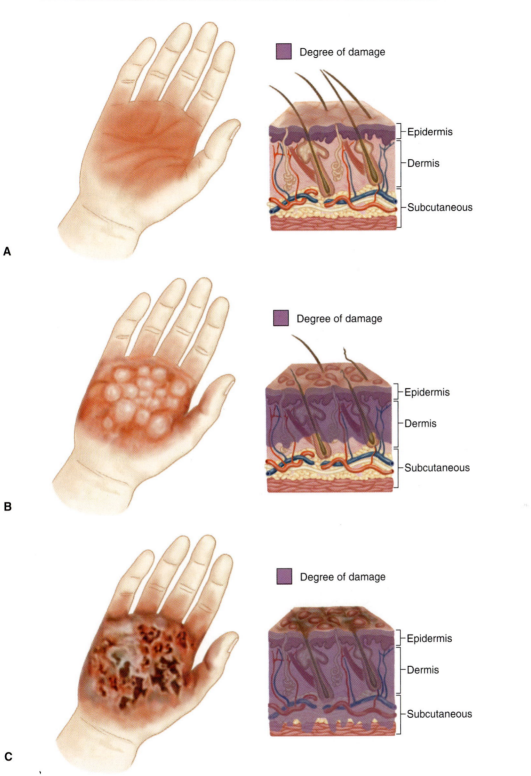

FIGURE 5-28 Classification of burns: (A) First-degree; (B) Second-degree; (C) Third-degree (From Eagle, S, et al. *The Professional Medical Assistant: An Integrative Teamwork-Based Approach.* 2009. Philadelphia: F.A. Davis Company, with permission.)

Treatment

First-degree burns usually heal without treatment (see Box 5-9). Patients with second- and third-degree burns should be seen by the physician immediately. Those with extensive second- and third-degree burns should be treated in an emergency room and will most likely require hospitalization, preferably at a hospital with a burn unit, because of risk of profound dehydration, shock, infection, septicemia, and other life-threatening complications (see Box 5-10).

Patients with burns covering less than 10% of the body can usually be treated as outpatients. Treatment is provided at the direction of the physician and may include cleansing the wound, applying silver sulfadiazine cream or another antibiotic ointment, and applying a nonadherent dressing. Medications include analgesics for pain and antibiotics.

Part of evaluating a patient with burns includes estimating the percentage of the body that has been affected. A commonly used tool for this process is a chart which divides the body up into 9% sections, called the rule of nines (see Fig. 5-29). By referring to this chart, a quick and fairly accurate estimation can be made. This data is vital to determining how critical the individual's condition is and making appropriate triage decisions.

Flashpoint

The rule of nines is used to estimate the percentage of the body that is burned.

Treatment of patients with third-degree burns includes intravenous fluid and electrolyte replacement, wound debridement, antibiotics, analgesics, a high-protein, high-calorie diet, and extensive rehabilitation. Patients may also be candidates for skin grafting and reconstructive surgery.

Appropriate treatment for burn injuries depends upon the severity and extent of the burn. Second-degree burns should be evaluated by a physician. Those covering a small area of the body may be treated in the outpatient setting; those covering extensive areas of the body may

---

Box 5-9 Wellness Promotion

FIRST AID FOR BURNS

First-degree burns (such as sunburns) can be treated at home. Simple treatment includes cooling the burn through application of a cool compress (but not ice) and use of over-the-counter analgesics such as ibuprofen or acetaminophen.

Blistering and skin sloughing indicate a second-degree burn. These burns should be evaluated and treated by a medical professional.

First Aid for Second- and Third-Degree Burns
- Loosely apply a sterile (or very clean) dressing to protect the burned tissue, but allow it to breathe.
- Take the patient with small-area burns to a medical facility for immediate evaluation.
- For severely burned patients, call 911 rather than trying to transport them yourself.
- Never apply home remedies such as lotions, ointments, oils, butter, or vinegar. They may hold in the heat (thus worsening the burn) and may promote the growth of infectious organisms.
- Never break blisters, because this allows pathogenic organisms to enter and may cause infection.

First Aid for Chemical Burns
- Remove clothing that has chemicals on it.
- Thoroughly rinse chemicals from the skin using large volumes of water for at least 15 minutes.
- If water is unavailable, brush dry chemicals from the skin using a clean, dry brush or cloth.
- Take the patient with small-area burns to a medical facility. Cover the burn with a sterile, loose bandage.
- For chemical splashes into the eyes, thoroughly irrigate the eyes with large volumes of sterile saline or clean water and seek immediate medical treatment.

Box 5-10 Wellness Promotion

PREVENTING INFECTION IN BURN WOUNDS

Patients suffering from second- and third-degree burns are at risk of infection. Therefore, patient education must include the following:

- Call the clinic if you observe the following signs of infection: increased pain, redness, swelling, fever, or yellow or green drainage.
- Do not break blisters. Intact skin helps keep bacteria out and prevents infection.
- Keep the wound clean.
- Wash hands thoroughly before providing wound care.
- Change the dressing as instructed.
- Do not apply anything to the wound unless it was prescribed by your physician.
- Avoid home remedies such as vitamin E oil, butter, or vinegar.
- Take antibiotics (if prescribed) until they are completely gone.
- Avoid the sun until the wound heals completely.
- Wear sunscreen for future sun exposure.
- Avoid suntanning for at least 1 year.

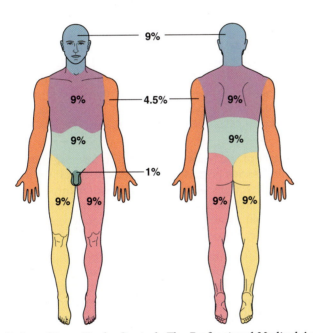

FIGURE 5-29 **Rule of nines** (From Eagle, S, et al. *The Professional Medical Assistant: An Integrative Teamwork-Based Approach.* 2009. Philadelphia: F.A. Davis Company, with permission.)

require hospitalization. Treatment usually includes cooling the burn with cold water or cold compresses. Ice should never be applied directly to the site, since it can cause frostbite. Any area where the skin is blistered or broken should be covered loosely with a sterile bandage. The physician may order topical or oral antibiotics to prevent or fight infection, and analgesics such as ibuprofen or acetaminophen to alleviate mild to moderate pain. Opiate analgesics may be required for severe pain.

Patients with third-degree burns usually require treatment in the hospital. Emergency treatment may include brief immersion in cool water to stop the burning process. Alternatively, cool compresses may be applied. As with other types of burns, ice and ice water should never be used. Care must be taken, however, to not overcool third-degree burns, since this can result in hypothermia. Blisters should not be broken. No topical ointments or lotions should be administered. A dry, sterile dressing, should be loosely applied.

In the hospital setting, the patient is given intravenous fluid replacement, help with breathing as needed, antibiotics to prevent or fight infection, and pain medication. For some third-degree burns, escharotomy may be necessary. This is a procedure in which the physician cuts through hardened, dead overlying tissue to maximize circulation to the living tissue beneath. The burn wounds are debrided as necessary to remove dead tissue. Antibiotic cream may be applied; Silvadene is commonly used. Sterile dressings are loosely applied. Regular debridement and dressing changes are needed to prevent infection and promote healing. Some third-degree burns require skin grafts for healing to occur.

Prognosis

Flashpoint

Preventing wound infection is critically important for the burn patient.

The prognosis for burns is variable, depending on the location and severity of the burn and the individual's underlying health status. Mild to moderate burn injuries generally heal fully with prompt and appropriate intervention. Severe burns may take months of treatment and physical therapy for healing to occur. Some burns result in permanent disability, disfigurement, and even death. Among those admitted to specialty burn centers, 94% survive.

Frostbite

ICD-9-CM: 991.0 (face), 991.1 (hand), 991.2 (foot), 991.3 (unspecified site)   **[ICD-10: T33.0 (face), T33.5 (hand), T33.8 (foot), T33.9 (unspecified site)]**

Frostbite develops when skin tissues are exposed to temperatures cold enough to cause them to freeze.

Incidence

The exact incidence of frostbite is unknown. It is most common in Canada and the northern United States, including Alaska. The most common victims of frostbite are males between the ages of 30 and 49. People who are most likely to suffer this type of injury are those who work outdoors, those who are homeless, and those who are outdoors for a prolonged period of time during freezing temperatures without appropriate clothing. Body parts most commonly affected are exposed parts such as the fingers, toes, ears, nose, and cheeks.

Etiology

Flashpoint

Frostbite typically affects the fingers, toes, ears, nose, and cheeks.

Frostbite occurs when parts of the body are exposed to freezing temperatures for prolonged periods of time. As tissues begin to freeze, ice crystals form in the extracellular spaces (fluid around the cells). Cells also tend to lose water into the extracellular spaces and become dehydrated, further compounding the problem. To make matters still worse, vessels in the area are injured as well. As rewarming occurs, cells swell, small blood clots develop, and the inflammatory process occurs.

Signs and Symptoms

Signs and symptoms of frostbite vary according to the severity of injury and whether the tissue is still frozen or has thawed and rewarmed. Very cold or frozen tissue on exposed body parts appears white or ashen (on dark-skinned people) and feels little pain until it thaws. Deep frostbite causes tissue to become stiff and have a waxy appearance. Symptoms of superficial frostbite include itching, numbness, burning, or cold sensations. When pressed, the tissue offers some resistance. Deep frostbite causes decreased sensation or even total loss of sensation; while still frozen, tissue will feel hard to the touch. When rewarmed, the affected tissue becomes edematous, and blood-filled blisters may be present over skin that appears yellow or white. The skin usually changes to a purple-blue color as it warms, and pain may be severe.

Diagnosis

Diagnosis is based upon physical examination and history. It can be initially difficult to distinguish superficial from deep frostbite and to identify the exact degree of tissue damage. Therefore, all individuals with suspected frostbite should be evaluated by a physician, including evaluation for possible hypothermia and dehydration.

Treatment

First aid for superficial frostbite includes moving the victim to a warm environment or warming the affected body part by covering it with another warm, dry body part. The frostbitten area should never be rubbed, as this causes further injury to the tissue. The tissue should not be allowed to refreeze; this will worsen the injury. Because of this, if refreezing is a risk, it is sometimes recommended to delay rewarming the frozen tissue until the victim is taken to the hospital. The injured body part should be moved as little as possible. The victim should not smoke or drink alcoholic beverages, since these worsen circulation.

In the medical setting, the individual will be evaluated for extent of the frostbite injury as well as possible hypothermia; vital signs will be monitored; analgesics may be given for pain; and the affected body part may be thawed in warm (but not hot) water.

Prognosis

Prognosis for frostbite depends upon the severity of injury and the appropriateness and timeliness of treatment. Death is rare except when hypothermia or wound sepsis are complicating factors. Potential complications include sensory deficits, infection and sepsis, and tissue death leading to the need for amputation.

Lacerations

ICD-9-CM: 879.8   [ICD-10: T14] (site unspecified for both codes)

A laceration, sometimes called a *cut* or *gash*, is a tear or break in the skin which may be jagged and irregular, but in which none of the skin is missing. It may bleed slightly or may hemorrhage profusely.

Incidence

The incidence of lacerations is unknown, since many minor ones go unreported. However, they are known to be extremely common.

Etiology

Lacerations are caused by many forms of trauma, such as falls, motor vehicle accidents, and blows to the body.

Signs and Symptoms

Lacerations usually result in some degree of bleeding and pain. Depending upon location and severity, they may result in loss of function of the affected body part. Flesh within the laceration may be visible (see Fig. 5-30).

Diagnosis

Diagnosis is easily made based upon the physical appearance of the wound.

Treatment

Minor lacerations may be treated at home by thoroughly washing the wound with soap and water and then applying an antibacterial ointment and a bandage. However, individuals suffering severe lacerations should be immediately taken to a medical facility. Bleeding can be stopped or slowed by direct application of pressure with a sterile (or very clean) absorbent material or, in extreme cases, of a constricting band (see Box 5-11). If necessary, 911 should be called to summon emergency help. At the medical facility, the health-care provider will apply direct pressure with absorbent dressing material and monitor the patient's vital signs. Intravenous fluids and blood products may be administered. Severe lacerations may require surgical repair; less-severe lacerations will be anesthetized, cleaned, and then closed with **sutures** (stitches used to hold tissue together), staples, butterfly closures, Steri-Strips, or a tissue adhesive. The patient may also be given a tetanus booster.

Flashpoint
Never rub frostbitten skin!

Flashpoint
Bleeding can usually be stopped with direct pressure.

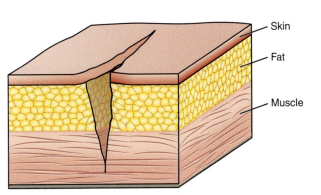

Skin

Fat

Muscle

FIGURE 5-30 Laceration

Box 5-11 Wellness Promotion

DON'T USE A TOURNIQUET

The use of tourniquets is no longer recommended, because a tightly applied tourniquet cuts off circulation to the distal extremity. As a result, tissue dies and the extremity may need to be amputated. Instead, hemorrhage should be controlled by using one of the following measures:

- Application of direct pressure with an absorbent dressing
- Application of direct pressure to the nearest pulse point
- Application of a constricting band tight enough to reduce, but not completely stop bleeding; this still allows some circulation to distal tissue

Prognosis

Prognosis for victims of laceration depends upon the severity of the injury, degree of blood loss, and timeliness and appropriateness of medical care. Most individuals recover fully. Potential complications include infection and, in extreme cases, hemorrhage, shock, and death.

Animal Bites

ICD-9-CM: 879.8   [ICD-10: T14.1] (uncomplicated, open wound for both codes)

An animal-bite injury is any injury caused by the bite of an animal or even another human.

Incidence

Because many bite injuries go unreported, the exact incidence is impossible to determine. However, an estimated five to six million animal-bite injuries are treated each year, the majority from dogs. Men are bitten more often by dogs and women more frequently by cats. The highest incidence of animal bites occurs among children between the ages of 5 and 9. Approximately 10 to 20 Americans (mostly children) die each year as a result of dog attacks.

Etiology

Because of their strong jaws (200 to 400 pounds per square inch) and rounded teeth, dogs create a crush type of injury that may damage deep structures such as muscles, nerves, tendons, vessels, and even bones. Cat bites commonly create smaller puncture wounds, but they become infected more commonly than dog bites. In any case, infection is a concern for all types of bites, since numerous species of bacteria are found in the mouths of animals.

Signs and Symptoms

Signs and symptoms of bite injury include bite marks that may include skin puncture, laceration, or tearing; pain; bleeding; and bruising of surrounding tissue.

Diagnosis

Diagnosis of a bite injury is based upon the victim's description of the event and the wound appearance. Infected bite wounds may be cultured to guide antibiotic therapy. Radiological tests such as x-rays or CT scan may be necessary if there is a concern about potential injury to deep structures.

Treatment

The wound is cleaned with sterile saline, antibacterial solution, or warm water and soap. An antibiotic ointment and dressing is then applied. More severe injuries may require surgical repair. The victim may be given a tetanus booster. An attempt will be made to identify the animal involved and determine whether rabies is a concern; if so, the individual must undergo rabies vaccination.

Prognosis

In most cases of bite injury, the prognosis is very good. However, some bite injuries carry greater risk of infection and the spread of infectious disease than others. Potential complications of bite injury include wound infection, cellulitis, sepsis, deformity, and loss of function.

Snakebites

ICD-9-CM: 989.5   [ICD-10: T63.0] (venomous snakes, lizards, and spiders for both codes)

A snakebite is a wound created by the fangs of a snake, regardless of whether venom has been injected. Most snakebites are relatively harmless; the only poisonous snakes found wild in North America are rattlesnakes, cottonmouths, copperheads, and coral snakes. In addition, zoos and some private collectors keep some of the more exotic species.

Incidence

The exact incidence of snakebites is uncertain, since they are often not reported. Approximately 4,000 to 7,000 snakebites are reported in the United States each year, with the highest incidence in North Carolina. Most bites are seasonal, occurring during the warmer months. Most victims are white males; half are between the ages of 18 and 28. The vast majority of bites are to an extremity.

Etiology

Most snakebites occur as a result of the individual attempting to handle or catch the snake. When a bite occurs, the snake may or may not inject venom; if it does, the amount may vary. The destructive effects of the venom vary depending upon the type of snake.

Signs and Symptoms

Nonvenomous snakebites may cause mild localized pain, discoloration, burning, edema, and inflammation. The symptoms of venomous snakebites vary with the type of snake and include local symptoms (as from nonvenomous snakebites) plus a variety of systemic symptoms; some of these are blurred vision, convulsions, diarrhea, dizziness, *diaphoresis* (profuse sweating), dyspnea, *syncope* (fainting), weakness, fever, thirst, loss of coordination, nausea, vomiting, tachycardia, hypotension, and heart failure.

Diagnosis

Diagnosis is based upon the victim's description of events and of the snake along with physical-examination findings. Since most snakebites result from the victim's attempting to handle the snake, the type of snake is often known. If it is not, it is helpful for someone to catch the snake and bring it in—however, risk of further bite injuries must be avoided. Identifying the time since the bite occurred is important to diagnosis and treatment, since early onset of intense pain indicates a probability of envenomation. Depending upon the type of snake involved, diagnostic testing may be done to identify and monitor complications of the kidneys, lungs, or blood.

Treatment

First aid for the snakebite victim includes offering reassurance, keeping the affected body part immobilized below heart level, and assisting the victim to rest in a position of comfort. Jewelry should be removed from the affected body part. In the medical setting, vital signs are monitored and the bite is washed with warm water and soap or antibacterial solution. The patient is treated as necessary for shock and other symptoms. An antibacterial ointment and dressing may be applied. *Antivenin* can be requested from a regional poison-control center.

> **Flashpoint**
>
> Most snakebites occur because the victim was attempting to handle the snake.

Prognosis

Snakebites are frightening to most people, but the mortality rate is low, with 97 deaths reported in the United States during a 20-year period (nearly half in the states of Texas, Florida, and Georgia).

Insect Stings and Bites

ICD-9-CM: 919.4   [ICD-10: W57] (nonvenomous insect bite for both codes)

An insect sting or bite may be a puncture of the skin by an insect stinger or a tiny bite. Some of the numerous types of insects that might bite humans include mosquitoes, ants, mites, spiders, and fleas. Insects that might sting humans include bees, ants, and wasps.

Incidence

Insect bites and stings are extremely common, but the exact incidence is unknown, since most go unreported. They occur most commonly during the warmer months. Individuals who spend time outdoors for work or recreational activities are most at risk of mosquito bites and bee stings.

Etiology

Insect bites and stings occur when an insect comes into contact with victims and either bites or stings them. When this occurs, venom is sometimes injected into the tissue, causing the characteristic signs and symptoms.

Signs and Symptoms

Signs and symptoms of insect bites and stings include a sharp stinging sensation, redness, itching, and localized edema. Symptoms generally last several hours to several days. Systemic allergic reactions may cause generalized edema, rash, itching, and respiratory problems.

Diagnosis

Diagnosis is based upon history and physical examination. In some cases the victim may have actually seen the insect and can describe it.

Treatment

To treat an insect sting, it is helpful to identify whether the stinger is still present. If so, it can be removed by scraping across it with a plastic card. Next, the site is cleansed with water and soap. Pain and inflammation can be relieved by application of a cold pack or anesthetic spray. The individual should be observed for signs of allergic reaction. If this is a concern, antihistamines, corticosteroids, and, if necessary, epinephrine may be administered.

Prognosis

The prognosis for most cases of insect sting or bite is excellent. Potential complications include allergic reactions and localized infection.

STOP HERE.

Select the flash cards for this chapter and run through them at least three times before moving on to the next chapter.

Student Resources

About.com Dermatology page: http://www.dermatology.about.com
Acne.com: http://www.acne.com
American Burn Association: http://www.ameriburn.org
DermIS (Dermatology Information System): http://dermis.net
HeadLice.org: http://www.headlice.org
Lyme Disease Foundation: http://www.lyme.org
Merck Manual Medical Library: http://www.merckmanuals.com/professional
National Eczema Association: http://www.nationaleczema.org
National Organization for Albinism and Hypopigmentation: http://www.albinism.org
National Psoriasis Foundation: http://www.psoriasis.org
Rosacea.org: http://www.rosacea.org

Chapter Activities

Learning Style Study Strategies

Try any or all of the following strategies as you study the content of this chapter:

Visual learners: Use your computer to find your own clip art, photos, or graphics to paste into your study notes. Create flash cards for diseases you don't have flash cards for.
Kinesthetic learners: Join a study group and actively participate. Have group members take turns presenting charades-like performances of key terms or diseases. Performances can be

improvisational or prepared ahead of time; they should be creative and fun. Give everyone permission to make mistakes and laugh. The sillier the performances are, the easier they will be to remember.

Auditory and verbal learners: Set content you need to remember—like disease descriptions and definitions of key terms—to simple, easily remembered tunes such as "Happy Birthday to You" or nursery-school songs.

Practice Exercises

Answers to Practice Exercises can be found in Appendix D.

Case Studies

CASE STUDY 1

A friend calls you with questions about her teenage son. She states that the skin on his feet is cracked, flaky, and red, especially between and around his toes. He complains of itching, stinging, and burning, and two of his toenails are soft and yellowish.

1. Based on this description, what disorder do you suspect he may have? (Your friend states that her son was playing with a stray cat recently, and she wonders if he caught ringworm from it.) What is your best response?

2. Your friend asks if there is any treatment that she can provide to her son at home. What is your best response?

CASE STUDY 2

An elderly woman is being cared for at home by her family members. Her adult daughter says she heard that bedsores can be a terrible problem for someone like her mother. She asks you what bedsores are and what causes them.

1. What is your best response?

2. The daughter asks what part of her mother's body is most vulnerable to ulcer formation. What do you tell her?

3. When she asks you what signs she should look for to catch an ulcer early, what do you tell her?

4. When she asks what measures she might take to prevent ulcer formation, what do you tell her?

CASE STUDY 3

A patient has come to see a health-care provider with complaints of calluses and corns on the feet. After providing treatment, the physician has asked you to educate the patient about measures that can reduce the risk of forming more calluses in the future. What will you tell the patient?

Multiple Choice

1. Which of the following terms is matched to the correct definition?

   a. Macule: small raised spot or bump on the skin, such as a mole

   b. Papule: clear, fluid-filled blister

   c. Wheal: rounded, temporary elevation in the skin that is white in the center with a red-pink periphery; accompanied by itching

   d. Nodule: large blister or skin vesicle filled with fluid

2. Which of the following is caused by a virus?

   a. Impetigo

   b. Warts

   c. Carbuncles

   d. Cellulitis

3. Which of the following disorders most affects skin pigmentation?

   a. Melasma

   b. Alopecia

   c. Paronychia

   d. Eczema

4. Which of the following is a bacterial infection transmitted by ticks?

   a. Scabies

   b. Pediculosis

   c. Tinea

   d. Lyme disease

5. A _____ is a thickened, hardened, toughened area of skin.

   a. Sebaceous cyst

   b. Callus

   c. Decubitus ulcer

   d. Paronychia

Short Answer

1. Explain the connection between chickenpox and shingles.

2. Describe the differences in signs and symptoms between decubitus ulcers of various stages.

3. Describe the differences between first-, second-, and third-degree burns.

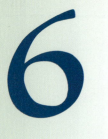

6 NEUROLOGICAL SYSTEM DISEASES AND DISORDERS

Learning Outcomes

Upon completion of this chapter, the student will be able to:

- Define and spell terms related to neurology
- Identify key structures of the neurological system
- Discuss the roles of structure and function played by the neurological system

- Identify characteristics of common neurological diseases and disorders, including:
  - description
  - incidence
  - etiology
  - signs and symptoms
  - diagnosis
  - treatment
  - prognosis

KEY TERMS	
ataxia	lack of coordination
aura	sensory warning prior to the onset of a migraine headache or a seizure
autonomic dysreflexia	serious nervous system response in those with spinal cord lesions to sensations that normally would be felt as painful; may progress to a stroke
bilateral	pertaining to both sides
bradykinesia	slow, hesitating pattern of movement
cognition	thinking that includes language use, calculation, perception, memory, awareness, reasoning, judgment, learning, intellect, social skills, and imagination
contrecoup	type of injury in which there is a rapid acceleration followed by deceleration, which throws the brain forward and backward within the skull
delirium	acute, reversible state of agitated confusion marked by disorientation, hallucinations, or delusions
dysphasia	difficulty speaking (expressive) or difficulty understanding (receptive) speech
exacerbation	aggravation of symptoms or increase in severity
hemiparalysis	one-sided paralysis
hemiparesis	altered sensation on one side of the body
ischemia	temporary deficiency in blood supply
neurotransmitter	chemical released by an axon terminal (end of a neuron) to inhibit or excite a target cell
nuchal rigidity	pain and stiffness of the neck with a resulting reluctance to flex the head forward
nystagmus	involuntary back-and-forth or circular eye movement

KEY TERMS—cont'd

paresthesia	altered sensation, such as numbness, stinging, or burning, that results from injury to nerves
phonophobia	sensitivity to sound
photophobia	sensitivity to light
tinnitus	ringing or other abnormal sounds in the ears
transient ischemic attacks (TIAs)	temporary strokelike symptoms caused by a brief interruption of blood supply to a part of the brain
unilateral	pertaining to one side

Abbreviations

Table 6-1 lists some of the most common abbreviations related to the neurological system.

Structures and Functions of the Nervous System

The nervous system plays a key role in maintaining homeostasis, the state of dynamic equilibrium in the internal environment of the body. More complex than the most advanced computer, the nervous system is capable of storing vast amounts of data as well as receiving and sending thousands of messages throughout the body instantly and simultaneously.

TABLE 6-1
ABBREVIATIONS

Abbreviation	Meaning	Abbreviation	Meaning
ALS	amyotrophic lateral sclerosis	HD	Huntington disease
ANS	autonomic nervous system	ICP	intracranial pressure
CNS	central nervous system	LP	lumbar puncture
CSF	cerebrospinal fluid	MMSE	Mini-Mental State Examination
CT	computed tomography	MS	multiple sclerosis
CTS	carpal tunnel syndrome	NCV	nerve conduction velocity
CVA	cerebrovascular accident	PNS	peripheral nervous system
EEG	electroencephalography	SCI	spinal cord injury
EMG	electromyography	TN	trigeminal neuralgia
GBS	Guillain-Barré syndrome		

Structures of the Nervous System

An understanding of the nervous system must begin with its most essential element, the neuron. While the nervous system functions as an integrated system, it is more easily understood when divided into its two major parts: the central nervous system (CNS) and the peripheral nervous system (PNS).

Flashpoint

The nervous system is divided into the central and peripheral nervous systems.

Neuron

A neuron includes a cell body, dendrites, and axons (see Fig. 6-1). The cell body houses the nucleus and organelles, which are a variety of specialized structures within the cell. Dendrites resemble branches coming off the cell body, much like the branches of a tree.

The axons of a neuron can be as short as a few millimeters or as long as a meter. They are cordlike projections sometimes covered in a myelin sheath made up of a specialized layer of cells. Neuron cell bodies grouped together form gray matter. Axons bundled together form white matter, named for the whitish hue of the myelin sheaths. Within the PNS, bundles of axons are called *nerves*.

Central Nervous System

The CNS comprises the brain and spinal cord. The brain weighs about 3 pounds and is divided into three major sections: the cerebrum, cerebellum, and brainstem (see Fig. 6-2). The cerebrum is the largest portion of the brain and lies within the forebrain. Its surface, called the *cortex*, is made up of gray matter and is characterized by deep folds and shallow grooves, which increase its surface area. The cerebral cortex, along with other areas of gray matter, is full of neurons as well as specialized

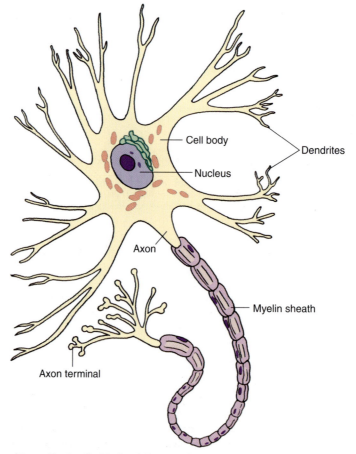

FIGURE 6-1 **Neuron** (From Eagle, S. *Medical Terminology in a Flash! An Interactive, Flash-Card Approach.* 2006. Philadelphia: F.A. Davis Company, with permission.)

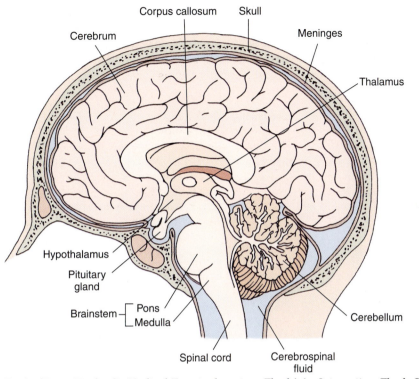

Corpus callosum   Skull

Cerebrum

Meninges

Thalamus

Hypothalamus

Pituitary
gland

Brainstem — Pons
            Medulla

Cerebellum

Spinal cord   Cerebrospinal
               fluid

FIGURE 6-2 Brain (From Eagle, S. *Medical Terminology in a Flash! An Interactive, Flash-Card Approach.* 2006. Philadelphia: F.A. Davis Company, with permission.)

support cells called *glia*. The cerebrum also contains white matter, which makes up the bulk of the tissue of the cerebral hemispheres. Buried in the white matter are special nuclei, called *basal ganglia*. The cerebrum is divided into two hemispheres, which are mostly separated by a deep groove but are joined by the corpus callosum.

The cerebellum is located in the lower posterior portion of the head. It is about the size of a fist and is shaped like a walnut. It is sometimes called the "little brain." Like that of the cerebrum, its surface has irregular ridges and folds. It has an outer cortex, inner white matter, and nuclei below the white matter. The brainstem runs from the forebrain to the spinal cord. Most of it is contained within the midbrain, which is located between the forebrain and the hindbrain. The brainstem includes the medulla oblongata and pons. The brain is enclosed and protected by the hard bones of the skull, known as the *cranium*.

The spinal cord extends from the base of the brain down to the second lumbar vertebra and is surrounded by the vertebral column. It is divided into sections that correspond to the vertebrae and paired spinal nerves. A cross section of the spinal cord reveals a butterfly-shaped inner core of gray matter, which contains nerve cell bodies. The gray matter is surrounded by white matter that forms ascending and descending pathways called *spinal tracts*.

The brain and the spinal cord are covered by three membranes called the *meninges*, which continue beyond the end of the spinal cord to the distal end of the sacrum. Cerebrospinal fluid—a colorless, clear fluid similar to blood plasma—is contained between layers of the meninges and circulates around the brain and spinal cord.

> **Flashpoint**
> The CNS includes the brain and spinal cord.

Peripheral Nervous System

The PNS includes 31 pairs of spinal nerves, 12 pairs of cranial nerves, and nerves in the arms and legs. (The cranial nerves are considered peripheral nerves.) Most are called *mixed* nerves because they are made up of sensory and motor neurons; however, some are only sensory or motor. The spinal nerves branch off from either side of the spinal cord between the vertebrae. Each spinal nerve is named for and corresponds to the vertebra above it. Spinal nerves are all mixed nerves.

An important part of the PNS is the autonomic nervous system (ANS), which controls involuntary functions. It consists of motor nerves leading to smooth muscle, cardiac muscle, and glands such as sweat and salivary glands. It is further divided into the sympathetic and parasympathetic nervous systems (see Fig. 6-3).

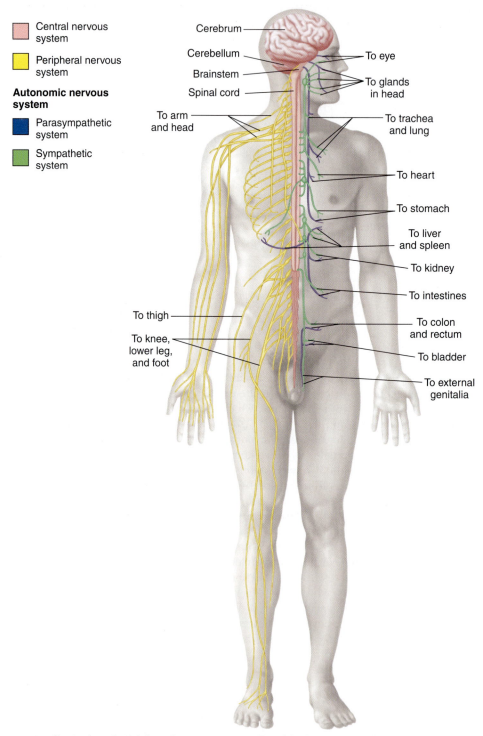

FIGURE 6-3 **Central and peripheral nervous systems with the autonomic nervous system** (From Eagle, S, et al. *The Professional Medical Assistant: An Integrative Teamwork-Based Approach.* 2009. Philadelphia: F.A. Davis Company, with permission.)

Functions of the Nervous System

The brain is a complex organ that allows humans to think, reason, express personality, and learn. It is an amazing organ capable of an incredible amount of multitasking. In simple terms, it stores a vast amount of data, processes a wealth of information, controls conscious thought, and keeps all autonomic (automatic) functions working all at the same time. The spinal cord acts as a messenger, sending information to the brain from the body and from the brain to the body. The functions of the nervous system are organized according to their location in the CNS or the PNS.

Neuron

Neurons work alone or in groups to sense internal and external environmental changes, transmit messages between the brain and body, initiate responses to help maintain the body's state of equilibrium, and facilitate voluntary movement. Dendrites of the neuron are actually extensions of the cell body, acting to sense changes in the body's internal environment by receiving information from other neurons or from sensory receptors and sending impulses to the main cell body. Axons are long, cordlike structures that transmit nerve impulses away from the cell body to other neurons, target organs, or muscles. The myelin sheath wrapped around each axon is composed of specialized cells made of a largely lipid substance that provides insulation to the axon, similar to the rubber covering on an electrical cord. The myelin sheath and the interspersed junctions, called *Ranvier's nodes*, allow the axon to function efficiently so that it can conduct impulses at an amazingly rapid rate.

Flashpoint
Neurons sense internal and external environmental changes.

Central Nervous System

The corpus callosum of the cerebrum serves to coordinate activity between the two hemispheres of the cerebrum. The convolutions of the cerebrum increase the surface area where nerve cell bodies are located, thus maximizing their function. The cerebral cortex, or gray matter, of the cerebrum is involved in sensory perception, emotions, and muscle control. The basal ganglia in the white matter of the cerebrum organize motor function. The cerebellum is responsible for posture, balance, and coordination. The brainstem is an essential pathway that conducts impulses between the brain and spinal cord. The cranium provides a strong, hard enclosure that protects the brain from injury.

The spinal cord is the pathway for sensory impulses to the brain from the rest of the body and motor impulses from the brain to the rest of the body. It also mediates the stretch, defecation, and urination reflexes. The vertebral column provides a bony structure to surround and protect the spinal cord. In conjunction with surrounding muscles, it also allows movement of the torso and provides an upright framework for the rest of the skeleton.

The meninges provide a supportive structure for many small blood vessels on the brain's surface. They also provide protection to the brain and spinal cord by housing the cerebrospinal fluid, which continuously circulates and provides a cushion to protect against injury from impact and sudden movement.

Flashpoint
The spinal cord acts as a pathway for information exchange between the brain and the body.

Peripheral Nervous System

In the PNS, the 12 pairs of cranial nerves originate in the brain and brainstem and innervate such structures as the eyes, ears, nose, face, tongue, and some muscles in the throat and neck (see Fig. 6-4).

A key function of the 31 pairs of spinal nerves is the innervation of the skin and muscles of the limbs. Specific areas of the skin associated with specific spinal nerves are called *dermatomes* (see Fig. 6-5). In some disorders, pain or other sensations caused by spinal-nerve injury are felt along the associated dermatome rather than at the actual site of injury. Thus, a patient suffering from spinal-nerve root compression sometimes feels pain or other symptoms in the arms or legs, rather than the back.

The ANS controls involuntary functions. Its motor nerves control smooth muscle, cardiac muscle, and glands such as sweat and salivary glands. Within the ANS, the sympathetic nervous system is responsible for the survival response known as the *fight-or-flight response.*

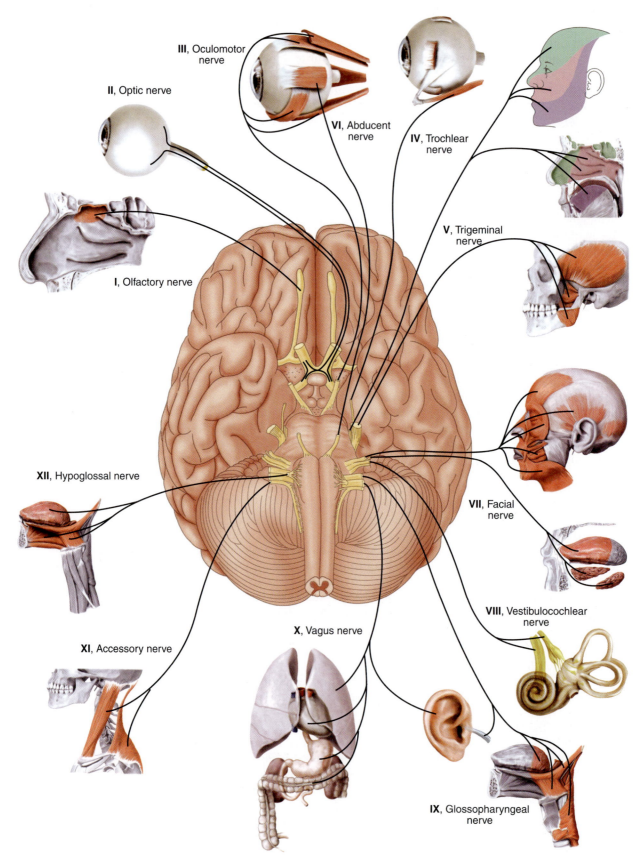

FIGURE 6-4 Cranial nerve locations and functions (From Eagle, S, et al. *The Professional Medical Assistant: An Integrative Teamwork-Based Approach.* 2009. Philadelphia: F.A. Davis Company, with permission.)

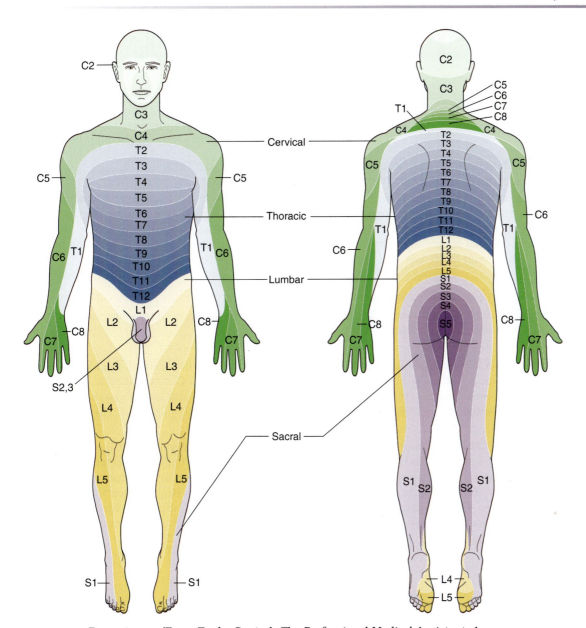

FIGURE 6-5 Dermatomes (From Eagle, S, et al. *The Professional Medical Assistant: An Integrative Teamwork-Based Approach.* 2009. Philadelphia: F.A. Davis Company, with permission.)

This response prepares a person for action, whether running from danger or responding in some other way. Physical changes within the body include increased heart rate and force, increased blood pressure, increased blood glucose levels, bronchodilation (expansion of airways), and decreased intestinal peristalsis (wavelike movement). These changes provide the body with increased energy and oxygen while slowing some functions (such as digestion) which are less important at the time. The parasympathetic nervous system essentially creates an opposite response and dominates during nonstressful times. Some of its effects include decreased heart rate, bronchoconstriction (narrowing of airways), and increased peristalsis.

Flashpoint

The autonomic nervous system controls automatic (involuntary) functions.

Diseases and Disorders of the Neurological System

This chapter discusses common disorders of the neurological system, which are grouped according to related causes or structures most commonly affected. In many cases, however, the causes are complex or not fully understood, and the disorders may affect multiple body systems.

Vascular Neurological System Diseases and Disorders

Vascular disorders are a major contributor to neurological dysfunction. They most commonly present in the form of a brain attack, commonly called a *stroke*. Less serious are *transient ischemic attacks* (TIAs), in which the person experiences temporary strokelike symptoms caused by a brief interruption of blood supply to a part of the brain. TIAs cause no permanent damage to the brain; however, they should be viewed as a warning sign that a future stroke is possible.

Stroke

ICD-9-CM: 434.91   [ICD-10: I61.9 (unspecified)]

A stroke, also called a *cerebrovascular accident (CVA)* or *brain attack,* is the sudden loss of neurological function due to vascular injury to the brain.

Incidence

More than 700,000 individuals suffer from strokes annually in the United States. At greatest risk are those over age 65 with a family history of cerebrovascular disease. Cerebrovascular disease is caused by atherosclerosis of cerebral arteries, which is the narrowing and loss of elasticity of vessels due to accumulation of fatty cholesterol deposits.

Etiology

Strokes are classified as hemorrhagic or ischemic. Hemorrhagic strokes occur when a vessel in the brain ruptures and bleeds. Risk factors for hemorrhagic strokes include hypertension; the presence of aneurysms, which are weak, bulging areas in a vessel; and arteriovenous malformations, which are abnormal clusters of tiny veins connected directly to tiny arteries without a capillary bed between. Strokes caused by *ischemia* (deficiency in blood supply) are further classified as thrombotic (caused by a blood clot—see Fig. 6-6) or embolic (caused by a substance in the

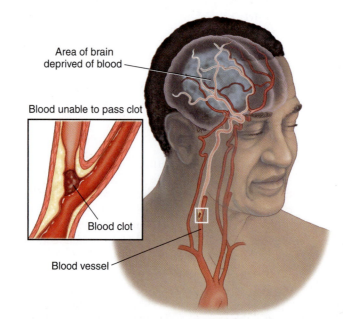

Area of brain
deprived of blood

Blood unable to pass clot

Blood clot

Blood vessel

FIGURE 6-6 Thrombotic stroke (From Eagle, S, et al. *The Professional Medical Assistant: An Integrative Teamwork-Based Approach.* 2009. Philadelphia: F.A. Davis Company, with permission.)

bloodstream that becomes lodged in a small vessel). Risk factors for ischemic stroke include cerebrovascular disease, atrial fibrillation (a type of heart irregularity), tobacco use, alcohol abuse, and clotting disorders.

Flashpoint
Strokes are either hemorrhagic or ischemic.

Signs and Symptoms

Signs and symptoms of stroke are variable depending on the extent of injury and the specific part of the brain affected. The patient usually exhibits symptoms on the opposite side of the body from the side of the brain injured. A left-sided stroke may cause right-sided paralysis or weakness, and a right-sided stroke may cause left-sided symptoms. Other symptoms are usually sudden in onset and may include vision loss or changes, *dysphasia* (difficulty speaking or understanding speech), dysphagia, severe headache, dizziness, confusion, altered consciousness, difficulty with gait (manner of walking) and balance, and *paresthesia* (altered sensation, such as numbness, stinging, or burning, that results from injury to nerves) and weakness on one side of the body.

Diagnosis

Diagnosis is suspected based on the patient's presenting signs and symptoms. Radiological studies such as computed tomography (CT), magnetic resonance imaging (MRI), and magnetic resonance angiography are used to confirm the diagnosis and differentiate hemorrhagic from ischemic strokes (see Box 6-1). In the case of a hemorrhagic stroke, a sample of cerebrospinal fluid (CSF) obtained by lumbar puncture (LP) may reveal the presence of blood.

Flashpoint
Signs and symptoms of stroke are highly variable.

Treatment

Treatment of ischemic strokes involves administration of thrombolytic and anticoagulant medications. Thrombolytics are powerful drugs that dissolve blood clots; anticoagulants are medications that delay or prevent blood-clot formation. Criteria for the use of thrombolytic agents are very strict: the drug must be started within a specific time frame, usually 3 hours or less from the onset of symptoms, and cannot be given to anyone at risk for hemorrhage. Anticoagulant medication protects the individual from another stroke while the body heals itself. Treatment of hemorrhagic stroke includes surgery to remove blood clots from the brain and repair identified aneurysms. Other treatment is individualized and depends on the type and severity of the stroke and on personal factors such as age and baseline health status. Extended hospitalization may be required. As the patient recovers and enters the rehabilitation phase, emphasis is placed on independent functioning in all activities of daily living, such as eating, bathing, toileting, dressing, and moving. The rehabilitation period commonly takes months.

Prognosis

Stroke is the third leading cause of death in the United States. It commonly produces long-term or permanent disability in those who survive. Common deficits include impairment of movement and speech. However, many individuals are able to recover significant function with the help of physical, occupational, and speech therapies.

Flashpoint
Stroke is a leading cause of death in the United States.

Transient Ischemic Attack

ICD-9-CM: 435.9 (transient cerebral ischemia, unspecified; various codes may be applicable, depending upon the specific site of the event)   **[ICD-10: G45.9 (unspecified)]**

A transient ischemic attack (TIA) is the temporary impairment of neurological functioning due to a brief interruption in blood supply to a part of the brain. Unlike with a stroke, impairment is only temporary in nature; neurological function is fully restored within minutes or hours.

Incidence

An estimated one-quarter of a million Americans experience a TIA each year. Rates are higher in Hispanic and African American populations.

Etiology

TIAs are commonly caused by tiny particles of atherosclerotic plaque or tiny blood clots that dislodge from a heart valve or artery wall and travel in the bloodstream to the brain. Because of their tiny size, they are quickly dissolved by the body's protective mechanisms before permanent damage results. Vascular spasm can also cause TIAs. Risk factors include cerebrovascular disease, tobacco use, alcohol abuse, hypertension, and clotting disorders.

(Text continued on page 144)

Box 6-1 Diagnostic Spotlight

COMPUTED TOMOGRAPHY, MAGNETIC RESONANCE IMAGING, AND LUMBAR PUNCTURE

Computed Tomography

Computed tomography (CT), sometimes called computed axial tomography (CAT) scanning, is a radiological imaging procedure that creates a three-dimensional image of the inner structures of a body part. It is based on the variable absorption of x-rays by different body tissues. During the test, the patient lies on a motorized table attached to the large, doughnut-shaped CT scanner. As the table slowly moves the patient through the large circular opening, the scanner creates thinly sliced images and saves them on a computer. Sometimes a contrast dye is administered to the patient by mouth, IV, or enema. The dye makes certain body structures stand out more clearly on the images.

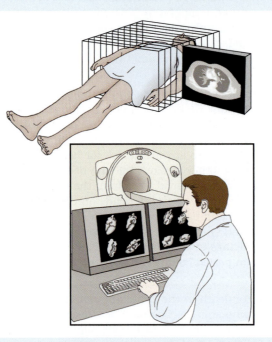

Computed tomography scan (From Eagle, S. *Medical Terminology in a Flash! An Interactive, Flash-Card Approach.* 2006. Philadelphia: F.A. Davis Company, with permission.)

Magnetic Resonance Imaging

Magnetic resonance imaging (MRI) is a radiological procedure that utilizes an electromagnetic field and radio waves to create visual images on a computer screen. This allows the creation of images of soft tissues of the central nervous and musculoskeletal systems that do not typically show up well on standard x-rays. During this procedure, the patient lies on a flat surface that moves inside a tube encompassing a large magnet. There is no discomfort for the patient other than the requirement to lie very still. The patient should be informed that hearing clicking and other sounds during the 60- to 90-minute procedure is normal. Note: This procedure may not be appropriate for patients with cardiac pacemakers or other devices in their bodies containing metal.

Box 6-1 Diagnostic Spotlight—cont'd

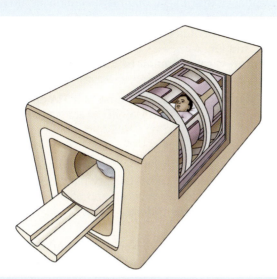

Patient undergoing an MRI scan (From Eagle, S, et al. *The Professional Medical Assistant: An Integrative Teamwork-Based Approach.* 2009. Philadelphia: F.A. Davis Company, with permission.)

Lumbar Puncture

Lumbar puncture (LP) is a procedure in which the physician punctures the subarachnoid space at the fourth intervertebral space. The procedure is done to obtain cerebrospinal fluid (CSF) for analysis or to administer drugs to the brain or spinal cord.

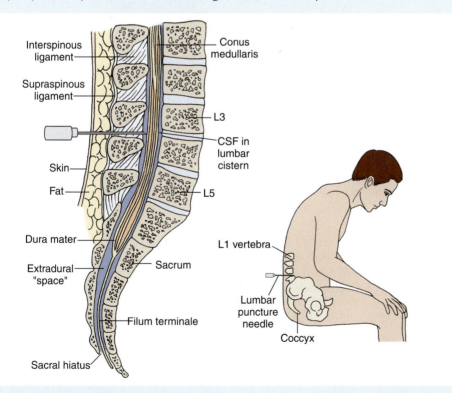

Lumbar puncture (From Eagle, S. *Medical Terminology in a Flash! An Interactive, Flash-Card Approach.* 2006. Philadelphia: F.A. Davis Company, with permission.)

Signs and Symptoms

Signs and symptoms of TIA are variable and temporary. They include one-sided weakness, paresthesia, vision changes or loss, dysphasia, dysphagia, dizziness, confusion, altered consciousness, and difficulty with gait and balance. Deficits usually resolve within minutes or hours; signs and symptoms may resolve by the time the patient is evaluated. Therefore, a careful history and description from the patient and any witnesses is essential. Because a TIA is viewed as a possible warning sign of a future stroke, it must be taken seriously.

Flashpoint

TIAs cause temporary stroke-like symptoms.

Diagnosis

Diagnostic testing is done to try to determine the cause of a TIA and may include MRI and CT scans to examine cerebral arteries. Carotid Doppler studies may identify carotid-artery narrowing.

Treatment

Treatment is aimed at preventing risk of stroke and may include anticoagulant medication, management of hypertension, and surgery to remove carotid-artery plaque. Patients are advised to reduce or eliminate modifiable risk factors such as tobacco and alcohol use, as well as lose weight and include regular exercise in their daily routine.

Prognosis

TIAs are self-limiting and resolve on their own. However, they should be viewed as a warning sign that the individual is at high risk of stroke—a leading cause of death in the United States.

Infectious Neurological System Diseases and Disorders

A variety of infectious disorders may impact the neurological system. In some cases they are contagious and directly caused by a known viral, bacterial, or other pathogenic agent; examples include meningitis, herpes zoster, and poliomyelitis. In other cases, such as with Guillain-Barré syndrome, the cause is less clear, but there is still compelling evidence that an infection of some type may play a role.

Encephalitis

ICD-9-CM: 323.01 (unspecified)   [ICD-10: A83.0–A86.0 (code by organism)]

Encephalitis is inflammation of the brain and is usually associated with meningitis, which is inflammation of the meninges. The two combined are known as *encephalomeningitis*.

Incidence

Encephalitis affects approximately 20,000 Americans each year.

Etiology

Encephalitis is most commonly caused by viruses, usually arboviruses (a group of viruses carried by insects, such as mosquitoes and ticks), herpesvirus, HIV, and viruses that cause influenza, measles, chickenpox, and rabies. Some types of fungi and protozoans may also be involved.

Flashpoint

Encephalitis is usually caused by a virus.

Signs and Symptoms

Patients with encephalitis may exhibit a wide variety of neurological symptoms, including seizures, fever, abnormal reflexes, muscle weakness, paralysis, and confusion. They may eventually lapse into a comatose state.

Diagnosis

Diagnosis is based on history and description of signs and symptoms. CSF is examined to determine the causative organism. Other diagnostic tests include CT and MRI scans.

Treatment

Treatment of encephalitis is aimed at the underlying cause. Antiviral medication is given for herpesvirus infections, and rabies is treated with rabies immune globulin and vaccine. In all cases treatment is supportive, focused on managing increased intracranial pressure (ICP) with diuretics and corticosteroids.

Prognosis

The prognosis for encephalitis depends on the timeliness of diagnosis and treatment. In many cases, rehabilitation and therapy is needed for the treatment of residual neurological deficits.

Meningitis

ICD-9-CM: 322.9 (unspecified)   [ICD-10: G00–G03 (code by organism)]

Meningitis is an infection of the meninges, the spinal cord, and CSF, and it is usually caused by an infectious illness.

Incidence

Between 5,000 and 15,000 Americans suffer from meningitis each year. Those at greatest risk include infants and children and those in the military or in dormitories. Other risk factors include a history of splenectomy, active and passive exposure to tobacco smoke, and exposure to those who are ill with meningitis.

Etiology

The cause of meningitis is usually viral or bacterial, although fungi, amoebas, and chemical irritation may also be causative factors. The most common infecting organisms include *Streptococcus pneumoniae* and *Neisseria meningitidis*. Fortunately, the practice of including the *Haemophilus influenzae (Hib)* vaccine with childhood immunizations has drastically reduced the incidence of *H. influenzae* meningitis. Some types of bacterial and viral meningitis are contagious and may be transmitted through exposure to large-droplet respiratory or oral secretions by coughing or kissing. Those who live in the same household or have close physical contact with infected people are at greatest risk; therefore, counseling about how to prevent disease transmission is important (see Box 6-2).

> **Flashpoint**
> Meningitis is usually caused by viral or bacterial infection.

Signs and Symptoms

Common signs and symptoms of meningitis include headache, high fever, **nuchal rigidity** (pain and stiffness of the neck with a resulting reluctance to flex the head forward), nausea, vomiting, **photophobia** (sensitivity to light), confusion, fatigue, and seizures. Many of these symptoms may not be obvious in infants, but notable symptoms may include loss of appetite, vomiting, irritability, and lethargy.

Diagnosis

Definitive diagnosis is based on examination of CSF, which may appear slightly cloudy due to increased white blood cells, protein, glucose, and bacteria. Most importantly, it will reveal the causative organism in cases of bacterial meningitis. Physical-examination findings may include signs and symptoms already described; a positive Kernig sign, which is

> **Flashpoint**
> Classic signs and symptoms of meningitis include headache, sensitivity to light, and a stiff, painful neck.

Box 6-2 Wellness Promotion

STOP THE BUGS

Those at risk for contracting or spreading infectious neurological diseases should be educated and reminded about the following precautions which will help to keep everyone healthier:

- Avoid intimate contact with anyone who has an infectious illness.
- Avoid areas with a high likelihood of infectious insects.
- Use insect repellent when in a high-risk area.
- Get the influenza vaccine every year.
- Stay at home if you have an infectious illness.
- Frequently and carefully clean areas in the home, such as the kitchen and bathroom, that are most likely to become contaminated.
- When you are ill, avoid public transportation where large numbers of people are confined to a small space, such as an airplane.

reflex contraction and pain in the hamstring muscles when attempting to extend the leg after flexing the hip; and a Brudzinski sign, in which neck flexion causes flexion of the hips when the patient is lying in a supine position. Deep-tendon reflexes are also increased.

Treatment

Treatment for meningitis must be aggressive to reduce the risk of death and disability. Differentiating bacterial from viral meningitis is important in determining the appropriate treatment and preventing transmission. Furthermore, identifying the specific causative organism in cases of bacterial meningitis is crucial in determining the appropriate antibiotic. Intravenous steroids reduce the risk of death and disability. Other medications may be given to reduce pain, fever, and seizure activity. The patient's room should be kept dark and quiet to reduce environmental stimuli. In the case of bacterial meningitis, those with close direct contact may be treated with antibiotics as a preventive measure.

Prognosis

Viral meningitis is usually less severe than bacterial meningitis, with a better prognosis. Bacterial meningitis has a greater risk of causing brain damage, disability, and even death. Mortality rates are between 10% and 40%, with the highest rates in the elderly. Between 11% and 19% of those who survive meningitis will suffer permanent deficits, such as hearing loss, mental retardation, and limb loss.

Brain Abscess

ICD-9-CM: 324.0   [ICD-10: G06.0]

A brain abscess is a collection of pus anywhere within the brain.

Incidence

Approximately 1,500 to 2,500 cases of brain abscess are reported annually in the United States. It most commonly occurs in people between the ages of 30 and 50, although it can happen to individuals of any age. At highest risk are those with weakened immune systems.

Etiology

Brain abscesses are caused by infection from a variety of sources and locations. Examples of local sources include infected head injuries and head-surgery sites, as well as infections in the ears, sinuses, and teeth; more distant sources can include infections within the lungs, heart, and kidneys. The causative organism is usually a streptococcus, but a variety of other bacteria, fungi, and even parasites may cause brain abscess.

Infection occurs when fungi or bacteria enter the brain tissue, usually through the bloodstream. Localized inflammation brings white blood cells to the site, and as they collect along with dead microorganisms and debris, the abscess grows. The area becomes enclosed within a membrane, which isolates the infection and protects the brain; however, the combination of the abscess with edema from inflammation increases pressure on the brain, which can impair circulation.

Flashpoint

Brain abscess is caused by infection within the brain.

Signs and Symptoms

Signs and symptoms of brain abscess may develop suddenly or slowly over 1 to 2 weeks. They include headache; aching and stiffness in the neck, shoulders, or back; vomiting; seizures; vision changes; fever and chills; weakness; *hemiparesis* (altered sensation on one side of the body); dysphasia; and changes in movement, coordination, and sensation. Mental-status changes include confusion, irritability, lethargy, and possible coma.

Diagnosis

Diagnosis of brain abscess is based upon the results of neurological examination and a variety of tests. Head CT and MRI will reveal a mass once the lesion has become encapsulated. Complete blood count may indicate an elevated white-blood-cell count. Blood cultures may reveal the causative organism if septicemia is the underlying cause; however, a needle biopsy of the abscess itself is the most accurate way to identify the organism involved.

Flashpoint

Brain abscess has a very high mortality rate and must be treated aggressively.

Treatment

Brain abscess is very serious and must be treated aggressively. Treatment includes intravenous antimicrobial medication and, in some cases, surgery to open and drain the infected material. Deep abscesses may be drained by needle aspiration. Increased ICP may be treated with corticosteroids and diuretics.

Prognosis

Untreated brain abscess has an extremely high mortality rate. However, those who receive appropriate treatment before coma occurs have an 80% to 95% chance of survival. Prognosis is poorer for those with multiple abscesses or abscess located deep within the brain. Possible complications include recurrent seizures, meningitis, recurrence of infection, and permanent neurological deficits.

Herpes Zoster
ICD-9-CM: 053.9   [ICD-10: B02.9] (without complications for both codes)

Outbreaks of herpes zoster, also called *shingles,* are caused by a reactivation of the varicella-zoster virus. After an initial outbreak of varicella (chickenpox), the varicella-zoster virus incorporates itself into nerve cells and lies dormant until it is reactivated years later. See Chapter 5 for a detailed description of herpes zoster.

Poliomyelitis
ICD-9-CM: 045.9   [ICD-10: A80.9 (acute unspecified)]

Poliomyelitis, also called *polio* and *infantile paralysis,* is an acute viral neurological infection. It has four variations, some of which lead to paralysis and some of which do not.

Incidence

Poliomyelitis was once common on a global level, with epidemics occurring during warm seasons. The number of poliomyelitis cases in the United States peaked during the 1950s. The disease has since essentially been eliminated within this country due to widespread vaccination programs. However, the continued importance of vaccination was highlighted by a case of imported polio in 2005 in an unvaccinated American who had traveled overseas. Small outbreaks continue to occur in countries throughout the world. Most vulnerable are those who are very young, very old, or pregnant, and those whose immune systems are suppressed. Global elimination of the disease is estimated to be 99% complete; the goal is total eradication.

Etiology

Poliomyelitis is caused by the poliovirus and is spread by direct contact with an infected person or contact with infected respiratory secretions or feces. The virus enters through the nose, mouth, and multiplies within the intestines. The virus is then absorbed through the intestinal wall into the bloodstream and travels to the central nervous system.

Signs and Symptoms

Most individuals infected with poliovirus are asymptomatic (free of symptoms), but some develop nausea, vomiting, anorexia, abdominal pain, fever, headache, or paralysis of one or more extremities. If respiratory muscles are affected, individuals may also experience respiratory failure. Some people develop postpolio syndrome as many as 20 to 40 years later. This syndrome is evidenced by a recurrence of fatigue and weakness that involves the same muscle groups originally affected. Individuals with nonparalytic poliomyelitis may also develop back and leg pain, nuchal rigidity, severe headache, and meningitis.

Flashpoint
Poliomyelitis causes paralysis in some individuals.

Diagnosis

Diagnosis of poliomyelitis is based on a combination of diagnostic tests, the patient's report of symptoms, and neurological-examination findings. Stool and throat cultures and specimens of CSF are tested for the presence of the virus. Serum is tested for the presence of antibodies.

Treatment

There is no cure for poliomyelitis; therefore, treatment is supportive. Analgesics are given for head and body aches. Respiratory function is supported as needed (some individuals may require mechanical ventilation). Physical therapy helps patients to maintain flexibility and muscle function. Other care is aimed at meeting nutritional needs and promoting bowel and bladder function.

Prognosis

Prognosis is generally good, depending upon how extensive the disease and symptoms are and whether diagnosis and treatment are timely and appropriate. Paralysis occurs in less than 5% of individuals, and full recovery may occur. Death is rare but possible.

Reye Syndrome
ICD-9-CM: 331.81   **[ICD-10: G93.7]**

Reye syndrome is a serious disease associated with aspirin use by children with viral illnesses. It can result in permanent brain damage or even death. See Chapter 4 for a detailed description of Reye syndrome.

Tetanus
ICD-9-CM: 037.9   **[ICD-10: A35] (tetanus for both codes)**

Tetanus, also known as *lockjaw*, is a noncontagious illness marked by severe, prolonged spasm of skeletal muscle fibers. See Chapter 4 for a detailed description of tetanus.

Guillain-Barré Syndrome
ICD-9-CM: 357.0   **[ICD-10: G61.0]**

Guillain-Barré syndrome (GBS), also known as *acute inflammatory demyelinating polyneuropathy*, is an acute inflammatory disorder causing rapidly progressing paralysis, which is usually temporary, and sometimes also sensory symptoms.

> **Flashpoint**
> GBS causes rapidly progressing paralysis that is usually temporary.

Incidence
Guillain-Barré syndrome is a rare disorder that affects as many as 6,000 Americans each year. It affects individuals of all ages and all races, men slightly more often than women.

Etiology
The exact cause of GBS is not well understood. In approximately 60% of cases, a viral infection such as influenza, the common cold, an intestinal viral infection, viral hepatitis, HIV, or mononucleosis precedes the disorder by 2 to 4 weeks, but the connection is not clear. Other possible triggers include Hodgkin disease and surgery. There is speculation that GBS may be related to an autoimmune response in which the myelin sheath becomes eroded.

Signs and Symptoms
The typical pattern of GBS includes onset and worsening of signs and symptoms over a period of approximately 2 weeks. These signs and symptoms include weakness, paresthesia, and ascending paralysis that may reach as high as the chest. This impairs the individual's ability to breathe in 30% of cases; these patients may require mechanical ventilation. Other signs and symptoms include difficulty speaking or swallowing, urinary retention, alteration in heart rate (rapid or slow), and alteration in blood pressure (high or low). Severe pain may be felt in the back, buttocks, thighs, or shoulder girdle. Less-common forms of GBS may cause descending paralysis or even **hemiparalysis** (one-sided paralysis). Symptoms usually peak within 3 to 4 weeks, plateau for several days, and then gradually improve.

> **Flashpoint**
> Some individuals with GBS require temporary mechanical ventilation.

Diagnosis
Diagnosis may be difficult, due to the different ways in which GBS can present and the variability of symptoms. Several different tests are performed to reach a diagnosis. Study of CSF reveals increased protein level in 90% of cases without an increase in white blood cells. This test may be repeated, since protein level generally peaks several weeks after the onset of symptoms. Electromyography (EMG) and nerve conduction-velocity (NCV) studies reveal a slowing of nerve impulses in muscle tissue (see Box 14-7 in Chapter 14). Respiratory function tests may be done to determine the degree of respiratory-muscle compromise and help determine whether mechanical ventilation is needed. Occasionally, muscle biopsy is done to differentiate GBS from other disorders.

Treatment
There is no known cure for GBS; however, treatment is available which reduces the severity and duration of symptoms. Plasmapheresis, also called plasma exchange, is a procedure in which the patient's blood is filtered or cleansed of the harmful antibodies. An alternative treatment is IV administration of immunoglobulin that contains healthy donor antibodies, which are thought to block the action of the patient's harmful antibodies. These treatments shorten peak symptom time by as much as 50%. Patients often require supportive care, which includes hospitalization for respiratory and nutritional care. Physical therapy may be initiated to preserve muscle function and joint mobility.

Prognosis

Approximately 80% to 85% of those with GBS recover fully within 6 to 18 months. Others suffer some degree of chronic weakness or altered sensation. Mortality rate is approximately 5%, usually related to respiratory complications. Relapse may occur in as many as 10% of cases.

Degenerative Neurological System Diseases and Disorders

A number of neurological diseases and disorders are chronic and degenerative. This means that there is no identified cure and that the signs and symptoms worsen over time. Examples include Parkinson disease, multiple sclerosis, amyotrophic lateral sclerosis (ALS), some forms of dementia, and Huntington disease.

Parkinson Disease
ICD-9-CM: 332.0   [ICD-10: G20.0]

Parkinson disease is a chronic degenerative disease of the central nervous system that results in movement disorders and changes in *cognition* and mood. Cognition is thinking that includes language use, calculation, perception, memory, awareness, reasoning, judgment, learning, intellect, social skills, and imagination.

Incidence

Parkinson disease affects 1.5 million Americans, is most common in patients over age 65, and is more common in men than women.

Etiology

The cause of Parkinson disease is not fully understood; however, the disease does tend to cluster in families. The symptoms are caused by a deficiency of dopamine, which is a type of *neurotransmitter,* a chemical released by an axon terminal (end of a neuron) to inhibit or excite a target cell. Neurotransmitters play an important role in nerve-impulse transmission. With a deficiency in these neurotransmitters, nerve impulses are transmitted less efficiently.

Flashpoint
Symptoms of Parkinson disease are caused by a deficiency in dopamine.

Signs and Symptoms

Early symptoms of Parkinson disease include gradual onset of aching and fatigue in the extremities, followed by resting hand tremor. Generalized muscle rigidity and classic, pill-rolling tremor of the hands becomes prominent. The face develops a masklike, inexpressive appearance and the voice becomes softer and quieter. *Bradykinesia,* a slow, hesitating pattern of movement, develops. In addition, the individual begins exhibiting a shuffling gait that tends to speed out of control. Posture becomes stooped, with the neck bent forward (see Fig. 6-7). The individual experiences difficulty initiating movements, such as standing up or turning over in bed. Dysphagia (difficulty swallowing) is common, and difficulty in managing oral secretions may eventually cause drooling. In some cases, mental slowing or even dementia also occurs.

Diagnosis

Diagnosis of Parkinson disease is based upon presenting signs and symptoms and neurological-evaluation findings. Dopamine levels in urine may be decreased.

Treatment

There is no known cure for Parkinson disease. Medical treatment includes dopamine agonists such as levodopa-carbidopa (Sinemet). Other medications may be given to reduce oral secretions, tremor, and muscle rigidity. A multidisciplinary team approach is required to help the patient and family cope with this disabling disease.

Prognosis

Because Parkinson disease is a progressive, degenerative disorder with no known cure, the outlook may be disheartening for those affected. Average life expectancy from the time of diagnosis is 10 years. However, many individuals live much longer and, with supportive care, are able to maintain a good quality of life.

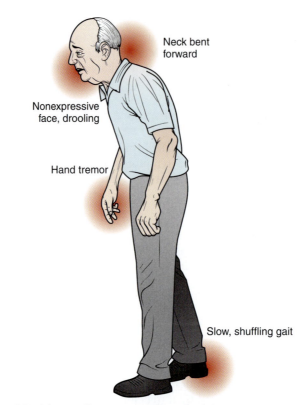

Neck bent forward

Nonexpressive face, drooling

Hand tremor

Slow, shuffling gait

FIGURE 6-7 **Effect of Parkinson disease on gait and posture**

Multiple Sclerosis
ICD-9-CM: 340   [ICD-10: G35]

Multiple sclerosis (MS) is a chronic autoimmune disease in which there is destruction of myelin and nerve axons within several regions of the brain and spinal cord. There are several different types of MS; the most common is the relapsing-remitting type, which affects 85% of patients with MS. It is characterized by increasingly frequent attacks in which the individual experiences *exacerbation* (aggravation of symptoms or increase in severity) of symptoms alternating with periods of remission.

Incidence

Approximately 500,000 people in the United States have been diagnosed with MS. It is twice as common in women than men, with typical onset between the ages of 20 and 40. It is more common among those living in cold climates.

Etiology

The cause of MS is not fully understood, although there is thought to be an autoimmune basis. Autoimmune diseases occur when the body's immune system loses the ability to distinguish self cells from nonself cells. As a result, the immune system attacks the body's own misidentified cells and tissues. In the case of multiple sclerosis, the central nervous system is affected, resulting in inflammation and degeneration of the myelin sheath that protects nerve fibers (see Fig. 6-8). Attacks are usually episodic, resulting in repetitive episodes of disrupted nerve-impulse conduction. Triggers for MS include infections, viruses, and pregnancy. There is a familial component; children of patients with MS are 15 times more likely to develop MS than the average person.

Signs and Symptoms

Symptoms of MS vary widely and may include weakness, fatigue, muscle spasms, altered gait, tremors, bowel and bladder dysfunction, sexual dysfunction, vertigo, *tinnitus* (ringing or other abnormal sounds in the ears), hearing loss, visual changes, altered sensation, dysphasia, dysphagia, anxiety, mood fluctuations, deficits in short-term memory, inattentiveness, and impaired judgment.

Flashpoint

The most common form of MS is the relapsing-remitting type.

Flashpoint

Symptoms of MS are caused by degeneration of the myelin sheath on nerves.

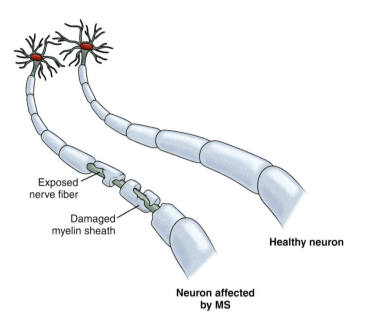

Exposed
nerve fiber

Damaged
myelin sheath

Healthy neuron

**Neuron affected
by MS**

FIGURE 6-8 **Damage to the myelin sheath on neurons causes many of the symptoms of multiple sclerosis.**

Diagnosis

Diagnosing MS commonly takes time because the symptoms are intermittent and variable, and other disorders must be ruled out. This process can feel frustrating to patients. Diagnostic studies include MRI and CT scans, which indicate the presence of MS plaques.

Treatment

There is currently no cure for MS. Acute exacerbations may be treated with corticosteroids. Some medications may reduce the frequency and severity of relapses for some types of MS; they are expensive, though, and not effective in every case. Therefore, therapy must be individualized. Patients with MS must develop a plan of self-care in which the focus is protection of the immune system. Regular, moderate exercise; good nutrition; adequate rest; and stress management are all key components of such a plan.

Prognosis

Prognosis for patients with MS varies and depends on the type of MS involved. Typically, life expectancy is 7 years less than that of the general population.

Amyotrophic Lateral Sclerosis
ICD-9-CM: 335.20   [ICD-10: G12.2]

Amyotrophic lateral sclerosis (ALS), also called *Lou Gehrig disease,* is a chronic, progressive, degenerative neuromuscular disorder that destroys motor neurons of the body.

Incidence

ALS affects approximately 30,000 Americans, with nearly 6,000 new cases diagnosed each year. Men are affected more than women, and whites are more commonly affected than other races. Typical onset is between the ages of 40 and 70.

Etiology

The cause of ALS is unclear, although there is one form of ALS, affecting approximately 10% of ALS patients, that is hereditary.

Signs and Symptoms

ALS affects the motor nerves of the body and usually leaves sensory nerves and cognitive function intact. The typical course involves muscle weakness and fatigue that begins in the extremities and progresses to the trunk and head. It eventually affects respiratory muscles and muscles of the head, neck, and face. As a result, individuals become progressively paralyzed and eventually experience difficulty with breathing, speech, and swallowing.

Flashpoint

Management of MS is focused on immune protection and health-maintenance activities.

Flashpoint

ALS causes progressive muscle weakness leading to eventual paralysis.

Diagnosis

There is no specific diagnostic test for ALS; the diagnosis is achieved by ruling out other disorders. A thorough neurological evaluation and medical history are required. EMG and NCV may reveal muscle fasciculation (visible, involuntary twitching of muscle fibers) and fibrillation (quivering or spontaneous contraction of muscle fibers). Muscle biopsy reveals atrophy (wasting).

Treatment

There is currently no cure for ALS. Survival time may be extended by the use of riluzole (Rilutek), a medication approved for the treatment of ALS. The focus of care is on support and palliation, with the goal of helping the individual to maintain an optimal level of independent function. Palliative care is care that attempts to relieve pain and suffering but does not provide a cure. Priority must be given to protecting respiratory function. Medications may be used to decrease muscle spasticity, relieve pain, and reduce oral secretions. A multidisciplinary approach to care is essential and should involve the patient, patient's family, physician, nurses, medical assistants, therapists, case managers, and hospice workers. The patient and family should be given information about community resources, support groups, and advance directives.

Prognosis

Flashpoint

Life expectancy for those with ALS is only about 5 years from diagnosis.

Life expectancy is only about 5 years from the time of diagnosis. Death is usually due to respiratory complications.

Dementia
ICD-9-CM: 290–294   [ICD-10: F00–F09 (code by complication, delirium, depression)]

Dementia, sometimes called *senility,* is a progressive neurological disorder with numerous causes, in which an individual suffers an irreversible decline in cognition due to disease or brain damage. Some forms of dementia are chronic, progressive, and ultimately fatal. Dementia is marked by deficits in reasoning and judgment, and it progressively impairs a person's ability to participate in occupational and social activities.

Incidence

Dementia has numerous causes, which makes it difficult to estimate the actual incidence. The most common type, Alzheimer dementia, is estimated to affect between four and five million Americans. However, experts estimate that by the year 2050, the number may increase to 14 million. This disorder costs nearly $100 billion each year in direct and indirect health-care costs.

Flashpoint

Alzheimer dementia is the most common form of dementia.

Dementia is most common among those over age 65, and prevalence approaches 40% to 50% among those over age 85. The early-onset type of Alzheimer dementia is familial and affects individuals between the ages of 30 and 60.

Etiology

Causes of dementia vary with the specific type. Alzheimer disease is responsible for over 60% of dementia cases. Its cause is not well understood, although it is known to involve progressive loss of brain-cell function. Contributing factors include advanced age, genetics, some viruses, previous brain injuries from head trauma or minor stroke, cardiovascular disease, severe deficiency of vitamin B_{12} and folate, brain infection, diabetes, and immunologic factors (see Box 6-3). Characteristic changes in the brain of those affected by Alzheimer disease include cerebral atrophy and degenerative changes to neurons. The affected neurons include *neuritic plaques,* which are accumulations of bundled fibers surrounding normal and damaged nerve cells in the brain, and *neurofibrillary tangles,* which are a distortion of neurofibrils that make up part of the nerve cell body. Patients with Alzheimer disease also experience a significant decrease in levels of neurotransmitters such as acetylcholine.

Flashpoint

Depression and delirium are sometimes confused with dementia.

Vascular dementia, also known as *multi-infarct dementia,* develops when brain cells die because of one or more infarcts (strokes). Other disorders that may cause dementia include alcoholism, Pick disease, Huntington disease, Parkinson disease, hypothyroidism, syphilis, and AIDS. In addition, some other disorders such as depression and ***delirium*** (acute, reversible state of agitated confusion marked by disorientation, hallucinations, or delusions) are commonly confused with dementia because the signs and symptoms are similar (see Box 6-4).

Box 6-3 Wellness Focus

PREVENTING ALZHEIMER DISEASE

You can preserve and protect your brain function and reduce your risk of developing Alzheimer disease by doing the following:

- Avoiding the use of tobacco and illicit drugs
- Avoiding lead exposure
- Avoiding chronically high levels of stress
- Maintaining a healthy blood pressure
- Managing diabetes effectively
- Following all recommended measures to prevent heart disease (which help protect the brain, too)
- Pursuing educational or mentally stimulating activities
- Exercising regularly
- Participating in social activities

Signs and Symptoms

The pattern of onset of dementia depends upon the type and cause. Signs and symptoms of Alzheimer dementia begin gradually and progress slowly. The following three stages have been identified:

- Stage I is characterized by progressive short-term memory loss.
- Stage II is characterized by deterioration of intellectual ability, personality changes, speech and language problems, impaired judgment, and continued worsening of memory, as well as possible paranoia, delusions, hallucinations, seizures, and depression.
- Stage III marks the patient's total dependence on others for care and can also include paranoia, delusions, hallucinations, seizures, and depression.

Diagnosis

Diagnosis of dementia is based upon history, neurological-examination findings, presenting signs and symptoms, and results of a variety of tests. Cognitive screening tests, such as the Mini-Mental State Examination (MMSE), may be used to evaluate short-term memory and reasoning. A variety of blood tests may be done to rule out treatable disorders such as those related to nutritional deficiencies. CT or MRI may be done to rule out stroke or brain lesions. There is no definitive test for Alzheimer disease other than autopsy; therefore, diagnosis is identified by noting the characteristic signs, symptoms, and progression and by ruling out all other causes.

Treatment

Treatment of dementia is aimed at the underlying cause, although in most cases there is no known cure. Cholinesterase inhibitors may temporarily enhance cognitive function by preventing the breakdown of acetylcholine. However, the effectiveness of these medications decreases after several months. Other medications including antipsychotics, antidepressants, anxiolytics, and benzodiazepines are sometimes used to help with behavioral problems associated with the disease.

Other treatment measures aim to maximize function and provide safety and comfort. Patients with early dementia may respond to efforts to reorient them to time and place; this strategy becomes less effective, though, as dementia progresses. Support resources for patients with Alzheimer disease and their families are available, including adult day services, respite care, support groups, and home health-care services. In addition, caregivers should be counseled on making the home environment safer for the patient with Alzheimer disease or other forms of dementia (see Box 6-5).

Flashpoint

Because there is no cure for dementia, treatment is aimed at promoting safety and quality of life.

Prognosis

There is no cure for Alzheimer disease or most other types of dementia. Therefore, care is focused on promoting safety and quality of life and on providing information and support to the

Box 6-4 Conditions Confused with Dementia

Dementia is sometimes confused with other states, including delirium and depression. Adverse effects of medications are also sometimes mistaken for signs of dementia. Therefore, careful evaluation is necessary to rule out other causes and determine an appropriate treatment plan.

By comparing features of delirium and depression, one can differentiate them from dementia. The table below outlines each disorder, along with its definition; onset, course, and duration; and effects on memory, thought processes, perception, psychomotor behaviors, and sleep patterns.

Disorder and Definition	Onset, Course, and Duration	Effects
dementia Neurological disorder characterized by chronic, progressive, irreversible decline in mental function	*Onset:* slow *Course:* long *Duration:* years	*Memory:* short-term memory loss in early stages and remote memory loss in later stages *Thought processes:* impaired judgment, difficulty finding words, difficulty performing familiar tasks *Perception:* usually no effects *Psychomotor behaviors:* usually no effects in the early stages *Sleep patterns:* impairment and fragmentation
delirium Acute, reversible state of agitated confusion marked by disorientation, hallucinations, or delusions	*Onset:* sudden *Course:* short, fluctuating, and commonly worse at night *Duration:* hours to days, usually less than 1 month	*Memory:* possible impairment of immediate and recent memory *Thought processes:* distortion and disorganization; easy distracting from tasks *Perception:* distortion, delusions, and hallucinations *Psychomotor behaviors:* possible alternation between hyperactivity (agitation, combative behavior) and hypoactivity (inattention, inability to follow directions or converse) *Sleep patterns:* impairment, with day and night cycles commonly reversed
depression Mood disorder marked by loss of interest or pleasure in living	*Onset:* slow *Course:* slow *Duration:* weeks to years	*Memory:* variable effect, with episodes of poor memory mixed with clear memory *Thought processes:* bleak outlook, apathy, difficulty focusing on tasks *Perception:* usually no effects *Psychomotor behaviors:* usually no effects *Sleep patterns:* impairment; possibly too little or too much sleep, commonly involving early morning awakenings

Box 6-5 Wellness Focus

HOME SAFETY FOR PATIENTS WITH DEMENTIA
Family members and caregivers of patients with dementia can follow these tips to provide a safe environment for their loved one:

- Keep doors and windows locked.
- Install safety latches on cabinets and drawers that contain objects such as knives.
- Lock up firearms or remove them from the home.
- Install protective gates at the top and bottom of stairs.
- Supervise the ingestion of all medications.
- Keep car keys in a locked cupboard.
- Place night-lights throughout the home, especially in the bedroom and bathroom.
- Keep walkways clear.

caregiver. Life expectancy for patients with Alzheimer disease is variable but averages 8 to 10 years from the onset of symptoms. Death is due not to the disease itself but to its complications, most commonly including infection of various types (such as pneumonia) and immobility and injury associated with falls.

Huntington Disease
ICD-9-CM: 333.4   [ICD-10: G10]
Huntington disease (HD), also called *Huntington chorea*, is an inherited progressive degenerative neurological disease that results in physical and mental decline. It was first studied in the late 1800s by a physician named George Huntington, who used the Greek term *chorea*, which means "dance," to refer to the typical involuntary, jerky movements made by individuals with this disease.

Incidence
Estimates of the incidence of HD vary widely between 1,500 and 30,000 for the United States. Incidence varies by region and ethnicity, with highest rate in those of Western European descent. Onset is usually in the mid-40s but may occur at any age.

Etiology
HD is inherited and is caused by an identified abnormal gene that is passed from either parent to the child. The likelihood of developing HD is 50% when one parent has the gene.

Signs and Symptoms
The first symptom of HD is difficulty controlling physical movements, which become progressively jerky and unpredictable. Gait and balance are increasingly impaired, and the individual walks in a progressively unsteady and staggering manner. Difficulties in speech, chewing, and swallowing begin to occur, putting the individual at risk of choking as well as nutritional deficits. Mental functioning becomes impaired, and as dementia progresses, memory and judgment become faulty. Psychiatric symptoms also develop, which may include depression, anxiety, irritability, aggressiveness, compulsiveness, and worsening of any addictive behaviors that might already be present.

Flashpoint

HD is inherited and is progressive, degenerative, and eventually fatal.

Diagnosis
The diagnostic process for HD includes a combination of medical history, neurological examination, and diagnostic tests. MRI or CT may reveal changes within the brain. DNA analysis may reveal the defective gene.

Treatment
There is no cure for Huntington disease. Treatment is therefore aimed at providing safety and promoting quality of life for the patient. Education and emotional support are important for both patient and caregivers. Medications including antipsychotics and antidepressants may be used to treat psychiatric symptoms and movement disorders. Nutritional needs must be met by ensuring adequate intake of calories, vitamins, and minerals, as well as adapting food to meet the individual's declining chewing and swallowing ability.

Prognosis

The prognosis for HD is extremely grim. Life expectancy from onset varies between 15 and 25 years. Symptoms progress until death, which is usually the result of a complication such as respiratory infection, choking, malnutrition, or injury from a fall. The suicide rate varies from 7% to 27%.

Neurological System Disorders Caused by Trauma

Traumatic injury is an all-too-common cause of neurological injury. Some injuries can cause death or leave the individual with profound, life-changing physical, mental, or emotional challenges. Examples include skull fractures that cause hematoma, concussion, or contusion and spinal cord injuries that may leave the victim with permanent paralysis. Other types of disorders caused by less traumatic events or by damage from repetitive activities, while rarely life-threatening, still pose significant challenges of chronic pain or dysfunction. Examples include carpal tunnel syndrome and herniated disks.

Cerebral Concussion and Contusion

ICD-9-CM: 850.00–850.91 (concussion; code by LOC and duration), 851.00–851.09 (contusion; code by wound site and LOC)   **[ICD-10: S06.0 (concussion), S06.2 (diffuse brain injury, NOS)]**

Cerebral concussion is a vague term which refers to a brief loss of consciousness or episode of disorientation or confusion following a head injury. Cerebral contusion refers to bruising of brain tissue and is therefore the more severe of the two injuries.

Flashpoint

More than 1.5 million Americans suffer traumatic brain injury each year.

Incidence

More than 1.5 million Americans suffer from traumatic brain injury each year. Fortunately, approximately 75% of these cases involve only mild concussion. The incidence of head injury is greatest in adolescents, elderly patients, men, and African Americans.

Etiology

The most common cause of cerebral concussion and contusion is a blow to the head or a ***contrecoup*** type of injury, in which there is rapid acceleration followed by deceleration, which throws the brain forward and backward within the skull (see Fig. 6-9). As a result, delicate brain tissue and small vessels may be torn by force or cut by sharp protrusions within parts of the skull.

Signs and Symptoms

Cerebral concussion usually results in a brief episode of loss of consciousness, confusion, or disorientation. Other temporary symptoms may include headache, drowsiness, and visual changes. The symptoms of contusion are generally more severe, due to tiny cerebral hemorrhages and edema, and include more prolonged loss of consciousness, vomiting, and memory problems.

Diagnosis

Diagnosis is based on neurological-evaluation findings and the patient's report of symptoms. A CT scan is recommended for those with loss of consciousness lasting more than 1 minute and those with deteriorating neurological status. A CT scan revealing a salt-and-pepper appearance caused by tiny hemorrhages confirms the diagnosis of cerebral contusion. Spinal films should also be done to rule out spinal injury.

Treatment

Treatment of mild concussion is conservative and usually involves rest and analgesics. Treatment of severe concussion and cerebral contusion is more aggressive; hospitalization is usually required. The focus of care is on reducing and managing ICP, which can contribute to further brain injury if it rises too high.

Flashpoint

Individuals suffering from postconcussion syndrome experience depression, dizziness, and memory difficulties.

Prognosis

Prognosis for those with mild concussion is good. Those with more severe concussion may develop postconcussion syndrome, which includes memory problems, depression, and dizziness. The prognosis for cerebral contusion is more guarded, with a risk of escalating ICP and microhemorrhages progressing to hematoma. In either case, compression of the brain increases the risk of further injury, with a higher likelihood of permanent neurological deficit.

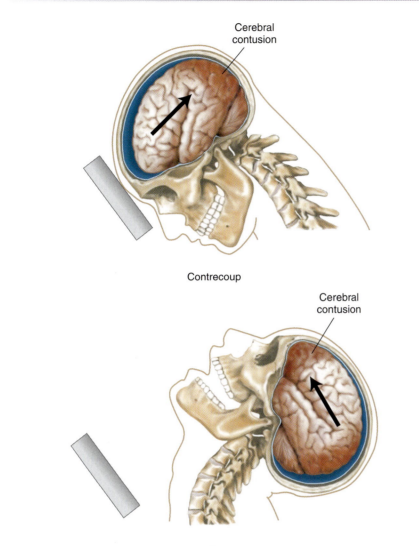

Cerebral
contusion

A

Contrecoup

Cerebral
contusion

B

Coup

FIGURE 6-9 Impact on the brain in a contrecoup injury (From Eagle, S, et al. *The Professional Medical Assistant: An Integrative Teamwork-Based Approach.* 2009. Philadelphia: F.A. Davis Company, with permission.)

Spinal Cord Injury

ICD-9-CM: 344.0 (quadriplegia,   [ICD-10: G82.2 (paraplegia, unspecified),
unspecified), 344.1   G82.5 (quadriplegia, unspecified)]

Spinal cord injury (SCI) involves traumatic bruising, crushing, or tearing of the spinal cord. Transection (cutting across) of the spinal cord may be partial or complete, depending on the mechanism of injury (means by which injury occurred).

Incidence

Approximately 14,000 individuals in the United States suffer from acute SCI each year, and another 300,000 to 400,000 are living with some degree of chronic disability as a result of SCI. More than 80% of acute SCI patients are young white men. Alcohol or mood-altering drugs are a factor in more than half of all spinal cord injuries.

Etiology

The cause of SCI is some type of traumatic force, most commonly a motor vehicle accident. Other causes include violence in the form of shootings and stabbings, falls, and injuries from sports such as diving and football.

Signs and Symptoms

Initial signs and symptoms of SCI include loss of function, sensation, and reflexes below the site of the injury. However, with time and medical care, some return of function may occur. The degree of permanent deficit is widely variable and depends on the location, extent, and nature of the injury. Some individuals with relatively minor injury may regain full function, while others may be left with permanent paralysis.

Diagnosis

Diagnosis of SCI is based upon neurological-evaluation findings and radiological studies, including x-rays of the spine, CT, or MRI, any of which may reveal vertebral fractures, hematoma, spinal cord compression, and other injuries.

Treatment

Treatment involves stabilization of the patient in the emergency department, followed by transfer to the critical-care unit. The spinal cord and vertebrae may require stabilization by application of Gardner-Wells tongs and traction (see Fig. 6-10). This protects the spinal cord from further damage until the patient is deemed stable enough for surgery. During surgery, bone fragments and hematomas are removed and the spine is stabilized through spinal fusion, which is the surgical immobilization of adjacent vertebrae by grafting of bone or insertion of hardware. Subsequently, application of a halo traction brace may enable increased mobility (see Fig. 6-11).

Prognosis

Victims of SCI often suffer profound, life-altering injury as well as severe emotional trauma. Long-term prognosis varies and depends on the location, type, and severity of injury. In general, the higher the injury on the spinal cord, the more severe the consequences and the grimmer the prognosis. As the patient moves into the rehabilitation phase, emphasis is placed on restoration of optimal function and independence. Rehabilitation takes many months. Many patients require special medical care and must pay careful attention to self-care for the remainder of their lives in order to avoid such complications as pressure ulcers and ***autonomic dysreflexia*** (see Box 6-6). This automatic response of functioning parts of the nervous system to sensations that normally would be felt as painful is a potentially life-threatening complication that can occur in those with spinal cord lesions above the sixth thoracic vertebra. It may be triggered by a number of things, but the most common are bowel distention (stretching) caused by constipation and bladder distention caused by urine retention or a blocked catheter. Other causes include rectal, pelvic, or urological examination, urinary tract infections, uterine contractions, pressure ulcers, and blood clots in the legs. The effects of autonomic dysreflexia are immediate and profound. Unless the patient gets immediate attention, it may progress to a stroke. The most common causes of death for those who survive the initial injury are pneumonia, pulmonary embolism, and kidney failure.

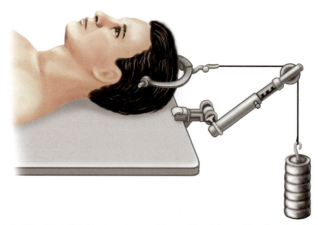

FIGURE 6-10 **Patient in Gardner-Wells tongs and traction** (From Eagle, S, et al. *The Professional Medical Assistant: An Integrative Teamwork-Based Approach.* 2009. Philadelphia: F.A. Davis Company, with permission.)

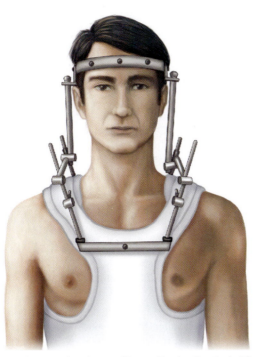

FIGURE 6-11 Patient with halo traction brace (From Eagle, S, et al. *The Professional Medical Assistant: An Integrative Teamwork-Based Approach.* 2009. Philadelphia: F.A. Davis Company, with permission.)

Box 6-6 Wellness Promotion

AUTONOMIC DYSREFLEXIA

The best way for individuals to avoid autonomic dysreflexia is to maintain regular and effective bowel and bladder elimination patterns. Common signs and symptoms associated with this condition are:

- hypertension
- profuse sweating above the spinal cord lesion
- severe, throbbing headache
- blurred vision
- apprehensiveness
- nausea

Herniated Disk

ICD-9-CM: 722.00–722.93   [ICD-10: M50.0–M53.9] (code by specific site and conditions for both codes)

A herniated disk, also called a *ruptured disk* or a *slipped disk*, occurs when the nucleus pulposus, the soft cushion between the vertebrae, bulges outward into the spinal canal. When this happens, the disk presses on nerves and causes pain in the back and legs. See Chapter 14 for a detailed description of a herniated disk.

Hematoma

**ICD-9-CM: 852.2 (subdural without mention   [ICD-10: I60.9 (subdural),
of open wound), 852.4 (unspecified, epidural)   I61.9 (epidural)]**

A hematoma is a collection of blood that results from internal bleeding (see Fig. 6-12). An epidural hematoma is a collection of blood between the dura mater (outer meningeal membrane of the

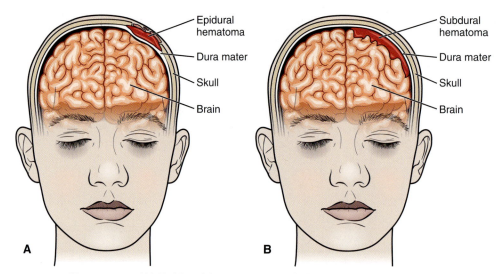

FIGURE 6-12 **Hematomas: (A) Epidural hematoma; (B) Subdural hematoma**

CNS) and skull. A subdural hematoma is a collection of blood between the dura mater and the arachnoid (middle or second layer of the meninges).

Incidence

Estimates of the incidence of epidural hematoma vary widely, from 40,000 to 200,000 cases per year. An estimated 30,000 individuals suffer from subdural hematoma each year. Both types occur in people of all ages, though infants and elderly people are more vulnerable to subdural hematoma than other age groups. Trauma caused by shaken-baby syndrome generally occurs before the age of 1 year. Traumatic head injury to the elderly often occurs due to falls.

Etiology

Both subdural and epidural hematomas are usually due to traumatic injury that causes tearing of blood vessels. Damage occurs when the head is subjected to high-velocity rotational or linear force, as happens with shaken-baby syndrome or contrecoup injuries. Movement of the brain and meningeal layers within the skull causes a shearing force which tears vessels and injures brain tissue. Epidural bleeding occurs rapidly because it usually involves arteries. The hematoma expands for 6 to 8 hours after the injury and strips the dura away from the inside of the skull.

Risk factors for both types of bleeding include age (very young and very old), alcohol abuse, and use of anticoagulant medication.

Flashpoint

Hematoma is usually caused by bleeding from the traumatic tearing of blood vessels.

Signs and Symptoms

Symptoms of epidural hematoma are often related to increased ICP and include loss of consciousness, abnormal pupil response, and decerebrate or decorticate posture (see Fig. 6-13). In decerebrate posture, the patient assumes a rigid position with arms stiff,

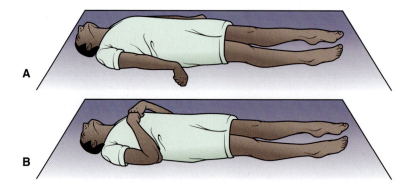

FIGURE 6-13 **Indicative postures with hematoma: (A) Decerebrate posture; (B) Decorticate posture**

extended, and pronated (turned downward). In decorticate posture, the patient assumes a rigid position with flexed arms, clenched fists, and extended legs. In either case, the posture is involuntary and indicates severe brain injury. Either type of hematoma may be visible on CT scan or MRI. Those with epidural hematoma may exhibit a lucid interval in which they briefly regain consciousness and then lose consciousness once more. This is an important clue that immediate surgical intervention is needed.

Individuals with subdural hematoma demonstrate a slower onset of symptoms. In fact, symptoms may be delayed by as much as 2 weeks. They include history of recent head injury, variable levels of consciousness, and assorted other neurological symptoms, such as headache, irritability, seizures, disorientation, amnesia, dizziness, nausea, vomiting, and difficulty walking or speaking.

Flashpoint

Symptoms may develop much more slowly in those with subdural hematoma than those with epidural hematoma.

Diagnosis

Both types of hematoma may be visible on CT scan, MRI, or cerebral arteriogram, although a chronic bleed may have a similar appearance to brain tissue, making it more difficult to identify.

Treatment

In either type of hematoma, surgery may be done to remove the hematoma and stop further bleeding. Potential complications include increased ICP from edema, further bleeding, infection, and seizures.

Prognosis

Prognosis for either type of bleed is variable and depends upon severity of injury, amount of bleeding, and timeliness of diagnosis and treatment. Epidural hematoma develops in up to 3% of head injuries and has a mortality rate of 15% to 20%. Acute subdural hematoma has a higher mortality rate, typically around 60%. Those with epidural hematoma who exhibit a lucid interval have a better prognosis (with prompt surgical intervention) than those who are comatose the entire time.

Skull Fracture

ICD-9-CM: 800–804   [ICD-10: S02.0–S02.9] (specify location and LOC for both codes)

A skull fracture is a break in any of the bones of the skull. There are several different types of fractures: linear (extending along the length of a bone), depressed (dented inward), comminuted (crushed into many pieces), and basilar (at the base of the skull) (see Fig. 6-14).

Incidence

An estimated 42,000 Americans suffer skull fracture each year. The majority of skull fractures are linear fractures.

Etiology

Skull fracture always results from some type of head trauma. Examples include falls, blows to the head from an object such as a rock, physical assault, athletic events, and motor vehicle accidents.

Flashpoint

Skull fracture is caused by traumatic injury such as in motor vehicle accidents, falls, or physical assault.

Signs and Symptoms

Individuals with linear skull fractures may be asymptomatic, or they may have swelling at the site. They rarely report loss of consciousness. Other types of fractures may cause variable signs and symptoms, including CSF or blood drainage from the ear or nose, loss of consciousness, temporary or permanent hearing loss, facial numbness, facial paralysis, *ataxia* (lack of coordination), vocal-cord paralysis, *nystagmus* (involuntary back-and-forth or circular eye movement), headaches, visual disturbances, nausea, vomiting, short-term memory loss, and seizures. Skull fractures are also known for causing typical patterns of bruising, including bruising around the eyes, sometimes called *raccoon eyes*, and behind the ears, sometimes called *Battle sign* (see Fig. 6-15).

Diagnosis

Diagnosis is based upon a thorough neurological examination and radiological studies, including skull x-rays, CT scan, and MRI. Drainage from the nose and ears is also tested for the presence of glucose, which indicates CSF.

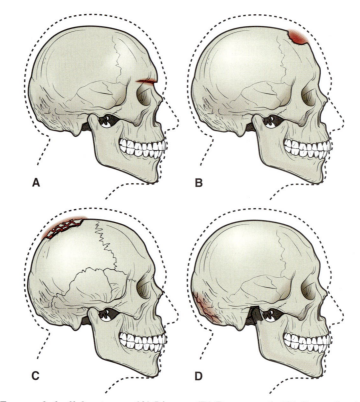

FIGURE 6-14 Types of skull fractures: (A) Linear; (B) Depressed; (C) Comminuted; (D) Basilar

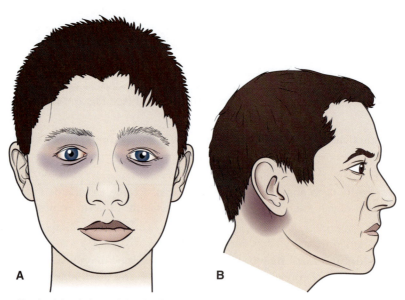

FIGURE 6-15 Typical bruising with skull fractures: (A) Bruising around the eyes known as raccoon eyes; (B) Bruising behind the ear known as Battle sign

Treatment

Individuals with simple, uncomplicated linear fractures may require no special treatment. Those with more complicated fractures are usually given antibiotics to prevent infection. Anticonvulsant medication may be given to prevent or manage seizures. Surgical intervention may be needed for infants or children with open depressed fractures and older individuals with significantly depressed skull fractures. Occasionally, craniotomy is performed to remove bone fragments, elevate the depressed bone, or remove hematoma.

Prognosis

Prognosis for individuals with skull fracture is quite variable. Those with a simple linear fracture usually recover fully with minimal treatment. The prognosis for others depends upon the severity of the injury to the brain and the timeliness of intervention. Potential complications include infection, abscess, meningitis, seizures, and permanent brain damage.

Carpal Tunnel Syndrome

ICD-9-CM: 354.0   [ICD-10: G56.0]

Carpal tunnel syndrome (CTS) is a common disorder that occurs when the median nerve in the forearm and hand becomes compressed or irritated as a result of inflammation. See Chapter 14 for a detailed description of carpal tunnel syndrome.

Chronic Neurological System Diseases and Disorders Caused by Degeneration of the Spine

Several diseases and disorders affect the structures within the vertebral column and spine. In many of these, compression of the spinal cord or spinal-nerve roots leads to acute and chronic pain and dysfunction. Common examples are degenerative disk disease, sciatica, and spinal stenosis.

Degenerative Disk Disease

ICD-9-CM: 722.6 (site unspecified) [ICD-10: M50.0–M51.1 (code by level)]

Degenerative disk disease is the deterioration of the disks between the vertebrae. Disks are cushionlike structures that absorb impact and help provide elasticity and flexibility for the spine. As aging occurs, the disks become thinner and less flexible and function less effectively.

Spinal Stenosis

ICD-9-CM: 724.00   [ICD-10: M48.0] (site unspecified for both codes)

Spinal stenosis is the narrowing of an area of the spine. It most typically affects the upper or lower back and puts pressure on the spinal cord and spinal-nerve roots.

Incidence

An estimated one-half million Americans suffer from spinal stenosis. It is most common in those over 50 years of age.

Etiology

In some cases, patients are born with spinal stenosis. However, it usually develops later in life, secondary to degenerative changes associated with aging. Primary contributors include osteoarthritis, disk herniation, ligament changes, misalignment of the vertebrae, spinal tumors, traumatic injuries, and disorders of bone-tissue formation. Any of these conditions can result in compression of the spinal cord or spinal-nerve roots, causing the associated symptoms (see Fig. 6-16).

Signs and Symptoms

Signs and symptoms of spinal stenosis vary depending on the severity and specific location. Patients commonly experience pain, numbness, or cramping in the legs, back, neck, shoulders, or arms. They may also complain of decreased sensation in the extremities, balance problems, and bowel and bladder dysfunction.

Diagnosis

Diagnosis of spinal stenosis is based on medical history, description of signs and symptoms, and a thorough examination of the spine. Radiological studies help confirm the diagnosis and may include spinal x-rays, MRI, CT scan, myelography (radiography of the spinal cord and associated nerves after injection of a contrast dye), and bone scan.

Treatment

Nonsurgical interventions for spinal stenosis include medications such as NSAIDs and analgesics for pain; rest; moderate exercise; physical therapy; use of a back brace or corset; epidural steroid injection; and an anesthetic injection known as *nerve block*. Surgical options, which usually provide long-term relief, include decompressive laminectomy, laminotomy, and spinal fusion.

> **Flashpoint**
> Spinal stenosis is caused by a narrowing of the spinal canal due to degenerative changes of the vertebrae and is most common in those over age 50.

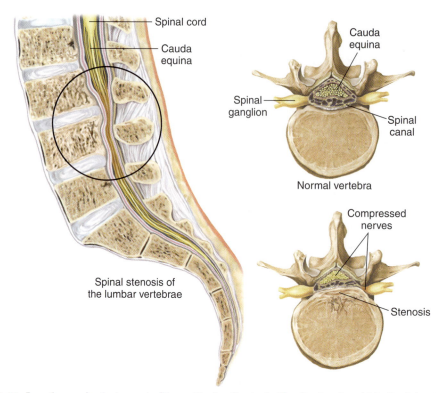

FIGURE 6-16 Lumbar spinal stenosis (From Eagle, S, et al. *The Professional Medical Assistant: An Integrative Teamwork-Based Approach.* 2009. Philadelphia: F.A. Davis Company, with permission.)

Prognosis

Prognosis is good with early detection and treatment. Surgical decompression usually provides long-term relief and improvement in quality of life.

Sciatica

ICD-9-CM: 724.3 [ICD-10: M54.3]

Sciatica is not a disorder in itself, but it is the term used for pain, numbness, weakness, or tingling that is felt from the lower back along the pathway of the sciatic nerve into the legs.

Incidence

It is estimated that up to 40% of the U.S. population will suffer from sciatica at some time during their lives. It affects men and women equally.

Etiology

Sciatica is a group of symptoms that have several different causes, including compression of lumbar-nerve roots or the spinal cord by herniated disks, tumors, spinal stenosis, and piriformis syndrome (compression by tension from the piriformis muscle). Other causes include pelvic injury, active trigger points (muscle ischemia from injury or chronic contraction), and uterine compression on the sciatic nerve in pregnancy.

Flashpoint

Symptoms of sciatica are related to compression of spinal-nerve roots or the spinal cord.

Signs and Symptoms

Symptoms of sciatica include pain, aching, tingling, and burning or numb sensations along the nerve path which runs through the buttocks, down the legs, and into the feet (see Fig. 6-17). Symptoms are usually *unilateral* (one-sided) but may affect both legs and may be mild or quite severe.

Diagnosis

Diagnosis is based upon presenting signs and symptoms along with physical-examination findings and possible radiological studies. Some individuals demonstrate weakness in one leg or abnormal reflexes. X-rays and MRI may be done to detect abnormalities within the lower spine.

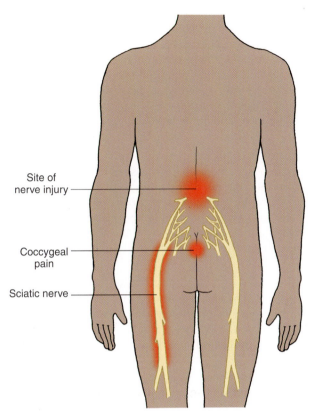

FIGURE 6-17 Sciatica (From Eagle, S. *Medical Terminology in a Flash! An Interactive, Flash-Card Approach.* 2006. Philadelphia: F.A. Davis Company, with permission.)

Treatment

Treatment for sciatica depends upon the underlying cause and is aimed at relieving symptoms and promoting function. Analgesics may be given for pain, and corticosteroid injections may relieve inflammation. Physical therapy may help reduce discomfort and maintain mobility and flexibility. Other treatments that may be helpful include acupuncture, chiropractic, osteopathy, stretching, yoga, and low-dose antidepressants or antiseizure medications. Some individuals also benefit from surgery to relieve compression of nerves.

Prognosis

Prognosis for sciatica is variable. In many cases, full recovery is achieved; in others, individuals may suffer some degree of disability. Potential complications include deficits in sensation and movement. For some individuals, sciatica becomes chronic.

Headaches

Few neurological disorders are as prevalent as headaches. Regardless of the many causes, headaches are a common source of pain, suffering, and, in some cases, temporary dysfunction. Two of the most common forms of headache are migraine and tension headaches.

Migraine Headache
ICD-9-CM: 346.9 (unspecified)   **[ICD-10: G43.0–G43.9 (with or without aura, complicated, and intractable)]**

Migraine headaches are a familial disorder marked by episodes of severe throbbing headache that is commonly unilateral and sometimes disabling.

Incidence

Migraines affect more than 28 million Americans and are three times as common in women as in men.

Flashpoint

Migraines are much more severe than typical tension headaches.

Etiology

The cause of migraine headaches is not fully understood, although they tend to run in families, be worse early in life, and generally improve in later years. Current theories about causes include involvement of the trigeminal nerve, imbalances in such chemicals as serotonin, and vascular dilation and inflammation. Many risk factors and potential triggers have also been identified, including hormonal changes and such foods as red wine, beer, aged cheese, chocolate, aspartame, and monosodium glutamate. Other triggers include stress, bright lights, fumes, perfumes, smoke, exertion, fatigue, environmental changes, and some medications.

Signs and Symptoms

Some individuals experience an *aura,* which is a type of sensory warning prior to the onset of the migraine headache or a seizure. Auras may include flashes of light, visual changes, or tingling in the arms or legs. Signs and symptoms of migraine headache vary somewhat with the individual but commonly include throbbing unilateral or *bilateral* (pertaining to both sides) pain, nausea with or without vomiting, and photophobia and *phonophobia* (sensitivity to sound). Untreated migraines usually last between 4 and 72 hours. They may occur as infrequently as once a year or as often as every week.

Flashpoint

Typical migraine symptoms include severe, throbbing pain; nausea; and sensitivity to light and sound.

Diagnosis

Diagnosis is nearly always based on the patient's description of symptoms and a physical examination. However, if the headaches have a sudden, severe onset or have changed significantly in frequency or character, more thorough neurological evaluation and diagnostic testing may be warranted. Such tests might include a CT or MRI scan and an LP so that cerebrospinal fluid can be evaluated.

Treatment

Treatment of migraine headaches has improved dramatically in recent years; numerous medications are now available, including NSAIDS and nonopiate and opiate analgesics, all of which help relieve pain. Triptans are a newer class of drugs that help to abort the migraine before it becomes severe. People who experience more than two migraines per month may benefit from preventive medications, such as antihypertensives, antidepressants, and antiseizure medications.

Prognosis

In most cases, migraines cannot be totally eliminated; however, the prognosis for most individuals is good. Effective management depends on identifying and eliminating or minimizing exposure to triggers and determining the most effective medication plan.

Tension Headache
ICD-9-CM: 307.81   [ICD-10: G44.0–G44.8 (code by type)]

A headache is a condition in which pain is felt in all or part of the head. While there are many types and causes, tension headache is by far the most common type of nonmigraine headache.

Incidence

Headaches are extremely common. In fact, 90% of the population of the United States reports at least one headache per year; an estimated 45 million Americans suffer chronic headaches. Headaches are known to cost billions of dollars each year in treatment costs and lost productivity. Tension headaches are experienced by people of all ages and races, male and female. However, they are most commonly reported by women over the age of 20.

Flashpoint

Tension headaches are extremely common, affecting 90% of the population.

Etiology

Tension headaches are caused by muscle tension in the scalp, neck, jaw, or upper shoulders. This tension is generally related to situational, physical, or emotional stress, anxiety, or depression. Examples of physical stress include certain types of manual labor and prolonged work at a desk or computer. Emotional stress is anything that causes feelings such as anxiety, anger, or frustration. Contributors to tension headaches include poor posture, lack of sleep, alcohol use, and missed meals. Pain may be worsened with noise.

Signs and Symptoms

Tension headaches may be chronic or episodic, lasting for minutes or days. They are experienced as a bilateral dull, aching sensation. Individuals may complain that the pain is centered in the forehead, base of the head, or neck. Individuals often describe a sensation of pressure or a bandlike tightness encircling the head. Episodic tension headaches are directly triggered by situational stress. Chronic tension headaches are present continuously or occur daily.

Diagnosis

Diagnosis of headaches depends largely upon the patient's medical history and description of symptoms. Therefore, the health-care provider carefully questions the patient about headache symptoms, including onset, location and duration of pain, character or quality of pain, and any other associated symptoms. Physical examination is done to rule out other causes.

Treatment

Most tension headaches can be treated at home with over-the-counter analgesics such as acetaminophen (Tylenol). Other treatments such as relaxation, massage, biofeedback, and stress-management activities are often helpful.

Prognosis

Prognosis for tension headache is good, since there is no underlying life-threatening pathology. However, for many people these types of headaches can have significant impact on quality of life and productivity. Individuals who do not experience relief or improvement with the treatment described here should see their health-care provider.

> **Flashpoint**
> Headaches of all kinds have a significant impact on quality of life and productivity of those who suffer from them.

Diseases and Disorders of the Peripheral Nervous System

Some common diseases and disorders primarily affect the peripheral rather than the central nervous system. Examples include peripheral neuropathy, Bell palsy, and trigeminal neuralgia.

Peripheral Neuropathy
ICD-9-CM: 356.9 (unspecified)   [ICD-10: G90.0 (idiopathic peripheral autonomic neuropathy)]

Peripheral neuropathy is a dysfunction of nerves that transmit information to and from the brain and spinal cord. It is characterized by pain, altered sensation, and muscle weakness, and it may affect a single nerve or nerve group or may affect multiple nerves.

Incidence

Experts do not agree about the definition of peripheral neuropathy, which makes its incidence difficult to estimate. However, they all agree that it is extremely common.

Etiology

The cause of peripheral neuropathy is not clear. A number of disorders are associated with it, though, including diabetes, alcoholism, AIDS, rheumatoid arthritis, systemic lupus erythematosus, ingestion of toxic substances and some drugs, and nerve injury from prolonged immobility or compression.

Signs and Symptoms

Symptoms of peripheral neuropathy may be motor, sensory, or both, and they vary widely depending on the nerve or nerves affected. The most common sensory symptoms are nerve pain and numbness. Motor symptoms include weakness, muscle twitching, atrophy, muscle cramps, loss of movement, and loss of coordination. Damage to autonomic nerves related to involuntary or semivoluntary functions may result in such symptoms as blurred vision, dizziness, diarrhea, constipation, urinary incontinence, and impotence, among others.

Diagnosis

Diagnosis is based on a detailed history and neurological examination. Tests may include an EMG, nerve conduction tests, and nerve biopsy. Blood tests may be done to identify or rule out underlying medical disorders, such as diabetes or nutritional deficits.

> **Flashpoint**
> Signs and symptoms of peripheral neuropathy vary widely and include pain, numbness, weakness, and loss of coordination.

Treatment

Therapy is individualized depending on the symptoms. One goal is treating underlying disorders or nutritional deficiencies. Physical and occupational therapy may help build muscle strength and coordination. Braces, splints, or mobility aids may improve independence. Emphasis is placed on safety, with a goal of preventing falls or injuries to extremities with decreased sensation. Medications such as analgesics, anticonvulsants, and antidepressants may help alleviate pain.

Prognosis

The prognosis for peripheral neuropathy is variable, depending on the specific cause. In cases where an underlying disorder can be cured or treated, the outlook is positive. However, in some cases nerve damage is permanent.

Bell Palsy

ICD-9-CM: 351.0   [ICD-10: G51.0]

Bell palsy is a disorder of the seventh cranial nerve that causes temporary weakness or paralysis of one side of the face. It usually develops suddenly and takes months to resolve.

Incidence

Bell palsy affects approximately 40,000 individuals each year in the United States. It is equally common in men and women and is most common between the ages of 15 and 60. It is more common among pregnant women and patients with diabetes or upper respiratory infections.

Etiology

Flashpoint

Bell palsy involves inflammation and compression of the seventh cranial nerve.

Bell palsy occurs when the seventh cranial nerve becomes inflamed, swollen, and compressed. The underlying cause is unknown, but a viral infection may serve as the triggering event.

Signs and Symptoms

Symptoms of Bell palsy vary somewhat. In most cases there is some degree of paralysis that causes drooping of the facial features on the affected side (see Fig. 6-18). Other symptoms may include twitching, weakness, drooling, eye dryness, impaired taste, excessive tearing, headache, ringing in the ears, and difficulty eating or drinking.

Diagnosis

Diagnosis of Bell palsy is based on the patient's signs and symptoms and neurological-examination findings. An EMG will detect nerve damage. CT scan, MRI, and skull x-rays may be done to rule out other disorders.

Treatment

There is no cure for Bell palsy. Corticosteroids may be given to decrease inflammation and swelling, and antiviral medications may be given if a viral cause is suspected. Analgesics and warm, moist compresses may help relieve pain. Because the individual may be unable to effectively blink or close the eye, measures must be taken to protect the eye and keep it moist, including using artificial tears or an eye patch.

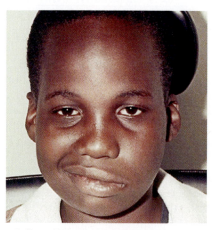

FIGURE 6-18 **Bell palsy** (From Dillon, PM. *Nursing Health Assessment: A Critical Thinking, Case Studies Approach,* 2nd edition. 2007. Philadelphia: F.A. Davis Company, with permission.)

Prognosis

The prognosis for those with Bell palsy is very good. Recovery is complete in most cases but may take as long as 6 months. In some cases the symptoms never fully resolve, and in a very small number of cases the paralysis may be permanent. Recurrences are rare.

Trigeminal Neuralgia
ICD-9-CM: 350.1   [ICD-10: G50.0]

Trigeminal neuralgia (TN), also called *tic douloureux*, is a neurological disorder that causes severe, episodic facial pain along the pathway of the fifth cranial (trigeminal) nerve.

Incidence

Onset of TN is most typical among those over the age of 50, although it can occur in younger individuals. An estimated 60,000 to 180,000 Americans suffer from TN, women more frequently than men.

Etiology

The exact cause of TN is not known. In many cases it has been attributed to compression of the trigeminal nerve root by blood vessels or lesions, resulting in hyperactive function of the nerve (see Fig. 6-19). In some cases it has also been connected with injury to the nerve or to multiple sclerosis. Events that may trigger pain include chewing, shaving, applying makeup, talking, drinking, brushing teeth, smiling, touching the face, and even feeling a cool breeze.

Signs and Symptoms

TN causes episodes of severe, sudden stabbing, shooting, or shocklike pain in the side of the face around the ears, jaw, cheeks, lips, nose, or eyes. Episodes may become increasingly frequent and intense over time. Atypical TN causes a less severe but constant aching or burning pain. Both types of TN usually affect just one side of the face, although bilateral TN occurs around 10% of the time. Many individuals experience disturbed sleep. Some suffer nutritional deficits due to difficulty chewing and swallowing.

Diagnosis

Diagnosis is based upon physical-examination findings and the patient's report of symptoms and description of pain patterns and typical triggers. There is no evidence of motor or sensory deficit (other than pain-related symptoms). MRI scan may be done to rule out multiple sclerosis and other disorders.

> **Flashpoint**
> TN is known for causing episodes of sudden, severe facial pain.

Treatment

There is no specific cure that works in all cases; however, a number of treatments are available which may provide resolution or improvement for most people. A number of medications are used to relieve or manage pain, including analgesics, anticonvulsants, antidepressants, and antispasmodics. Medication may also be injected to numb or disable the nerve. Surgical procedures may be done to relieve pressure on the trigeminal nerve or even disable it

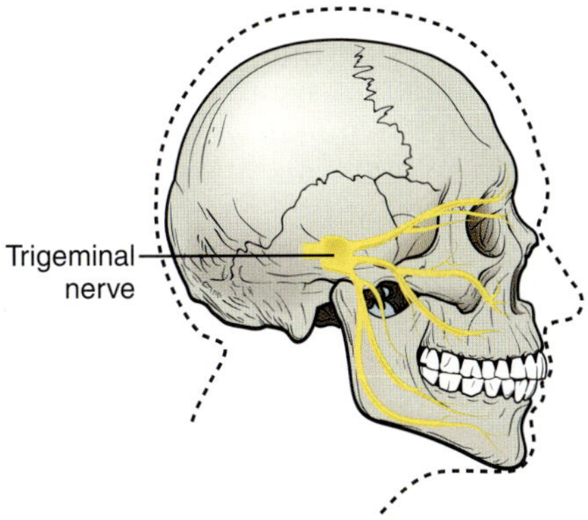

Trigeminal nerve

FIGURE 6-19 Trigeminal neuralgia

temporarily or permanently. Some individuals find that direct application of heat or cold is helpful. Complementary therapies such as chiropractic treatments, acupuncture, meditation, and hypnosis may also helpful.

Prognosis

TN is one of the most painful conditions known and can have a significant impact on quality of life. Some patients find help and encouragement through support groups. In some cases the disorder resolves spontaneously; in others, medication or surgery provides partial or complete relief. For some, the pain recurs at a later time, necessitating repeated treatments. Possible side effects from some procedures include facial weakness, numbness, or paralysis, which may be temporary or permanent.

Sleep Disorders

> **ICD-9-CM: 780.50–780.59 (sleep disturbances)**   **[ICD-10: F51.0–F51.8 (code by hypersomnia or insomnia)]**

A sleep disorder is a disruption of the normal human sleep patterns; types and causes are numerous. Some sleep disorders are mild and others are serious enough to disrupt health and the ability to function in daily life. See Chapter 18 for detailed descriptions of sleep disorders.

Epilepsy

> **ICD-9-CM: 345.90   [ICD-10: G40.9] (unspecified for both codes)**

Epilepsy is a chronic disorder of the brain marked by recurrent seizures, which are repetitive abnormal electrical discharges within the brain. Epilepsy seizure types are categorized as *partial, generalized,* and *unclassified.* In generalized seizures, the electrical nervous activity affects both sides of the brain. In partial seizures, also called *focal* or *local* seizures, activity begins in one part of the brain, but these seizures may occasionally evolve into generalized ones.

Flashpoint

Seizures are repetitive, abnormal electrical activity within the brain.

Incidence

An estimated three million Americans have epilepsy, and 200,000 new cases are diagnosed each year. Those most commonly affected are children and those over age 70.

Etiology

The cause of epilepsy is not clear, but the disorder is thought to result from congenital (present at birth) or acquired brain disease. Various types of stimuli may trigger a seizure, including withdrawal from antiseizure medication, head trauma, illness, emotional or physical stress, fatigue, specific foods or chemicals, and flickering or flashing lights.

Signs and Symptoms

Signs and symptoms of epilepsy depend on the type of seizure involved (see Table 6-2).

Diagnosis

Diagnosis is based on a history and description of symptoms and a description of the seizure activity. A thorough neurological evaluation is required. A number of diagnostic studies may be done, including electroencephalogram (EEG), CT scan, MRI scan, and LP (see Box 6-7).

Treatment

Treatment of epilepsy is aimed at reducing the number and severity of seizures. A variety of antiseizure medications are available; a certain amount of trial and error may be required to find the one that works best for a given individual. For patients whose epilepsy does not respond to medication, surgical options may be considered, including implantation of a vagal-nerve stimulator, excision of the brain tissue responsible for triggering the seizures, and corpus callosotomy, in which the corpus callosum is partially divided in two. These surgical procedures effectively reduce the severity and frequency of seizure activity and make the individual more responsive to antiseizure medication. Treatment during an actual seizure should focus on protecting the individual from injury and providing privacy (when possible). Nothing should be inserted in the individual's mouth.

Flashpoint

Treatment of the patient experiencing a seizure should be aimed at providing safety and privacy.

TABLE 6-2
TYPES OF SEIZURES

Generalized Seizures

tonic-clonic (formerly called *grand mal*)	• Duration: 2–5 minutes • Intense muscle tension followed by jerking movements • Loss of consciousness • Bowel and bladder incontinence • Postictal state for up to an hour characterized by fatigue, lethargy, and confusion
tonic	• Duration: 30 seconds to several minutes • Intense muscle tension • Loss of consciousness
clonic	• Duration: several minutes • Muscle contraction alternating with relaxation
absence	• Duration: several seconds • Possible staring off into space • No postictal state • More common in children, with a familial tendency
myoclonic	• Duration: several seconds • Brief jerking or stiffening of extremities
atonic	• Sudden loss of muscle tone, which may cause the individual to fall • Postictal state characterized by confusion
complex partial (also called *psychomotor* or *temporal lobe*)	• Duration: 1–3 minutes • Loss of consciousness that involves automatisms, which are specific behaviors such as lip smacking, patting, or picking at clothing or other items • No recall of the event afterwards
simple partial	• Duration: 1–2 minutes • No loss of consciousness • Possible aura prior to seizure, which might include a feeling of déjà vu, an offensive smell, or a painful sensation • Unilateral extremity movement • Unusual sensations • Possible autonomic symptoms including change in heart rate, flushing, and epigastric discomfort

Prognosis

The prognosis for epilepsy is generally good, depending on the severity of the disorder and the patient's responsiveness to treatment. In some cases the seizures cannot be totally eliminated; in most cases, though, the severity and frequency can be reduced, resulting in an improved quality of life for the patient. A life-threatening complication of epilepsy is status epilepticus, in which the individual experiences continuous or recurrent seizure activity.

Transient Global Amnesia

ICD-9-CM: 437.7   [ICD-10: G45.4]

Transient global amnesia (TGA) is a rare disorder, not caused by a neurological event or injury, which involves the sudden, temporary loss of recent memory.

Box 6-7 Diagnostic Spotlight

ELECTROENCEPHALOGRAPHY

Electroencephalography is a diagnostic test in which electrical brain activity is amplified and recorded. The printed record obtained is called an electroencephalogram (EEG). In this test, a variety of electrodes are placed at specific locations on the patient's scalp. The machine records electrical activity at each site and measures the difference in activity between various sites. In resting adults, the most common waveform is called the alpha wave; it has 8½ to 12 cycles per second. Characteristic waveform changes occur with sleep, waking rest, and concentration. In some cases, neurological diseases may cause waveform changes.

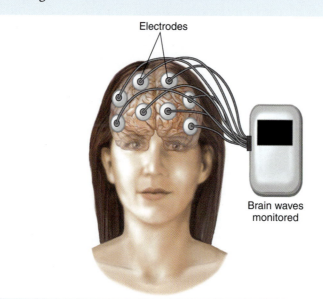

Patient undergoing EEG testing (From Eagle, S, et al. *The Professional Medical Assistant: An Integrative Teamwork-Based Approach.* 2009. Philadelphia: F.A. Davis Company, with permission.)

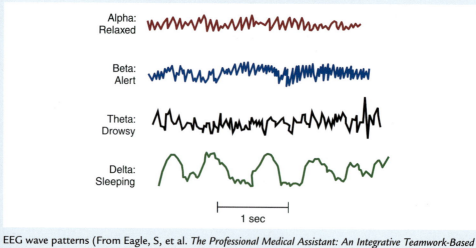

EEG wave patterns (From Eagle, S, et al. *The Professional Medical Assistant: An Integrative Teamwork-Based Approach.* 2009. Philadelphia: F.A. Davis Company, with permission.)

Incidence

An estimated 15,000 to 70,000 Americans suffer from TGA annually. The typical age of those affected is greater than 50. TGA occurs equally in men and women.

Etiology

The exact cause of TGA is unknown. A variety of theories include temporarily disrupted blood flow to parts of the brain and possible triggering events such as cold-water immersion, severe emotional or physical stress, sexual activity, recent migraine headache, and medical procedures.

Signs and Symptoms

The primary symptom of TGA is loss of recent memory (covering days, weeks, or months) with retention of personal identity and distant memory. The episode generally lasts less than 24 hours. Of note is the absence of neurological deficits such as paralysis, weakness, numbness, loss of consciousness, seizures, or history of recent head injury. During the event, individuals retain the ability to function normally, including using language and social skills, following directions, and recognizing familiar objects. They may experience headache or anxiety-related symptoms such as trembling, sweating, increased heart rate, and emotional distress or agitation. Symptoms generally resolve within 12 to 24 hours, after which the individual returns to a normal state with the usual ability to remember events.

> **Flashpoint**
> The key symptom of TGA is loss of recent memory with retention of personal identity and distant memory.

Diagnosis

Diagnosis of TGA is based upon a witnessed description of the event and the individual's report of recent memory loss and other symptoms (as described). Neurological-examination results are notable for an absence of deficits during or after the event. Diagnostic tests such as EEG and CT scan are done to rule out other neurological events, such as stroke or seizures.

Treatment

TGA is self-limiting, and symptoms completely resolve within 24 hours. Therefore, no treatment is needed.

Prognosis

Prognosis for TGA is excellent because it causes no residual physical deficits, and recurrence is very uncommon. However, a thorough evaluation should be done to rule out any concerns about stroke, transient ischemic attack (TIA), or seizure disorder. TGA is a frightening and distressing event for the patient; emotional support and even counseling may be helpful.

STOP HERE.
Select the flash cards for this chapter and run through them at least three times before moving on to the next chapter.

Student Resources

ALS Association: http://www.alsa.org
Alzheimer's Association: http://www.alz.org
Bell's Palsy Information Site: http://www.bellspalsy.ws
Epilepsy Foundation: http://www.epilepsyfoundation.org
Huntington's Disease Society of America: http://www.hdsa.org
National Headache Foundation: http://www.headaches.org
National Multiple Sclerosis Society: http://www.nationalmssociety.org
National Parkinson Foundation: http://www.parkinson.org
National Spinal Cord Injury Association: http://www.spinalcord.org
National Stroke Association: http://www.stroke.org
TNA The Facial Pain Association: http://www.endthepain.org

Chapter Activities

Learning Style Study Strategies

Try any or all of the following strategies as you study the content of this chapter:

Visual and kinesthetic learners: Create a table to line up and compare features of disorders that are similar. This will help you to easily spot features that are similar as well as those that are uniquely different. For example, you might create a table with Parkinson disease, multiple sclerosis, ALS, and Huntington disease. As you review your table, color-code commonalities with a colored highlighter. Then use a different color to highlight items that are uniquely different about each one.

Auditory learners: With your instructor's permission, record lectures so that you can play them back later. Listening as you review class notes will help you to fill in details. Listening while doing household chores helps you to maximize your time by completing two tasks at once.

Verbal learners: Play instrumental music (without lyrics) when you study, and sing terms and definitions aloud to yourself over and over until you can remember them.

Practice Exercises

Answers to Practice Exercises can be found in Appendix D.

Case Studies

CASE STUDY 1

Burt O'Connor is a 70-year-old man with Alzheimer dementia. His wife, Hilda, brings him to the medical clinic for his regular health checkups, as well as when he is ill or injured. She has been struggling to understand his disease and provide the best care for him that she can, but she confesses to feeling overwhelmed at times. One day, while her husband is with the physician, she asks the nurse the following questions. How should the nurse respond?

1. What exactly causes Alzheimer dementia?

2. My son says that he thinks Burt is just depressed. How can you tell the difference?

3. I'm not sure how long I can continue to provide care for my husband, but I hate the idea of putting him in a nursing home. Can you give me any ideas for keeping him safer at home?

4. What other suggestions do you have for me?

CASE STUDY 2

A 46-year-old man named Martino Silva is a patient in the family medicine clinic today. When he awoke this morning he was dismayed to find the entire left side of his face paralyzed. After evaluating him, the physician makes the diagnosis of Bell palsy. Mr. Silva has several questions; how should they be answered?.

1. What is Bell palsy?

2. How did I catch this?

3. Besides not being able to move half of my face, are there any other symptoms that I should expect?

4. Is there anything you can do about it?

5. Is this ever going to go away?

CASE STUDY 3

Vaishali Patel is a 28-year-old woman who has come to the medical clinic with complaints of headaches. She reports that they have been slowly getting worse and more frequent over the past year, and she wants to know what might be done about them. The health-care provider completes a physical examination and asks some questions to determine the most likely cause of her headaches.

1. Which signs and symptoms would most likely indicate that Ms. Patel's headaches are migraines?

2. Which signs and symptoms would most likely indicate that her headaches are tension headaches?

3. How do migraine and tension headaches differ in cause?

4. How do treatment methods differ for migraines and tension headaches?

Multiple Choice

1. Which of the following terms is matched with the correct definition?

   a. Unilateral: pertaining to both sides

   b. Aura: sensory warning prior to the onset of a migraine headache or a seizure

   c. Dysphagia: lack of coordination

   d. Nuchal rigidity: ringing or other abnormal sounds in the ears

2. Which of the following is the correct definition of *paresthesia*?

   a. Altered sensation, such as numbness, stinging, or burning, that results from injury to nerves

   b. Aggravation of symptoms or increase in severity

   c. Sensitivity to sound

   d. Sensory warning prior to the onset of a migraine headache or a seizure

3. All of the following statements are true regarding migraine headache **except:**

   a. They are a familial disorder.

   b. Common triggers include red wine, beer, aged cheese, chocolate, and aspartame.

   c. Some individuals experience an aura prior to the onset of headache.

   d. Migraines can be cured with the use of medications called triptans.

4. All of the following statements are true regarding Alzheimer dementia **except:**

   a. Life expectancy averages 8 to 10 years from the onset of symptoms.

   b. Education and emotional support are important for the caregiver.

   c. It is definitively diagnosed with MRI.

   d. It has a slow onset and long, progressive course, and it lasts for a number of years.

5. Which of the following statements is true regarding stroke?

   a. It is always caused by a blood clot in the brain.

   b. Signs and symptoms are present on the same side of the body as the stroke.

   c. Rehabilitation is rarely needed.

   d. Treatment may include the use of thrombolytic and anticoagulant medications.

Short Answer

1. **Describe the differences between a stroke and a TIA with regard to cause and signs and symptoms.**

2. **List the movement disorders caused by Parkinson disease.**

3. **Describe the measures individuals can take to promote healthy brain function and help prevent dementia.**

URINARY SYSTEM DISEASES AND DISORDERS

7

Learning Outcomes

Upon completion of this chapter, the student will be able to:

- Define and spell terms related to urology
- Identify key structures of the urinary system
- Discuss functions of the kidneys, ureter, and bladder

- Identify characteristics of common diseases and disorders of the urinary system, including:
  - description
  - incidence
  - etiology
  - signs and symptoms
  - diagnosis
  - treatment
  - prognosis

KEY TERMS	
anuria	absence of urine production
culture	laboratory examination of growing microorganisms
diuresis	abnormal increase in urine production and excretion
dysuria	pain, burning, or other discomfort during urination
frequency	need to urinate frequently
hematuria	presence of blood in the urine
hemodialysis	filtration of wastes and fluid from blood as it passes through selectively permeable membranes; also called *dialysis*
ischemia	temporary deficiency in blood supply
lithotripsy	procedure in which shock waves or sound waves crush stones in the kidneys or urinary tract
micturition reflex	urge to urinate
nocturia	frequent need to urinate during the night
oliguria	deficient urine production
peritoneal dialysis	filtration of fluid and wastes from the blood using the lining of the patient's peritoneal cavity as a dialyzing membrane
proteinuria	presence of protein in urine
renal colic	severe, intermittent pain caused by spasm of the ureter
stress incontinence	leakage of urine with minor physical stress, such as coughing, sneezing, lifting, or laughing
uremia	presence of increased nitrogenous waste products, especially urea, in the blood

Continued

KEY TERMS—cont'd	
urge incontinence	leakage of urine with the urge to void
urgency	need to urinate urgently
urinalysis	laboratory analysis of the urine

Abbreviations

Table 7-1 lists some of the most common abbreviations related to the urinary system.

Structures and Functions of the Urinary System

The urinary system consists of the kidneys, ureters, bladder, and urethra. It facilitates filtration of the blood, excretion of wastes, and regulation of fluid, electrolytes, acids, and bases.

Structures of the Urinary System

The structures of the urinary system include two kidneys, two ureters, the bladder, and the urethra (see Fig. 7-1).

Kidneys

The key organs of the urinary system are the kidneys, which are located in the retroperitoneal space in the back of the abdominal cavity, to either side of the vertebral column. The right kidney is slightly lower than the left. Each kidney is surrounded by a renal capsule made up of connective tissue and a thick layer of fat. The renal artery, vein, nerves, and ureter exit the kidney on the medial side, at the hilum. The kidneys are highly vascular organs made up of an outer cortex and an inner medulla. Within the medulla are several oval-shaped renal pyramids, which point inward. Cupping the tip of each renal pyramid is a calyx. The area where all the calyces join is called the renal pelvis. The renal pelvis narrows and joins the ureter.

TABLE 7-1			
ABBREVIATIONS			
Abbreviation	**Meaning**	**Abbreviation**	**Meaning**
ARF	acute renal failure	IVP	intravenous pyelography
ATN	acute tubular necrosis	KUB	kidney, ureter, bladder
BUN	blood urea nitrogen	PKD	polycystic kidney disease
CRF	chronic renal failure	RP	retrograde pyelogram
ESRD	end-stage renal disease	STI	sexually transmitted infection
GFR	glomerular filtration rate	UA	urinalysis
IC	interstitial cystitis	UTI	urinary tract infection

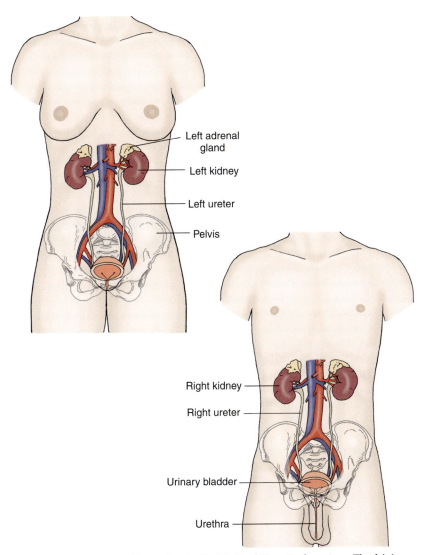

FIGURE 7-1 The urinary system (From Eagle, S. *Medical Terminology in a Flash! An Interactive, Flash-Card Approach.* 2006. Philadelphia: F.A. Davis Company, with permission.)

Nephrons

Located primarily within the outer cortex of the kidney are the nephrons. There are more than one million nephrons in each kidney. Each one is a complex microscopic structure composed of an arteriole, venule, glomerulus (capillary cluster within the Bowman capsule), proximal tubule, loop of Henle, distal tubule, and capillary bed (see Fig. 7-2).

Ureters, Urinary Bladder, and Urethra

The ureters are long, narrow tubes that connect the renal pelvis to the urinary bladder. The bladder is a flexible, muscular container for urine. The lining of the ureters and the bladder is uniquely designed to be flexible in accommodating varying amounts of fluid. At the base of the bladder is the exit into the urethra, a tube that varies in length by sex; the male urethra is approximately 20 centimeters long and the female urethra is approximately 4 centimeters long.

> *Flashpoint*
> Each kidney contains more than one million nephrons.

Functions of the Urinary System

Each structure of the urinary system is uniquely designed and suited to its purpose. The urinary system's main functions are filtering and excreting the waste products of digestion and metabolism from the body, helping to regulate blood pressure, and maintaining an optimal level of fluid and electrolytes within the body.

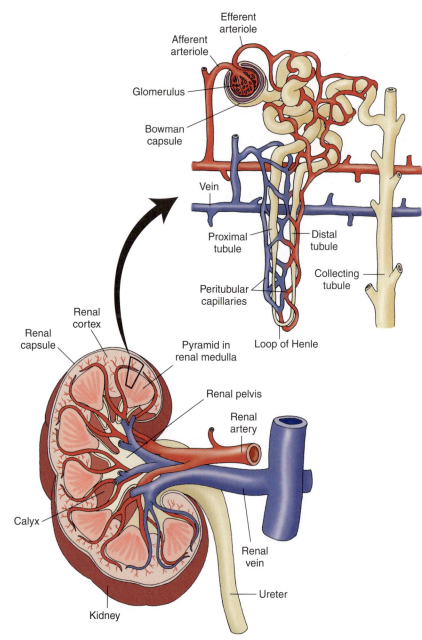

FIGURE 7-2 The kidney and nephron (From Eagle, S. *Medical Terminology in a Flash! An Interactive, Flash-Card Approach.* 2006. Philadelphia: F.A. Davis Company, with permission.)

Kidneys

The thick layer of fat in the renal capsule that surrounds each kidney acts as a shock absorber to cushion and protect the kidneys, so that they may perform a key function of the urinary system— the filtration of blood and regulation of electrolytes. The highly vascular nature of the kidneys lends itself to this function. Over 20% of the blood pumped by the heart each minute passes through the kidneys. When urine is formed, it drains into the calyces, which funnel the urine inward through the renal pelvis and into the ureter, which in turn drains urine from the kidney to the urinary bladder. In addition to filtering fluid and wastes from the body, the kidneys play an active role in maintaining blood pressure and blood pH (acidity or alkalinity); regulating blood pressure by retaining or excreting more fluid and electrolytes (especially sodium); and maintaining an optimal acid-base balance by retaining or excreting buffers and acids as needed.

Flashpoint

More than 20% of the body's blood is pumped through the kidneys every minute.

Nephrons

The nephron has long been called the functional unit of the kidney, because it is where most of the action takes place. To begin the filtration process, blood passes from a tiny arteriole into the glomerulus. The walls of the glomerulus and Bowman capsule are designed to permit optimal filtration of water, electrolytes, urea, and other small molecules. A large amount of this fluid (approximately 180 liters), called filtrate, is created each day. As the filtrate moves on through the proximal tubule, loop of Henle, and distal tubule, a majority (99%) of the water and useful solutes is reabsorbed and additional wastes are excreted. After the kidneys make final adjustments in the composition of the fluid, it is called urine. The kidneys produce and excrete an average of 1 to 2 liters of urine each day.

Ureters, Urinary Bladder, and Urethra

Urine drains from the kidneys to the bladder via the two long, narrow ureters. In the bladder, urine accumulates until the volume stimulates stretch receptors. These receptors initiate the **micturition reflex,** which is the urge to urinate. A person may temporarily ignore this urge, but eventually the increased urine volume stimulates the stretch receptors again and the urge to urinate becomes even stronger. The urethra functions as a passageway for final urine elimination and emptying of the bladder. It serves a dual role in the male as a passageway for urine and for sperm mixed with seminal fluid when ejaculation occurs.

> **Flashpoint**
> The kidneys produce approximately 180 liters of filtrate each day!

Diseases and Disorders of the Urinary System

This chapter discusses many disorders of the urinary system. An attempt has been made to group disorders according to common causes or to structures most commonly affected. However, this poses a challenge because in many cases the causes are complex or not fully understood, and the disorders may affect multiple body systems.

Conditions of Inflammation or Infection

Some diseases and disorders of the urinary system are caused by bacterial infection or inflammatory changes. Common examples include bacterial cystitis and urethritis, pyelonephritis, acute and chronic glomerulonephritis, interstitial cystitis, and interstitial nephritis.

Bacterial Cystitis and Urethritis

ICD-9-CM: 595.9 (cystitis, unspecified), 595.0 (cystitis, acute), 595.1 (cystitis, chronic) (use additional code to identify organism), 597.80 (urethritis, unspecified) (use additional code to identify organism) **[ICD-10: N39.0 (cystitis; use additional code to identify organism: B95–B97), N34 (urethritis; use additional code to identify organism: B95–B97)]**

Cystitis is an inflammation of the bladder. Urethritis is an inflammation of the urethra. These conditions commonly coexist and together constitute a urinary tract infection (UTI), sometimes referred to as a *bladder infection.*

Incidence

UTIs are more common in women than men, because women have a short urethra (about 4 cm long), which allows microorganisms to ascend the urethra into the bladder more easily. Men, however, have a higher incidence of urethritis, which is the most common type of sexually transmitted infection (STI) in men.

Etiology

Cystitis and urethritis (UTIs) are most commonly caused by bacterial invasion, particularly *Escherichia coli, Enterobacter, Klebsiella, Proteus,* and *Pseudomonas.* Other causes include such organisms as *Chlamydia trachomatis, Neisseria gonorrhoeae,* and the herpes simplex virus, as well as other viruses, parasites, and fungi. Contributors to the development of

> **Flashpoint**
> UTIs are much more common in women than in men.

cystitis and urethritis include sexual activity and poor hygiene, both of which increase the likelihood of microorganisms entering the urinary tract.

Signs and Symptoms

Common symptoms of bladder infection include **urgency** (need to urinate urgently), **frequency** (need to urinate frequently), and **dysuria** (pain, burning, or other discomfort during urination). Other symptoms include fever, malaise, bladder spasms, pelvic or low back pain, and cloudy, pink, or foul-smelling urine. When urethritis is caused by an STI, urethral discharge may also be present. In the elderly, the most common sign associated with UTI or kidney infection is new onset of confusion.

> **Flashpoint**
>
> Classic symptoms of UTI are urgency, frequency, and dysuria.

Diagnosis

Diagnosis of UTI is usually based on the results of a **urinalysis** (laboratory analysis of the urine), which reveals bacteria and increased numbers of white and red blood cells (see Box 7-1). A urine **culture,** in which a laboratory examines the growth of microorganisms in a urine specimen under a microscope, may identify the causative organism. A culture of urethral discharge may also identify whether an STI is involved.

Treatment

Treatment of UTI depends on the underlying cause. In the case of bacterial infection, the physician will prescribe antibiotics. Other treatment includes phenazopyridine (Pyridium), which is a urinary tract analgesic; general analgesics; and fluids to help flush the urinary tract. To help prevent recurrence, the female patient should empty her bladder soon after sexual intercourse and drink plenty of water (six to eight glasses each day) and fluids that acidify the urine and inhibit bacterial growth, such as cranberry juice. Other measures include wiping from front to back after defecation, avoiding tight-fitting clothing (which harbors moisture), and conducting routine daily hygiene (see Box 7-2).

> **Flashpoint**
>
> Individuals with a UTI should drink lots of water.

Prognosis

Prognosis for UTIs is good, with timely diagnosis and treatment. Complications develop when bacterial organisms enter other parts of the urinary tract, causing prostatitis, kidney infection, and other types of infection.

Pyelonephritis

ICD-9-CM: 590.80 (unspecified)   **[ICD-10: N10–N12 (code as acute, chronic, or obstructive)]**

Pyelonephritis, sometimes called *pyelitis*, is a bacterial infection of the kidney and renal pelvis. It may affect one or both kidneys.

Box 7-1 Diagnostic Spotlight

URINALYSIS

Urinalysis (UA), the laboratory analysis of the urine, is among the most commonly performed laboratory tests. It is useful in the diagnosis of urinary tract infections as well as a variety of other disorders. Normal UA values are:

Appearance: clear	Crystals: negative
Color: yellow	Casts: negative
pH: 4.6–8.0	Glucose: negative
Protein: under 8 mg/dl	White blood cells: under four per low-power field
Specific gravity: 1.005–1.030	
Leukocyte esterase: negative	Red blood cells: under two per low-power field
Nitrites: negative	
Ketones: negative	

Box 7-2 Wellness Promotion

TREATING AND PREVENTING URINARY TRACT INFECTION

If you think you may have a UTI, see your health-care provider. He or she will take a brief health history, will collect a urine specimen, and may conduct an exam.

What Else Can You Do?

- Drink lots of healthy fluids, like water and juice. This helps keep you well hydrated and helps flush your urinary tract.
- Drink cranberry juice; it helps to make your urine more acidic and therefore less hospitable to bacteria.
- Take medications as prescribed by your health-care provider. Be sure to take anti-infective medication until it is gone—don't stop taking it early just because you feel better.

What Can You Do to Help Prevent Recurrent UTIs?

- Continue drinking lots of fluids daily, unless told otherwise by your physician.
- Urinate soon after sexual intercourse.
- Wipe from front to back after bowel movements.
- Avoid wearing tight-fitting undergarments that harbor moisture.
- Follow additional advice from your physician.

Incidence

More than 250,000 individuals are diagnosed with pyelonephritis in the United States each year; nearly 80% require hospitalization for treatment. Women are affected much more frequently than men (85% of cases versus 15%), and elderly men are more prone to pyelonephritis than are younger men.

Etiology

In most cases, pyelonephritis is caused by organisms common to the gastrointestinal system that gain entry to the urinary tract; *E. coli* causes up to 90% of all cases. As pathogens grow within the lower urinary tract, the individual may experience signs and symptoms of bladder infection. Left untreated, pathogens may ascend the ureters to the kidneys and cause infection there. In most people this is prevented by the normal one-way flow of urine from the kidneys, down the ureters, and out of the bladder. However, some conditions, such as calculi (kidney stones), pregnancy, or enlarged prostate, may disrupt this flow and increase risk of infection. Other risk factors include catheterization, diabetes, immune suppression, multiple sexual partners, family history of pyelonephritis, and vesicoureteral reflux (backward flow of urine up the ureters). Less commonly, infection may spread from other parts of the body via the bloodstream.

Flashpoint

Most people with pyelonephritis require hospitalization.

Signs and Symptoms

Classic signs and symptoms of pyelonephritis include dysuria, abdominal pain, flank pain over the costovertebral angle, fever, shaking chills, headache, malaise, nausea, and vomiting. These symptoms may be preceded by those commonly associated with UTI, such as frequency, urgency, dysuria, and pelvic or low back pain.

Diagnosis

Physical examination reveals tenderness of the costovertebral angle over the area of the involved kidney. Testing of the urine with a urine dipstick test indicates nitrite and white blood cells. Urinalysis reveals the presence of bacteria, casts, and white and red blood cells. Urine culture and blood culture may also be done to identify the causative organism.

Flashpoint

Classic symptoms of pyelonephritis include dysuria, flank pain, fever, shaking chills, and malaise.

Treatment

Pyelonephritis is usually treated with 14 days of antibiotics, rest, and fluids; complicated cases may require longer treatment. Pregnant women and people who have severe symptoms or are unable to tolerate oral intake are admitted to the hospital for IV antibiotics and fluid hydration.

Prognosis

Most people fully recover from pyelonephritis. Delayed recovery and complications are more likely if the person needs hospitalization, the infecting organism is resistant to commonly used antibiotics, or the person has a disorder that weakens the immune system (such as certain cancers, diabetes mellitus, and AIDS) or has a kidney stone.

Glomerulonephritis

ICD-9-CM: 580.0–580.9 (acute; code by underlying disease and lesion), 582.0–582.9 (chronic; code by lesion and underlying pathology)

[ICD-10: N00–N03 (code as acute, chronic, diffuse, or focal)]

Acute glomerulonephritis, also called *acute nephritic syndrome,* is a type of nephritis (kidney infection) in which the glomeruli are the key structures affected. Chronic glomerulonephritis, also called *chronic nephritis,* is a condition in which the glomeruli suffer gradual, progressive, destructive changes, with a resulting loss of kidney function.

Incidence

Acute glomerulonephritis most commonly affects individuals between ages 5 and 15, although it can occur at any age. It is twice as common in men as in women. Incidence has declined in western countries in recent years. Chronic glomerulonephritis is currently the third leading cause of kidney failure.

Flashpoint

Acute glomerulonephritis is more common in men than in women.

Etiology

The cause of acute glomerulonephritis is not clear in every case; however, it has been noted to most commonly follow infection of the upper respiratory tract by specific strains of streptococci. It has also been caused by disorders such as systemic lupus erythematosus, subacute bacterial endocarditis (infection of heart muscle), and others. In many cases, chronic glomerulonephritis develops after the onset of acute glomerulonephritis.

Signs and Symptoms

Signs and symptoms of acute glomerulonephritis include rust-colored or bloody urine, **oliguria** (deficient urine production), facial edema, itching, nausea, constipation, and high blood pressure. Other possible symptoms include malaise, fever, weakness, and pain in the abdomen or flank. Symptoms typically follow a streptococcal upper respiratory or skin infection by 1 to 4 weeks.

Those with chronic glomerulonephritis are often asymptomatic in the early stages. As the disease progresses, they exhibit similar signs and symptoms to those of acute glomerulonephritis. As kidney function worsens, they also begin to experience chronic kidney failure.

Flashpoint

Glomerulonephritis can lead to renal failure.

Diagnosis

Diagnosis of both types of glomerulonephritis is based upon a combination of data, including the patient's presenting signs and symptoms and the results of urinalysis and renal biopsy. Urinalysis indicates abnormally large numbers of red and white blood cells and protein. It also reveals renal tubular cells and casts, which both suggest injury to the renal tubules. Kidney biopsy is important for confirming diagnosis and identifying the severity of inflammation and fibrosis (development of fibrous, scar-like tissue). Serum complement (important immune-related proteins) testing may also be done. Because small kidneys may indicate irreversible disease, a renal ultrasound is useful in detecting renal size and ruling out any structural abnormalities. The presence of protein in the urine, especially albumin, is useful in predicting prognosis and risk of progression to complete renal failure.

Treatment

Treatment of both forms of glomerulonephritis is similar: Inflammation and related fibrosis are minimized with immunosuppressive medications such as corticosteroids. Management of hypertension is critical and includes the use of various classes of antihypertensive medications and diuretics. Dietary restrictions include reduction in the intake of salt, fluids, and protein. Hemodialysis (filtration of wastes and fluid from blood as it passes through selectively permeable membranes) may be needed on a temporary basis for those with acute disease; those with chronic disease may require ongoing dialysis or kidney transplantation. Creatinine clearance rate is monitored in those with chronic disease to determine response to therapy.

Prognosis

Prognosis is generally good for those with acute disease; the majority achieve a full recovery. However, some cases may progress to a chronic form, which may in turn lead to chronic renal failure and even death. The mortality rate among pediatric patients with acute glomerulonephritis may be as high as 7%.

Interstitial Cystitis

ICD-9-CM: 595.0 (acute), 595.1 (chronic)   [ICD-10: N30.0 (acute), N30.1 (chronic)]

Interstitial cystitis (IC), sometimes called *painful bladder syndrome* and *chronic pelvic pain*, is a chronic inflammatory condition of the bladder lining not caused by infection or other identified pathology.

Flashpoint
Interstitial cystitis is not caused by infection.

Incidence

IC affects an estimated one million Americans. Most commonly diagnosed are women in their 30s or 40s, although men and children may also develop this disorder.

Etiology

The cause of IC is not fully understood. Most individuals are found to have tiny lesions or ulcerations in the lining of the bladder. Because urine is often acidic, its presence may cause pain. Theorized causes of IC include heredity, allergies, and autoimmune response.

Signs and Symptoms

Symptoms vary, since most individuals report periods of remission and exacerbation. During a flare-up, most people report frequency, urgency, and feelings of pressure, aching, or severe pain in the pelvis or low back area. Some individuals also report pain in the urethra, vulva, or scrotum, and pain with intercourse. For many, pain is most severe during the early morning hours.

Flashpoint
Symptoms of IC may fluctuate unpredictably.

Diagnosis

Because symptoms of IC are sometimes similar to those associated with bladder infection, urinalysis is done to rule out UTI. Other disorders that must also be ruled out include prostatitis and bladder cancer. Cystoscopy is often done under general anesthesia so that the bladder can be visually examined and biopsy tissue obtained (see Box 7-3).

Box 7-3 Diagnostic Spotlight

CYSTOSCOPY

Cystoscopy is a procedure in which the physician performs a visual examination of the bladder. It may be done in a procedure room of the medical office or under general anesthesia as a same-day surgical procedure, depending upon whether additional procedures such as distention and biopsy are planned. Cystoscopy helps the physician diagnose disorders such as interstitial cystitis and bladder cancer.

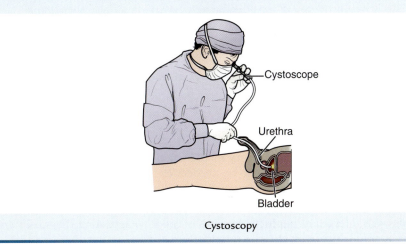

Cystoscopy

Treatment

Common signs and symptoms of IC mimic those of bladder infection, which may lead individuals to believe they have a UTI; however, if standard therapy for UTI (antibiotics and analgesics) does not bring relief, then individuals should be evaluated for IC. There is no cure for IC. A variety of treatment options can be used to manage pain and minimize flare-ups, but individual response varies, so a certain amount of trial and error is needed for most individuals to create an effective management plan. Thus far, just one oral medication has been approved specifically for the treatment of IC: Pentosan (Elmiron) is thought to help the bladder resurface itself. Results are variable, and it may take several months for maximal effect.

Other medications that may relieve or reduce symptoms include analgesics, antihistamines, and antidepressants.

Bladder distention may be done to increase bladder capacity; for some individuals this also reduces pain for a time. Instillation of medications such as dimethyl sulfoxide and heparin into the bladder is also sometimes helpful. Approximately 5% to 10% of IC patients who have Hunner ulcers within their bladder experience improvement of symptoms with laser surgery. Some individuals also respond to diet modification; recommendations are numerous, including eliminating or reducing intake of acidic or spicy foods such as tomatoes, citrus fruit, and chocolate as well as eliminating alcoholic and caffeinated beverages.

Flashpoint
There is no cure for IC, but there are a number of treatments.

Prognosis

IC is a chronic disorder which affects individuals to varying degrees. For some it is a minor annoyance; for others it has a devastating impact on quality of life. Complications include sleep disruption and reduced bladder capacity, resulting in the need for frequent urination (which can interfere with work and social activities). Relationships may also suffer due to the impact on sexual intimacy.

Interstitial Nephritis
ICD-9-CM: 580.89 [ICD-10: N10 (acute), N11 (chronic)]

Interstitial nephritis is a condition of inflammation of the interstitium, which is the area between and around the glomeruli and tubules of the kidneys. It may be acute or chronic and may result in kidney failure.

Incidence

Interstitial nephritis affects approximately 1,200 Americans each year. The acute form is more common than the chronic form and contributes to as many as 15% of all cases of kidney failure.

Etiology

Interstitial nephritis is most commonly caused by an allergic reaction or otherwise toxic effect of certain drugs. Medications implicated include some antimicrobials, NSAIDs, and diuretics. Less common causes include infection, immune disorders, and transplant rejection.

Flashpoint
Interstitial nephritis is usually caused by a reaction to medication.

Signs and Symptoms

Common signs and symptoms of interstitial nephritis include fever, edema, **hematuria** (blood in the urine), nausea, vomiting, oliguria, and mental status changes such as confusion. The individual may have a recent history of infection or may be taking a new medication.

Diagnosis

Interstitial nephritis is diagnosed based upon signs and symptoms and the results of diagnostic tests. Urinalysis may indicate protein, red and white blood cells, casts, renal tubule cells, decreased specific gravity, and increased pH. Diagnosis is confirmed with kidney biopsy, which reveals inflammation within the tissue.

Treatment

Treatment of interstitial nephritis is aimed at relieving symptoms and addressing the underlying cause. Offending medications are discontinued. The use of corticosteroid or anti-inflammatory medications may be useful for several months. Dietary modifications may include fluid, sodium, and protein restriction. Short-term dialysis may also be needed. Hemodialysis is a procedure in which wastes and excess fluid are filtered from the patient's blood (see Box 7-4).

Prognosis

Prognosis for individuals with interstitial nephritis is usually good, with prompt diagnosis and treatment. Complications include acute or chronic renal failure.

Box 7-4 Diagnostic Spotlight

HEMODIALYSIS

Hemodialysis is filtration of wastes and fluid from blood as it passes through selectively permeable membranes.

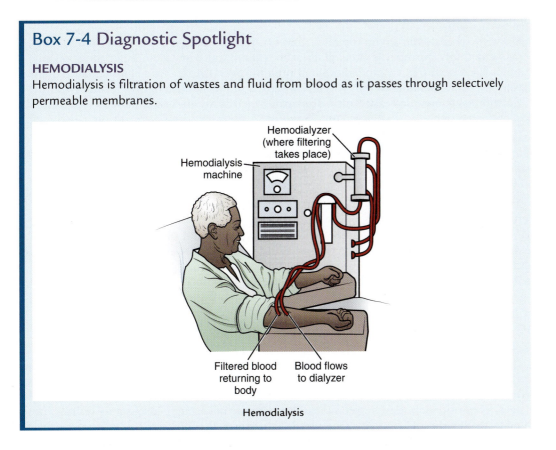

Hemodialysis

Renal Failure

Among the more serious disorders of the urinary system are various forms of renal failure. The ones discussed here are acute tubular necrosis, acute renal failure, and chronic renal failure.

Acute Tubular Necrosis
ICD-9-CM: 584.5   [ICD-10: N17.0]

Acute tubular necrosis (ATN) is a type of renal failure in which the renal tubules have suffered acute injury. Because the tubules play such a critical role in the reabsorption of fluid and adjustment of electrolytes, their injury can result in renal impairment or failure.

Incidence

ATN is the most common cause of acute renal failure in hospitalized patients. It is noted in approximately 5% of all patients admitted to the hospital and as many as 30% of those admitted to intensive care units.

Etiology

ATN has two general causes: *ischemia* (temporary deficiency in blood supply) and toxic injury. Conditions that lead to tubular ischemia include episodes of very low blood pressure associated with hemorrhage from trauma or vascular surgery (such as open heart surgery or aneurysm repair), and complications associated with sepsis and birth-related obstetric complications.

Toxic injury to renal tubules is commonly caused by antimicrobial drugs such gentamicin, amphotericin B, and streptomycin; some chemotherapeutic drugs; and radiocontrast media used in some radiological studies. In some situations, the body may also produce certain substances that are toxic to the renal tubules. For example, severe crush injuries can cause injured muscle tissue to release the enzyme creatinine phosphokinase into the blood. Large amounts of this enzyme may cause damage as it is filtered through the glomeruli and tubules.

Flashpoint
ATN is usually caused by ischemia or toxic injury.

Signs and Symptoms

Individuals with ATN are often asymptomatic. However, if they develop acute renal failure, oliguria becomes apparent. During this time, diagnostic tests reveal a low glomerular filtration rate (GFR) and increased serum creatinine and blood urea nitrogen (BUN). These levels may remain abnormal for several weeks, followed by a gradual return to normal as oliguria resolves. During recovery, individuals sometimes experience **diuresis,** which is an abnormal increase in urine production and excretion.

Diagnosis

Diagnosis of ATN is based upon elevated serum creatinine after exposure to a toxin or a hypotensive event, as well as evidence of oliguria. Other diagnostic tests which may reveal abnormal values include BUN, urine osmolality, and urine sodium. Renal ultrasound may be done to rule out obstruction.

Treatment

Treatment of ATN is supportive. It includes elimination of toxins and support of normal blood pressure. Rehydration with IV fluids is given and is especially important in those with ATN associated with radiocontrast media or elevated creatinine phosphokinase. Transfusion of blood products may be given if hemorrhage is a causative factor. Infection is treated if necessary, and diuretic medications are sometimes given to promote urine output in patients experiencing oliguria. Any medications that are potentially nephrotoxic or eliminated by the kidneys must be used carefully, so as not to further exacerbate the ATN.

Prognosis

Prognosis is good if ATN is diagnosed and treated early. Recovery usually occurs within 3 weeks. However, the overall mortality rate is approximately 50%. This may be largely due to the underlying illness or event that causes the ATN. Prognosis is worse for those with immune suppression, seizures, poor nutrition, and severe illness such as cardiovascular disease, as well as those who demonstrate oliguria and rapidly rising serum creatinine. Prognosis is better for those with better underlying health status. Among those who survive ATN, half have some degree of permanent renal deficit, and up to 10% experience renal failure and eventually require dialysis.

Acute Renal Failure

ICD-9-CM: 584.0–584.9   [ICD-10: N17.0–N17.9] (code by site and lesions for both codes)

Acute renal failure (ARF) is defined as an acute rise of 25% or more in serum creatinine and decreased GFR. It may last days or weeks or develop into acute renal disease.

Incidence

Approximately three million people develop community-acquired ARF, meaning that it develops prior to hospitalization. A larger number of hospitalized patients develop hospital-acquired ARF. The highest rates are among those admitted to critical care and are related to advanced age, severity of illness, volume depletion, and exposure to nephrotoxic substances such as medications. Men and women are affected equally.

Etiology

ARF occurs when the kidneys rapidly lose function due to some type of damage. As a result, the body retains waste products, such as urea and creatinine, that are normally excreted. There are many causes of ARF, categorized as *prerenal, renal,* and *postrenal* depending on the physical location of the problem. Prerenal failure involves inadequate blood flow to the kidneys. Causes include hypotension caused by hemorrhage, severe burns, shock, or severe dehydration; liver failure; and renal vein thrombosis secondary to nephrotic syndrome. In renal failure, injury occurs to the kidney, glomeruli, or tubules. Causes of renal failure include pyelonephritis, some medications or toxins, and diseases that may damage the kidneys, such as sickle cell disease, systemic lupus erythematosus, and multiple myeloma. In postrenal failure, urine outflow is obstructed; causes include prostatic enlargement, kidney stones, and prostate cancer.

> **Flashpoint**
> ARF is often caused by an episode of inadequate blood supply to the kidneys.

Signs and Symptoms

Common symptoms of ARF include oliguria or **anuria** (absence of urine production), generalized edema, altered mental status, tremors, anorexia, a metallic taste in the mouth, easy bruising or bleeding, flank pain, fatigue, hypertension, and seizures.

Diagnosis

Diagnosis is based on elevated creatinine or blood urea nitrogen (BUN) values in an ill, oliguric patient. Abdominal or kidney ultrasounds are the most common radiological tests, but others may include x-ray, CT scan, and MRI, which would rule out obstruction.

Treatment

Treatment of ARF is aimed at identification and treatment of the underlying cause. In many cases, the condition resolves spontaneously after the underlying cause is alleviated, as with removal, destruction, or passage of a kidney stone. Treatment also includes careful monitoring of fluid intake and output and electrolytes, and administration of diuretic medications. The physician may also order diet modifications to increase carbohydrates and limit protein, sodium, and potassium intake while ensuring adequate calories and nutrients. In some cases, temporary dialysis is also necessary.

There are two forms of dialysis: hemodialysis and peritoneal dialysis. *Hemodialysis* involves sending a patient's blood through tubes within a dialysis machine comprising selectively permeable membranes. Just outside of the tubes is dialysis fluid, which is somewhat similar in composition to human blood without the blood cells or waste products. Wastes, along with excess fluid and electrolytes, move from the blood across the membrane into the dialysis fluid, and the machine returns the clean blood to the patient's body. *Peritoneal dialysis* is similar to hemodialysis except that the lining of the patient's peritoneal cavity (abdomen) is used as the dialyzing membrane. In this process, dialysis fluid is infused through a tube inserted in the patient's abdomen. Wastes then diffuse from the patient's blood vessels beneath the peritoneum, across the membrane, and into the dialysis fluid. After a specified period of time, usually 1 to 2 hours, the fluid is removed.

Flashpoint

Treatment of ARF may include hemodialysis.

Prognosis

Acute renal failure requires careful treatment and is potentially life-threatening. The mortality rate for hospital-acquired ARF is as high as 70%. Infants and children with ARF have a 25% mortality rate. Some individuals may develop chronic renal failure, requiring ongoing dialysis or a kidney transplant; however, most individuals recover within several weeks or months.

Chronic Renal Failure

ICD-9-CM: 585.1–585.9   [ICD-10: N18.0–N18.9] (code by stage for both codes)

Chronic renal failure (CRF), also called *chronic kidney disease*, is defined as the progressive loss of the kidney's effectiveness in excreting waste products and regulating fluid and electrolytes.

Incidence

In 2002, an estimated 20 million individuals in the United States suffered from some degree of CRF. Since that time the numbers have steadily increased, largely due to increased prevalence of hypertension and diabetes. The United States has the highest rates of end-stage renal disease (ESRD), with the highest rates in the African American population; Japan follows in second place. At increased risk are elderly patients and those with diabetes or hypertension.

Etiology

CRF develops slowly over a period of years and may result from any number of diseases that cause kidney damage. The most common causes are diabetes and hypertension, which cause at least two-thirds of all cases (see Box 7-5). Other causes include polycystic kidney disease, glomerulonephritis, analgesic nephropathy (damage caused by long-term use of analgesics), and various types of urine outflow obstruction. Risk factors include a family history of diabetes or renal failure. Also at increased risk are the elderly and African American, Hispanic, Native American, and Pacific Islander populations.

Flashpoint

More than 20 million people in the United States have CRF, and numbers are on the rise.

Signs and Symptoms

The progression of CRF is usually so gradual that symptoms are not evident until 90% of kidney function is lost. Symptoms are related to *uremia,* which is the increased nitrogenous waste products, especially urea, in the blood. Initial symptoms include nausea, vomiting, weight loss, fatigue, malaise, generalized pruritus, headache, and frequent hiccups; later ones include oliguria, *nocturia* (frequent need to urinate during the night), easy bleeding or bruising, lethargy, diminished sensation in the extremities, muscle twitching, and seizures. Other symptoms might include polydipsia (increased thirst), pallor, hypertension, agitation, and changes in skin tone (darker or lighter).

Flashpoint

Patients with CRF are often symptom-free until they have lost 90% of kidney function.

> ## Box 7-5 Wellness Promotion
>
> ### BE KIND TO YOUR KIDNEYS
> Because most people are symptom-free during the early stages of kidney failure, they may be unaware of progressing damage. Therefore, everyone—especially those with hypertension or diabetes—should take good care of their kidneys. Measures include:
>
> - preventing or treating high blood pressure through weight loss, regular exercise, healthy diet, and, if necessary, prescription medication
> - for diabetics, keeping blood glucose level within recommended ranges through regular glucose checks, diet, exercise, and, if needed, medication
> - following instructions when using over-the-counter analgesics and other medications

Diagnosis

According to the National Kidney Foundation, diagnosis of CRF is determined by checking blood pressure, urine albumin, and serum creatinine, all three of which will be elevated. GFR, considered the most reliable indicator of renal function, is used to track the disease. Normal GFR varies by age, from 116 milliliters per minute for patients around age 20 to 75 milliliters per minute for those aged 70 or older. The National Kidney Foundation has categorized the severity of chronic kidney disease in five stages:

- *Stage 1:* kidney damage with GFR that is normal or increased to greater than 90 milliliters per minute
- *Stage 2:* GFR of 60 to 89 milliliters per minute
- *Stage 3:* GFR of 30 to 59 milliliters per minute
- *Stage 4:* GFR of 15 to 29 milliliters per minute
- *Stage 5:* kidney failure with GFR less than 15 milliliters per minute; or dialysis

Other findings may include progressively increasing creatinine and BUN levels with decreasing creatinine clearance, ***proteinuria*** (protein in the urine), hyperkalemia (high blood potassium), hypertension, neuropathy (disease of the nerves), fluid retention, metabolic acidosis (decreased pH related to retention of acids or loss of buffers), and abnormally small kidneys (noted via x-ray, ultrasound, MRI, or CT scan).

Treatment

Treatment of CRF is aimed at managing symptoms, slowing disease progression, and reducing the risk of complications. In addition, careful management of related disorders—such as heart failure, chronic UTI, kidney stones, and anemia—is essential. The physician will prescribe dietary changes, usually including restriction of fluid, protein, and electrolytes.

For individuals with ESRD, the physician will prescribe long-term dialysis and may consider kidney transplantation.

Flashpoint

Many patients with CRF eventually require hemodialysis or kidney transplantation.

Prognosis

The mortality rate is highest among those with CRF severe enough to require chronic dialysis. The 5-year survival rate for this population is approximately 35%; it is even lower—25%—for those with underlying diabetes. Death is usually related to cardiovascular disease.

Diabetic Nephropathy

ICD-9-CM: 250.4 (use additional codes 580–585 to identify manifestations)	[ICD-10: E10.3–E14.3 (the third digit identifies nephropathy; E10–E14 identify the type of diabetes)]

Diabetic nephropathy is a disease of the kidneys associated with diabetes. It results in inflammation, degeneration, and sclerosis of the kidneys.

Incidence

Diabetic nephropathy is one of the most devastating long-term complications of diabetes and is the most common cause of CRF in the United States and other industrialized countries. Incidence is higher in those with type 1, insulin-dependent diabetes mellitus than in those with type 2, non–insulin-dependent diabetes mellitus. Onset usually occurs among those who have had type 1 diabetes for 10 or more years. Some degree of nephropathy may already be present in those diagnosed with type 2 diabetes, since they often have diabetes for several years before they are diagnosed.

Etiology

The exact cause of diabetic nephropathy is unclear, but it is thought to develop as damage to the glomerulus and tiny blood vessels within the kidneys is caused by inflammation and injury from hyperfiltration brought on by hyperglycemia. Patients are also often prone to hypertension, which further worsens the condition by adding to vascular injury. In addition to diabetes, other risk factors for nephropathy include hypertension, high cholesterol, smoking, and Native American, African American, or Mexican American descent.

> **Flashpoint**
> Nephropathy may already be present in those diagnosed with type 2 diabetes.

Signs and Symptoms

Individuals in the early stages of diabetic nephropathy are usually asymptomatic. The earliest sign may be small amounts of protein in the urine. As the disease progresses, individuals may experience more severe proteinuria, worsening hypertension, and high cholesterol and triglyceride levels. As renal failure develops, signs and symptoms may include anorexia, weight loss, edema, fatigue, weakness, nausea, and insomnia.

Diagnosis

Diagnostic criteria for diabetic nephropathy in a patient with diabetes include albuminuria (presence of albumin in urine) on at least two separate tests 3 to 6 months apart, declining GFR, and hypertension. Yearly testing is recommended for those who have had type 1 diabetes for 5 or more years and upon diagnosis of type 2 diabetes. Creatinine and BUN may also be tested to monitor kidney function, and renal ultrasound may be done to determine kidney size and rule out obstruction. Diagnosis may be confirmed with kidney biopsy.

Treatment

Treatment of diabetic nephropathy is individualized and generally includes measures to lower blood pressure and achieve optimal control of blood glucose. A variety of antihypertensive medications may be used, but angiotensin-converting enzyme inhibitors have been found to be especially effective in delaying the progression of nephropathy. Aggressive control of blood glucose has been found to partially reverse some of the damage to kidneys and delay the development of proteinuria. A low-fat, low-salt, low-protein diet is recommended to minimize progression and cardiovascular complications. Protein should comprise no more than 10% of calorie intake. Other possible treatment options are discussed in the section on chronic renal failure.

> **Flashpoint**
> Aggressive control of blood glucose may partially reverse kidney damage.

Prognosis

Prognosis for those with diabetic nephropathy is variable and depends upon the individual's other health factors, the type of diabetes, and the timeliness of diagnosis and treatment. At one time, as many as 50% of diabetic patients developed nephropathy; however, early treatment has been found to delay and even prevent this complication. In some individuals, nephropathy may progress to renal failure and risk of death.

Neurogenic Bladder

ICD-9-CM: 596.54   [ICD-10: N31.9] (unspecified for both codes)

Neurogenic bladder is a condition of bladder dysfunction related to disease or injury of the central nervous system or certain peripheral nerves.

Incidence

The exact incidence of neurogenic bladder is not known. Because neurogenic bladder is a neurological disorder, at risk are those who have suffered traumatic injury to the spinal cord or brain.

Etiology

Neurogenic bladder is caused by neurological disease or damage to the central nervous system or peripheral nerves involved in bladder function, as is caused by brain injury, stroke, and spinal-cord tumors or trauma. Other diseases and disorders that can lead to neurogenic bladder include Alzheimer disease, multiple sclerosis, diabetes, Parkinson disease, and cerebral palsy.

Signs and Symptoms

Flashpoint

Urge incontinence causes urine leakage with the urge to void.

Signs and symptoms associated with neurogenic bladder include various forms of incontinence. ***Urge incontinence*** is the leakage of urine with the urge to void; individuals may not make it to the toilet in time. ***Stress incontinence*** is the leakage of urine with minor physical stress, such as coughing, sneezing, lifting, or laughing (see Fig. 7-3). Urinary retention may also occur; this is the inability to empty the bladder when desired. Individuals may experience loss of bladder sensation and increased incidence of urinary tract infections.

Flashpoint

Stress incontinence causes urine leakage with minor physical stress.

Diagnosis

Diagnosis is based upon neurological evaluation, examination of the bladder, patient's description of symptoms, and results of urodynamic studies. Postvoid residual is a measurement of the amount of urine remaining in the bladder after urination; increased volumes indicate urinary retention. A cystogram is useful to confirm stress incontinence. Cystoscopy allows the physician to visualize the inner bladder. Other tests may be done to identify urine-flow rate and bladder capacity.

Treatment

Treatment for neurogenic bladder is individualized and depends upon the cause, severity of symptoms, and type of dysfunction present. Injection of botulinum toxin into one of the urinary sphincters may allow urination for those with urinary retention. Intermittent or chronic use of a urinary catheter may be used to empty the bladder. A suprapubic catheter may also be placed through a surgically created hole into the bladder through the pelvic wall. Incontinence briefs or pads, while not a form of treatment, can be used if needed to protect skin integrity and clothing. These products should not be used instead of treatment, however. Urethral occlusive devices may be inserted into the urethra to prevent urine leakage; however, they must be removed regularly for bladder emptying, are difficult for some individuals to place, and have the potential to become dislodged. Surgical procedures may increase bladder volume or the effectiveness of the urethral outlet. Individuals with stress or urge incontinence may benefit from exercises designed to strengthen the muscles of the pelvic floor and increase bladder capacity. These same individuals may also benefit from urinary antispasmodics, which are medications that promote urinary retention.

Flashpoint

Medications called urinary antispasmodics may help promote urine retention.

Prognosis

There is usually no cure for the underlying nervous system disorders that cause neurogenic bladder. In most cases, though, prognosis for those with the disorder is very good. Complications of incontinence include skin breakdown and the associated emotional

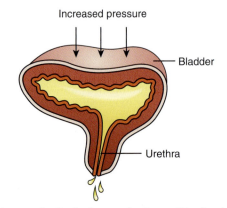

FIGURE 7-3 Stress incontinence is the leakage of urine with physical stress, such as coughing, sneezing, lifting, or laughing.

distress. The most common complications associated with intermittent or chronic catheterization are bladder and kidney infection.

Nephrotic Syndrome

ICD-9-CM: 581.9 (unspecified)   [ICD-10: N04.0–N04.9 (code as diffuse versus focal and by degree of damage)]

Nephrotic syndrome is an uncommon disorder marked by increased glomerular permeability to proteins, resulting in massive protein loss in the urine, edema, hypoalbuminemia (low blood albumin), hyperlipidemia (high blood lipids), and hypercoagulability (tendency to form blood clots).

Incidence

More than 39,000 people die each year from nephrotic syndrome. Incidence is greater in men than women. Adolescents and adults between the ages of 15 and 59 are most commonly affected, with the average age in the early 30s. Around 20% of cases are in those over age 75. More severe and rapidly progressing cases are most common in the older population.

Etiology

There are several causes of nephrotic syndrome; all include injury to the glomerulus or other parts of the kidneys. Some are drug toxicity, diabetes, complications of systemic lupus erythematosus, and AIDS. When known causes have been ruled out, the individual is diagnosed with idiopathic nephrotic syndrome, which means the cause is uncertain.

Flashpoint
More than 39,000 people die each year from nephrotic syndrome.

Signs and Symptoms

A common symptom of nephrotic syndrome is peripheral edema that is usually worse in the legs and increases throughout the day. Children with nephrotic syndrome may exhibit facial edema. In severe cases, individuals may retain 10 to 20 liters of excess fluid; such cases may also result in ascites and pleural effusion. Patients may note frothy urine and complain of fatigue and lethargy. Other symptoms include complications associated with blood-clot formation in renal or leg veins, which may include leg pain, chest pain with breathing, and shortness of breath. Hyperlipidemia may result in symptoms associated with atherosclerosis. Anorexia and proteinuria may result in symptoms associated with protein-calorie malnutrition, such as muscle wasting and white fingernails.

Flashpoint
Nephrotic syndrome may cause severe edema.

Diagnosis

Definitive diagnosis of nephrotic syndrome usually requires a renal biopsy. Among other tests, GFR and serum albumin can be measured.

Treatment

Treatment of nephrotic syndrome is based upon the underlying cause. Daily weight monitoring and administration of diuretics is used to reduce and manage edema. Electrolytes such as sodium and potassium must be monitored. Anticoagulants are used to treat or prevent clotting complications, lipid-lowering agents minimize atherosclerosis, and a special diet limits quantities of fluid, sodium, potassium, and protein. Medications may include corticosteroids and other immunosuppressive agents. Dialysis may be required if renal failure develops.

Prognosis

Complications of nephrotic syndrome include infections such as peritonitis (which affects the membrane that lines the abdomen) and cellulitis (infection of the subcutaneous layer of the skin) as well as thromboembolism (blood clots). Prognosis depends upon the underlying cause. In cases of drug toxicity, discontinuation of the drug may result in complete recovery. When AIDS is the cause, death may result within a few months.

Hydronephrosis

ICD-9-CM: 591   [ICD-10: N13.0–N13.9 (code by location)]

Hydronephrosis is a condition in which the renal pelvis and calyces of the kidneys become distended and dilated and begin to atrophy due to urine outflow obstruction.

Incidence

Incidence of hydronephrosis varies with the type. An estimated 3 million Americans suffer from unilateral hydronephrosis at some point during their lives.

Etiology

Hydronephrosis is caused by obstructed urinary outflow, which stretches tissues of the renal pelvis due to pressure from urine accumulation (see Fig. 7-4). Thus, it may be caused by anything that obstructs urine outflow. Obstruction may be complete or partial, unilateral or bilateral. Hydronephrosis occurs in infants and children due to congenital (existing at birth) defects. It occurs in adults due to prostate enlargement or complications of pregnancy, or to kidney stones, tumors, ureteral strictures, or other malformations. Other contributors include parasitic infestations, neurogenic bladder, bladder cancer, and urinary tract inflammation.

> **Flashpoint**
>
> Hydronephrosis is caused by anything that blocks urine flow from the kidneys.

Signs and Symptoms

Patients with hydronephrosis are commonly asymptomatic, unless kidney stones are the cause. Those with kidney stones complain of severe flank pain that may radiate into the lower abdomen or groin. If kidney failure develops, associated symptoms are present.

Diagnosis

Radiological tests, which may include ultrasound, intravenous pyelography (IVP), and occasionally MRI, reveal dilation of the renal pelvis and obstruction (see Box 7-6). Blood tests may reveal creatinine and electrolyte imbalances. Urine pH may become more alkaline. In cases of complete obstruction, the kidney may be palpable (capable of being felt) on physical examination, due to enlargement.

Treatment

Treatment of hydronephrosis is aimed at the underlying cause, with an emphasis on restoring urine flow. The physician may order renal-function studies to monitor kidney function. In the case of kidney stones, the physician may perform **lithotripsy,** a procedure in which shock waves or sound waves crush stones in the kidneys or urinary tract. The physician may also prescribe surgery to remove lodged stones or tumors or to place a stent (device used to hold tissue in place and maintain an opening) for urine drainage. Treatment for obstruction of the bladder outlet may include insertion of a urinary or suprapubic catheter (tube), or prostate surgery, if benign prostatic hypertrophy (BPH) is the cause.

> **Flashpoint**
>
> Treatment of hydronephrosis is aimed at restoring urine outflow.

Prognosis

If removal of the obstruction occurs in a timely manner, hydronephrosis resolves spontaneously. If restoration of urinary flow does not occur, kidney tissues dilate and atrophy, and chronic renal failure may occur.

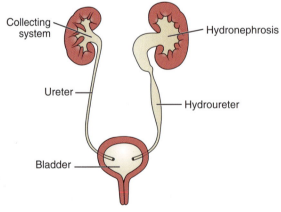

FIGURE 7-4 **Hydronephrosis**

Box 7-6 Diagnostic Spotlight

INTRAVENOUS PYELOGRAPHY

Intravenous pyelography (IVP) is a procedure in which a series of x-rays are taken of the kidneys, ureters, and bladder after IV injection of a dye.

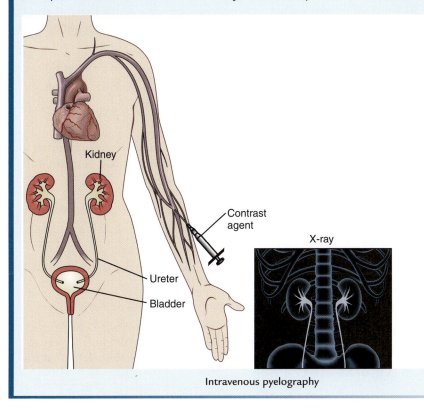

Intravenous pyelography

Polycystic Kidney Disease

ICD-9-CM: 753.12–753.19 (code as congenital, autosomal dominant, or autosomal recessive)	[ICD-10: Q61.0–Q61.9 (code as congenital, autosomal dominant, or autosomal recessive)]

Polycystic kidney disease (PKD) is a group of hereditary, progressive disorders in which cysts (small sacs of fluid) form in the kidneys, eventually destroying them. Other organs may also be affected, including the liver, heart, pancreas, and brain.

Incidence

One form of PKD usually appears early in childhood and is more severe than other forms, which develop later in life. PKD is the most common life-threatening hereditary disease in the United States, affecting approximately 600,000 people. Approximately 12.5 million are affected worldwide. Incidence is higher in men, African Americans, and people with sickle cell disease.

Etiology

PKD is inherited. Autosomal recessive PKD is rarer and deadlier than autosomal dominant PKD. Children of parents with PKD have a 50% chance of getting the disease. Onset of autosomal dominant PKD is usually in middle age.

Flashpoint

PKD is the most common life-threatening hereditary disease in the United States.

Signs and Symptoms

Signs and symptoms of autosomal recessive PKD are commonly present at birth or become apparent in early infancy. The most common signs of PKD include hypertension, hematuria, frequent kidney infections, and back or side pain.

Diagnosis

Diagnosis usually occurs after the individual begins to experience symptoms. Ultrasound and CT scan create images of the kidneys and detect the presence of cysts. Genetic testing helps definitively diagnose PKD.

Flashpoint

Genetic testing is used to diagnose PKD.

Treatment

There is no cure for PKD. Treatment includes measures to improve comfort, possibly kidney dialysis and transplant.

Prognosis

Many adults with PKD may be able to lead normal or near-normal lives. However, complications can occur, including hypertension, cerebral aneurysm, and renal failure. About half of those with autosomal dominant PKD will develop ESRD by the age of 60.

Renal Calculi

ICD-9-CM: 592.0	[ICD-10: N20.0]

Renal calculi, also called *kidney stones,* are composed of mineral salts and cause problems when they obstruct portions of the kidney or, more likely, ureter (see Fig. 7-5).

Incidence

An estimated 2% to 5% of Americans develop kidney stones at some time in their lives. White males between the ages of 40 and 70 are most commonly affected. People with gout, hypercalcemia (high blood calcium), hyperparathyroidism (overactive parathyroid), and inflammatory bowel disease are at increased risk.

Flashpoint

Kidney stones are most common among middle-aged white males.

Etiology

Causes of renal calculi are not fully understood, but some include hypercalciuria, gout, hyperparathyroidism, and Crohn disease. One cause is hypercalciuria, an

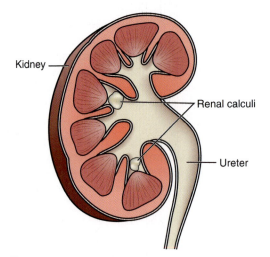

FIGURE 7-5 **Renal calculi**

inherited condition in which excessive calcium is excreted into the urine. Another is gout, which causes abnormal metabolism of uric acid. Other contributors include hyperparathyroidism and Crohn disease. Hyperparathyroidism affects serum calcium levels, increasing the likelihood of calcium stones. Crohn disease is a chronic inflammatory condition of the colon; it can cause malabsorption of bile salts and fat, increasing the likelihood of calcium oxalate kidney stones. Risk factors for kidney-stone formation include immobilization, prolonged dehydration, urine stasis caused by obstruction, and prolonged use of some medications.

Signs and Symptoms

Patients with renal calculi are commonly asymptomatic when stones remain in the kidneys. However, when a stone moves into and obstructs a ureter, the patient experiences a sudden onset of severe, intermittent pain caused by spasm of the involved ureter. This pain, commonly called **renal colic,** radiates downward from the flank into the abdomen or groin area. Other symptoms include chills, fever, hematuria, and urinary frequency.

Diagnosis

Preliminary diagnosis is based on the patient's signs and symptoms and the presence of blood in the urine. The presence of renal stones is confirmed by such radiological tests as CT scan, ultrasound, IVP, MRI, and abdominal x-rays.

Treatment

Conservative treatment of renal calculi includes opiate analgesics for pain; fluids; and smooth-muscle relaxants. The goal is to support the patient in passing the stone in the urine. If the stone is too large or the ureter is completely blocked, the surgeon may perform surgery to remove the stone. Lithotripsy is another treatment option (see Fig. 7-6 and Box 7-7).

Prognosis

Most patients are able to pass kidney stones without permanent damage. However, complete obstruction may result in hydronephrosis and potential failure of the involved kidney. The risk of recurrence is estimated at 50%.

Flashpoint
A classic symptom of kidney stones is intermittent, severe flank pain.

Flashpoint
Lithotripsy breaks up kidney stones into smaller pieces.

STOP HERE.
Select the flash cards for this chapter and run through them at least three times before moving on to the next chapter.

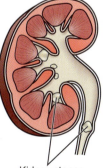
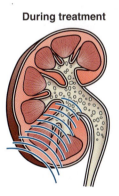
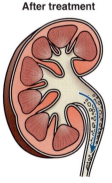

Before treatment

During treatment

After treatment

Kidney stones

Shock waves crush stones

Smaller pieces pass out of body in urine

FIGURE 7-6 Kidney stones may be dissolved with lithotripsy.

Box 7-7 Diagnostic Spotlight

LITHOTRIPSY

Extracorporeal shock wave lithotripsy is a procedure in which a device called a lithotriptor breaks up stones in a sedated patient with an external, high-intensity acoustic pulse after the stones are located with an ultrasound device. The procedure takes about an hour, after which the crushed stone is then passed out of the ureters (kidney stone) or cystic duct (gallstone).

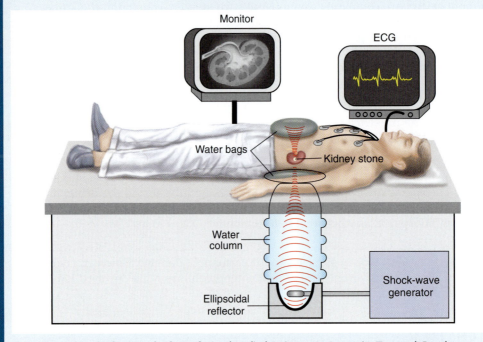

Lithotripsy (From Eagle, S, et al. *The Professional Medical Assistant: An Integrative Teamwork-Based Approach.* 2009. Philadelphia: F.A. Davis Company, with permission.)

Student Resources

American Urological Association: http://www.auanet.org
Healthcommunities.com Urology Channel: http://www.urologychannel.com
Interstitial Cystitis Association: http://www.ichelp.org
Kidney Cancer Association: http://www.kidneycancer.org
Mayo Clinic: http://www.mayoclinic.com
National Kidney and Urologic Diseases Information Clearinghouse: http://www.kidney.niddk.nih.gov
National Kidney Foundation: http://www.kidney.org
Nephrology Channel: http://www.nephrologychannel.com/atn/index.shtml

Chapter Activities

Learning Style Study Strategies

Try any or all of the following strategies as you study the content of this chapter:

Visual learners: Write terms and definitions on sticky notes and place them around your house on mirrors and cupboard doors and anywhere else you will see them. This supports you in reviewing them multiple times throughout the day while going about your regular activities.

Kinesthetic learners: Use arts-and-crafts supplies (colored paper, glue, clay, stickers, yarn, etc.) to create models of the things you are studying (such as the heart, bones, cells, etc.).

Auditory learners: Be sure to attend class, where you can listen to lecture and ask questions about anything you find confusing. Listening to your instructor's explanations will be helpful for you.

Verbal learners: Create silly rhymes to help you remember terms and definitions.

Practice Exercises

Answers to Practice Exercises can be found in Appendix D.

Case Studies

CASE STUDY 1

Stephanie Bell is a 34-year-old patient. She came in 10 days ago with complaints of pelvic discomfort, frequency, urgency, and dysuria. The physician ordered a urinalysis, which was nearly normal except for a trace amount of blood. The physician gave Ms. Bell a prescription for an antibiotic for possible UTI and told her to drink lots of fluids. She has returned to the clinic stating that her symptoms did not improve. After another urinalysis shows the same results, the physician decides to refer Ms. Bell to the urologist.

1. If Ms. Bell does not have a UTI, what other disorder might explain her symptoms?

2. Besides the symptoms reported by this patient, what other symptoms are associated with this disorder?

3. How might the diagnosis in question 1 be confirmed?

4. List at least two types of treatment that might be used for Ms. Bell's condition.

5. When Ms. Bell asks how long it will take for her bladder to be healed so she won't be bothered with her symptoms anymore, how should the nurse answer this question?

CASE STUDY 2

Robert Nyle is a 50-year-old white man who presents to the clinic with complaints of severe, intermittent right-flank pain that started several hours earlier. His temperature is 100.4°F, and he complains that he is beginning to feel chilled. Urine chem stick testing indicates the presence of blood. The physician suspects that Mr. Nyle has a renal calculus.

1. What is the common name for this disorder?

2. How will the physician confirm the diagnosis?

3. Is Mr. Nyle typical of patients who commonly get this disorder? Why or why not?

4. Describe the typical treatment plan for someone with this disorder.

5. What disorder might Mr. Nyle be at risk for if the calculus lodges in and obstructs his ureter?

CASE STUDY 3

Kwahu Hinto is a 54-year-old Native American patient at Valley Medical Center. He has had type 2 diabetes for approximately 10 years. He also has moderate hypertension and smokes one pack of cigarettes per day. He has recently been diagnosed with diabetic nephropathy and wants to know what this means for him. How will you answer his questions listed here?

1. What is nephropathy, and how did I get it?

2. Why didn't I know that I had this? I felt fine until recently.

3. What kinds of symptoms will I have in the future?

4. What kind of treatment can I have to cure this condition?

Multiple Choice

1. Which of the following terms is **not** matched with the correct definition?

   a. Dysuria: pain, burning, or other discomfort during urination

   b. Anuria: need to urinate frequently

   c. Nocturia: frequent need to urinate during the night

   d. Oliguria: deficient urine production

2. Which of the following terms is **not** matched with the correct definition?

   a. Hematuria: presence of blood in the urine

   b. Proteinuria: presence of protein in the urine

   c. Diuresis: abnormal increase in urine production and excretion

   d. Uremia: temporary deficiency in blood supply

3. The kidneys produce and excrete an average of ____ of urine each day.

    a.   500 to 750 milliliters

    b.   1 to 2 liters

    c.   2 to 3 liters

    d.   3 to 4 liters

4. Which of the following statements is true regarding urinary tract infections?

    a.   They are usually caused by a virus.

    b.   They are more common in men than women.

    c.   Common symptoms include frequency, urgency, and dysuria.

    d.   Patients are encouraged to drink fluids that make the urine more alkaline.

5. Which of the following statements is true regarding nephrotic syndrome?

    a.   It is marked by large amounts of glucose in the urine.

    b.   Individuals with this disorder often experience dehydration.

    c.   It is most common in children under age 8.

    d.   Definitive diagnosis usually requires a biopsy.

Short Answer

1. **What causes prerenal acute renal failure? List three specific examples of triggering events.**

2. **Describe the common symptoms of acute renal failure.**

3. **List the two most common causes of chronic renal failure.**

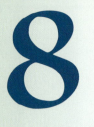

8 REPRODUCTIVE SYSTEM DISEASES AND DISORDERS

Learning Outcomes

Upon completion of this chapter, the student will be able to:

- Define and spell key terms related to the reproductive system
- Identify key structures of the male and female reproductive systems and their functions
- Discuss the roles played by the male and female reproductive systems in the process of procreation

- Identify characteristics of common reproductive system diseases and disorders, including:
  - description
  - incidence
  - etiology
  - signs and symptoms
  - diagnosis
  - treatment
  - prognosis

KEY TERMS	
circumcision	procedure in which part or all of the foreskin of the penis is removed
cryptorchidism	undescended testicle(s)
dyspareunia	pain with intercourse
gestation	time from conception to birth
lactation	production of breast milk
menorrhagia	excessive menstrual flow
orchiectomy	surgical removal of one or both testes
phimosis	stenosis of the foreskin opening so that it cannot be pushed back over the glans penis
rape	forced vaginal, anal, or oral penetration
uteropexy	surgical fixation of the uterus

Abbreviations

Tables 8-1, 8-2, and 8-3 list some of the most common abbreviations related to reproductive system diseases and disorders.

TABLE 8-1

ABBREVIATIONS RELATED TO THE MALE REPRODUCTIVE SYSTEM

Abbreviation	Meaning	Abbreviation	Meaning
♂	male	PSA	prostate-specific antigen
BPH	benign prostatic hypertrophy (hyperplasia)	TSE	testicular self-examination
DRE	digital rectal examination	TUNA	transurethral needle ablation
ED	erectile dysfunction	TURP	transurethral resection of the prostate

Structures and Functions of the Male Reproductive System

Structures of the Male Reproductive System

The male reproductive system shares some structures with other body systems, such as the penis and urethra (shared by the urinary system) and the testes (shared by the endocrine system). Other structures of the male reproductive system include the prostate gland, the scrotum, and a series of ducts and glands (see Fig. 8-1).

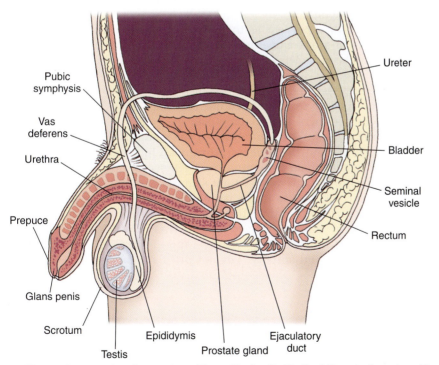

FIGURE 8-1 **The male reproductive system** (From Eagle, S. *Medical Terminology in a Flash! An Interactive, Flash-Card Approach.* 2006. Philadelphia: F.A. Davis Company, with permission.)

The scrotum is composed of two internal compartments surrounded by loose connective tissue and a smooth muscle layer. A second muscle group, the *cremasters*, extends from the abdomen into the scrotum. Within the compartments of the scrotum are the testes, oval-shaped organs comprising an outer capsule of thick, white connective tissue and an inner part divided into 200 to 300 lobules, which contain the seminiferous tubules. The area from the posterior portion of the scrotum to the anus is called the perineum.

From the testes to the urethra, a series of ducts connect to each other, beginning with the seminiferous tubules, then the rete testis, efferent ductules, epididymis, vas deferens, and finally the ejaculatory duct, which joins with the urethra.

The urethra begins at the exit of the bladder and passes through the penis, ending at its tip. The penis is composed of three sections of erectile tissue and a distal, rounded end, the glans penis. A fold of skin commonly called the *foreskin* covers the glans penis. In many cultures, a procedure called **circumcision** is commonly practiced. In this procedure, part or all of the foreskin is removed.

Functions of the Male Reproductive System

A primary function of the male reproductive system is reproduction. Sperm cells vital to this process are created and stored within the testes. They are sensitive to heat and must live in an environment at slightly less than normal body temperature. Therefore, prior to birth, the testes in the male fetus normally descend from the lower abdomen into the scrotum. The structures of the scrotum are designed to maintain an optimal temperature for spermatogenesis (sperm production). In a cold environment, the smooth muscle of the scrotum and the cremaster muscles contract, bringing the scrotum and testes closer to the body to keep them warmer. In a warm environment, the same muscles relax and allow the scrotum and testes to descend away from the body to keep them cooler.

Flashpoint

Sperm cells are heat sensitive and must live in an environment at slightly less than normal body temperature.

Spermatogenesis takes place within the seminiferous tubules of the testes. When the spermatocytes have reached maturity, they exit the testes through a series of ducts and leave the body during ejaculation.

The urethra serves a dual purpose as the exit passageway for both urine and semen; however, both do not exit at the same time. During sexual activity, the internal urinary sphincter contracts to keep semen from entering the bladder and urine from exiting the bladder.

During arousal, the erectile tissue of the penis becomes engorged with blood and the penis becomes firm and erect, to facilitate sexual intercourse and ejaculation. The state of erection ends with ejaculation or diminishment of sexual arousal.

Secretions from a variety of sources contribute to the seminal fluid. Mucous secretions from the bulbourethral glands and the inner urethral wall lubricate the urethra and neutralize its normally acidic environment. Seminal vesicles secrete fructose and other nutrients for sperm cells, as well prostaglandin, which stimulates smooth-muscle contractions in the female reproductive tract; this is thought to help move sperm through that environment. The prostate gland secretes prostatic fluid that flows through a number of ducts to the urethra and contributes an alkaline pH, to help further neutralize the environment. A neutral environment is important to sperm motility—sperm need an environment with a pH between 6.0 and 6.5 for optimal activity. Vaginal pH, by comparison, is normally between 3.5 and 4.0.

Common Male Reproductive System Diseases and Disorders

There are innumerable diseases and disorders of the male reproductive system. Common ones include benign prostatic hypertrophy, sexually transmitted diseases, and erectile dysfunction.

Common Conditions of Inflammation and Infection

Numerous disorders of the male reproductive tract are caused by inflammation, infection, or both. The most common ones, discussed here, are balanoposthitis, prostatitis, epididymitis, and orchitis.

Balanoposthitis

ICD-9-CM: 607.1   [ICD-10: N48.1]

Balanoposthitis, also called *balanitis*, is the inflammation of the glans penis and foreskin covering the glans penis.

Incidence

The general incidence of this disorder is unknown. One study found that 11% of male visitors to genitourinary clinics had this disorder.

Etiology

Balanoposthitis is most commonly caused by fungal infection, but bacterial pathogens may also be involved. Organisms include the *Candida* species, *Bacteroides, Gardnerella,* and beta-hemolytic streptococci. They proliferate (grow rapidly) in the presence of smegma (a thick, cheesy, malodorous secretion). The result is localized inflammation and edema. It develops most commonly in uncircumcised men with poor hygiene.

Signs and Symptoms

Signs and symptoms of balanoposthitis include tenderness, itching, redness, edema, and ulceration of the glans penis and foreskin; stenosis of the urethral meatus (opening); and **phimosis** (stenosis of the foreskin opening so that it cannot be pushed back over the glans penis).

> **Flashpoint**
>
> Balanoposthitis is most common among uncircumcised men with poor hygiene.

Diagnosis

Diagnosis is usually based on physical-examination findings. Laboratory studies may include culture of urethral discharge and microscopic evaluation to identify the pathogen involved.

Treatment

Treatment depends on the cause and usually includes daily retraction and cleaning of the foreskin with application of antibiotic or antifungal cream. The physician may prescribe oral antibiotics and may also recommend circumcision for those patients with phimosis, to prevent recurrence.

Prognosis

Prognosis for balanoposthitis is good with proper treatment. Individuals with chronic or recurring inflammation may require circumcision.

Prostatitis

ICD-9-CM: 601.0 (acute), 601.1 (chronic)   [ICD-10: N41.0 (acute), N41.1 (chronic)]

Prostatitis is the inflammation of the prostate gland. It is categorized as acute or chronic, and it includes conditions known previously as *prostatodynia, chronic pelvic pain syndrome,* and *abacterial prostatitis,* regardless of whether the individual is symptomatic.

Incidence

Prostatitis is most common in men over the age of 50.

Etiology

Prostatitis usually develops secondary to bacterial growth after the development of a urinary tract infection. Causative organisms include *Neisseria gonorrhoeae, Escherichia coli, Staphylococcus, Pseudomonas,* and *Streptococcus.*

Signs and Symptoms

Signs and symptoms of prostatitis include fever, chills, urethral discharge, dysuria, malaise, myalgia (muscle aches), and perineal discomfort. Upon examination, the prostate gland is tender and enlarged.

Diagnosis

Culture of prostatic secretions helps identify the causative organism so that appropriate antibiotics can be selected.

Treatment

Treatment includes an extended course of antibiotics, opiate analgesics, and antispasmodics to relieve discomfort.

Prognosis

Prognosis is very good for acute prostatitis. The prognosis for chronic prostatitis is less certain, because complications may occur, including urethritis, epididymitis, and cystitis.

Epididymitis

ICD-9-CM: 604.0 (with abscess),   [ICD-10: N45.0 (with abscess),
604.9 (without mention of abscess)   N45.9 (without abscess)]

Epididymitis is the inflammation or infection of the epididymis, a tubular structure on the posterior surface of the testicle. The condition may be acute or chronic.

Incidence

Epididymitis is the most common cause of scrotal inflammation, affecting nearly 140,000 American men each year. Most are between the ages of 20 and 40, although younger or older males may also be affected.

Etiology

Epididymitis is commonly caused by a sexually transmitted infection. Causative organisms typically include *N. gonorrhoeae* and *Chlamydia trachomatis,* but *Staphylococcus* and *E. coli* may also be involved. Epididymitis can also result as a complication of mumps, a urinary tract infection, prostatitis, or injury associated with surgery, the presence of a urinary catheter, or other trauma. Risk factors include frequent urinary tract infections, untreated bacterial prostatitis, unprotected sex, immune suppression, and bladder obstruction.

Signs and Symptoms

Signs and symptoms of epididymitis include abdominal or flank pain or more localized pain in the testicle or scrotum. Other manifestations may include edema, dysuria, urinary frequency and urgency, urinary retention, fever, chills, malaise, discharge, and symptoms of urethritis. The individual may also have difficulty walking due to scrotal pain and tenderness.

Diagnosis

Diagnosis of epididymitis is based on physical-examination finding of an enlarged, tender, firm epididymis. Lymph nodes in the groin area, and the prostate, may also be tender and enlarged. Urinalysis and urine culture reveal the presence of bacteria and increased white blood cells. Blood tests may also indicate an elevated white blood cell count. In some cases, regular or color-coded Doppler ultrasonography reveals a thickened, enlarged epididymis and increased Doppler wave pulsation.

Treatment

Treatment of epididymitis is aimed at the underlying cause. Antibiotics are given for bacterial infection. Sexual partners are treated if the infection is sexually transmitted. Cases caused by mumps or trauma are treated symptomatically. Pain and inflammation are managed with analgesic medication, rest, cold compresses, and scrotal support. Surgery is reserved for severe, complicated cases where abscess or necrosis (tissue death) are complicating factors.

Flashpoint

Untreated epididymitis can result in scarring and sterility.

Prognosis

Potential complications of epididymitis are scarring and sterility, especially if the condition is bilateral. However, the prognosis is usually good with timely diagnosis and treatment.

Orchitis

ICD-9-CM: 604.90 (unspecified)   [ICD-10: N45.0–N45.0 (use additional codes
B95–B97 to identify infectious organism)]

Orchitis is a condition of inflammation of one or both testicles caused by infection, usually viral. It may be acute or chronic.

Incidence

Orchitis often occurs in young men or boys who are infected with the mumps. It also occurs in those suffering from epididymitis, which is often related to sexually transmitted infections.

Etiology

Nearly 70% of orchitis cases develop when the testicles become inflamed secondary to infection with the mumps virus. The next most common cause is complication of a sexually transmitted infection. Less commonly, orchitis results from other viruses, traumatic injury, or damaged circulation.

Signs and Symptoms

Patients with orchitis usually complain of unilateral testicular pain, which may arise gradually but more commonly develops fairly abruptly. It may be located initially in the back of one testicle but then spread throughout the scrotal and then pelvic area. Other signs and symptoms may include edema, redness, warmth, malaise, dysuria, frequency, urethral discharge, and fever. The patient may also experience ejaculation of blood and hematuria. Current or very recent edema and pain of the parotid gland, in the jaw region, will also be apparent in those with mumps.

Diagnosis

Initial diagnosis of orchitis is often based upon a recent history of mumps infection, along with presenting signs and symptoms. Testing of urine and blood and culturing of urethral discharge may be done to identify a potential sexually transmitted infection. Ultrasound may be done to rule out testicular torsion or other structural problems.

Treatment

Treatment of bacterial infection involves the use of antibiotics. Mumps- and trauma-related orchitis are treated symptomatically, with analgesic medication, rest, cold compresses, and scrotal support.

Prognosis

Prognosis for orchitis is generally very good. Cases caused by mumps usually resolve within several days without any special treatment. In approximately 60% of cases some testicular atrophy occurs. Atrophy is the shrinkage or wasting away of tissue due to impaired circulation or another cause. Although deficient testosterone production and fertility problems are possible, sterility is rare; these problems are more likely when both testicles are involved. Also rarely, chronic orchitis may develop, leading to chronic pain.

Other Disorders of the Male Reproductive System

Numerous noncancerous disorders affect the male reproductive system. Some of the most common include benign prostatic hypertrophy, testicular torsion, varicocele, and erectile dysfunction.

Benign Prostatic Hypertrophy

ICD-9-CM: 600.20 (without urinary obstruction),   [ICD-10: N40]
600.21 (with urinary obstruction)

Benign prostatic hypertrophy (BPH), also called *benign prostatic hyperplasia,* is a noncancerous growth and enlargement of the prostate gland in men (see Fig. 8-2).

Incidence

BPH is rare in younger men but becomes increasingly common as men age, because the prostate gland increases in size with age. Incidence of symptomatic BPH is greatest in men over age 40 and is estimated at 50% for men over age 50. This rises proportionally to 80% for men over age 80; however, only a quarter of all men, approximately 300,000 per year, will seek treatment.

Etiology

The cause of BPH is not fully understood; however, BPH develops in men who have elevated estrogen levels compared with relatively low testosterone levels. A substance known as dihydrotestosterone may be a factor. Dihydrotestosterone is synthesized from testosterone but is much more potent, and it plays an important role in prostate growth. As the prostate gland enlarges, it compresses the lumen, or passage, of the urethra, making it increasingly difficult for the patient to pass urine. Incomplete emptying of the bladder increases the risk of infection and other inflammatory changes to urinary-tract structures.

Flashpoint

The incidence of BPH rises significantly as men age.

Signs and Symptoms

Common symptoms of BPH are related to urethral obstruction and difficulty emptying the bladder. As a result, individuals usually complain of urgency, frequency, hesitancy, and nocturia. Patients may also notice a decrease in the force and consistency of the urinary stream. Urinary

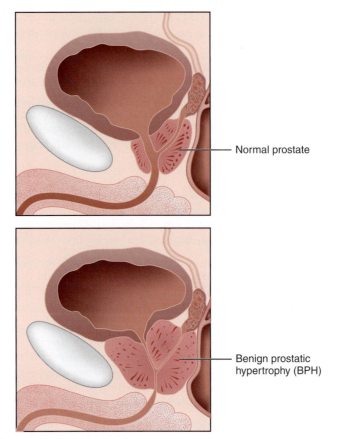

Normal prostate

Benign prostatic hypertrophy (BPH)

FIGURE 8-2 **Benign prostatic hypertrophy**

retention causes some individuals to become prone to urinary tract infections, kidney problems, and incontinence.

Diagnosis

Diagnosis of BPH is based on the patient's description of signs and symptoms and is confirmed by digital rectal examination (DRE), which reveals an enlarged prostate that is rubbery in texture. (A swollen, tender prostate indicates prostatitis; a hard or nodular prostate may indicate cancer.) A prostate-specific antigen (PSA) blood test reveals an elevated level of prostate-specific antigen in 30% to 50% of individuals with BPH. Other diagnostic tests include rectal ultrasound, urine flow study, IVP, and cystoscopy, which help identify the degree of prostate enlargement and impedance of urine flow, and differentiate benign prostatic enlargement from prostate cancer.

Treatment

In some cases, initial treatment for BPH involves stabilization of kidney function by discontinuing anticholinergic drugs, treating infection, and emptying the bladder via catheterization. Further treatment for BPH aims to shrink or remove all or part of the prostate gland. For some men, the drug finasteride helps shrink the prostate gland. Other medications may act to improve urine flow and more complete emptying of the bladder in some patients. Transurethral microwave procedures may destroy prostate tissue. Such procedures can usually be done in the medical office without general anesthesia. In a procedure called *transurethral needle ablation* (TUNA), low-level radiofrequency energy burns away part of the prostate. Prostate tissue can be removed with more invasive forms of surgery, including transurethral resection of the prostate (TURP), in which a surgeon inserts tiny surgical instruments via the urinary tract and uses them to remove prostate tissue. There are no external incisions or scars with this form of surgery. A urinary catheter must be in place for 1 to 5 days after surgery to enable bladder irrigation and monitor urine output. Other options for surgery include laparoscopic prostatectomy, open prostatectomy, and radical prostatectomy. These are all more invasive and are generally reserved for patients with prostate cancer. They also require hospitalization and a longer recovery time.

Prognosis

Prognosis for BPH is generally good with adequate diagnosis and treatment. Around 5% to 10% of patients may experience some postoperative problems with sexual function and incontinence. In cases of extreme, prolonged obstruction, the ureters may dilate and hydronephrosis may develop.

Testicular Torsion

ICD-9-CM: 608.2   [ICD-10: N44]

Testicular torsion is a condition in which the testicles become twisted and the spermatic cord, blood vessels, nerves, and vas deferens become strangled (see Fig. 8-3).

Incidence

Testicular torsion primarily affects infants in the first year of life and adolescent boys between 12 and 18 years old, although it can occur at any age. Males with cryptorchidism (undescended testicles) develop testicular torsion more often than the general population.

Etiology

The cause of testicular torsion is often unclear. It may be related to vigorous physical activity or scrotal injury, though it frequently occurs during sleep.

Signs and Symptoms

Signs and symptoms of testicular torsion include sudden, intense testicular pain, lower abdominal pain, edema, redness, a lump in the testicle, and blood in the semen. Pain may be severe enough to also cause nausea and vomiting.

Diagnosis

Diagnosis is usually based upon the patient's presenting signs and symptoms and physical-examination findings. Color Doppler sonography may identify lack of circulation to the testicle, which is characteristic of torsion and is useful in ruling out epididymitis.

Treatment

Treatment of testicular torsion includes an attempt at manual detorsion (untwisting) of the testicle. Surgical intervention may be necessary if this is not successful. **Orchiectomy** (surgical removal of one or both testes) is necessary if necrosis has occurred. If the testicle can be saved, it is sutured to the wall of the scrotum to secure it.

Prognosis

Testicular torsion is a medical emergency and must be treated immediately. If it is diagnosed and treated within 6 hours, prognosis is good. Complications include necrosis and subsequent loss of the affected testicle.

Flashpoint

Testicular torsion is a medical emergency and must be treated immediately.

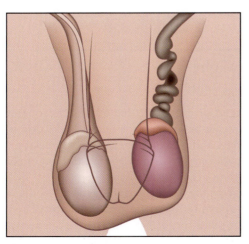

FIGURE 8-3 **Testicular torsion**

Varicocele

ICD-9-CM: 456.4   [ICD-10: I86.1]

Varicocele is the enlargement and dilation of the veins of the spermatic cord that drain the testes. Distention of veins surrounding the testes raises testicular temperature by several degrees, which can have a negative impact on fertility.

Incidence

The majority of the time, varicocele develops in the left testicle. It develops in 15% to 20% of the male population between ages 15 and 25; it is rare in older men, but possible. It is a common finding in men with fertility problems.

Etiology

Varicocele develops when the drainage of blood from the testes becomes disrupted. Normally the blood flows away from the testes through veins that run alongside the spermatic cord. One-way valves within the veins ensure the efficiency of blood flow. However, if the valves are defective or if the veins become compressed by a nearby structure, the vessels may become distended from blood congestion. The process usually occurs slowly. Varicocele in men over age 40 may be caused by abdominal or pelvic malignancy and should be carefully investigated.

Signs and Symptoms

Most men with varicocele are symptom free, and the condition is usually noted during a routine physical examination. However, some men may experience a feeling of testicular heaviness or aching, or they may note a vein that is enlarged enough to see or feel. They may also experience shrinkage of the affected testicle, due to atrophy, and possible fertility problems.

Diagnosis

Moderate-sized varicoceles may be palpable during physical examination as a twisted mass alongside the spermatic cord. The patient is examined while standing, because this increases pressure within the abdomen and produces greater venous dilation. Several diagnostic methods may be used to confirm diagnosis: Doppler ultrasonography may detect blood backflow through the valves, thermography detects heat pockets caused by pooling blood, and venogram allows the physician to inspect anatomical structures radiologically (see Box 8-1). If fertility is a concern, semen samples may also be analyzed.

Treatment

Men who are symptom free may require no treatment. Those with minor symptoms may alleviate them by using scrotal support such as briefs or a jockstrap. Patients who are concerned about fertility or are experiencing pain or other symptoms may need to undergo surgical repair to have the vessels ligated (tied off). Open surgery is usually done on an outpatient, same-day basis. Most individuals are able to resume light physical activities after 2 days and strenuous activities after 2 to 6 weeks. A treatment alternative is embolization, a procedure in which the doctor inserts tiny coils or injects a substance into the problematic veins to cause them to become non-functional. Blood then flows from the testes through other smaller veins. The patient is able to resume normal activities within 2 days after this procedure.

Box 8-1 Diagnostic Spotlight

DOPPLER ULTRASONOGRAPHY

Doppler ultrasonography is a diagnostic procedure that transforms sound waves into a real-time visual image. It is noninvasive and painless. It allows evaluation of the direction, speed, and turbulence of blood flow and is useful for evaluating circulation in the heart, legs, and other locations. Recent advances have allowed the addition of color, which reveals images even more clearly than in black and white.

During the procedure, a technician applies a gel to the patient's skin and then uses a transducer to collect the data and send it to a monitor, which displays it in the form of a moving image. The images may be saved for further study by the physician.

Prognosis

Individuals with varicocele may experience testicular atrophy. It is unclear what effect this condition has on fertility, since fertility doesn't always improve after surgery. The general prognosis is very good; most varicoceles are easily diagnosed and repaired. A small percentage of surgical patients develop fluid accumulation around the testicle. This can be corrected with minor surgery. Between 10% and 20% of individuals may experience a recurrence of varicocele and require a second repair.

Erectile Dysfunction

ICD-9-CM code: 607.84 (organic origin), [ICD-10: N48.4 (organic origin),
302.72 (inhibited sexual excitement)   F52.2 (inhibited sexual excitement)]

Erectile dysfunction (ED), also called *impotence*, is a general term that describes a number of disorders that all impact a man's ability to attain an erection adequate to achieve a satisfactory sexual experience. Episodic ED occurs at some time to most men and is not considered problematic from a medical standpoint. As men age, some changes in erectile function are common, including loss of rigidity, need for more stimulation, less intense orgasm, and need for increased recovery time between erections. However, when problems with ED become chronic or recur frequently, they can be a sign of a physical or emotional problem. Men who experience ED that lasts longer than 2 months are encouraged to see their health-care provider.

Incidence

ED is most common in men over the age of 65 but can occur at any age. Incidence is higher in men who smoke or abuse alcohol or other drugs and in those with diabetes or cardiovascular disease.

Etiology

Causes of ED fall into two categories: physical and psychological. Common physical causes include disorders that affect nerve function, such as diabetes, spinal-cord injury, and multiple sclerosis. Other disorders may cause ED from cardiovascular disease or hormonal problems. ED may also be caused by adverse effects of medication, surgical complications, and drug or alcohol abuse. Psychological causes include fatigue, depression, stress, anxiety, and negative feelings toward or lack of interest in the sexual partner.

> **Flashpoint**
> Episodic ED occurs at some time to most men and is not considered problematic from a medical standpoint.

Signs and Symptoms

The main symptom of ED is difficulty developing or maintaining a full erection throughout intercourse.

Diagnosis

In order to diagnose ED, the physician must gather a health history, including a description of symptom onset and pattern and information about other medical conditions, medications, and recent physical and emotional events. Blood tests check hormone levels, such as testosterone, and help rule out underlying disorders such as diabetes. The physician may adjust current medications to determine whether they are a factor. Ultrasonography can evaluate circulation; neurological evaluation checks for nerve damage. Other tests include cavernosography, to visualize the corpus cavernosum, and dynamic infusion caverosometry, to measure vascular pressure in the penis.

Treatment

Treatment of ED depends on the underlying cause. Psychological causes are treated with counseling and, in some cases, medication. When ED is caused by medications, a change in dose or a switch to another medication may resolve the problem. Treatment of physical causes is tailored to the individual disorder. There are numerous medications on the market for the treatment of ED. These drugs relax smooth muscle in the penis, enabling greater blood flow, which results in increased quality of an erection when physical and psychological stimulation occur. Other treatments include testosterone replacement therapy, surgery, penile implants, and needle-injection therapy.

Prognosis

Prognosis for ED is variable. In many cases, it may resolve completely with appropriate treatment. In other cases, it may not fully resolve but can be lessened (see Box 8-2).

Box 8-2 Wellness Promotion

SAFE TREATMENT FOR ED

Erectile dysfunction (ED) is a personal subject that many men feel embarrassed to discuss. However, many men deal with it at some time in their lives; they should be encouraged to discuss their concerns with their physician so they can identify safe solutions. Important points for these men to know include:

- Many forms of treatment for ED are available. A treatment plan can be designed for each individual's unique needs.
- Many unapproved treatments are promoted on television and the Internet. Many of them do not work, and some can actually cause harm.
- Even approved treatment methods are not right for everyone. For example, someone with a history of stroke, heart attack, or heart rhythm problems within the past 6 months should not take certain medications.
- Medications such as sildenafil (Viagra), tadalafil (Cialis), and vardenafil (Levitra) should not be combined with nitrate medications such as nitroglycerine, because of the risk of heart and blood pressure problems.
- It may take time to experience the full benefit of some medications, so patience is needed.
- The key to a mutually satisfying sexual relationship is communication. Therefore, men should discuss their concerns with their partners and seek counseling if needed.

Sexually Transmitted Infections

STIs, formerly called *sexually transmitted diseases,* are a group of infections transmitted through sexual intercourse or other intimate contact with infected individuals. Viruses that most commonly cause STIs include human papillomavirus (HPV) and herpes simplex virus (HSV). HPV is actually a group of more than 100 tumor viruses which can cause tissue growths on the surface of the skin and mucous membranes, and in some cases, is responsible for cervical cancer in women. Other organisms that often cause STIs include *C. trachomatis* and *N. gonorrhoeae.* In nearly all cases, infection is spread through direct contact with lesions or other body fluids. While some STIs, such as syphilis, are becoming less common, others have become epidemic.

Herpes Simplex

ICD-9-CM: 054.10 (genital herpes simplex) [ICD-10: A60.0]

Herpes simplex, commonly called *genital herpes,* is a sexually transmitted infection. There are many variations of the herpesvirus. Herpes simplex virus type 2 (HSV-2) most commonly causes lesions on the genitals (see Fig. 8-4). The virus causes repeated eruptions of acutely painful vesicles and then spreads along nerve pathways, where it lies dormant between outbreaks.

Flashpoint

Infection is most contagious when vesicles rupture, but transmission can still occur even in the absence of an outbreak.

Incidence

An estimated 90 million people worldwide are infected with HSV-2.

Etiology

HSV-2 is a virus spread by sexual contact with an infected person. All forms of herpes are contagious and spread via direct contact with secretions. Once an individual has herpes, certain triggers may precipitate repeated outbreaks, including stress, illness, and immunosuppressive medications.

TABLE 8-2			
ABBREVIATIONS RELATED TO SEXUALLY TRANSMITTED INFECTIONS			
Abbreviation	**Meaning**	**Abbreviation**	**Meaning**
GC	gonorrhea	STI	sexually transmitted infection
HPV	human papillomavirus	Trich	trichomoniasis
HSV	herpes simplex virus		

Signs and Symptoms

Symptoms of genital herpes include local pain and itching, burning, dysuria, and tingling or shooting pains 1 to 2 days before eruption of a rash. The rash is characterized by reddened patches with small vesicles in the anogenital region. Some patients complain of fever and malaise during an outbreak. The rash lasts for approximately 10 days, and the infection is most contagious when the vesicles rupture during this time; however, asymptomatic shedding of the virus can cause transmission in the absence of an outbreak.

Diagnosis

Diagnosis is based on the characteristic appearance and may be confirmed by a culture of secretions or, more rarely, by the detection of antibodies in the blood.

Tests used to confirm HSV diagnosis use a sample of cells or fluid, most commonly from lesions in the genital area but sometimes from spinal fluid, blood, urine, or tears. There are two tests that confirm HSV infection:

- A herpes viral culture tests cells or fluid from a fresh lesion. The physician collects the sample with a cotton swab and places it in a culture cup. This is the most specific method of determining infection and is, therefore, the most common test performed.
- Herpesvirus antigen detection tests cells from a fresh lesion. The physician scrapes some cells from the lesion and smears them on a microscope slide. Herpesvirus antigens are visible through the microscope on the surface of cells infected with the virus. The physician may order this test along with a viral culture.

Treatment

Treatment usually includes antiviral medications, which reduce viral shedding and shorten outbreaks if given early. Analgesics may help reduce pain and tenderness caused by the lesions. Other medications may include corticosteroids and antipruritics (anti-itching medication). Patients should be counseled on safe sexual practices to reduce the risk of transmission.

There is no cure for genital herpes; antiviral medication can be used for the initial outbreak and subsequent outbreaks. Although these antivirals shorten the duration of the lesions, patients must

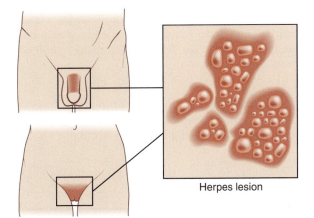

Herpes lesion

FIGURE 8-4 HSV 2 - Genital herpes

be aware that the outbreak can return. Patients should be advised to abstain from sexual contact during an outbreak, to prevent transmission to their partners. Genital herpes can also be transmitted from mother to fetus during delivery and can cause respiratory illnesses, retinal infection, encephalitis (brain infection), and death of the neonate. Pregnant women with genital herpes can schedule a cesarean delivery or take acyclovir to suppress the infection until after birth. Women with genital herpes have an increased risk of cervical cancer and should get yearly Papanicolaou (Pap) tests.

Prognosis

There is no cure for herpes; once acquired, the virus lies dormant in the body until something triggers another outbreak. Individuals should learn to identify their most common triggers and avoid them if possible. They should also take precautions to avoid transmission of the virus to others. Women who are pregnant or considering becoming pregnant should inform their healthcare provider if they have genital herpes, because transmission during childbirth can result in serious complications for the newborn. The duration of outbreaks may range from 10 days to 5 weeks. A potential complication of herpes zoster is postherpetic neuralgia, persistent nerve pain that lasts for months after lesions disappear.

Chlamydia

ICD-9-CM: 079.98   [ICD-10: A56.0]

Chlamydia is a sexually transmitted infection caused by the pathogen *C. trachomatis.*

Incidence

Chlamydia is one of the most commonly transmitted STIs in North America, affecting three to nine million people per year. It is thought to be present in 10% of all college students and half of all patients with pelvic inflammatory disease (PID). The CDC recommends yearly chlamydia screenings for sexually active women under age 26.

Etiology

C. trachomatis is spread through sexual contact.

Signs and Symptoms

Up to 75% of females are asymptomatic, giving chlamydia its name as the "silent" STI. Individuals who experience symptoms generally do so within 1 to 3 weeks of exposure. Women may complain of dysuria, itching, **dyspareunia** (pain with intercourse), and abnormal vaginal discharge. If the infection ascends into the fallopian tubes, they may complain of low back pain, lower abdominal pain, fever, nausea, and bloody spotting between menstrual periods. Men may experience urethral discharge and dysuria. Those who have receptive anal intercourse may complain of rectal pain, bleeding, or discharge.

Diagnosis

Diagnosis can be confirmed by cultures of cervical or urethral discharge and urine testing.

Treatment

Treatment may include antibiotic therapy for a minimum of 1 week. If acquired during pregnancy, chlamydia will also spread from the mother to the fetus during delivery and can cause conjunctivitis, pneumonia, or even blindness in the baby.

Prognosis

If left untreated, chlamydia can migrate up the reproductive tract, causing inflammation and scarring of the fallopian tubes and resulting in permanent infertility. In addition, women with an active chlamydia infection are more susceptible to infection with HIV.

Genital Warts

ICD-9-CM: 078.11   [ICD-10: A63.0]

Genital warts are small, raised, pink, soft, painless growths caused by HPV (see Fig. 8-5).

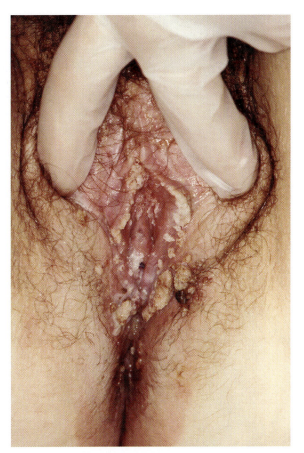

FIGURE 8-5 Genital warts caused by the human papillomavirus (Photo courtesy of the Centers for Disease Control and Prevention/Joe Millar.)

Incidence
HPV has become the most common STI in the United States today, with more than 50% of all sexually active men and women becoming infected at some time. An estimated 20 million Americans between the ages of 15 and 49 are currently infected, and over six million become newly infected each year.

Etiology
Unlike warts that can appear on the hands or the feet, genital warts are sexually transmitted. In most cases they are caused by one or more strains of the human papillomavirus (HPV).

Signs and Symptoms
A wart may be a single growth that develops into a cauliflower-like growth and can spread to the perianal area. Most patients are asymptomatic, but some will report itching and burning.

Diagnosis
The physician diagnoses genital warts primarily by visual inspection. If the warts turn whitish in color when swabbed with acetic acid (vinegar), the diagnosis is confirmed.

Treatment
There is no complete cure for genital warts. Although topical podophyllin or laser surgery can be used to destroy genital warts, they may return after treatment. Treatment should be administered weekly until all warts are removed. After successful treatment, the patient should schedule a follow-up examination in 3 months. Patients should be instructed to abstain from intercourse, or use condoms, to prevent infecting partners.

Flashpoint
There is no complete cure for genital warts.

Prognosis
The lesions may disappear without treatment; however, active infection may still be present, and transmission to a partner is possible. The patient should undergo testing for HIV and other STIs.

Women should undergo regular Pap tests, because genital warts increase risk of cervical cancer.

Gonorrhea

ICD-9-CM: 098.0   [ICD-10: A54.0]

Gonorrhea is a sexually transmitted infection caused by the pathogen *N. gonorrhoeae.*

Incidence

Sexually active teens are at the highest risk of contracting gonorrhea. Co-infection with chlamydia is common, occurring in an estimated 30% of patients with gonorrhea. The CDC estimates that more than 700,000 people in the United States newly acquire gonorrhea infections each year. Only about half of these infections are reported to the CDC. Young inner-city teens are most at risk for contracting gonorrhea and nearly 400,000 cases are reported annually in the United States.

Etiology

Because the *N. gonorrhoeae* bacteria die with exposure to air, gonorrhea is spread only through direct sexual contact.

Signs and Symptoms

Men are more likely than women to be symptomatic with gonorrhea. They usually experience white, yellow, or green urethral discharge, burning with urination, and swollen testicles. Women with gonorrhea may be symptom free or may experience a greenish-yellow discharge from the cervix. If the fallopian tubes are affected, women may experience lower abdominal pain. Symptoms can also include swollen glands and a milky discharge from the anus.

Diagnosis

Diagnosis is based upon examination findings and the results of culture. Urine kits are also available for initial screening.

Treatment

Because of increasing resistance of gonorrhea to fluoroquinolone antimicrobial medication, the CDC currently recommends that gonorrhea be treated only with cephalosporins, as either a single injection or a single-dose pill. All people who have had sexual contact with the patient should be tested and treated if necessary.

Prognosis

Pregnant patients with a known case of gonorrhea cannot deliver vaginally, because the bacteria can cause blindness in the neonate. Since many women are asymptomatic, routine treatment of newborns includes administration of silver nitrate solution to their eyes immediately after birth to kill the bacteria that may be present. If left untreated, gonorrhea can cause PID and permanent sterility.

Syphilis

ICD-9-CM: 091.0 (primary),   [ICD-10: A51.0 (primary), A51.3 (secondary,
091.1 (secondary, unspecified),   unspecified), A52.9 (late, unspecified)]
097.1 (latent, unspecified)

Syphilis is a multistage infection caused by the spirochete *Treponema pallidum.*

Incidence

Syphilis is a sexually transmitted infection that is most commonly seen in sexually active teens, young adults, illicit drug abusers, and patients with HIV infection. In the United States, health officials reported over 36,000 cases in 2006, including nearly 10,000 cases of primary and secondary syphilis.

Etiology

Syphilis is transmitted from person to person by direct contact with skin and mucous membranes. The spirochetes can penetrate the skin and enter regional lymph nodes, spreading to the entire body.

Signs and Symptoms

After an incubation period of 10 days to 2 months, painless ulcers, or *chancres*, appear in the primary stage of syphilis (see Fig. 8-6). The chancres are highly infectious and mostly appear on the genitals.

In the secondary stage, a widespread body rash appears with symptoms of fever, headaches, malaise, and inflammation of the lymph nodes. Moist, broad papules (bumps) filled with infectious fluid appear along the perineum. Shallow ulcerations in the mouth can also appear. If left untreated, secondary syphilis can progress to the third (late) stage.

Tertiary syphilis includes tissue damage to the aorta, central nervous system, bones, and skin. Permanent damage may include aortic aneurysm, meningitis, sensory and gait deficits, and damage to the optic nerve, causing blindness.

> **Flashpoint**
> Tertiary syphilis can lead to serious complications, including blindness.

Diagnosis

Diagnosis is made by the polymerase chain reaction test, available mostly at research hospitals. This test detects antibodies to *T. pallidum* in blood, body fluid, or tissue. It can be used to screen for or confirm syphilis infection.

Treatment

Treatment consists of long-acting preparations of penicillin. The duration of treatment depends on the stage of syphilis and any co-infections, such as HIV. Other antibiotics may be used for individuals allergic to penicillin.

Prognosis

If diagnosed and treated during the primary or secondary stage, the patient will suffer no permanent damage. Late-stage syphilis can lead to long-term health problems, such as damage to the heart and blood vessels, skin, and bones.

Trichomoniasis

ICD-9-CM: 553.3   **[ICD-10: A59.0 (unspecified)]**

Trichomoniasis, sometimes called *trich*, is a sexually transmitted infection with the protozoan *Trichomonas vaginalis.*

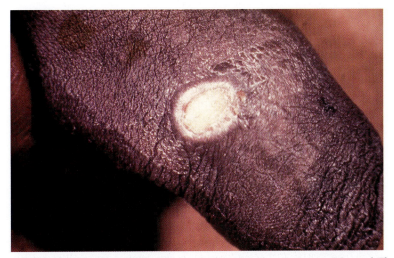

FIGURE 8-6 Chancre caused by syphilis (From Goldsmith, LA, Lazarus, GS, and Tharp, MD. *Adult and Pediatric Dermatology: A Color Guide to Diagnosis and Treatment.* 1997. Philadelphia: F.A. Davis Company, with permission.)

Incidence

Trichomoniasis is considered the most common curable STI in the world. Incidence is estimated at 5 to 7 million cases annually in the United States and more than 180 million cases globally.

Etiology

Trichomoniasis is spread through sexual intercourse or other direct genital-to-genital contact. Risk factors include infection with other STIs, multiple sexual partners, and African descent. Approximately 5% of infants born to infected mothers also acquire the infection.

Signs and Symptoms

Some individuals with trichomoniasis are symptom free. This is especially true for men, although they may complain of burning with urination or ejaculation, and of urethral discharge. Women experience frothy white, gray, or yellow-green vaginal discharge with a characteristic foul, fishy odor; pain with urination and intercourse; and genital irritation or itching and swelling.

Diagnosis

Culture is the most accurate means of diagnosis, but it takes 10 days for results. Therefore, many physicians examine a wet preparation, which indicates the presence of *T. vaginalis.* Urinalysis and Pap test may also be done. Because this infection often occurs along with others, patients are also screened for gonorrhea, chlamydia, syphilis, and HIV.

Treatment

Treatment should include any sexual partners, since the infection is easily spread back and forth, and symptom-free individuals may not even know they are infected. Patients are treated with antiprotozoal medication.

Prognosis

With treatment, a full recovery from infection is common. Previous infections can increase the risk of HIV transmission and delivery of a baby with low birth weight. In addition, the patient with trichomoniasis is at greater risk for cervical cancer because of the damage to cervical cells.

Chancroid

ICD-9-CM: 099.0   [ICD-10: A57]

Chancroid is a bacterial infectious disease transmitted through sexual contact.

Incidence

Annual global incidence of chancroid is estimated at six million. The disorder is rare in the United States, with an estimated annual incidence of about 150. Incidence is higher among populations with high-risk lifestyles, such as those who engage in prostitution or have sexual contact with prostitutes. Chancroid is also often contracted by individuals who engage in unprotected sex while traveling to high-risk areas abroad. It is most common in low-income groups in Asia, Africa, and the Caribbean, especially those who participate in high-risk sexual practices. It is more common in men than in women; uncircumcised men are three times more likely to contract chancroid from an infected partner than are circumcised men.

Etiology

Chancroid is caused by the bacterium *Haemophilus ducreyi,* which gains entry to the skin or mucous membranes through minor trauma such as that caused by sexual intercourse.

Signs and Symptoms

Within 2 weeks of exposure, infected people develop a small bump on their genitals which quickly progresses to an ulcer (see Fig. 8-7). Lesions range in size from a few millimeters to 5 centimeters; have sharply defined, irregular borders and a base covered with yellowish-gray material; are painful; and bleed easily. Women are more likely than men to develop multiple lesions, typically

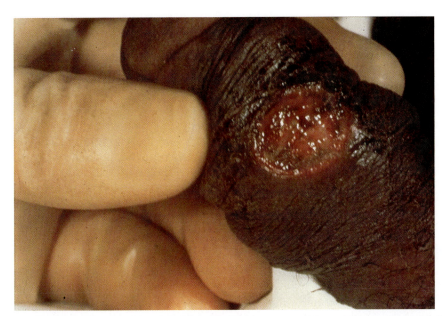

FIGURE 8-7 Chancroid lesion (From Goldsmith, LA, Lazarus, GS, and Tharp, MD. *Adult and Pediatric Dermatology: A Color Guide to Diagnosis and Treatment.* 1997. Philadelphia: F.A. Davis Company, with permission.)

located on the labia majora, labia minora, perineum, and even the inner thighs. Ulcerations in men typically develop anywhere on the penis or scrotum. Nearby inguinal lymph nodes may become enlarged and even rupture and drain. Individuals commonly complain of painful urination and pain with intercourse, vaginal discharge, fever, and weakness.

Diagnosis

Chancroid is diagnosed through history and physical examination of lesions. Because lesions are somewhat similar in appearance to the chancre lesion caused by syphilis, serological tests are done to rule out syphilis (see Box 8-3). Lesions may also be cultured, but this has proven unreliable. The World Health Organization and the CDC recommend that diagnosis be based upon the presence of one or more painful ulcers, especially when inguinal lymphadenopathy (tender, enlarged lymph nodes) is present and syphilis and herpes simplex have been ruled out.

Box 8-3 Differentiating Chancroid from Chancre

Chancroid and chancre lesions, caused by different bacteria, have some similarities in appearance, sometimes leading to confusion. Here are the key differences.

Chancroids:

- are painful
- have grey or yellow exudate
- have a soft border

Chancres:

- are not painful
- are usually nonexudative
- have a hard border
- heal spontaneously within 6 weeks, even with no treatment
- may develop in the throat as well as the genitals

Treatment

The CDC recommends treatment of chancroid with antibiotic medication such as an oral macrolide, or cephalosporin for 7 days or in a single intramuscular injection. HIV-positive patients may require extended treatment. Those with infected inguinal lymph nodes may require incision and drainage. Partners of infected individuals should also be treated; sexual activity should be avoided until lesions have healed.

Prognosis

Flashpoint

With early diagnosis and treatment, most individuals are cured.

Prognosis is excellent with early diagnosis and treatment; most individuals are cured. Potential complications of chancroid include painful inguinal lymphadenopathy, sometimes called buboes, which may rupture and drain. Healing may leave scars. Open lesions increase the risk of HIV transmission. Individuals with weakened immune systems experience more complications and reduced cure rates.

Structures and Functions of the Female Reproductive System

The female reproductive system includes the ovaries, fallopian tubes, uterus, vagina, vulva, clitoris, labia, and perineum. The female reproductive system houses the organs necessary for the reproduction of another human. It also manufactures hormones, which are chemicals secreted into the bloodstream that cause reactions. The female reproductive system produces the hormones that are necessary for the development and functioning of reproductive organs.

Structures of the Female Reproductive System

The female reproductive system is made of both internal and external structures.

Internal Structures

Internal organs and structures of the female reproductive system include the ovaries, fallopian tubes, fimbriae, uterus, cervix, vagina, endometrium, and myometrium (see Fig. 8-8).

The ovaries are flat, oval-shaped structures located in the lower abdominal cavity on both sides of the uterus, attached to the broad ligament. The ovaries contain the graafian follicles,

TABLE 8-3			
ABBREVIATIONS RELATED TO THE FEMALE REPRODUCTIVE SYSTEM			
Abbreviation	Meaning	Abbreviation	Meaning
♀	female	LMP	last menstrual period
BSE	breast self-examination	OB	obstetrics
C-section	cesarean section	OC	oral contraceptives
D&C	dilation and curettage	PAP, Pap	Papanicolaou test
GYN, gyn	gynecology	PCOS	polycystic ovary syndrome
HCG, hCG	human chorionic gonadotropin	PID	pelvic inflammatory disease
HRT	hormone replacement therapy	PMS	premenstrual syndrome
IUD	intrauterine device	TAH	total abdominal hysterectomy
IVF	in vitro fertilization	TSS	toxic shock syndrome

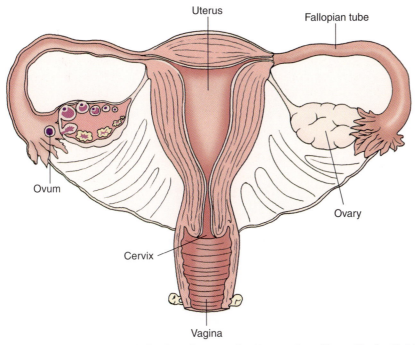

FIGURE 8-8 Internal structures of the female reproductive system (From Eagle, S. *Medical Terminology in a Flash! An Interactive, Flash-Card Approach.* 2006. Philadelphia: F.A. Davis Company, with permission.)

in which are the immature ova, or eggs. The two fallopian tubes extend approximately 10 cm from the sides of the superior lateral surface of the uterus toward the ovaries. The fallopian tubes do not connect to the ovary directly; they are attached to the broad ligament for stability. Each fallopian tube ends in wavelike structures called *fimbriae.*

The uterus is a thick-walled, muscular organ located posterior to the urinary bladder and anterior to the rectum. It consists of the fundus, the rounded upper portion; the corpus, the body of the uterus; and the cervix, the narrowed section that opens into the vagina. The cavity of the uterus is triangular, and its innermost lining is called the *endometrium.* The *myometrium,* or muscular tissue of the uterus, consists of muscle fibers that run in many directions, including circular, longitudinal, and diagonal.

External Structures

The external structures of the female reproductive system, also called the *vulva,* include the clitoris, urethral meatus, labia, mons pubis, and Bartholin glands (see Fig. 8-9). The area between the vagina and the anus is the *perineum.*

The clitoris, made up of elongated erectile tissue, is located beneath the anterior aspect of the labia. The urethral meatus, located posterior to the clitoris and anterior to the vaginal opening, is the opening to the urinary bladder. The labia, which cover the clitoris, urethral meatus, and vaginal opening, consist of two layers: The labia minora are thin layers of tissue that extend from the anterior clitoris to the posterior aspect of the vaginal opening; the labia majora lie on both sides of the labia minora and form the lateral borders of the vulva. In the adult female, the labia majora and mons pubis, the pad of fatty tissue that covers the pubic symphysis (or *pubic bone*), are covered in coarse hair.

Breasts

During puberty, increased secretion of estrogen causes the breasts to develop (see Fig. 8-10). The center of each breast has a region of pigmented tissue called the *areola.* At the center of the areola is the nipple. Inside each breast are 15 to 20 lobes of glandular tissue including mammary glands, which are the milk-producing glands. This glandular tissue is surrounded by connective and adipose tissue.

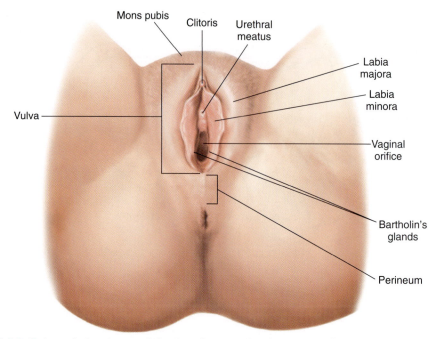
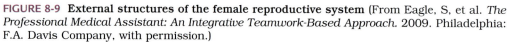

FIGURE 8-9 **External structures of the female reproductive system** (From Eagle, S, et al. *The Professional Medical Assistant: An Integrative Teamwork-Based Approach.* 2009. Philadelphia: F.A. Davis Company, with permission.)

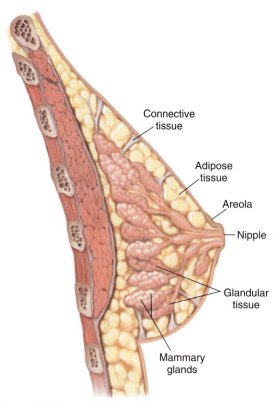

FIGURE 8-10 **Cross section of the female breast** (From Eagle, S, et al. *The Professional Medical Assistant: An Integrative Teamwork-Based Approach.* 2009. Philadelphia: F.A. Davis Company, with permission.)

Functions of the Female Reproductive System

The primary function of the female reproductive system is to produce offspring. The internal and external organs and structures of the female reproductive system all function toward achieving this ultimate goal.

Internal Structures

Ovaries are the primary sex organs in females. Ovaries produce ova, one-half of the necessary components of a new life. They also produce two female hormones:

- Estrogen acts to develop the female reproductive organs during puberty, produces secondary sexual characteristics such as breasts and pubic hair, and prepares the uterus for a fertilized egg.
- Progesterone is responsible for the changes in the endometrium that allow for implantation of the blastocyst (the developing embryo).

The fallopian tubes are the pathways an ovum travels from the ovary to the uterus. The wavelike fimbriae on the ends of the fallopian tubes help direct the ovum from the ovary into the tube. As the ovum travels down the tube, the ovary secretes estrogen and progesterone to change the endometrial tissue to be more receptive to implantation of the ovum.

The cervix and uterus house and protect the developing fetus. The muscular tissue of the uterus is able to expand during pregnancy to accommodate the growing fetus. The cervix will dilate during the birth process to allow delivery of the fetus. The multidirectional muscles of the myometrium also enable forceful contraction of the uterus during the birth process.

External Structures

The labia protect other external and internal structures. The clitoris responds to stimulation, causing orgasm. The vagina acts as the passageway for the penis during sexual intercourse and the birth canal during the birth process.

Breasts

The connective tissue of the breasts provides support and the adipose tissue provides insulation. The amount and distribution of the adipose tissue determines the size and shape of the breasts. The role of the breasts in reproduction is nourishing the newborn infant by producing breast milk, a process called **lactation** (see Box 8-4).

The mammary glands of the breasts are the organs of milk production, which occurs in response to the later part of pregnancy and after childbirth. During pregnancy, the breasts respond to four hormones:

- Estrogen increases the size of the breasts.
- Progesterone stimulates the development of the duct system (for lactation).
- Prolactin stimulates the production of milk.
- Oxytocin promotes the ejection of milk from the glands.

Flashpoint

The ovaries produce the two female hormones estrogen and progesterone.

Flashpoint

Fimbriae help direct the ovum from the ovary into the fallopian tube.

Common Female Reproductive System Diseases and Disorders

There are innumerable diseases and disorders of the female reproductive system. Some of the most common include vaginal disorders, menstrual disorders, uterine disorders, complications of pregnancy, infertility, and fibrocystic breast disease.

Vaginal Disorders

Infections of the vagina, or *vaginitis,* may be acquired through sexual contact or as an adverse effect of medications, such as antibiotics or steroids. If left untreated, many vaginal infections can migrate up the reproductive tract and cause further infection and possible infertility. Common vaginal infections include candidiasis and Bartholin gland cysts.

Box 8-4 Wellness Promotion

BREASTFEEDING FOR A HEALTHY BABY AND MOTHER

The American Academy of Pediatrics (AAP) recommends breastfeeding exclusively for the first 6 months of an infant's life. At 6 months of age, solid food can be introduced; however, the AAP recommends that breastfeeding continue to age 12 months. The health benefits associated with breastfeeding for this length of time or longer are significant for the baby and the mother.

Benefits for Baby

Research shows that babies who are exclusively breastfed for 6 months are less likely to develop certain infections, diabetes, sudden infant death syndrome, asthma, allergies, some cancers, and possibly even childhood obesity. Benefits of breastfeeding for babies include:

- emotional bonding between the infant and mother
- easier digestion
- all needed nutrients, calories, and fluids
- needed growth factors for organ development
- many substances (not present in formula) that help protect the infant from conditions such as ear infection, diarrhea, respiratory disorders such as pneumonia and bronchiolitis, and bacterial and viral infections such as meningitis.

Benefits for Mother

Benefits of breastfeeding for the mother include:

- release of hormones that promote mothering behaviors
- faster return of the uterus to its pre-pregnancy size
- help with weight loss
- delayed return of menses (which helps keep iron in the body)
- reduced risk of ovarian and breast cancers

Candidiasis
ICD-9-CM: 112.1   [ICD-10: B37.3] (vulva and vagina for both codes)

Vaginal candidiasis, also known as a vaginal *yeast infection,* is infection of the vagina by the pathogen *Candida albicans.*

Flashpoint

Vaginal candidiasis is known by most women as a vaginal *yeast infection.*

Incidence

Nearly 75% of all adult women have experienced symptoms of a yeast infection. In addition, studies show that up to 19% of women may have experienced a yeast infection without symptoms (see Fig. 8-11).

Etiology

Infection with *C. albicans* can occur in other areas, such as the mouth (where it is frequently known as thrush), but when the normal flora (helpful bacteria) of the vaginal area have been disrupted, vaginal candidiasis usually occurs. The most common cause of candidiasis is antibiotic use. Although the intended effect of antibiotic therapy is to kill harmful bacteria, it kills helpful bacteria as well. The resulting disruption of normal flora allows *C. albicans* to overgrow, possibly leading to infection. Other contributing factors include oral contraceptives, diabetes, tight clothing or undergarments, and steroid therapy. Vaginal candidiasis during pregnancy is common, possibly as a result of increased estrogen levels.

Signs and Symptoms

Signs and symptoms of vaginal candidiasis include pruritus and an odorless, white vaginal discharge that may be described as cottage cheese–like. Other patients may complain of burning with urination.

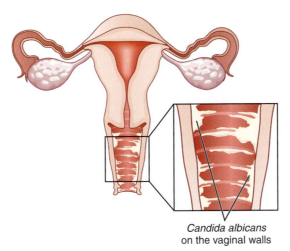

Candida albicans
on the vaginal walls

FIGURE 8-11 *Candida albicans* (vaginal yeast infection)

Diagnosis

The physician determines a diagnosis using a procedure called a *wet preparation* or *wet prep*. A speculum is used to open the vagina and a wooden applicator is used to obtain a specimen from the vagina. The specimen is placed on a clean glass slide and 10% potassium hydroxide is added before the application of a glass cover slip. Positive results reveal groups of *C. albicans* cells, which have a characteristic appearance when viewed with a microscope.

Treatment

Treatment for vaginal candidiasis includes the use of vaginal antifungal drugs in oral form or vaginal cream or suppositories. Topical creams can also be applied to the outer area, if irritation is present. Typically, treatment is restricted to the female patient; however, if the infection recurs, treatment of a sexual partner may be necessary. To prevent recurrence of candidiasis while taking antibiotics, patients should eat active yogurt cultures and drink acidophilus milk to replenish "good" bacteria in the vagina.

Prognosis

With treatment, 90% of *C. albicans* infection resolve. Patients who are immune suppressed, such as those with cancer or HIV, and those with diabetes may require a longer treatment regimen.

Bartholin Gland Cyst
ICD-9-CM: 616.2   [ICD-10: N75.0]

The Bartholin glands are two small mucous glands located in the lateral walls of the vestibule of the vagina. These glands secrete a lubricating fluid for intercourse.

Incidence

Approximately 2% of women develop a Bartholin gland cyst, and 85% of those cases occur during a woman's reproductive years.

Etiology

Occasionally, the ducts of one or both of the Bartholin glands become blocked, although the cause of blockage is unknown. If blockage occurs, the lubricating fluid cannot leave the gland, causing it to become inflamed and tender, forming a cyst (see Fig. 8-12).

Signs and Symptoms

Signs and symptoms of a Bartholin gland cyst include a tender or painful lump near the vaginal opening, discomfort while walking or sitting, pain during intercourse, and fever.

Diagnosis

Visual inspection reveals an inflamed gland, which confirms the diagnosis.

Treatment

Treatment includes application of warm compresses to the area in an effort to open the duct and express the fluid. If this treatment is unsuccessful, the physician may lance the gland with a

Flashpoint

Patients who are immune suppressed may require a longer course of treatment.

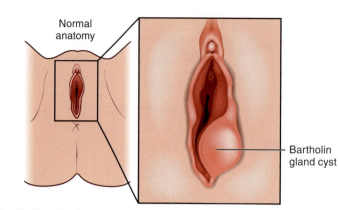

Normal anatomy

Bartholin gland cyst

FIGURE 8-12 Bartholin gland cyst

scalpel and insert a small rubber tube to facilitate drainage. The patient must leave the drain in for a prescribed period of time, which varies with the severity of the occlusion to the duct. The patient must then return to the office so that the physician can remove the drain.

Prognosis

The cyst should not return, because the duct remains open after removal of the drain. The patient should be instructed to abstain from intercourse until the drain is removed.

Menstrual Disorders

Many women experience symptoms related to menstruation. The intensity of the symptoms varies greatly. Treatments are directed at decreasing symptoms without disrupting fertility. Common menstrual disorders include dysmenorrhea, amenorrhea, ovarian cysts, premenstrual syndrome, and toxic shock syndrome.

Dysmenorrhea

> *Flashpoint*
>
> Dysmenorrhea commonly causes pelvic and back pain.

ICD-9-CM: 625.3   **[ICD-10: N94.4]**

Dysmenorrhea is pain in the lower abdominal and pelvic area and other discomfort associated with menses.

Incidence

Dysmenorrhea is most common in women in their 20s and early 30s, although it can affect menstruating women of any age.

Etiology

Causes of dysmenorrhea include hormonal imbalances, endometriosis, uterine fibroids, pelvic inflammatory disease (PID), and uterine malposition.

Signs and Symptoms

Signs and symptoms of dysmenorrhea include pelvic and back pain, headache, nausea, vomiting, fatigue, and diarrhea. Symptoms typically begin 12 to 24 hours before menstruation begins and continue for 3 to 5 days.

Diagnosis

Diagnosis of dysmenorrhea depends on the health history. The patient suffering from dysmenorrhea will report an inability to go to work or school on some days during menses each month, due to the described symptoms. She may also report a flow that is unmanageable even with a combination of extra-absorbent tampons and overnight sanitary pads.

Treatment

Treatment may include analgesics, warm or cold compresses, medications to reduce uterine contractions, and oral contraceptives, which suppress ovulation and therefore decrease symptoms. Patients are advised to get plenty of rest and avoid caffeine and alcohol. A healthy diet and moderate physical exercise have also been shown to lessen symptoms of dysmenorrhea.

Prognosis

Some women experience a significant decrease in dysmenorrheal symptoms after pregnancy. Others experience a more gradual decrease with increasing age.

Amenorrhea
ICD-9-CM: 626.0   [ICD-10: N91.2 (unspecified)]

Amenorrhea is the absence of menses in a woman between the ages of 16 and 40.

Incidence

Amenorrhea affects 2% to 5% of all women of childbearing age in the United States.

Etiology

Causes of amenorrhea include hypothalamic, pituitary, and endocrine dysfunction; congenital or acquired abnormalities of the reproductive tract; and eating disorders that cause extreme weight loss.

> **Flashpoint**
> Amenorrhea can be caused by extreme weight loss.

Signs and Symptoms

Symptoms of amenorrhea include absent menses for 3 or more consecutive months.

Diagnosis

Diagnosis is based on the patient's report of a lack of menses for 3 or more consecutive months (in the absence of pregnancy or breastfeeding).

Treatment

Treatment of amenorrhea is directed at the cause. Hormone therapy can regulate hormonal disruptions. In the case of eating disorders, the patient is referred for psychotherapy.

Prognosis

Amenorrhea is reversible with treatment.

Ovarian Cysts
ICD-9-CM: 616.2   [ICD-10: N83.0]

Ovarian cysts are sacs of fluid or semisolid masses that grow within the ovary (see Fig. 8-13). A related condition, polycystic ovary syndrome (PCOS), is an endocrine disorder that causes irregular ovulation, lack of menses, and secretion of excessive amounts of androgens (male hormones). The suppression of ovulation makes this syndrome a major cause of infertility.

Incidence

Ovarian cysts can form at any time between puberty and menopause, including during pregnancy. In the United States, nearly all premenopausal women have ovarian cysts and around 14% of postmenopausal women have them. PCOS affects approximately 10% of all women in the United States.

Etiology

The definitive cause of ovarian cysts is unknown. Hypothyroidism and early age of menarche may contribute to their development. The cause of PCOS is also unclear; however, it is linked to a decrease in

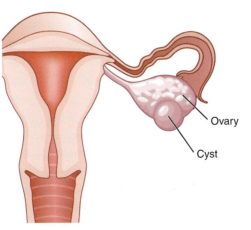

FIGURE 8-13 Ovarian cyst

follicle-stimulating hormone as well as abnormally high levels of testosterone, estrogen, and luteinizing hormone.

Signs and Symptoms

Most women with ovarian cysts are asymptomatic, and the cysts are not considered a problem. Larger cysts or cysts that occur in groups on the ovary can produce symptoms of low back pain, nausea, vomiting, and abnormal uterine bleeding. Women with PCOS are commonly diagnosed while being evaluated for infertility or absence of menses. Symptoms of this syndrome include acne, hyperinsulinemia (excessive production of insulin), obesity, type 2 diabetes, male pattern baldness, and hirsutism (excessive body hair). Because the follicles of the ovaries are not stimulated each month, absent menses is a common sign.

Flashpoint

Ovarian cysts can cause low back pain, nausea, vomiting, and abnormal uterine bleeding.

Diagnosis

Ultrasound confirms the diagnosis by revealing cysts.

Treatment

Treatment with oral contraceptives slows the growth of ovarian cysts and reduces symptoms by suppressing ovulation and changes to the ovary. If oral contraceptives do not control symptoms, the physician may perform a laparoscopic procedure to drain or remove the cysts. Emergency surgical removal is indicated if a large cyst ruptures or the ovary twists and its blood supply is compromised. Symptoms of this emergency condition include acute abdominal pain and massive internal hemorrhage. Treatment of PCOS is directed at normalizing hormone ratios and reestablishing normal menstrual cycles. Treatment for diabetes and obesity should accompany hormone therapy. With hormone therapy, problems of baldness and hirsutism will also decrease.

Prognosis

Prognosis for ovarian cysts varies with age. Around 66% of women under age 20 who undergo treatment for ovarian cysts experience a reduction in cyst size and symptoms. About 75% of patients ages 21 to 49 experience a reduction in symptoms and ovary size without treatment; 7% of women in this age group are diagnosed with ovarian cancer. The rate of cancer increases with age, so surgical removal is recommended for postmenopausal women.

With proper treatment to balance hormones, pregnancy is possible for patients with PCOS. Increased body hair and skin eruptions may adversely affect body image in young women, producing emotional effects.

Premenstrual Syndrome
ICD-9-CM: 625.4   [ICD-10: N94.3]

Premenstrual syndrome (PMS) includes a range of symptoms that generally occur 7 to 14 days before menstruation begins.

Incidence

About 30% to 50% of women ages 22 to 40 suffer premenstrual syndrome.

Flashpoint

Up to 50% of women ages 22 to 40 suffer from PMS.

Etiology

The exact cause of premenstrual syndrome is unknown. Increased levels of antidiuretic hormone may be a factor.

Signs and Symptoms

Women with PMS may experience a wide variety of symptoms, including fluid retention, bloating, temporary weight gain, headaches, depression, irritability, lethargy, nervousness, diarrhea, constipation, and appetite changes. They may also experience an increase in acne, and pain, tenderness, or enlargement of the breasts.

Diagnosis

Diagnosis is based on the patient's report of a cyclical pattern of symptoms that develop prior to menstruation and resolve when menstrual flow begins or shortly thereafter.

Treatment

Treatment is directed at reducing symptoms. The only definitive cure for PMS is hysterectomy, including removal of the ovaries; thus, most patients manage symptoms with over-the-counter medications, diet, and exercise. Medications can include diuretics, analgesics, stimulants such as caffeine, and antihistamines. Over-the-counter combination products contain various combinations of medications which may help reduce or relieve symptoms.

Prognosis

Women with PMS generally experience no long-term complications from the disorder, other than the continuing cycle of symptoms near the onset of menses. PMS alone is not linked to a decrease in fertility.

Toxic Shock Syndrome
ICD-9-CM: 040.82   [ICD-10: A43.8]

Toxic shock syndrome (TSS) is a rare disorder caused by an exotoxin, a dangerous substance produced by bacteria. The causative agents are *Staphylococcus aureus* and *Streptococcus pyogenes.*

Incidence

Approximately 55% to 75% of patients who develop TSS are female. The Centers for Disease Control and Prevention (CDC) estimates that between one and 17 out of 100,000 menstruating females will develop TSS.

> **Flashpoint**
> Up to 75% of patients with TSS are female.

Etiology

TSS is caused by toxins produced by certain strains of bacteria. The release of the toxins into the blood produces an overreaction of the immune system, which leads to the symptoms of TSS. The most common form of TSS occurs in young women who use tampons during menstruation. The toxin produced by *S. aureus* and *S. pyogenes* requires a neutral pH and protein-rich environment, which is provided by menstrual blood. The insertion of a tampon allows air to enter, making the normally anaerobic vagina aerobic. This air provides oxygen for further growth of the toxin. TSS may also develop from other sources (and in men and children), such as infection from cuts, surgical incisions, or burns in the skin. However, most people exposed to the toxin-producing strains of *S. aureus* and *S. pyogenes* do not develop TSS, because of antibodies to these toxins produced by the normal flora of the skin.

Signs and Symptoms

Symptoms include fever of 102°F or greater and diffuse, erythematous rash followed 1 to 2 weeks later by peeling of the skin. The patient may experience hypotension and syncope (fainting), gastrointestinal disturbances such as diarrhea and vomiting, and muscle aches and pains. Symptoms may progress to renal and hepatic failure.

Diagnosis

There is no single diagnostic test for TSS; diagnosis is determined from a variety of information, including the patient's description of symptoms, fever, low blood pressure, skin rash that eventually peels, white blood cell count, blood cultures which may indicate the causative organism, and evidence of multiple organ dysfunction.

Treatment

Treatment includes hospitalization for IV fluids and antibiotics. Patients who use tampons should be instructed to change them often and discontinue their use if fever develops during use.

Prognosis

About 5% to 15% of TSS cases are fatal. Women who have been successfully treated for TSS should never use tampons again, because they are at an increased risk for recurrence.

Uterine Disorders

The healthy uterus has the ability to cleanse itself with menstrual flow and secretion of normal mucus. Infections of the uterus can be caused by sexually transmitted infections, poor hygiene, and untreated vaginal infection. Uterine disorders may also be caused by the growth of abnormal tissues and uterine malposition. Common uterine disorders include endometriosis, pelvic inflammatory disease, uterine fibroids, and uterine prolapse.

Endometriosis
ICD-9-CM: 617.9   [ICD-10: N80.9] (site unspecified for both codes)

Endometriosis is the growth of endometrial tissue outside of the uterus. Normally, the endometrium grows thicker in response to hormonal changes during the menstrual cycle. The uterus sheds the active endometrial layer during menses. In women with endometriosis, the endometrial tissue grows

Flashpoint

Endometrial tissue growing outside of the uterus causes pain in the abdomen, pelvis, and vagina.

outside of the uterus, affecting the structures that it adheres to, such as ovaries, ligaments, and peritoneal tissues (see Fig. 8-14).

Incidence

Endometriosis occurs in 7% to 10% of menstruating women worldwide. It can persist, though rarely, in postmenopausal women.

Etiology

Although the cause of endometriosis is unknown, it is thought either that endometrial cells migrate during fetal development or that the cells that are shed during menstruation are possibly expelled out of the fallopian tubes during menses. Recent trauma or uterine surgery are possible causes. Endometrial tissue that grows outside of the uterus is not shed, and causes pain in the abdomen, pelvis, and vagina.

Signs and Symptoms

The most common symptom of endometriosis is pain that ensues 5 to 6 days before menses and lasts until 3 to 4 days after the menstrual period, although it may arise at other times as well. The degree of pain and discomfort varies depending on the quantity of tissue growth and the location. Other possible symptoms include fatigue, irregular or heavy menstrual flow, abdominal bloating, and diarrhea or constipation.

Diagnosis

Diagnosis is based on visual examination via laparoscopy or biopsy, which reveals endometrial tissue outside of the uterus (see Box 8-5).

Treatment

Treatment options vary based on the patient's age and desire to preserve her fertility. Surgical removal of endometrial cysts can clear ovaries and fallopian tubes, restoring fertility. Oral

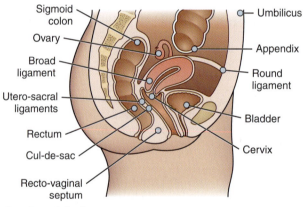

FIGURE 8-14 Sites of endometriosis

Box 8-5 Diagnostic Spotlight

LAPAROSCOPY

Laparoscopy is a procedure in which the health-care provider visualizes the contents of the patient's pelvis or abdomen through a laparoscope. Structures typically examined include the gallbladder, liver, large and small intestines, appendix, uterus, ovaries, and fallopian tubes. This procedure may be used for either diagnostic or treatment purposes.

Laparoscopy is done in the hospital or an outpatient surgical center. The patient is usually under general anesthesia, but the procedure may also be done with local anesthesia. The laparoscope is inserted through a very small incision. A tiny video camera is included. An additional incision may be needed if more instruments are required for a procedure. After the procedure is completed, only a bandage is required to cover the incisions.

contraceptives can suppress ovulation and therefore reduce symptoms. If fertility is not desired, the physician may prescribe medication to inhibit the pituitary release of gonadotropins or to suppress production of gonadotropin-releasing hormone. These medications cause the decline of follicle-stimulating hormone and luteinizing hormone, which decreases ovarian function and can induce early menopause. If the patient decides that she no longer wants to bear children, severe cases of endometriosis are treated with complete hysterectomy, including the removal of the uterus, fallopian tubes, and ovaries.

Prognosis
The main complication of endometriosis is impaired fertility. Around 30% to 50% of women who experience infertility are diagnosed with endometriosis. For patients who are able to decrease the amount of endometrial tissue growth outside the uterus, pregnancy may be possible. Severe endometriosis can cause bowel and urethral obstructions.

> **Flashpoint**
> The main complication of endometriosis is impaired fertility.

Pelvic Inflammatory Disease
ICD-9-CM: 614.9   [ICD-10: N70.9] (unspecified for both codes)
Pelvic inflammatory disease (PID) is any acute or chronic infection of the female reproductive system, including the uterus, fallopian tubes, and ovaries.

Incidence
More than one million women in the United States are affected by PID each year. It is most common in teenagers.

Etiology
PID can be caused by an untreated vaginal infection that ascends into the internal reproductive organs. The longer the infection goes untreated, the further it ascends, affecting more of the reproductive tract. The fallopian tubes may become blocked with pus or scar tissue, causing infertility. Common pathogens that cause PID include *N. gonorrhoeae* and *C. trachomatis*.

Signs and Symptoms
The patient may be asymptomatic or may experience such signs and symptoms as purulent vaginal discharge, odor, fever, malaise, lower abdominal pain, dysuria, nausea, vomiting, and heavy bleeding.

Diagnosis
Diagnosis is based upon pelvic examination and culturing the discharge to identify the causative organism. Testing for sexually transmitted infections (STIs) may also be done.

Treatment
Treatment includes antibiotic or antifungal medications as indicated by the causative organism. If the patient is diagnosed with a STI, sexual partners should also be treated.

Prognosis
Because patients with PID may be asymptomatic, infection may progress untreated. Prolonged infection causes sterility through scarring of the fallopian tubes, ovaries, and uterus. The infection also increases the chances of an ectopic pregnancy.

> **Flashpoint**
> PID can cause sterility.

Uterine Fibroids
ICD-9-CM: 218.9   [ICD-10: D25.9] (unspecified for both codes)
Uterine fibroids are benign, smooth tumors made of muscle and fat, also called *leiomyomas*. They grow in size during the reproductive years and may regress after menopause (see Fig. 8-15).

Incidence
Noncancerous tumors of the uterus are the most common tumor found in women. In the United States, about 20% to 40% of women age 35 and older have uterine fibroids. African American women are at greater risk. Fibroids are the most common cause of hysterectomy in premenopausal women.

Etiology
The cause of uterine fibroids is unknown. Risk factors include age of at least 30, obesity, family history of fibroids, African Caribbean descent, and not having had children.

Signs and Symptoms
Women are typically asymptomatic until age 30, but symptoms may eventually develop as tumors grow in size and number. Uterine fibroids most commonly occur in clusters; symptoms

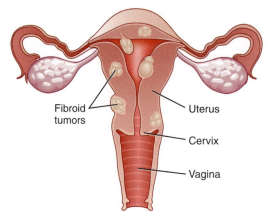

FIGURE 8-15 Uterine fibroids

are related to their specific location. Fibroids that encroach on the bladder region will produce urinary frequency and dysuria; those that encroach on the rectum can cause spasms of the anal sphincter. The patient may feel abdominal fullness due to enlargement of the uterus. The most common site of uterine fibroids is within the endometrium. These fibroids can cause **menorrhagia** (excessive menstrual flow) and dysmenorrhea. If the fibroid is attached to the uterus by a stalk, pain is caused by uterine contractions attempting to expel the fibroid.

Flashpoint

Uterine fibroids can cause symptoms of urinary frequency and dysuria, as well as menorrhagia.

Diagnosis

Diagnosis is suspected based on the patient's report of symptoms. Visualization by ultrasound confirms the diagnosis; it is the most common diagnostic tool, because it is minimally invasive and available in most medical offices. Less commonly, MRI or hysteroscopy can confirm the presence of fibroids. Ultrasound may also serve as an assessment tool to determine if fibroids are growing in size and number.

Treatment

Asymptomatic fibroids should be left untreated and observed for changes throughout the patient's life. Treatment of fibroids that cause symptoms includes oral administration of luteinizing hormone-releasing hormone, which causes the fibroids to shrink. If the patient no longer wants to preserve fertility, uterine ablation can debulk endometrial fibroids. The ablation procedure is a one-day surgery done under general anesthesia, in which the surgeon fills the uterine cavity with heated fluid that destroys the active layer of the endometrium. If uterine fibroids are connected by a stalk, the surgeon removes them before the ablation. As a result of ablation, the fibroid's blood supply is diminished and the fibroid tumor will shrink.

Prognosis

Treatment of uterine fibroids is commonly successful. Depending on their location, fibroids may impact fertility. Most women who experience uterine fibroids and infertility also suffer from other disorders, such as decreased production of ova.

Uterine Prolapse
ICD-9-CM: 618.1   [ICD-10: N81.4] (unspecified for both codes)

Uterine prolapse is the displacement of the uterus downward into the vagina (see Fig. 8-16).

Incidence

In the United States, approximately 14% of women who have given birth at least once have some degree of uterine prolapse. African American women have the lowest risk; Hispanic women have the highest risk. Other risk factors include history of multiple pregnancies and obesity.

Etiology

Uterine prolapse develops when pelvic floor muscles become weakened and supporting ligaments become overstretched. Contributors include advanced age, pelvic tumors (which create pressure on the uterus), traumatic vaginal delivery, multiple pregnancies, obesity, decreased estrogen, and chronic constipation.

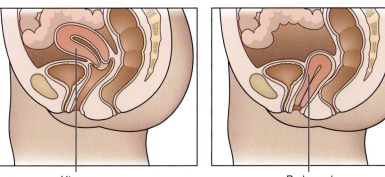

Uterus   Prolapsed
uterus

FIGURE 8-16 **Uterine prolapse**

Signs and Symptoms

Some women are symptom free; others may experience a variety of symptoms that usually improve with rest and are worsened by prolonged standing or walking. Symptoms may include a sensation of pressure or heaviness, low back or pelvic pain, sexual dysfunction, difficulty walking or urinating, urinary frequency, urgency or incontinence, or constipation.

Diagnosis

Diagnosis is based on physical examination. During the examination, the physician asks the patient to bear down. This pressure causes the cervix to protrude out through the vaginal opening. There are three stages of uterine prolapse:

- mild: protrusion of the cervix into the lower portion of the vagina
- moderate: protrusion past the vaginal opening
- severe: protrusion of the entire uterus past the opening of the vagina

Treatment

Surgical correction, called **_uteropexy,_** can lift the uterus, fix it in its normal position, and repair weakened support structures. A device called a pessary may also be used to provide temporary relief by holding the uterus in place; it is usually a ring-shaped structure that must be inserted by a physician.

Prognosis

After surgical correction, most patients experience no further problems. However, some women suffer from recurrent prolapse and require additional surgical correction.

Flashpoint

Severe uterine prolapse can cause total protrusion of the uterus past the vaginal opening.

Complications of Pregnancy

Many women enjoy a healthy pregnancy and deliver a child without complication. Unfortunately, some pregnancies are difficult for the mother, fetus, or both. Some pregnancies are unsuccessful and the patient does not deliver a live infant. Common complications of pregnancy include ectopic pregnancy, abortion, gestational (pregnancy-related) diabetes, placenta previa, abruptio placentae, and eclampsia.

Ectopic Pregnancy
ICD-9-CM: 633.9   [ICD-10: O00.9] (unspecified for both codes)

Ectopic pregnancy involves the implantation of a fertilized ovum somewhere other than in the uterus. Most commonly it implants in the wall of the fallopian tube, but it may implant at any number of sites (see Fig. 8-17).

Incidence

Ectopic pregnancy occurs in approximately 1% of all pregnancies. About 98% of these cases involve implantation in the fallopian tube.

Flashpoint

Ectopic pregnancy is sometimes called tubal pregnancy because it usually occurs in the fallopian tube.

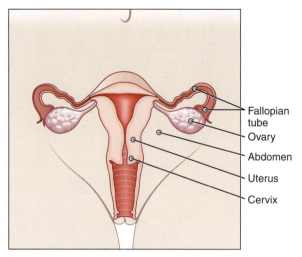

FIGURE 8-17 **Implantation sites of ectopic pregnancy**

Etiology

Normally, fertilization occurs in the outer one-third of the fallopian tube. The corpus luteum releases secretions from the glands within the tubes. The fertilized cell, now called a zygote, must move from the fallopian tube into the uterus for implantation. If the zygote does not move into the uterus, and instead begins to implant in the wall of the fallopian tube, it will not be able to grow and develop in the narrow space of the tube.

Signs and Symptoms

As the zygote grows in size, the patient may experience sharp pelvic pain, fever, and bleeding.

Diagnosis

Diagnosis is based on a positive urine pregnancy test and a blood test, which both indicate elevated human chorionic gonadotropin (hCG). Abdominal ultrasound shows an empty uterus and possibly a gestational sac with a fetal heart within the fallopian tube.

Treatment

Approximately 50% of ectopic pregnancies result in miscarriage and require no surgical intervention. The other 50% require surgical removal of the embryo to prevent rupture of the tube, hemorrhage, and infection.

Prognosis

Rupture can result in hemorrhage, shock, and death; however, the mortality rate has dropped significantly in the past 30 years and is currently less than 0.1%. The patient may be able to conceive again if no damage exists to the other fallopian tube. Infertility occurs in 10% to 15% of women. Repeated ectopic pregnancies occur in as many as 20% of women.

> **Flashpoint**
> Rupture of ectopic pregnancy can result in hemorrhage, shock, and death.

Abortion

ICD-9-CM: 779.6   [ICD-10: O03.9 (unspecified)]

Abortion, also called *miscarriage,* is the spontaneous or therapeutic loss of a pregnancy at less than 20 weeks' *gestation* (time between conception and birth).

Incidence

Spontaneous abortion occurs in 30% of all first pregnancies and up to 15% of all pregnancies. Some miscarriages occur so early in gestation that the patient is unaware that she was ever pregnant.

> **Flashpoint**
> Some miscarriages occur in which patients are unaware they were ever pregnant.

Etiology

The most common cause of spontaneous abortion is an error in fetal development that is incompatible with life. Other causes include abnormalities of the placenta, endocrine disturbances, acute infectious disease, severe shock, and trauma.

Signs and Symptoms

Signs and symptoms of a spontaneous abortion include abdominal cramps, vaginal bleeding, and passage of clots of tissue.

Diagnosis

If the patient is aware of the pregnancy, diagnosis is confirmed by examination of expelled fetal tissue. Ultrasound may confirm complete expulsion of tissue.

Treatment

If the abortion is incomplete and fetal tissue is still present in the uterus, the patient must undergo dilation and curettage (D&C), a procedure that removes any remaining tissue that could cause infection.

Prognosis

Prognosis for surgical and spontaneous abortion in the first trimester of gestation is usually good. The patient should recover and, if no underlying fertility issues are present, should be able to become pregnant again in the future. Women experiencing second- or third-trimester abortions may have complications resulting from hemorrhage and damage to internal organs. This could lead to an inability to become pregnant. Unsafe abortions, performed illegally and commonly by unqualified individuals, are a public health concern worldwide, due to the high incidence of incomplete abortion, sepsis, hemorrhage, and damage to internal organs. The World Health Organization estimates that 19 million unsafe abortions are performed annually, with 68,000 resultant deaths (see Box 8-6).

> **Flashpoint**
> Unsafe abortions often lead to incomplete abortion, sepsis, hemorrhage, and damage to internal organs.

Gestational Diabetes
ICD-9-CM: 648.80   [ICD-10: O24.9] (unspecified for both codes)

Gestational diabetes is the development of type 2 diabetes mellitus in a woman during pregnancy who did not have diabetes before becoming pregnant. In the United States, gestational diabetes occurs in about 4% to 8% of pregnancies and usually resolves after the woman gives birth. See Chapter 13 for a detailed description of gestational diabetes.

Placenta Previa
ICD-9-CM: 641.00   [ICD-10: O44.0] (unspecified for both codes)

Placenta previa is the implantation of the placenta in the lower uterine segment rather than the central or upper portion of the uterine wall. During labor, the fetus normally leaves the uterus before the placenta is delivered. However, if the placenta implants in the lower uterine segment, it can obstruct delivery of the fetus. There are three degrees of placenta previa:

- centralis: the placenta completely covers the cervix
- marginalis: the placenta partially obstructs the cervix
- lateralis: the placenta does not obstruct the cervix but is low enough to possibly obstruct a vaginal delivery of the fetus (see Fig. 8-18)

> **Flashpoint**
> Placenta previa causes recurrent bleeding that increases in severity during the seventh or eighth month of pregnancy.

Incidence

Placenta previa occurs in approximately one out of every 200 pregnancies.

Etiology

The cause of placenta previa is unknown, but advanced maternal age (35 or older), increased number of previous pregnancies, and previous uterine surgery (including cesarean section) increase the risk.

Signs and Symptoms

Signs and symptoms of placenta previa include slight hemorrhage with recurrent severity in the seventh or eighth month of pregnancy. Gradually, the patient will experience anemia, pallor, rapid weak pulse, shortness of breath, and low blood pressure.

Diagnosis

Diagnosis of placenta previa is made using ultrasound. This may occur during a regular prenatal visit or after the woman has noticed vaginal bleeding.

Treatment

Treatment prior to delivery should include hospital bedrest and treatment of anemia. Vaginal examination is deferred, if possible, until 36 weeks' gestation, to prevent infection. Vaginal delivery may be attempted in cases of placenta previa marginalis and lateralis, but not for the

Box 8-6 Wellness Promotion

EMOTIONAL SUPPORT AFTER ABORTION

Health-care providers caring for a patient who has experienced a spontaneous or elective abortion must try to ease the patient's anxiety and help her cope with the loss of the pregnancy. Whether she has miscarried or has elected to end the pregnancy for physical, economic, or other personal reasons, the patient must process the experience emotionally. Emotional responses may vary among grief, anger, guilt, depression, sadness, or even relief. Many support groups are available online and through local organizations to help women cope. Some other resources are:

- Fertility Plus's Miscarriage Support and Information Resources list: http://www.fertilityplus.org/faq/miscarriage/resources.html
- BellaOnline's Miscarriage Site: http://www.bellaonline.com/subjects/6461.asp
- Cohen, J. *Coming to Term: Uncovering the Truth about Miscarriage.* New Brunswick, NJ: Rutgers University Press, 2007.
- McLaughlin, S. *Surviving Miscarriage: You Are Not Alone.* Bloomington, IN: iUniverse, Inc., 2005.

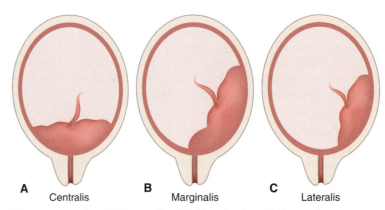

A Centralis   **B** Marginalis   **C** Lateralis

FIGURE 8-18 Placenta previa: (A) Centralis; (B) Marginalis; (C) Lateralis

centralis form. If vaginal delivery is attempted, the obstetrician will order a "double setup," where all equipment and personnel are available for emergency cesarean delivery. Immediate postpartum care includes monitoring the mother closely for continued bleeding and administering antibiotics to lessen the high risk of infection.

Prognosis

The risk of complications increases with the severity of placenta previa. Complications can include medical problems for the infant secondary to blood loss, small birth weight (due to restricted growing space in utero), and increased incidence of congenital anomalies. Risks to the mother include life-threatening hemorrhage, cesarean delivery, increased risk of postpartum hemorrhage, and increased risk of placenta accreta (in which the placenta attaches directly to uterine muscle, requiring surgical removal).

Abruptio Placentae
ICD-9-CM: 641.20   [ICD-10: O45.9] (unspecified for both codes)
Abruptio placentae is the sudden, premature detachment of the placenta from the uterine wall. There are three levels of abruption (see Fig. 8-19):

- grade 1: detachment of less than 20% of the placental surface
- grade 2: detachment of 20% to 50% of the placental surface
- grade 3: detachment of more than 50% of the placental surface

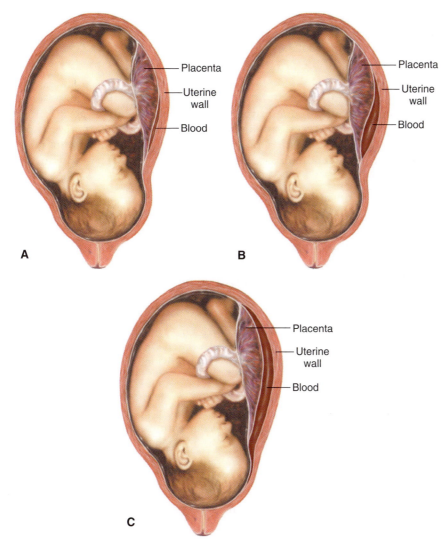

FIGURE 8-19 **Abruptio placentae: (A) Grade 1; (B) Grade 2; (C) Grade 3** (From Eagle, S, et al. *The Professional Medical Assistant: An Integrative Teamwork-Based Approach.* 2009. Philadelphia: F.A. Davis Company, with permission.)

Incidence
It is estimated that one in 120 births are complicated by placental abruption.

Etiology
The cause of abruptio placentae is unknown; however, cocaine abuse and toxemia increase the risk.

Signs and Symptoms
Symptoms of mild abruption (grade 1) include vaginal bleeding, uterine tenderness, and mild tetany (muscular spasm). Grade 2 symptoms include those of grade 1 as well as fetal distress, because the fetus is not getting enough oxygen and nutrition. In grade 3, uterine tetany is severe, the mother is in shock, and the fetus dies from lack of oxygen.

Diagnosis
Diagnosis is usually made when the patient reports painless bleeding during the third trimester. Ultrasound provides a visual confirmation of the diagnosis.

Treatment
Treatment of abruptio placentae varies with the severity of detachment. Women with grade 1 detachment may be restricted to bedrest and may be monitored to prolong the pregnancy to a safe gestational age for the fetus. Administration of betamethasone, a drug that expedites the development of

fetal lungs, may be necessary if the fetus must be delivered early. Grade 2 detachment at or near term is treated by delivery of the fetus, by either vaginal induction or cesarean section. Because grade 3 detachment results in the death of the fetus, treatment is aimed at caring for the mother.

Prognosis

Depending on the degree of separation, abruptio placentae causes fetal death in 20% to 40% of cases. It can also cause maternal death due to shock and hemorrhage. In cases of hemorrhage, an emergency hysterectomy may be necessary to save the mother's life. About 40% to 50% of infants who survive abruptio placentae experience complications, which range from mild to severe. Women who have had the condition are more likely to have recurrences in subsequent pregnancies.

Eclampsia

ICD-9-CM: 642.60   [ICD-10: O51.9] (unspecified for both codes)

A condition called *preeclampsia* is characterized by severe hypertension in pregnancy. If left untreated, preeclampsia can progress to eclampsia, which includes convulsions and coma.

Incidence

About 3% to 5% of all pregnant women suffer from preeclampsia. Of those women, one in 20 progress to eclampsia.

Etiology

The causes of preeclampsia and eclampsia are unknown; however, the risk is greater in teens, women age 35 and older, African American women, and women who are pregnant for the first time or have multiple fetuses or a history of diabetes, hypertension, or renal disease.

Signs and Symptoms

Signs and symptoms of preeclampsia include hypertension, proteinuria, and edema. Progression to eclampsia is indicated by severe muscle aches, severe agitation, one or more generalized seizures, and coma. Without treatment, seizures may recur within minutes. Severe pain in the right upper quadrant, indicative of hepatic (liver) edema, and generalized abdominal pain may also be present.

Diagnosis

Diagnostic findings include new onset of high blood pressure and protein in the urine after 20 weeks' pregnancy. Testing is also done to evaluate kidney and liver function.

Treatment

Treatment is directed at managing seizures, monitoring blood pressure, and continuing the pregnancy for as long as possible. The patient must be hospitalized and have an indwelling catheter inserted. Hourly monitoring of urinary output is necessary to diagnose renal failure. The hospitalized patient is given IV magnesium sulfate in an attempt to stop seizures. Induction of labor and cesarean section are necessary if blood pressure becomes dangerously high.

Prognosis

Eclampsia is the most serious complication of pregnancy and can lead to maternal and fetal death. Organ damage can involve the kidneys, liver, brain, and placenta. Damage to the placenta includes infarcts, thromboses, and hemorrhages. The developing fetus may suffer severe developmental delays due to inadequate supplies of blood, oxygen, and nutrition from the damaged placenta.

Other Disorders of the Female Reproductive System

Other disorders of the female reproductive system include infertility and fibrocystic breast disease. Other conditions seen all too often in the medical office include physical and emotional trauma related to sexual assault and sexual abuse.

Infertility

**ICD-9-CM: 628.9 (female, unspecified),   [ICD-10: N97.7 (female, unspecified),
606.9 (male, unspecified)   N46.9 (male, unspecified)**

Infertility is an inability to achieve pregnancy after trying to conceive for a period of 1 year or more. Infertility can be either primary, which is an inability of a woman to conceive her first child, or secondary, which is infertility in a woman who has previously conceived.

Incidence

The condition is found in 20% of all couples and may be caused by problems in men or in women.

Etiology

Causes of female infertility vary from hormonal imbalances that suppress ovulation to structural problems, such as blocked fallopian tubes or uterine malposition. Eating disorders and nutritional disorders may also decrease the chance of successful conception. Causes of male infertility are numerous and generally involve problems with sperm count, sperm mobility, or impaired ability to fertilize the egg. These may result from structural defects in male anatomy, such as undescended testicles or varicocele. Other contributors may include scarring from STIs and underlying disorders such as diabetes or testosterone deficiency. General lifestyle factors may also impair fertility. Examples include emotional stress; obesity; malnutrition; alcohol, tobacco, or drug misuse; cancer; and cancer treatment.

Signs and Symptoms

The primary symptom of infertility is the inability to achieve pregnancy after trying for a period of 1 year or more.

Diagnosis

Diagnosis of the cause of infertility is obtained by a comprehensive health history of both partners, with an assessment of their usual timing for intercourse. Female assessment includes evaluation of ovulation by charting basal body temperature. Laparoscopic examination of the ovaries, fallopian tubes, and uterus may reveal structural abnormalities. Blood tests include an evaluation of hormone levels that may indicate under- or overproduction of one or more of the female hormones. Hormonal balance is necessary for normal ovulation, implantation of the ova, and successful pregnancy. The most common diagnostic test for males is semen analysis. This involves the study of one or more ejaculated specimens. Semen are analyzed for color, quantity, number, shape, motility, and presence of any infectious material such as bacteria or blood. Other testing includes measurement of male hormone levels, especially testosterone, and ultrasound examination for structural defects such as obstructed ducts.

Treatment

Treatments for infertility vary. Nonsurgical treatments are directed at correcting hormonal imbalances that suppress ovulation or cause an inability of the embryo to implant in the uterus. Surgical treatments include in vitro fertilization, where ova are harvested and fertilized outside of the mother's body and then implanted into the uterus. Treatment for the male partner may involve behavioral therapy to remedy impotence or premature ejaculation. Hormone therapy will increase testosterone level. Surgery may be done to correct structural problems.

Prognosis

Treatments for infertility are expensive and often not covered by medical insurance. Patients who are experiencing infertility may be depressed and extremely emotional. The rates of successful treatment for infertility depend on the cause, the age of the patient(s), and underlying health problems that may impact fertility. The CDC reports that assisted reproductive therapy is successful in 38% of women under age 35, 30% of women age 35 to 37, 20% of women age 38 to 40, and only 11% of women age 41 and older.

Fibrocystic Breast Disease
ICD-9-CM: 610.1　　[ICD-10: N60.1]

Fibrocystic breast disease is the presence of multiple lumps in the breast, consisting of fibrous tumors or fluid-filled cysts (see Fig. 8-20).

Incidence

About 33% of women age 30 to 50, and 50% of all women at some point their lifetime, develop fibrocystic breast disease.

Etiology

Causes of fibrocystic breast disease are unknown but may be related to normal aging.

Signs and Symptoms

Symptoms include palpable, firm, well-defined, painless nodules in the breast. The cysts may be more tender than the fibroids, and tenderness may increase in relation to the menstrual cycle. Over time, the fluid-filled cysts enlarge and become fibrous, increasing in density and firmness.

Flashpoint

Twenty percent of all couples experience infertility.

Flashpoint

Treatments for infertility are expensive and often not covered by medical insurance.

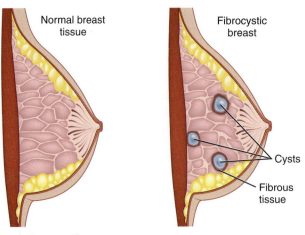

FIGURE 8-20 Fibrocystic breast disease

Diagnosis

Diagnosis is confirmed by a manual breast examination and mammography (see Box 8-7).

Treatment

Treatments for fibroids include needle aspiration of fluid-filled cysts. After aspiration, the cysts rarely refill with fluid. Patients should be advised to reduce intake of caffeine and dietary fat, which are known to cause exacerbations of fibrocystic breast disease.

Flashpoint

Patients may be advised to reduce intake of caffeine and dietary fat.

Prognosis

If dietary changes decrease the symptoms and the patient can maintain these changes, recurrence of cysts may be avoided. Although the presence of fibroids does not increase the risk of breast cancer, their presence may interfere with the diagnosis of breast cancer by mammogram.

Sexual Assault

ICD-9-CM: E960.1 [ICD-10: Y05.9 (unspecified place of occurence)]

Sexual assault is a broader term than **rape** (forced vaginal, anal, or oral penetration) and is therefore more useful for conveying the scope of the problem of sexual attack. Sexual assault is defined as any form of unwanted sexual contact forced upon an individual. The victim may or may not be known to the perpetrator and may even be a friend, date, or spouse. Victims may be subdued by chemical means through drugs or alcohol, physically restrained or overpowered, or coerced to cooperate though threats of harm. Forms of sexual contact vary and include, but are not limited to, forced vaginal, anal, or oral penetration; touching of the breasts or genitalia; and masturbation. Assault may also take the form of forced nudity and photography or video recording.

Box 8-7 Diagnostic Spotlight

MAMMOGRAPHY

Mammography is a radiological procedure in which images of breast tissue are created and evaluated by a radiologist. It successfully detects 85% to 90% of existing breast cancers and has been shown to reduce mortality from breast cancer in women age 40 to 69.

In this procedure the breasts are compressed, one at a time, between two plastic plates while a picture is taken. The compression may cause mild discomfort but lasts only a few seconds. Usually two pictures are taken of each breast; the entire procedure takes less than 15 minutes.

Incidence

More than 200,000 sexual assaults are reported in the United States each year. Given that this statistic does not include victims under the age of 12 and that most sexual assaults go unreported, one can only speculate as to the actual numbers, but they are surely much higher.

Etiology

Sexual assault is a crime of power and control. It is not so much about sex or meeting sexual needs as about the offender's desire to use sex as a weapon to dominate and humiliate the victim.

> **Flashpoint**
> Sexual assault is a crime of power and control.

Signs and Symptoms

Signs and symptoms vary widely depending upon the individual situation and timeliness of the report. They may include obvious injury in the form of bruises and lacerations to the genitalia or other parts of the body. If the victim seeks help immediately, there may be evidence of torn or stained clothing as well as possible biological evidence (semen, blood, hair, etc). For this reason, victims are strongly encouraged to contact the police and seek professional care immediately, without bathing, showering, douching, or changing clothing beforehand. Such evidence is critical to any legal action that may follow. However, the absence of such evidence does not disprove sexual assault. Victims who cooperate out of fear of physical harm may escape with fewer physical wounds but may be just as emotionally traumatized. The victim's emotional responses are variable and may include tearfulness, anxiety, anger, or withdrawal. Some may seem to handle the event well at the time but experience psychological effects later.

Diagnosis

Diagnosis is based upon the victim's report of the incident, presenting signs and symptoms, and reports of any witnesses (although most events are not witnessed).

Treatment

Treatment of sexual assault includes carefully collecting any evidence as well as addressing the victim's physical and emotional needs. Evidence collection must be done by a properly trained health-care provider. Improperly collected, labeled, or managed evidence will not be admissible in a court of law. If necessary, the victim is tested and treated for sexually transmitted infection (including HIV) and potential pregnancy. Treatment of physical wounds (lacerations, bruises, etc.) is provided as needed. Counseling from a rape crisis center or other counseling service should be offered. Health-care providers should take care to treat the victim with nonjudgmental sensitivity.

> **Flashpoint**
> Improperly managed evidence will not be admissible in a court of law.

Prognosis

For those who seek professional medical and psychological help, the prognosis is good. However, sexual assault is a horrific crime that often leaves invisible yet destructive effects in its wake. Victims and their loved ones may continue to suffer physical and emotional effects for a very long time. Many individuals report experiencing flashbacks, post-traumatic stress disorder, depression, suicidal thoughts, and other psychological problems. Anyone who has suffered sexual assault should be encouraged to seek professional help in coping with the aftermath.

Sexual Abuse

ICD-9-CM: 995.53 (child sexual abuse),   [ICD-10: Z61.4]
995.54 (child physical abuse)

Sexual abuse of children includes any sexual act between a child and adult or older child. The act may or may not involve physical contact. Signs of sexual abuse in a child are subtle and may include difficulty sitting or walking, hesitance to remove clothing for examination, sleep disturbance, bedwetting, inappropriate sexual knowledge for the child's age, bruising or injuries to the genitalia, and the presence of sexually transmitted disease. See Chapter 4 for a detailed description of child abuse (including sexual abuse).

STOP HERE.
Select the flash cards for this chapter and run through them at least three times before moving on to the next chapter.

Student Resources

Endometriosis.org: http://www.endometriosis.org
Healthcommunities.com Urology Channel: http://www.urologychannel.com
Mission Pharmacal's Trichomoniasis Site: http://www.trichomoniasis.org
Planned Parenthood: http://www.plannedparenthood.org
Rape, Abuse and Incest National Network (RAINN): http://www.rainn.org

Chapter Activities

Learning Style Study Strategies

Try any or all of the following strategies as you study the content of this chapter:

Visual learners: Make a collage with photos and illustrations related to diseases that you need to learn about. You can find them in medical journals or on the Internet. Label each one with the correct term, a very brief definition, and just a few key facts that you need to remember.

Kinesthetic learners: Visit a family planning or family practice clinic in your town and ask for literature regarding sexually transmitted infections and any diseases described in this chapter that you need to learn about. Patient education literature is usually well written, easy to read, and easy to understand.

Auditory and verbal learners: Study with a buddy. Take turns looking up pathological conditions in a medical dictionary and reading them aloud.

Practice Exercises

Answers to Practice Exercises can be found in Appendix D.

Case Studies

CASE STUDY 1

A 20-year-old woman named Jamie has just been diagnosed with genital warts. She has a number of questions about it; what will you tell her?

1. How can I have gotten this? I've only ever had sex with one person, and I've been going steady with him for the past year.

2. Can't you just give me some antibiotics or something to get rid of this?

3. My boyfriend said that he noticed a few small warts over a year ago, but they went away and so he didn't think he had it anymore. This doesn't make any sense.

4. What other advice can you give me?

CASE STUDY 2

Manuel is a 14-year-old who awakens early one morning with sudden, severe testicular pain. His father takes him to the urgent-care center, where he is evaluated and diagnosed with testicular torsion. His father has questions about this painful disorder. Answer them for him.

1. What is this, and what caused it?

2. How will the doctor diagnose this so I know that it's not something else, like cancer or a tumor?

3. How can this be fixed?

CASE STUDY 3

Guadalupe is a 27-year-old woman who is visiting her health-care provider with complaints of painful menses. She has noticed that her pain has increased in severity, and her menstrual flow has become heavier since she stopped taking her birth control pills 3 months ago. She states that she and her husband are now trying to start their family.

1. What is the correct term for her physical complaint?

2. What disorders discussed in this chapter might account for her menstrual pain?

3. Given that Guadalupe is trying to become pregnant, what measures might she take to alleviate or reduce her pain?

4. She asks if she might have fertility problems, since she has been trying to get pregnant for 3 months without success. How might the health-care provider respond?

Multiple Choice

1. Cryptorchidism is:

   a. Undescended testicle(s)

   b. Pain with intercourse

   c. Surgical removal of one or both testes

   d. Surgical fixation of the uterus

2. Stenosis of the foreskin opening so that it cannot be pushed back over the glans penis is called:

   a. Cryptorchidism

   b. Circumcision

   c. Orchiectomy

   d. Phimosis

3. Which of the following statements regarding balanoposthitis is true?

    a. It is most commonly caused by a fungal infection.

    b. It is most common in circumcised men.

    c. Phimosis is a common contributing factor.

    d. It usually leads to the need for orchiectomy.

4. Which of the following statements regarding abruptio placentae is not true?

    a. Grade 3 is the most severe.

    b. It is defined as the sudden premature detachment of the placenta from the uterine wall.

    c. A classic symptom is high maternal blood pressure.

    d. Prognosis for mother and infant is usually excellent.

5. All of the following statements are true regarding toxic shock syndrome **except:**

    a. It is caused by a bacterial toxin.

    b. Patients are always female.

    c. Common symptoms include fever, rash, and low blood pressure.

    d. Patients are usually hospitalized for treatment.

Short Answer

1. **Describe fibrocystic breast disease and how a diagnosis of it is made.**

2. **List the sexually transmitted infections discussed in this chapter. Place an asterisk next to the one that is known for causing cervical cancer in women. Place a circle next to the one that might be confused with syphilis. Place a square next to the one that is caused by a spirochete. Place a triangle next to the one that is caused by protozoan. Place a check mark next to the one that causes an outbreak of painful vesicles.**

3. **Describe the definition of sexual assault and how it differs from the definition of rape.**

IMMUNE SYSTEM DISEASES AND DISORDERS

Learning Outcomes

Upon completion of this chapter, the student will be able to:

- Define and spell terms related to the immune system
- Identify key structures of the immune system
- Discuss the roles of the thymus and spleen as part of the immune system

- Identify characteristics of common immune system diseases and disorders, including:
  - description
  - incidence
  - etiology
  - signs and symptoms
  - diagnosis
  - treatment
  - prognosis

KEY TERMS	
antibody	substance produced by white blood cells in response to a specific antigen that then acts to destroy a pathogen
lymph	clear, colorless, alkaline fluid found within lymph vessels; made up of water, protein, salts, urea, fats, and white blood cells
lymphadenopathy	enlarged, tender lymph nodes
lymphocyte	a type of white blood cell responsible for much of the body's immune protection
opportunistic infections	infections by pathogens that do not normally cause disease unless the immune system is impaired
phagocytosis	process in which specialized white blood cells engulf and destroy microorganisms, foreign antigens, and cell debris
sepsis	systemic infection

Abbreviations

Table 9-1 lists some of the most common abbreviations related to the immune system.

TABLE 9-1

ABBREVIATIONS

Abbreviation	Meaning	Abbreviation	Meaning
AIDS	acquired immune deficiency syndrome	HIV	human immunodeficiency virus
AS	ankylosing spondylitis	ITP	idiopathic thromboycytopenic purpura
CFIDS	chronic fatigue and immune dysfunction syndrome	PCP	*Pneumocystis carinii* pneumonia
CFS	chronic fatigue syndrome	PM	Polymyositis
CMC	chronic mucocutaneous candidiasis	RBC	red blood cells
EBV	Epstein-Barr virus	SLE	systemic lupus erythematosus
ESR or Sed rate	erythrocyte sedimentation rate	SS	Sjögren syndrome
GVHD	graft-versus-host disease	WBC	white blood cell
HAART	highly active antiretroviral therapy		

Structures and Functions of the Immune System

The lymphatic system includes an intricate network of lymph vessels that collect excess tissue fluid and return it to circulation. It plays a major role in the immune system as it cleanses the collected fluid, now called **lymph.** Lymph is a clear, colorless, alkaline fluid made up mostly of water, along with some protein, salts, urea, fats, and white blood cells. Lymph enters lymph capillaries and makes its way into larger lymph vessels. Lymphatic vessels are found throughout the body alongside arteries, veins, and capillaries. While blood vessels rely on the pumping action of the heart, there is no pump for lymphatic vessels; instead, lymph flow is facilitated by the pumping action of skeletal muscle contraction. The lymphatic system includes *lymph nodes,* commonly called *glands,* which serve as filters to clean debris from lymph and also to produce some white blood cells. Because of these functions, the lymphatic system is also considered part of the immune system.

Flashpoint

Lymph nodes act like filters to clean debris from lymph fluid.

Structures of the Immune System

Lymph is excess fluid from tissues that is eventually returned to the circulatory system via lymphatic vessels. While located in tissue spaces, it is called *interstitial fluid* or *intercellular fluid.* When located within lymphatic vessels, it is called lymph. Lymphatic vessels are located throughout the body and are connected to the superior vena cava, which is where lymph enters the circulatory system and is combined with blood (see Fig. 9-1). Lymph nodes are distributed along lymphatic vessels, with higher concentrations in the neck, axillae, groin, and the mesentery of the abdomen. There are two sets of lymph nodes in the oropharynx, commonly known as the *tonsils* and *adenoids.* These nodes can become tender and swollen when an individual has an upper respiratory infection. This occurs when lymph nodes which have been working to filter bacteria, viruses, or other substances from lymph become overwhelmed and inflamed. An inflamed gland may be referred to as adenitis or adenopathy. Other organs of the lymphatic system include the thymus gland and spleen.

Thymus

The thymus gland is located in the mediastinum (central chest area) above the heart. It consists of two fused lobes and is divided into an outer cortex, mostly composed of immature T **lymphocytes**

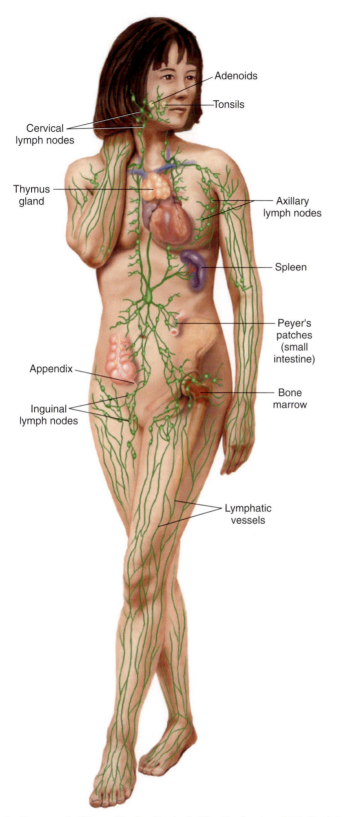

FIGURE 9-1 Lymphatic vessels (From Eagle, S, et al. *The Professional Medical Assistant: An Integrative Teamwork-Based Approach.* 2009. Philadelphia: F.A. Davis Company, with permission.)

(a type of white blood cell), and an inner medulla. The thymus grows until puberty and then gradually shrinks in size as we age.

Spleen

The spleen is a dark-red, oval-shaped lymphoid organ located in the left upper quadrant of the abdomen, just under the ribs. It is surrounded by an outer capsule of connective tissue and is divided into compartments.

Functions of the Immune System

The lymphatic system includes an intricate network of lymph vessels that collect and filter excess tissue fluid and return it to circulation. This system plays a major role in the immune system, because lymph nodes are rich in white blood cells, which engulf bacteria and cellular debris in a process known as *phagocytosis.* The body responds to infection and inflammation by increasing production of phagocytes.

Flashpoint

WBCs engulf and eliminate bacteria and debris in phagocytosis.

Thymus

The thymus is most active during the prenatal (before birth) period and early years of life. It plays a role in cellular immunity and is believed to play a role in protecting the body against cancer. T lymphocytes, also known as *killer T cells,* mature in the thymus and then circulate to the spleen, lymph nodes, and other lymphoid tissue, where they are involved in cell-mediated immune responses.

Spleen

The spleen contains a supply of 100 to 300 milliliters (roughly one-half to one and one-quarter cups) of blood. It also contains about 30% of the body's total platelets, specialized cell fragments that help form blood clots. These substances can be returned to circulation in the event of hemorrhage. Because of its location and rich blood supply, the spleen may be injured if the individual experiences a blow to the abdomen. Such an injury may require a splenectomy (surgical removal of the spleen) to stop internal bleeding. Fortunately, most people can survive without their spleen, although their immune system will be slightly weakened and they will be more vulnerable to infection.

During prenatal development, the spleen forms red and white blood cells (RBCs and WBCs). After birth, RBCs are produced by the spleen only in cases of severe need; however, the spleen continues creating WBCs as well as *antibodies* as part of its role in the immune system. Antibodies are a substance produced by white blood cells in response to a specific antigen that then acts to destroy a pathogen. Those antibodies later combine with that antigen when it presents itself again (during a second exposure) to mark the microorganism for destruction by macrophages, a type of WBC designed for phagocytosis. The process of phagocytosis removes microorganisms, cell debris, and blood cells that are damaged, old, abnormal, or marked by antibodies.

Immune System Diseases and Disorders

There are many diseases and disorders of the immune system. Some of the more common ones are discussed in this chapter: AIDS, chronic mucocutaneous candidiasis, chronic fatigue syndrome (CFS), graft-versus-host disease, transfusion incompatibility reaction, transplant rejection, and anaphylaxis. Autoimmune diseases discussed in this chapter are autoimmune hemolytic anemia, pernicious anemia, idiopathic thrombocytopenic purpura, systemic lupus erythematosus, scleroderma, Sjögren syndrome, and polymyositis.

AIDS

ICD-9-CM: 042   **[ICD-10: B24]**

AIDS is a late-stage infection with HIV which progressively weakens the immune system. It was first reported in the United States in 1981 and has since become a pandemic.

Incidence

AIDS is the fourth-most common cause of death worldwide and the leading cause of death in Africa. Worldwide, those most commonly affected are age 15 to 44, poor, and heterosexual, with inadequate access to health care. Within the United States, although heterosexuals are affected, the highest incidence continues to be among young men who have sex with men. African Americans, Hispanics, and Latinos are disproportionately affected compared to whites. More than one million cases of AIDS have been reported in the United States, and about half of those individuals have died. It is estimated that only about 10% of those infected have been diagnosed. Approximately 56,000 Americans are newly infected each year, more than 40 million individuals are currently infected worldwide, and more than 25 million people have died from AIDS, making it the worst pandemic in history.

Etiology

HIV is a retrovirus that cannot survive on its own but invades human CD-4 lymphocytes and uses them as its host cells. As the virus proliferates and destroys the lymphocytes, it leaves the body vulnerable to infection. It is spread from person to person via direct contact with blood, semen, vaginal secretions, or breast milk. The most common means of HIV transmission are unprotected sexual intercourse, injection drug use, men having sex with men, and childbirth; it is not spread through casual contact such as shaking hands or hugging. Health-care workers may contract the virus through needlestick injuries and major exposure to mucous membranes, such as the splashing of blood or bodily fluids into the eyes and nose (see Box 9-1).

> **Flashpoint**
> HIV is not spread through casual contact such as hugging.

Signs and Symptoms

Within 1 to 2 weeks after exposure, individuals often experience flu-like symptoms of fever, body aches, and sore throat. However, few people recognize this as a warning that they have contracted HIV. For the most part, individuals are asymptomatic (symptom free) in the early stages and may unwittingly transmit the virus to others. As the disease progresses and the immune system weakens, **opportunistic infections** become common. These are infections by pathogens that do not normally cause disease unless the immune system is impaired; common examples include *Pneumocystis carinii* pneumonia, cytomegalovirus infection, infections with *Candida albicans*, and a type of cancer called Kaposi sarcoma (see Fig. 9-2). These infections cause anorexia, weight loss, fatigue, fevers, chills, sweats, breathlessness, pneumonia, diarrhea, **lymphadenopathy** (enlarged, tender lymph nodes), and skin rashes. In some cases dementia also develops.

> **Flashpoint**
> People with weak immune systems are more vulnerable to opportunistic infections.

Diagnosis

AIDS is diagnosed as a later stage of HIV infection. HIV infection is diagnosed by detection of HIV antibodies in the blood with the enzyme-linked immunosorbent assay (ELISA) and Western blot tests. If the ELISA test is positive, it is repeated; confirmation of diagnosis is made

---

Box 9-1 Wellness Promotion

REDUCE YOUR RISK
The following self-care habits will help reduce your risk of contracting HIV:

Avoid
- Unprotected sex
- Multiple sexual partners
- IV drug use or sharing of needles

Practice
- Safer sex
- Monogamous sexual relationships
- Use of personal protective devices on the job, such as gloves, goggles, and masks
- Good self-care (healthy diet, adequate sleep, etc.) to keep your immune system strong

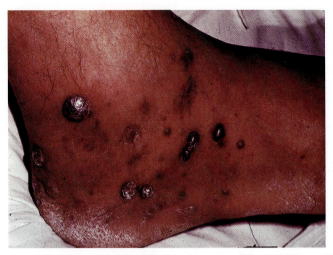

FIGURE 9-2 **Kaposi sarcoma** (From Goldsmith, LA, Lazarus, GS, and Tharp, MD. *Adult and Pediatric Dermatology: A Color Guide to Diagnosis and Treatment.* 1997. Philadelphia: F.A. Davis Company, with permission.)

with the Western blot test. Newer testing methods produce results within 60 minutes and involve testing either blood or a swab from inside the mouth, around the gums.

A home test for HIV is also available. Instructions are included for obtaining a drop of blood by pricking the finger and applying it to a card, which is mailed to a laboratory for testing. Because the individual uses an identification number, this system provides privacy and confidentiality. As with other HIV testing, positive results must be confirmed with a Western blot test. Disease progression is monitored by checking CD-4 lymphocyte count and viral load (see Box 9-2). As the disease progresses and the immune system weakens, CD-4 count decreases and viral load increases.

Besides confirmation of HIV, other diagnostic criteria for AIDS include a CD-4 lymphocyte count of less than 200 (normal value is 600 to 1,500), presence of an opportunistic infection, or the presence of an AIDS-defining malignancy.

Box 9-2 CD-4 Lymphocyte Count and Viral Load

CD-4 lymphocytes, sometimes called *helper T cells,* are a special type of white blood cell that help fight infection. As an HIV infection worsens, CD-4 lymphocyte count decreases and the immune system weakens. CD-4 cell count is usually reported as the number of CD-4 lymphocytes in a cubic millimeter of blood. Normal values range between 600 and 1,500. If the level drops below 200, the individual with HIV is diagnosed with AIDS. CD-4 count is also sometimes reported as a percentage of the total lymphocyte count. Normal CD-4 percentage is between 20% and 40%; a value that drops below 14% indicates probable AIDS. CD-4 cell count is evaluated along with viral load to monitor disease progression and prognosis.

Viral load is a test which measures copies of HIV in one milliliter of blood. It is a valuable tool for monitoring HIV and AIDS. A test showing stable numbers indicates that the disease has stabilized; however, growing numbers indicate that the virus is reproducing and the disease will likely worsen. This test is also a good predictor of the risk of transmission to others and an indicator of how responsive an individual is to therapy. A variety of tests can measure viral load; for consistency, the same type of test should be used each time for a given individual. The result may be as low as 20 copies per milliliter (using ultra-sensitive methods) or as high as one million or more.

Treatment

There is currently no cure for HIV or AIDS. Treatment includes the use of highly active antiretro-viral therapy (HAART), which includes a drug that inhibits HIV-1 protease and drugs that block viral reverse transcriptase, which prevents replication of the virus. General measures that protect the immune system and protect against other infections are advised, including immunizations, use of anti-infective medications as needed, avoidance of high-risk behaviors, good nutrition, adequate sleep, moderate exercise as tolerated, and avoidance of others who are ill with communicable diseases or infections.

Prognosis

AIDS is ultimately a fatal disease. However, individuals with AIDS are living much longer, health-ier lives than in the past, due to advances in treatment. Current life expectancy with HIV infec-tion is 10 to 20 years, depending upon the individual's self-care practices and access to health-care resources. Once the illness has progressed to AIDS, prognosis is poorer, but some may continue to live for several more years with a T-cell count of less than 200.

> **Flashpoint**
> There is still no cure for HIV and AIDS.

Chronic Mucocutaneous Candidiasis

ICD-9-CM: 112   [ICD-10: B37.0–B37.9 (code by site)]

Chronic mucocutaneous candidiasis (CMC) is a group of disorders in which persistent or recur-rent infections of *Candida* fungi develop on the skin, nails, or mucous membranes. *C. albicans* is the most common offender.

Incidence

CMC affects males and females equally. It is more common among the Iranian, Jewish, Finnish, and Sardinian populations. Approximately 60% to 80% of cases develop during infancy or tod-dlerhood. Onset during adulthood, however, is also possible and is sometimes associated with myasthenia gravis, thymoma (tumor of the thymus), and bone-marrow deficits.

Etiology

CMC is not one specific disease but rather a group of disorders; some variations are associated with problems of the endocrine system, and others with thymoma. A common character-istic of all seems to be faulty T-cell-mediated immunity, which results in the develop-ment of autoantibodies against the *Candida* species.

> **Flashpoint**
> Most cases of CMC develop during infancy or toddlerhood.

Signs and Symptoms

Symptoms may develop around age two or three or, with late-onset CMC, during young adulthood. Large, circular skin lesions manifest on the skin, nails, mucous membranes, or vagina. Infants generally develop recurrent diaper rash or oral thrush as their first symptoms. With older children, lesions often begin on the scalp or fingernails. Those in the later stages may develop recurring respiratory infections. Endocrine system involvement manifests as hypoparathyroidism, hypocalcemia (low blood calcium), and pernicious anemia (a form of anemia caused by vitamin B_{12} deficiency), which is discussed later in this chapter. There is also a ten-dency to be more vulnerable to bacterial, viral, and other fungal infections.

Diagnosis

A patient history is done to identify the pattern and prevalence of infections, and a physical examination is performed. Diagnosis is confirmed with a KOH test (see Box 9-3). A fungal cul-ture may also be done. Other immunodeficiency disorders, such as HIV, must be ruled out.

Treatment

This disorder is treated with antifungal medication, immunosuppressive therapy, or a combination of the two. Topical antifungals are generally not helpful, but oral antifungals are useful in treating oral thrush, and systemic antifungals are usually effective against all forms. Symptoms tend to recur once medication is stopped. Therapy aimed at correcting the immune deficit involves the administration of *transfer factor,* which is small proteins taken from the T lymphocytes of donors who are immune to *Candida.* This has not been found effective in every case but may result in long-term remission if combined with antifungal medication.

Box 9-3 Diagnostic Spotlight

THE KOH TEST

The KOH (potassium hydroxide) test is often used to confirm the presence of fungi. The physician scrapes cells from the margin of a lesion, places them on a glass slide, adds a few drops of a 10% KOH solution, and then examines the slide under a microscope. Because the KOH dissolves normal body cells, the fungal cells that remain are easily observed. This test is useful for confirming the presence of many types of fungal infection, such as tinea pedis (athlete's foot) and candidal (yeast) infections.

Prognosis

CMC is chronic and recurrent. Symptoms generally respond well to antifungal medications but recur after the drugs are discontinued. Life expectancy is usually normal; however, death can occur in rare cases due to disseminated infection (scattered throughout the body), *sepsis* (systemic infection), pneumonia, and other complications.

Chronic Fatigue Syndrome

ICD-9-CM: 780.71   [ICD-10: G93.3]

Chronic fatigue syndrome (CFS), sometimes called *chronic fatigue and immune dysfunction syndrome (CFIDS)*, is a complex chronic disorder that may last for years. It is marked by severe fatigue that is not relieved by rest and is often worsened by mental or physical activity.

Flashpoint

The key feature of CFS is unusual fatigue that is not relieved by rest.

Incidence

CFS is known to affect over one million Americans in all age, socioeconomic, racial, and ethnic groups. However, the CDC estimates that less than 20% of all people with CFS in the United States have been diagnosed, which suggests that as many as five million may actually have the disorder. In addition, it is estimated that tens of millions more suffer from severe fatigue but do not meet the diagnostic criteria for CFS. It affects women four times more often than men.

Etiology

The cause of CFS is not clear. Various theories have suggested endocrine, immune, and nervous system involvement. Environmental and genetic factors may also be involved. Depression has been identified as a common coexisting disorder but not a cause.

Signs and Symptoms

The main symptom of CFS is pronounced fatigue, unrelieved by rest, that causes a significant reduction in the ability to perform activities of daily living. In addition, physical exertion is followed by extreme fatigue that lasts for 24 hours or more. Other symptoms vary greatly in type and severity. They include insomnia, unrefreshing sleep, weakness, muscle aches, and difficulty with concentration and memory.

Diagnosis

There are no definitive diagnostic tests for CFS; therefore, the diagnosis is not made until other possibilities have been excluded. Currently, the key diagnostic criteria include severe fatigue for more than 6 months along with at least four of the following: short-term memory deficit or difficulty concentrating, lymph-node tenderness, sore throat, joint or muscle pain without redness or swelling, unrefreshing sleep, postexertion malaise of greater than 24 hours, and onset of headaches of a new type, severity, or pattern.

Treatment

There is no known cure for CFS. Treatment is aimed at relieving symptoms and maximizing function. Medications to provide symptom relief may include those that help with pain, anxiety, gastrointestinal complaints, and insomnia. Lifestyle recommendations include stress-reduction strategies and dietary modification. Other measures that may be helpful include nutritional supplementation (under a physician's direction), massage, meditation, and acupuncture. Moderate exercise and careful physical therapy are aimed at maintaining strength and health without causing undue fatigue.

Prognosis
According to the CDC, a delay of more than 2 years in accurate diagnosis is a predictor of a more complicated course and less-favorable outcomes. CFS affects individuals differently; some improve enough to resume work and other activities, while others are confined to their homes. Full recovery is uncommon, but an average of 40% of patients report improvement.

> **Flashpoint**
> There is currently no cure for CFS.

Diseases and Disorders Related to Rejection by the Immune System

Some immune system disorders develop when the immune system responds to transplanted tissue. Examples include graft-versus-host disease, transfusion incompatibility reaction, and transplant rejection.

Graft-Versus-Host Disease
ICD-9-CM: 279.50   [ICD-10: T86.0]
Graft-versus-host disease (GVHD) is a complication of bone-marrow transplantation. Acute GVHD develops during the first 100 days after the transplant and chronic GVHD develops after day 100.

Incidence
The incidence and severity of GVHD are related to how well the tissues of donor and recipient are matched. The greater the degree of mismatch, the greater the likelihood of this complication. Risk increases with age; patients younger than 20 experience a 20% risk, while those older than 50 have an 80% risk.

Etiology
Although many types of transplantation occur on a daily basis, GVHD is most commonly associated with blood and bone-marrow transplantation, because of the high numbers of immune cells those tissues contain. Blood transfusions are commonplace and are done for many reasons; a typical example is the patient who suffers severe blood loss due to traumatic injury and is then given a transfusion. Bone-marrow transplants are done to replace immune cells and blood-forming cells that were destroyed during chemotherapy or radiation treatment for cancer or leukemia. In either case, immune cells in the transplanted tissue identify tissue in the recipient as foreign and begin to attack it.

> **Flashpoint**
> GVHD occurs when transplanted immune cells attack body tissue.

Signs and Symptoms
Acute GVHD primarily affects the skin, gastrointestinal tract, and liver. Early symptoms include the development of skin lesions such as redness, red macules, papules, and bullae. Gastrointestinal symptoms include diarrhea, abdominal pain, vomiting, and weight loss. Liver involvement often causes jaundice (yellowing of the skin and mucous membranes).

Chronic GVHD can affect multiple organs but primarily affects the skin, which develops changes resembling lichen planus. These are lesions in the form of shiny, flat-topped papules, usually pink or lavender, sometimes with fine white lines, and usually itchy. In some individuals, the skin changes manifest in the form of scleroderma (discussed later in this chapter), which is an autoimmune disorder affecting the skin as well as other connective tissues in the body. Other symptoms of chronic GVHD include hair loss, dry mouth and eyes, and hepatitis.

Signs and symptoms associated with a blood transfusion usually occur between 4 and 30 days afterward and are related to the key functions of blood: clotting, transporting oxygen, and fighting infection. The individual may manifest evidence of anemia due to lack of healthy RBCs, a tendency to bleed, and increased vulnerability to infection. To reduce the risk of this type of reaction, blood is often irradiated (using x-rays) before transfusion. This leaves the RBCs intact but eliminates the threat from the immune cells.

Diagnosis

A diagnosis of GVHD can be difficult to sort out from the many other potential complications suffered by transplant recipients. Testing may include liver function tests, skin biopsy, and endoscopy (visualization inside of a part of the body). Diagnosis may be confirmed by identification of lymphocytes with a different human leukocyte antigen type than those of the host (recipient) cells. (Human leukocyte antigen is a type of genetic material involved in the immune response and other functions.)

Treatment

The mainstay of treatment is administration of immunosuppressive medications. Antibiotics may be given to treat infection.

Prognosis

Complications of GVHD include liver failure and infection. Infection may be an ongoing problem, because of the underlying disease being treated, immunosuppressive medications, and prior chemotherapy or radiation. Mortality rates vary with the type and severity of GVHD, from 22% to 90%.

The good news is that those who survive GVHD related to leukemia treatment seem to be less likely to suffer a recurrence of the type of leukemia that was being treated. Furthermore, grafted cells often develop a tolerance to the recipient after 6 to 12 months, and immunosuppressive medications can then be decreased or even discontinued.

Transfusion Incompatibility Reaction

ICD-9-CM: 999.6 (ABO incompatibility), 999.7 (Rh incompatibility reaction), 999.8 (other transfusion reaction)   **[ICD-10: T80.3 (ABO incompatibility), T80.4 (Rh incompatibility reaction), T80.9 (other transfusion reaction)]**

A transfusion incompatibility reaction occurs when antibodies present in transfused blood react to RBCs in the recipient's blood, or when antibodies in the recipient's blood react to RBCs in the transfused blood.

Incidence

As many as 50,000 transfusion incompatibility reactions occur each year in the United States, although the majority of them are mild. Milder reactions include nonfatal allergic reactions, febrile (having a fever) reactions, and others. Transfusion reactions can occur in patients of any age, but they are most common among those over 60.

Etiology

An acute hemolytic (blood-destroying) reaction occurs when a recipient is transfused with blood of a different type from the recipient's own. When this occurs, the recipient's immune system attacks the RBCs in the transfused blood, causing them to hemolyze (rupture) or agglutinate (clump together), which can result in obstruction of capillaries. This can lead to kidney failure, shock, and even death.

Flashpoint

An acute hemolytic reaction occurs when a patient is transfused with blood of a different type from the patient's own.

Signs and Symptoms

Signs and symptoms of transfusion reaction depend upon the specific type and severity of the reaction. Symptoms usually appear during or immediately after the transfusion, although delayed reactions can occur. By far the most common—and often the only—symptom is fever. Other symptoms include hypotension, chills, rash, wheezing, anxiety, vomiting, flank or back pain, hematuria, dizziness, and fainting. Generalized bleeding may be a late sign and indicates a complication called disseminated intravascular coagulation, in which hemorrhage develops due to microvascular blood clotting. Allergic reactions produce a typical maculopapular urticaria rash. Severe allergic reactions may cause dyspnea and other signs of anaphylaxis.

Diagnosis

The health-care provider should suspect a transfusion reaction if the patient experiences dyspnea, back pain, fever, chills, and hives during the transfusion. Blood samples from the donor blood and the recipient must be collected right away for testing and retyping. An acute hemolytic reaction is identified by a positive Coombs' test (which identifies antibodies bound to RBCs that cause hemolysis) and by examination of the individual's urine and plasma for indication of hemolysis.

Treatment

Treatment of a transfusion reaction includes immediately stopping the transfusion, if it is still in progress, while maintaining intravenous access. Blood and urine specimens must be obtained and sent to the laboratory, along with the remainder of the untransfused blood. Treatment measures depend upon the type of symptoms manifested. Allergic reactions are treated with antihistamines; fever and discomfort are treated with analgesic/antipyretic medication. Corticosteroids are used to suppress the body's immune response. For severe reactions, intravenous fluids and other medications may be administered to treat kidney failure or shock.

Prognosis

The prognosis for individuals experiencing transfusion reaction is usually good, depending upon the type and severity of reaction. Potential complications include discomfort, kidney failure, anemia, lung problems, and shock.

Flashpoint
If the patient has a reaction, the transfusion should be stopped immediately.

Transplant Rejection

ICD-9-CM: 996.80–996.89   [ICD-10: T86.0–T86.9] (code by organ or tissue for both codes)

Transplant rejection occurs when a recipient's immune system identifies transplanted tissue as foreign and responds by attacking it. Rejection is classified as hyperacute, acute, or chronic.

Incidence

The incidence of transplant rejection varies by transplant organ or tissue type. It occurs in 60% to 75% of first kidney transplants and up to 60% of liver transplants.

Etiology

Hyperacute rejection develops within minutes of transplant and is caused by the immediate reaction of preexisting antibodies in the donor to the transplanted tissue. Acute rejection is caused by T-cell responses to donor proteins; it develops several days after the transplant if the recipient is not taking immunosuppressive medications. Chronic rejection is caused by a chronic immune response against the organ.

Signs and Symptoms

The signs and symptoms of transplant rejection depend upon the type of tissue or organ transplanted. The most common signs and symptoms, by organ, are:

- Kidney: hypertension, decreased urine output, fever, flu-like symptoms (body aches, fatigue, nausea, vomiting, chills, headache), increased pain over the transplant site, and fluid retention (indicated by swollen ankles, fingers, etc.)
- Heart: fever, shortness of breath, irregular heartbeat, flu-like symptoms, hypotension, and fluid retention
- Lung: chest pain, shortness of breath, cough, and malaise
- Liver: itching, yellow skin or eyes, darkened urine, light-colored stool, fatigue, weight gain, and abdominal swelling

Diagnosis

Acute rejection is diagnosed based upon patient signs and symptoms and laboratory testing, which varies depending upon the type of transplanted organ or tissue. In some cases, tissue biopsy of the transplanted organ is done.

Treatment

Hyperacute rejection is usually prevented by careful crossmatching before surgery to identify antibodies. However, should rejection occur, the transplanted organ or tissue must be immediately removed to prevent a severe systemic inflammatory response.

Acute organ rejection may be prevented by the use of immunosuppressive medications; however, rejection can occur after months or even years. Acute rejection is treated with high doses of IV corticosteroids. In some cases, plasma exchange may be done to remove antibodies that are attacking the transplanted tissue. Chronic rejection cannot be treated; re-transplantation is necessary.

Flashpoint
Reaction is usually prevented by careful crossmatching.

Prognosis

Acute rejection can damage or even destroy the transplanted organ; however, if it is recognized and treated promptly, the organ may be saved. In some cases recurrent episodes may lead to chronic rejection.

Ankylosing Spondylitis

ICD-9-CM: 720.0   [ICD-10: M45]

Ankylosing spondylitis (AS) is a type of inflammatory arthritis that causes degenerative changes in the spinal vertebrae and sacroiliac joints. It also causes inflammatory changes in connective tissues such as tendons and ligaments, and it can affect joints of the hips, shoulders, knees, feet, and ribs. Tissues of the lungs, eyes, and heart valves may be affected as well. AS manifests as an episodic pattern or in a severe chronic form.

Incidence

AS affects nearly 400,000 Americans, men more than women and Native Americans more than other ethnic groups. Age of onset is usually between 16 and 40.

Etiology

The specific cause of AS has not been determined; however, genetics is a known risk factor, since most people with AS have been identified as carrying the HLA-B27 gene. This does not mean that everyone with this gene will develop AS—in fact, the risk is quite low. However, those with this gene seem to be more susceptible.

Signs and Symptoms

The signs and symptoms associated with AS are related to the degenerative changes that occur in the spine and other structures (see Fig. 9-3). As the disease progresses, new bone tissue develops in response to inflammation. This results in the fusing of many of the bones and joints. Fusion decreases the range of motion of joints and results in feelings of stiffness and difficulty moving. When bones of the thorax are affected, a result is decreased lung capacity. Pain and stiffness become more pronounced with time, especially in the morning and after periods of inactivity. As the condition becomes more severe, individuals experience chronic stooping, fatigue, difficulty breathing, spinal stiffness, anorexia, weight loss, and inflammation of the eyes and bowels.

Flashpoint

The signs and symptoms of AS are caused by degenerative changes of the spine and fusing of joints.

Diagnosis

Diagnosis is sometimes delayed when symptoms are mistakenly identified as resulting from other, more common back disorders. An early sign of AS is a significant loss in lumbar spine flexibility. As the disease progresses, stiffness may be felt in the sacroiliac area, neck, upper back, shoulders, hips, and feet. Some individuals develop eye inflammation, and those with severe cases may have heart involvement as well.

The erythrocyte sedimentation rate (ESR) and C-reactive protein tests indicate the presence of inflammation (see Box 9-4). Other tests may reveal the presence of anemia or the HLA-B27 gene. Arthritic changes will be evident on x-rays and bone scans. Other tests may include computerized tomography (CT) or magnetic resonance imaging (MRI) scans.

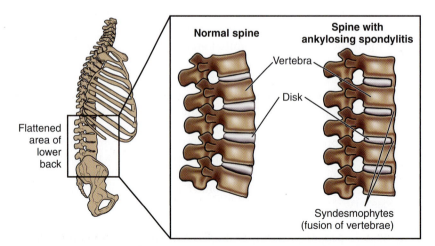

FIGURE 9-3 Ankylosing spondylitis causes vertebrae to fuse together, which results in the loss of normal curvature.

Box 9-4 Diagnostic Spotlight

ERYTHROCYTE SEDIMENTATION RATE

The erythrocyte sedimentation rate, often abbreviated as *ESR* or *Sed rate,* is a nonspecific test used in the diagnosis and monitoring of many diseases that cause acute or chronic inflammation, including many autoimmune disorders. It measures the rate at which red blood cells settle in plasma or saline over a specific period of time. The normal value is around 15 (men) to 20 (women) millimeters per hour. This test is considered nonspecific because it does not identify the exact cause or source of the inflammation; however, it is useful in helping the physician identify whether inflammation is a key feature of an illness, and it is often used to track the patient's response to treatment. Increasing values may indicate worsening disease. Decreasing values may indicate improvement in the disease or a positive response to treatment.

Treatment

Treatment is aimed at preventing pain and stiffness and minimizing spinal deformity and other complications. NSAIDs are used to reduce inflammation. Corticosteroids are used to suppress inflammation by suppressing the body's immune response. Tumor necrosis factor blockers may be used to reduce the pain and stiffness associated with inflammation and swelling. Measures which help to reduce stiffness and promote function are also helpful, including physical therapy to improve positioning for walking and sleeping, exercises and stretching to promote flexibility, and breathing exercises to increase lung capacity and function.

Prognosis

The course and severity of AS varies with each individual. Complications can include difficulty walking or standing, difficulty breathing, lung infections, heart-valve dysfunction, anemia, inflammatory bowel disease, and iritis (eye inflammation).

Anaphylaxis

ICD-9-CM: 995.0   [ICD-10: T78.2]

Anaphylaxis is a life-threatening systemic allergic reaction to a substance that the body was previously sensitized to. An anaphylactic reaction differs from lesser forms of sensitivities; hypersensitivity is a general term used to refer to a reaction of the immune system to an antigen, resulting in inflammation and organ dysfunction. The term *allergy* has traditionally been used, but it is now recognized that there are five separate types of reactions. Therefore the term *allergy* is now reserved for *type 1 hypersensitivity* reactions (see Table 9-2).

Flashpoint

Anaphylaxis is a life-threatening allergic reaction.

Incidence

General allergies are experienced by an estimated 50 million Americans. It is further estimated that 82,000 episodes of anaphylaxis are experienced by Americans each year, resulting in 6,000 deaths. Most are due to penicillin reactions, but others are caused by insect stings and food allergies.

Etiology

Anaphylaxis is caused by an overreaction of the immune system to a substance. As a result, histamine and other substances are released, causing a systemic inflammatory response. This causes blood vessels to dilate and become more permeable, as well as the other physical changes commonly seen. Risk factors include a history of allergies and previous severe reactions.

Signs and Symptoms

The symptoms of anaphylaxis are sudden and severe. They include feelings of apprehension followed by difficulty breathing, rapid pulse, hypotension, urticaria (hives), itching, nausea, vomiting, and shock.

TABLE 9-2

HYPERSENSITIVITY REACTIONS

Type	Description	Examples
Type 1	Reexposure to an antigen via direct contact, inhalation, ingestion, or injection causes the release of the chemicals histamine, leukotriene, and prostaglandin, which results in localized or systemic effects including vasodilation and smooth-muscle contraction.	Hay fever, anaphylaxis
Type 2	Autoantibodies are produced by the person's immune system and bind to antigens on their own cells. As a result, these cells are then identified as foreign and are attacked by the immune system.	Autoimmune hemolytic anemia
Type 3	Antigens and antibodies link to form large immune complexes that lodge in vessel walls and cause an inflammatory response. This causes the key symptoms of many connective-tissue diseases.	Rheumatoid arthritis, systemic lupus erythematosus (SLE)
Type 4	This is a delayed, cell-mediated reaction that occurs up to 3 days after exposure.	Positive purified protein derivative (PPD)(tuberculosis reaction), chronic transplant rejection, contact dermatitis
Type 5	Normal cell surfaces are continuously stimulated by an autoantibody, causing the affected tissue to be hyper-responsive.	Graves disease, myasthenia gravis

Diagnosis

Diagnosis is based upon a rapid physical assessment, description of signs and symptoms from the patient (if the patient is able to talk), and information from family or friends who may be familiar with the patient's allergies. A quick search for medical-alert jewelry may give health-care providers important clues about what triggered the event.

Treatment

Anaphylaxis requires emergency intervention. An adequate airway is the top priority, followed by assuring that breathing is adequate. If it is not, the patient must be given ventilatory support, which may mean the insertion of an endotracheal tube, use of a ventilator, or supplemental oxygen. Medication includes epinephrine, antihistamines, and corticosteroids, which must be given immediately. If necessary, blood pressure is supported with IV fluids and vasoactive medications.

Individuals who are known to have severe allergies should wear medical-alert identification and talk with their health-care provider about carrying an emergency kit (see Box 9-5).

Flashpoint

The patient with anaphylaxis must be given immediate help.

Prognosis

Prognosis is generally good if appropriate treatment is instituted immediately. However, anaphylaxis is a life-threatening event: Death may occur without proper treatment.

Diseases and Disorders Related to Autoimmune Responses

Many immune system disorders are related to a faulty response of the immune system in which the body's normally protective defense mechanisms misidentify body tissues as foreign. The immune system then attacks those tissues as it might a threatening pathogen. Some conditions that have been classified as probably autoimmune in nature are autoimmune hemolytic anemia,

Box 9-5 Wellness Promotion

BE PREPARED

Many patients have chronic conditions, such as severe allergies, that can result in life-threatening emergencies. Because altered consciousness may occur as a result of many of these conditions, individuals should wear a medical-alert bracelet or necklace. This can provide essential information to a health-care provider in the event that the person is unable to provide the information personally. Data may include:

- nature of the condition, such as allergy and diabetes
- person's name
- code status
- emergency contact number

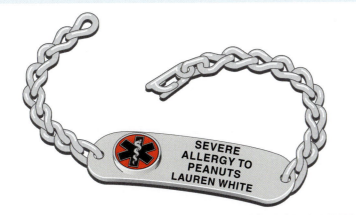

Medical-alert bracelet (From Eagle, S, et al. *The Professional Medical Assistant: An Integrative Teamwork-Based Approach.* 2009. Philadelphia: F.A. Davis Company, with permission.)

Individuals with known severe allergies should talk with their health-care provider about keeping an emergency kit on hand. This kit is sometimes called a "bee-sting kit," although individuals may react to things other than bee stings. The kit may contain the following items:

- EpiPen, an autoinjector containing epinephrine. It may be purchased with a prescription and is available in adult and child doses. It contains a spring-loaded needle and is very easy to self-administer. Its shelf life is usually around 20 months; it should be replaced regularly.
- Some type of antihistamine, such as diphenhydramine (Benadryl). The standard dose is 50 milligrams by mouth for adults (check with your health-care provider for the most appropriate medication and dose for you).
- Information card that includes your identification, allergies, medications, and contact information for your health-care provider and family members.

pernicious anemia, idiopathic thrombocytopenic purpura, systemic lupus erythematosus, scleroderma, Sjögren syndrome, and polymyositis.

Autoimmune Hemolytic Anemia
ICD-9-CM: 283.0   [ICD-10: D59.1] (anemias for both codes)

Autoimmune hemolytic anemia is a group of disorders caused when the immune system misidentifies red blood cells as foreign and creates autoantibodies that attack them. It is classified as either warm-antibody or cold-antibody hemolytic anemia.

Flashpoint

In autoimmune disorders the immune system attacks the body's own tissues.

Incidence

This group of disorders comprises approximately 5% of all anemias and affects between 4,000 and 8,000 people in the United States. It affects women more than men and may strike at any age, although it is more common in middle-aged and elderly populations. It does not affect any one race more than any other.

Etiology

The cause of autoimmune hemolytic anemia is often unclear. It is sometimes triggered by other diseases, such as systemic lupus erythematosus, or may occur as a complication of some medications (such as penicillin). Warm-antibody autoimmune hemolytic anemia develops at normal or higher-than-normal body temperatures; the cold-antibody variation is triggered by colder-than-normal body temperatures.

Signs and Symptoms

Some individuals may be asymptomatic, especially those with mild cases. Others develop symptoms commonly seen with other types of anemia, especially those with severe illness. These include jaundice, fatigue, pallor, tachycardia, darkened urine, dyspnea, splenomegaly (enlarged spleen), and abdominal discomfort.

Diagnosis

Diagnosis is based upon a finding of decreased numbers of healthy RBCs; decreased hemoglobin and haptoglobin (a serum protein); and increased reticulocytes (immature RBCs), bilirubin, urine hemoglobin, and levels of some antibodies identified on a Coombs' test.

Treatment

Mild forms may not be treated. Disease that is severe or worsening is usually treated with corticosteroids and other immunosuppressive medications. Splenectomy may also be performed. Plasmapheresis, which is a filtration process done to remove antibodies from the blood, may be performed as well. In severe cases blood transfusions may be given, but they provide only temporary relief.

Prognosis

Children generally recover from this disease, but adults are more likely to have a chronic course and relapses. Complications include severe anemia.

Pernicious Anemia
ICD-9-CM: 281.0   [ICD-10: D51.0–D51.9 (code by type)]

Pernicious anemia is a form of megaloblastic anemia (it produces many large, immature, dysfunctional RBCs). It has a number of other names, including *congenital pernicious anemia, juvenile pernicious anemia, macrocytic achylic anemia,* and *vitamin B$_{12}$ deficiency anemia.* It is a chronic disease caused by a deficit in the absorption of vitamin B$_{12}$. This, in turn, reduces the body's ability to produce sufficient numbers of healthy RBCs.

Flashpoint

Pernicious anemia is caused by inadequate absorption of vitamin B$_{12}$.

Incidence

Approximately 400,000 individuals in the United States are affected with pernicious anemia. A congenital form occurs in children, but the average age of patients is 60.

Etiology

Vitamin B$_{12}$ is required for the production of healthy RBCs. It cannot be produced by the body, so it must be obtained through the diet. Intrinsic factor is a protein produced by the parietal cells of the stomach lining that is necessary for the absorption of vitamin B$_{12}$. Pernicious anemia is caused when the stomach loses the ability to produce intrinsic factor, which then results in the ineffective utilization of B$_{12}$.

Pernicious anemia is considered an autoimmune disorder because approximately 90% of those affected are found to have autoantibodies against their stomach's parietal cells. Risk factors for pernicious anemia include family history of the disease, northern European or Scandinavian ancestry, and a history of other autoimmune endocrine disorders, such as myasthenia gravis, Graves disease, Addison disease, type 1 diabetes, and hypoparathryoidism.

Signs and Symptoms

There are many potential signs and symptoms of pernicious anemia, including fatigue, malaise, pallor, shortness of breath, and tachycardia. Gastrointestinal symptoms include diarrhea, nausea, constipation, abdominal pain, and anorexia. These lead to a common problem with weight loss. The desire or ability to eat is also affected by common mouth problems, including sore, red tongue, burning tongue, and bleeding gums. The sense of smell may be impaired. Abnormal neuromuscular symptoms include paresthesia (abnormal sensation) of the hands and feet, muscle spasms, weakness, difficulty moving, and impaired reflexes. Other effects include fever, confusion, and memory deficits.

Diagnosis

Diagnosis is based upon history, physical examination, and a variety of tests including vitamin B_{12} level, complete blood count, reticulocyte count, and a Schilling test (used to determine whether the body is absorbing vitamin B_{12} normally). Gastroscopy and biopsy of the stomach mucosa may confirm a diagnosis of atrophic gastritis, a condition in which chronic inflammation leads to fibrous changes, resulting in the insufficient production of intrinsic factor as well as certain acids and enzymes.

Treatment

The mainstay of treatment is the administration of monthly vitamin B_{12} injections. In some cases, B_{12} may also be taken by mouth. A well-balanced diet is important to ensure that the individual is receiving adequate amounts of folic acid, vitamin C, iron, and other essential nutrients.

Flashpoint

The key treatment of pernicious anemia is supplemental vitamin B_{12}.

Prognosis

The prognosis for individuals with pernicious anemia is excellent if treatment is instituted in a timely manner. Potential complications of the disorder include the development of gastric polyps (abnormal growths projecting from mucous membranes) and chronic neurological deficits if treatment is not initiated soon enough. The incidence of gastric cancer in those with pernicious anemia is twice that of the general population.

Idiopathic Thrombocytopenic Purpura
ICD-9-CM: 287.31   [ICD-10: D69.3]

Idiopathic thrombocytopenic purpura (ITP) is a disorder in which a deficiency of platelets results in abnormal blood clotting. It is characterized by tiny purple bruises (purpura) that form under the skin.

Incidence

ITP affects approximately 15,000 children and 20,000 adults in the United States each year. Chronic ITP most commonly affects adults 20 to 50 years old, women nearly three times as often as men. Acute ITP commonly affects children under the age of 10, boys and girls in equal proportion.

Etiology

The term "idiopathic" indicates that the cause of ITP is not fully understood. However, because an autoantibody called immunoglobulin G has been identified on the surface of platelets in people with this disorder, ITP is believed to be the result of an autoimmune response in which the body's own platelets are attacked and destroyed. Acute forms of ITP in children have been linked to recent viral infections or immunization with live virus; however, the same connection has not been identified in adults.

Signs and Symptoms

The onset of illness in children is rapid; in adults it is more gradual. Common signs and symptoms include purpura, or tiny purple bruises, and a tendency to bleed more easily than normal. This is evidenced by epistaxis (nosebleeds), gingival (gum) bleeding, menorrhagia (heavy menstrual flow), and easy bruising.

Flashpoint

Key symptoms of ITP include tiny purple bruises and bleeding.

Diagnosis

Diagnosis of ITP includes a complete physical examination and history. Other bleeding disorders must be ruled out. A complete blood count in which platelets are very low while other factors are normal is the most definitive finding.

Treatment

Treatment is usually initiated for symptomatic children whose platelet count falls below 30,000, symptomatic adults whose platelet count falls below 50,000, and those with very high-risk factors for bleeding. Administration of immunoglobulins (proteins that help the immune system) and high doses of corticosteroids are the mainstays of treatment. Transfusion of platelets and other blood products is given as needed. In some cases splenectomy may be done.

Prognosis

The prognosis for children with ITP is very good: Over 80% experience spontaneous remissions and nearly 90% eventually recover. Approximately 2% die. The prognosis for adults is not as optimistic. Only about 2% experience spontaneous recovery, about 65% eventually recover, and around 30% develop a chronic form of the disease. About 5% die from intracranial hemorrhage, the most life-threatening complication of ITP, and the 5-year mortality rate among those over age 60 with severe disease is nearly 50%.

Systemic Lupus Erythematosus
ICD-9-CM: 710.0   [ICD-10: L93]

Systemic lupus erythematosus (SLE) is a chronic autoimmune disorder that causes inflammation and degeneration of various connective tissues and organs in the body, such as the skin, lungs, heart, joints, kidneys, blood, and nervous system (see Fig. 9-4). Lupus that affects only the skin is called discoid lupus. SLE, on the other hand, is considered systemic because it can target any number of tissues or organs within the body.

Flashpoint

SLE affects many body systems in addition to the skin.

Incidence

SLE affects up to 1.5 million Americans and is eight times more common in women than men. It can occur at any age but is most common in women between the ages of 15 and 45. It is also more common in African Americans, Latinos, Native Americans, and those of Japanese or Chinese descent.

Etiology

SLE is an autoimmune disorder, in which the body produces antibodies that target "self" tissues, resulting in inflammation and degeneration. The exact cause of the autoimmune response is not fully understood. There is some thought that genetics, viruses, some drugs, female hormones, stress, and ultraviolet light (sunlight, fluorescent lights, and tanning beds) may play a role.

Signs and Symptoms

Lupus is marked by exacerbations (periods of illness) and remissions (periods of wellness). One of the most prominent features of both discoid lupus and SLE is the skin rash that may develop anywhere on the body but is most obvious on the face and scalp. It is generally red and flat—but may have raised borders—and painless, and it doesn't itch. Other symptoms of SLE depend upon the body system affected. General whole-body symptoms include mild fever, fatigue,

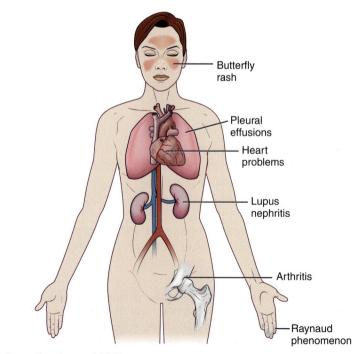

FIGURE 9-4 **Complications of SLE**

anorexia, and weight loss. Other symptoms include myalgia (muscle aches), arthralgia (aching joints), photosensitivity, splenomegaly, lympadenopathy, and Raynaud phenomenon (a circulatory disorder of the fingers and toes). Arthritic changes develop in 90% of those with SLE and cause joint pain, stiffness, edema, and possible joint deformity.

Diagnosis

There is no single test that definitively diagnoses SLE. Instead, 11 criteria are used to confirm diagnosis. Identification of four or more suggests a diagnosis of SLE. They are the classic "butterfly" rash across the cheeks and nose; discoid skin rash; photosensitivity; ulcerations in the mouth, nose, or throat; arthritis; pleuritis (inflammation in the lining of the lungs) or pericarditis (inflammation in the lining of the heart); kidney abnormalities; brain irritation; abnormal blood count; positive antinuclear antibody test; and immunologic disorder characterized by abnormal immune tests, including anti-DNA or anti-Sm (Smith) antibodies, false-positive blood test for syphilis, anticardiolipin antibodies, lupus anticoagulant, and positive lupus erythematosus cell preparation (LE) test. The ESR test, while not a conclusive diagnostic test, can be very helpful in monitoring an individual's response to therapy. Other testing that may be helpful includes blood-chemistry testing, tissue biopsies, and fluid specimen analysis.

Treatment

There is no cure for SLE. Treatment goals are relief of symptoms and prevention or minimization of complications. A variety of medications may be used to prevent or treat inflammation, including NSAIDS. Severe exacerbations may be treated with corticosteroids. Other immunosuppressive medications may be used as well. Hydroxychloroquine is helpful for treating SLE patients suffering from skin and joint disease and fatigue. Those with severe kidney or brain disease may benefit from plasmapheresis. General recommendations also include rest and regular, moderate exercise.

> *Flashpoint*
> Erythrocyte sedimentation rate (ESR) is often used to monitor the patient's response to therapy.

Prognosis

Complications of SLE include some forms of cancer, pleuritis, pericarditis, cardiovascular disease, heart attack, kidney failure, stroke, Raynaud phenomenon, and brain damage. Some patients go into remission for up to a year and require no treatment during that time. Survival and longevity varies depending upon how many of the 11 diagnostic criteria are present and which organs are affected. Self-care practices can help to prevent or minimize disease exacerbations (see Box 9-6). Those with SLE limited to the skin and joints have the best prognosis; those with disease of the kidneys or central nervous system have a poorer prognosis.

Scleroderma
ICD-9-CM: 710.1   [ICD-10: L94.0 (code by type)]

Scleroderma is a group of uncommon chronic autoimmune diseases. The name comes from the Greek words *skleros* (hard) and *derma* (skin), and it refers to the skin changes caused by the condition. It has also been known as *progressive systemic sclerosis*, but this name has fallen out of favor as it became clear that the disease is not always progressive in nature. Scleroderma is considered a rheumatic disease because it causes inflammation and pain in muscles, joints, and fibrous tissues. It is also considered a connective-tissue disease because of fibrotic changes that occur in affected connective tissues, such as tendons, cartilage and skin. Variations of scleroderma include localized and diffuse forms.

> *Flashpoint*
> Patients with SLE should take measures to protect their immune system and keep it strong.

Incidence

Scleroderma affects up to a half a million Americans, predominantly women between the ages of 30 and 50. Localized scleroderma is more common in children and those of European descent. Systemic scleroderma is more common among adults and women of African American descent.

> *Flashpoint*
> Scleroderma causes fibrous changes to many tissues in the body.

Etiology

The cause of scleroderma is not fully understood. However, it is thought to be an autoimmune disease in which the immune system stimulates cells known as fibroblasts to produce excessive amounts of collagen, a substance that normally adds strength to the skin. Risk factors include a family history of rheumatic disease. Because scleroderma is much more common in women than men, hormones may play a role as well, although this has not been proven.

Box 9-6 Wellness Promotion

BE KIND TO YOUR IMMUNE SYSTEM
Self-care is critically important for individuals with autoimmune disorders. Many of the activities that help to keep the immune system strong are simple, commonsense measures that everyone should take:

Avoid
- Exposure to individuals with known infectious disease
- Smoking or use of any tobacco products
- Unnecessary exposure to pollution
- Extreme physical or emotional stress
- Excessive fatigue

Make Time For
- Moderate exercise
- Adequate sleep and rest
- Stress-management activities
- Positive, supportive relationships

Report to Your Health-Care Provider
- Unusual fatigue
- Unexplained cough
- New or increased allergy reactions
- New or worsened skin conditions

Signs and Symptoms

Localized scleroderma affects areas of the skin and related tissue. It is classified as either morphea or linear. Morphea refers to localized patches of reddish or light-purple skin with light-colored centers that develop a thickened, firm texture. These patches are usually located on the stomach, back, or chest but can also develop on the arms, legs, and face. Linear scleroderma is characterized by a band or line of abnormally colored, thickened skin, usually on the arm, leg, or forehead.

The systemic form of scleroderma affects approximately one-third of those with the disorder. In this case it affects not only the skin but also deeper tissues, blood vessels, major organs, and organ systems. There are two subtypes of systemic scleroderma: limited and diffuse cutaneous scleroderma. Limited cutaneous scleroderma develops gradually and affects the skin in specific areas of the body, such as the arms, legs, hands, fingers, or face. Individuals with this form of scleroderma usually also have Raynaud disease, which most likely manifests before the onset of scleroderma symptoms. Individuals with limited scleroderma may develop gastrointestinal and lung problems and may develop some or all of the features of CREST syndrome:

Flashpoint

CREST syndrome is associated with a poorer prognosis.

- **C**alcinosis: Calcium is deposited in connective tissues of the hands, fingers, face, elbows, knees, or trunk.
- **R**aynaud phenomenon: Small vessels of the hands or feet spasm in response to triggers such as cold temperatures or anxiety. The impaired circulation may result in the fingers or toes becoming white and cold, then blue, and then, as circulation is restored, red. This can be painful; depending upon the severity of circulatory compromise, ulcerations or even gangrene may result.
- **E**sophageal dysfunction: Swallowing difficulties and heartburn may result from smooth-muscle dysfunction.
- **S**clerodactyly: Skin on the fingers and hands becomes thickened, tight, and shiny, resulting in loss of motion and function.
- **T**elangiectasia: Painless, tiny red spots appear on the hands and face, caused by the swelling of tiny blood vessels.

Diffuse cutaneous scleroderma develops suddenly and is characterized by skin changes which begin on the hands and spread over the body in a symmetrical fashion. Internal organs such as the heart, lungs, kidneys, and intestines may also suffer damage. Affected skin typically appears swollen, tight, and shiny, and it may be itchy. Individuals typically complain of joint pain and may struggle with anorexia and weight loss. Symptoms of diffuse cutaneous scleroderma tend to peak in the first 3 to 5 years. The disease may then stabilize for a period of time, during which the individual experiences a lessening of symptoms.

Diagnosis

Diagnosis is based upon physical-examination findings, the patient's report of symptoms, and laboratory tests. The presence of antibodies called anti-topoisomerase I (or anti-scl-70) and anticentromere help to confirm the diagnosis, although they are not found in all people with scleroderma. Skin biopsy may also be done. Other diagnostics may be done to evaluate for systemic complications of scleroderma; for example, imaging studies may include chest x-ray and CT scan to identify pulmonary fibrosis, echocardiography and heart catheterization to identify heart dysfunction, and esophagography to identify esophageal dysfunction and incompetence of the lower esophageal sphincter.

Treatment

There is no cure for scleroderma; treatment is therefore focused on relieving symptoms and maximizing function. Because there are several variations of scleroderma and they can all affect people differently, treatment must be individualized. Patients are typically referred to a rheumatologist for management. Other specialists are consulted as needed. Pain and inflammation are treated with analgesics and corticosteroids. Specific medications and other treatments are aimed at individual symptoms and disease complications.

Patients are advised to follow a number of nonpharmaceutical measures to alleviate or minimize symptoms. Those with Raynaud phenomenon are cautioned to avoid smoking, to dress warmly, and to avoid the cold. Biofeedback training can help individuals improve circulation to the hands and feet. Medications which improve circulation may also be used. To maintain or improve joint flexibility, individuals are advised to perform specified stretches and exercises. Consultation with a physical or occupational therapist may be helpful in this regard. Skin should be protected from sun and wind damage by use of sunscreens, moisturizing creams, humidification of the air at home or work, and avoidance of harsh soaps or chemicals. Regular oral and dental care can help minimize tooth and gum problems. Gastrointestinal problems may be minimized by eating small, frequent meals, avoiding late-night eating, and taking medications to reduce heartburn and diarrhea. Pulmonary fibrosis and pulmonary hypertension may be treated with prescription medications. Patients are cautioned to report breathing difficulties and to get regular pneumonia and influenza vaccinations. Heart problems may be treated with medications or even surgery, depending upon the individual need. Kidney problems can be minimized or detected with regular blood-pressure screening and reporting of specific symptoms to the health-care provider as instructed.

Prognosis

Prognosis for individuals with scleroderma is quite variable, depending upon the type and complications. Approximately one third of those with diffuse scleroderma suffer heart, lung, digestive, or kidney complications. Life expectancy is quite variable but averages 12 years from diagnosis. The most common causes of scleroderma-related death are renal failure and pulmonary hypertension.

> **Flashpoint**
>
> Because there is no cure for scleroderma, patients must practice careful self-care.

Sjögren Syndrome
ICD-9-CM: 710.2   [ICD-10: M35.0]

Sjögren syndrome is an autoimmune disorder that affects the mucous membranes of the eyes, mouth, and other areas of the body. Dysfunction of salivary and lacrimal glands accounts for the majority of symptoms.

Incidence

Approximately 1.5 million Americans are affected by this disorder. Women, particularly those who are postmenopausal, are affected nine times more often than are men, although the disorder can also strike younger individuals.

Etiology

Primary Sjögren syndrome occurs alone. Secondary Sjögren syndrome affects individuals with another immune system disorder, usually rheumatoid arthritis, although SLE, scleroderma, and other autoimmune disorders may be seen. There is also a possible link with the Epstein-Barr virus (EBV).

Signs and Symptoms

Signs and symptoms of Sjögren syndrome include eye fatigue, photophobia, and eye irritation. Eyes may feel especially dry during the night or in the morning, when tear production is lowest. Eyelids may be swollen and inflamed, and the eyes may produce a mucous discharge. Many individuals also complain of dry mouth.

Diagnosis

Diagnosis is based upon presenting signs and symptoms (particularly dry eyes and dry mouth) and the presence of another autoimmune disease. Test findings include a low Schirmer test (which determines whether the eye produces enough tears to keep it moist), decreased salivary-gland flow, absence of nasolacrimal-reflex tearing, autoantibodies in the serum, and lymphocytic infiltration revealed by salivary-gland biopsy.

Treatment

Symptoms are relieved with the use of artificial tears and lubricating ointments. Drying is minimized by wearing glasses or goggles, modifying temperature and humidity in the home and work environment, avoiding environmental irritants, and avoiding use of medications that dry the eyes.

Prognosis

Prognosis is generally good. Complications may include corneal scarring, infection, ulceration, and possible perforation. Patients with Sjögren syndrome may experience lung and kidney complications, and they also may have an increased risk of developing lymphatic disorders such as lymphoma.

Polymyositis
ICD-9-CM: 710.4   [ICD-10: M33.2]

Polymyositis is a disorder that causes the slow onset of muscle weakness and pain in muscles of the trunk and progresses to affect muscles of the neck, shoulders, back, and hip, and possibly the hands and fingers.

Incidence

Polymyositis affects approximately 15,000 to 30,000 Americans of middle age, women more often than men and African Americans more often than whites.

Etiology

The exact cause of polymyositis is not understood. However, it is thought be an autoimmune response in which the body begins attacking its own muscles.

Signs and Symptoms

Common signs and symptoms of polymyositis include the gradual or sudden onset of muscle weakness in the trunk that progresses to affect muscles of the neck, shoulders, back, and hip, and possibly the hands and fingers. Affected individuals may experience muscle pain and difficulty with activities such as standing, climbing stairs, reaching overhead, and lifting objects. They may be at risk of falling. They may also notice dysphagia, fatigue, and thickening of the skin on their hands.

Diagnosis

Diagnosis is based on history and physical examination. Tests include creatine phosphokinase (muscle enzymes), ESR, and muscle-tissue and skin biopsy. MRI scans indicate muscle inflammation, electromyograms identify changes in muscle function, and antibody testing reveals the presence of antinuclear antibodies or myositis-associated antibodies.

Treatment

The treatment of polymyositis must be individualized for each person. Medications usually include high doses of IV corticosteroids followed by the same drug in a lower-dose oral form or other immunosuppressant medications. This reduces inflammation and alleviates many of the symptoms. IV immunoglobulin therapy may also be given. Physical therapy will help prevent muscle atrophy and help individuals regain range of motion and strength.

Prognosis

The prognosis is variable depending upon the severity of the disease and the patient's responsiveness to therapy. Complications may include respiratory difficulties due to weakening respiratory muscles and potential aspiration from dysphagia. This can lead to pneumonia and respiratory failure. Weight loss and malnutrition can also become a problem.

> **Flashpoint**
> Polymyositis is usually treated with high-dose corticosteroids.

 STOP HERE.
Select the flash cards for this chapter and run through them at least three times before moving on to the next chapter.

Student Resources

Aids.org: http://www.aids.org
Arthritis Foundation: http://www.arthritis.org
CFIDS Association of America: http://www.cfids.org/
Lupus Foundation of Minnesota: http://www.lupusmn.org
The Myositis Association: http://www.myositis.org
Scleroderma Foundation: http://www.scleroderma.org
Sjögren's Syndrome Foundation: http://www.sjogrens.org
WebMD: http://www.webmd.com
American Society of Transplantation: http://www.healthytransplant.com

Chapter Activities

Learning Style Study Strategies

Try any or all of the following strategies as you study the content of this chapter:

Visual and kinesthetic learners: After you read a paragraph, write one sentence that summarizes key points. Then create an illustration or flowchart that visually represents these points.

Kinesthetic and verbal learners: Write summaries of each of the diseases you need to learn about and then read them aloud to yourself each morning and evening.

Auditory and verbal learners: Ask your study buddy to verbally explain (in simple terms) a complex concept that you may be struggling to understand. Now take your turn providing a simplified explanation of a concept that your study buddy is struggling to understand. Work together to create simplified explanations or translations of any concepts that you are both struggling with. This technique using verbal and auditory strategies will help both of you.

Practice Exercises

Answers to Practice Exercises can be found in Appendix D.

Case Studies

CASE STUDY 1

Ilka is a medical assistant who works in a family medicine clinic. During a coffee break one morning, one of her coworkers states that she heard there was a new patient diagnosed with chronic mucocutaneous candidiasis (CMC) and she is curious about it.

1. How might Ilka respond to her coworker's question?

2. What might Ilka share about the cause of CMC?

3. How might Ilka describe the most common signs and symptoms?

4. How might Ilka describe the typical treatment for CMC?

CASE STUDY 2

Marguerite Muller is a 45-year-old woman who was recently diagnosed with chronic fatigue syndrome (CFS). Today she brought her adult daughter to the family medical clinic with her because they both want to better understand this disorder. How might a health-care provider answer the following questions?

1. What causes CFS?

2. What are the typical signs and symptoms of CFS?

3. Can CFS be cured?

CASE STUDY 3

Robert Jordan is a 59-year-old man who has been on kidney dialysis for the past year because of kidney failure. He is currently undergoing evaluation for a possible kidney transplant. In one of his conversations, the physician mentions the risk of transplant rejection. Mr. Jordan wants to learn more about this complication. How should the health-care provider answer his questions?

1. What causes transplant rejection, and how often does it occur?

2. What signs or symptoms might a patient experience if his or her body rejects the transplanted kidney?

3. Is there a way that rejection can be prevented or treated?

Multiple Choice

1. Which of the following statements is true regarding the lymphatic system?

   a. Lymph is a milky, tan-colored, acidic fluid made up mostly of water and carbohydrates.

   b. Lymph nodes are distributed along lymphatic vessels, with higher concentrations in the neck, axillae, groin, and the mesentery of the abdomen.

   c. The thymus is most active during the teen years.

   d. The spleen contains a supply of 400 to 700 milliliters of blood and 50% of the body's total platelets, most of which can be returned to circulation in the event of hemorrhage.

2. Which of the following statements is true regarding AIDS?

   a. Diagnostic criteria includes a CD-4 helper T count of less than 400.

   b. The most common victims are homosexual.

   c. AIDS may be spread by shaking hands and hugging.

   d. Current life expectancy is 10 to 20 years from the time of diagnosis.

3. Which of the following statements is **not** true regarding chronic fatigue syndrome?

   a. It affects women four times more often than men.

   b. It is commonly triggered by depression.

   c. The main symptom is pronounced fatigue unrelieved by rest.

   d. There is no known cure for CFS.

4. Which of the following is **not** true regarding transplant rejection?

   a. Transplant rejection occurs in 25% of first kidney transplants.

   b. Hyperacute rejection develops within minutes of transplant.

   c. Signs and symptoms of lung-transplant rejection include chest pain, shortness of breath, cough, and malaise.

   d. Acute organ rejection may be prevented by the use of immunosuppressive medications.

5. Which of the following is **not** true regarding scleroderma?

   a. Scleroderma is considered a rheumatic disease because it causes inflammation and pain in muscles, joints, and fibrous tissues.

   b. Morphea is localized patches of reddish or light-purple skin with light-colored centers that develop a thickened, firm texture.

   c. The skin should be treated with sunlight or tanning beds.

   d. Sclerodactyly is when skin on the fingers and hands becomes thickened, tight, and shiny, resulting in loss of motion and function.

Short Answer

1. What are the common signs and symptoms of polymyositis?

2. Polymyositis may be treated with what classification of medications?

3. Sjögren syndrome is an autoimmune disorder that affects what part of the body?

4. What population is most often affected by Sjögren syndrome?

5. What virus has been linked with Sjögren syndrome?

6. What is considered the primary cause of SLE?

7. Describe the typical signs and symptoms of SLE.

8. What is the protein produced by cells in the stomach lining that is necessary for the absorption of vitamin B_{12}?

9. Describe the signs and symptoms of pernicious anemia.

10. What is the typical treatment for pernicious anemia?

11. Define ankylosing spondylitis, and describe its signs and symptoms.

10 CARDIOVASCULAR SYSTEM DISEASES AND DISORDERS

Learning Outcomes

Upon completion of this chapter, the student will be able to:

- Define and spell terms related to the cardiovascular system
- Identify key structures of the cardiovascular system
- Discuss the roles of the heart, arteries, and veins as part of the cardiovascular system

- Identify characteristics of common cardiovascular system diseases and disorders, including:
  - description
  - incidence
  - etiology
  - signs and symptoms
  - diagnosis
  - treatment
  - prognosis

KEY TERMS

ablation	destruction of electrical conduction pathways of the AV node
angioplasty	surgical repair of a vessel by insertion of a stent or balloon inflation
apical pulse	heartbeat heard over the apex of the heart, best for auscultating sounds from the mitral valve
arrhythmia	irregularity or loss of rhythm of the heartbeat; also called dysrhythmia
ascites	abnormal fluid accumulation in the abdominal space between organs
blood pressure	pressure created by pumping blood
bruit	abnormal swooshing sound
cardiac cycle	contraction and relaxation of all chambers of the heart
cardiac output	volume of blood pumped by the heart each minute
cardiomegaly	enlargement of the heart
cardioversion	synchronized shock of electrical current delivered to the chest wall while the patient is under sedation and analgesia
claudication	sensation of tiredness, aching, cramping, pain, tightness, heaviness, or weakness in the leg (usually the calf) with exercise that is relieved with rest
crackles	abnormal lung sound heard on auscultation that indicates fluid in the alveoli
depolarization	electrical change in cardiac muscle cells that causes them to contract
diastolic pressure	lower blood-pressure number, which measures the lowest pressure exerted against artery walls during ventricular relaxation

KEY TERMS—cont'd

mitral valve prolapse	abnormal displacement of the mitral valve into the atrium each time it attempts to close
palpitation	sensation of rapid or irregular beating of the heart
paroxysmal-nocturnal dyspnea	episodes of dyspnea at night that occur repeatedly and without warning
perfusion	circulation of blood, nutrients, and oxygen through tissues and organs
pericardial effusion	increased fluid collection between the heart and pericardium
postphlebitic syndrome	chronic condition, marked by edema and aching, that may develop after an episode of phlebitis
prehypertension	blood pressure in which the systolic pressure is between 120 and 140 or the diastolic pressure is between 80 and 90
pulmonary embolism	obstruction by a blood clot of vessels in the lungs
pulse points	points on the body where large arteries are near the surface, making the pulse easily palpated; also called *pressure points*
stasis	sluggish blood flow
systolic pressure	upper blood-pressure number, which measures the highest pressure exerted against artery walls during ventricular contraction

Abbreviations

Table 10-1 lists some of the most common abbreviations related to the cardiovascular system.

TABLE 10-1
ABBREVIATIONS

Abbreviation	Meaning	Abbreviation	Meaning
AAA	abdominal aortic aneurysm	HDL	high-density lipoprotein
ACE	angiotensin converting enzyme	INR	international normalized ratio
AV	atrioventricular	IV	intravenous
BP	blood pressure	JVD	jugular-vein distention
CAD	coronary artery disease	LA	left atrium
CBC	complete blood count	LDL	low-density lipoprotein
CPR	cardiopulmonary resuscitation	LV	left ventricle
DIC	disseminated intravascular coagulation	MI	myocardial infarction
DVT	deep vein thrombosis	NSR	normal sinus rhythm
ECG	electrocardiography	PAC	premature atrial contraction
ESR	erythrocyte sedimentation rate	PAD	peripheral artery disease

Continued

TABLE 10-1			
ABBREVIATIONS—cont'd			
Abbreviation	Meaning	Abbreviation	Meaning
PND	paroxysmal-nocturnal dyspnea	RBC	red blood cell
PT	prothrombin time	RV	right ventricle
PTT	partial thromboplastin time	SA	sinoatrial
PVC	premature ventricular contraction	TAO	thromboangiitis obliterans
PVD	peripheral vascular disease	VLDL	very low-density lipoprotein
RA	right atrium	WBC	white blood cell

Structures and Functions of the Cardiovascular System

The cardiovascular system is made up of the heart and the circulatory system, including arteries, veins, and capillaries. It provides oxygen and nutrients to the entire body.

Structures of the Cardiovascular System

The structures of the cardiovascular system are the heart, located in the center of the chest, and the complex system of arteries, veins, and capillaries distributed throughout the entire body.

Heart

The heart is a muscular organ about the size of a closed fist (see Fig. 10-1). It is located in the center of the chest, slightly to the left, in an area called the mediastinum. The heart has three layers: the outer lining, called the epicardium; the middle, muscular layer, called the myocardium; and the inner lining, called the endocardium. The heart is enclosed in a fibrous membrane called the pericardium, or pericardial sac, which also contains a small amount of fluid called pericardial fluid.

Flashpoint
Your heart is about the same size as your closed fist.

The heart has two upper chambers, the right and left atria, and two larger lower chambers, the right and left ventricles. The left ventricle is larger and more muscular than the right because of its greater workload. The right and left sides of the heart are divided by a thick layer of muscle tissue called the septum.

There are four valves in the heart. The tricuspid valve exits the right atrium into the right ventricle and the mitral, or bicuspid, valve exits the left atrium into the left ventricle. The pulmonary valve exits the right ventricle into the pulmonary arteries, and the aortic valve exits the left ventricle into the aorta.

Flashpoint
Your heart has four chambers and four valves.

The largest part of the heart, the lower left, is known as the apex. This site is best for auscultating sounds from the mitral valve and is where the **apical pulse** is best heard. Auscultating the apical pulse for one full minute is considered the most accurate method of measuring heart rate and is the preferred method in situations where accuracy is critically important.

Circulatory System

The circulatory system is composed of all the blood vessels of the body (see Fig. 10-2). The major vessels entering and exiting the heart are the aorta, which is the largest artery in the body; the right and left pulmonary arteries, which connect the right ventricle to the lungs; the superior and inferior venae cavae, which are the largest veins in the body; and the right and left pulmonary veins, which connect the lungs to the left atrium. Blood flows from the heart to the body through smaller and smaller arteries, eventually ending in capillary beds. Capillaries are the tiniest blood vessels in the

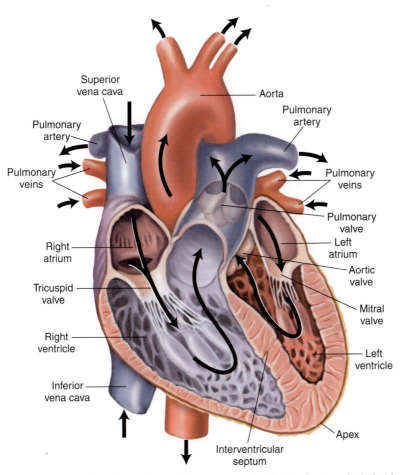

FIGURE 10-1 Structures of the heart (From Eagle, S, et al. *The Professional Medical Assistant: An Integrative Teamwork-Based Approach.* 2009. Philadelphia: F.A. Davis Company, with permission.)

body; they connect arteries and veins. Blood leaves capillary beds and is returned to the heart by way of larger and larger veins.

Functions of the Cardiovascular System

The heart serves as a pump that propels blood throughout the entire circulatory system. The heart and the circulatory system deliver much-needed oxygen and nutrients to all parts of the body.

Heart

The heart generates its own contractions approximately 60 to 100 times per minute throughout a person's entire life span. At an average rate of 72 beats per minute, the heart beats about 104,000 times per day and about 38,000,000 times per year. The pericardial fluid acts as a type of lubricant to reduce friction as the heart repeatedly contracts and relaxes.

Blood flows through both sides of the heart simultaneously; each side pumps blood to different parts of the body. Blood that is low in oxygen but high in carbon dioxide returns from the body to the right atrium via the inferior and superior venae cavae. The atria are smaller than the ventricles and do approximately 30% of the heart's workload, while the larger, more muscular ventricles do the other 70%. Both atria contract at the same time, each pumping blood to a different area. As the right atrium contracts, blood is forced downward through the tricuspid valve into the right ventricle. As the right ventricle contracts, it forces blood up and out through the pulmonary valve into the pulmonary arteries. The pulmonary

Flashpoint
Your heart beats an average of 60 to 100 times each minute for your entire life.

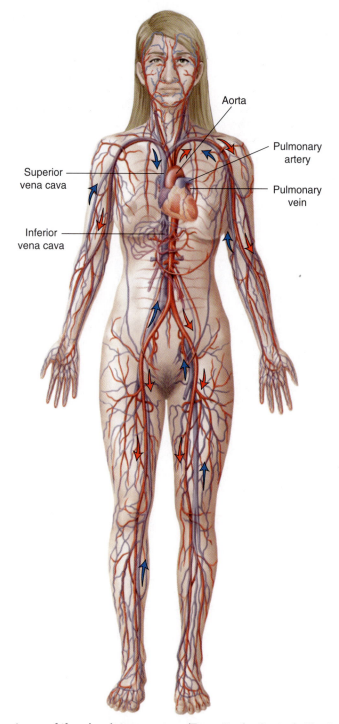

FIGURE 10-2 **Structures of the circulatory system** (From Eagle, S, et al. *The Professional Medical Assistant: An Integrative Teamwork-Based Approach.* 2009. Philadelphia: F.A. Davis Company, with permission.)

arteries lead to the lungs, where carbon dioxide is exchanged for oxygen—the pulmonary arteries are the only arteries in the body that transport deoxygenated blood. Oxygen-enriched blood then returns through the pulmonary veins—the only veins in the body that transport oxygenated blood—to the left atrium. As the left atrium contracts, it forces blood downward through the mitral valve into the left ventricle. As the left ventricle contracts, it forces blood upward and out through the aortic valve into the aorta and out to various parts of the body. Branching off the base of the aorta are the right and left coronary arteries, which provide the heart with its own blood supply, ensuring that it always receives a generous share of richly oxygenated blood.

Conduction System

A cluster of specialized cells in the right atrium called the *sinoatrial (SA) node* serves as a natural pacemaker for the heart, initiating an electrical impulse about 60 to 100 times per minute. Each of these impulses is transmitted throughout all muscle cells of the heart, resulting in electrical **depolarization.** Depolarization is an electrical change in cardiac muscle cells in which the inside of the cells become positive in relation to the outside. This depolarization causes individual cardiac muscle cells in the atria to contract in unison.

Within the floor of the right atrium is a backup pacemaker, the *atrioventricular (AV) node.* It receives the impulse from the SA node and transmits it onward to both ventricles via the bundle of His and the Purkinje fibers. From there it is distributed throughout the septum and ventricles. As the electrical impulse is transmitted throughout the ventricles, all ventricular muscle fibers contract in unison. This contraction occurs just slightly after the contraction of the atria; the combination of the two results in one complete heartbeat. This entire process is repeated with each heartbeat (see Fig. 10-3).

Flashpoint

The pulmonary veins are the only veins in the body that carry oxygen-rich blood.

Flashpoint

The SA node is your heart's natural pacemaker.

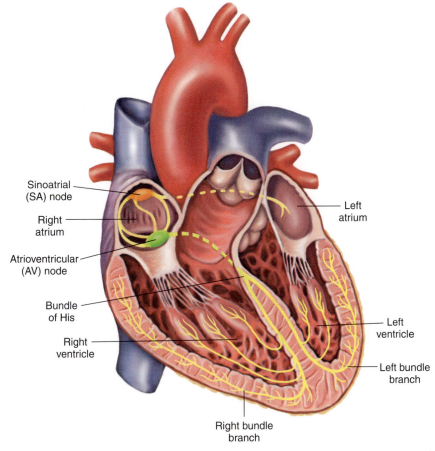

FIGURE 10-3 **Electrical conduction system of the heart** (From Eagle, S, et al. *The Professional Medical Assistant: An Integrative Teamwork-Based Approach.* 2009. Philadelphia: F.A. Davis Company, with permission.)

Cardiac Cycle

The contraction and relaxation of the four heart chambers creates each heartbeat and is known as the **cardiac cycle.** Each cardiac cycle takes approximately 0.8 seconds. The pressure created by pumping blood, known as **blood pressure,** is written as one number over another, such as 120/80. The upper number, called the **systolic pressure,** is a measurement of the highest pressure exerted against artery walls during ventricular contraction or *systole.* The lower number, called the **diastolic pressure,** measures the lowest pressure exerted against artery walls during ventricular relaxation, or *diastole.*

Flashpoint

Blood pressure is the force exerted against your artery walls by your blood as it is pumped by your heart.

Large arteries in the body that have a strong pulse and are easily palpated are known as **pulse points.** These points, sometimes called *pressure points*, may be compressed to slow bleeding in the case of hemorrhage.

Circulatory System

The aorta, the largest artery of the body, delivers oxygen-rich blood from the heart to various parts of the body via systemic circulation. As blood leaves the aorta, it moves through smaller and smaller arteries, all of which have thick, muscular walls because they carry blood under high pressure. The tiniest arteries, called arterioles, terminate in capillary beds. Capillaries are the tiniest blood vessels in the body and are where the exchange of gases and nutrients occurs. Capillary walls are only one cell thick, making them semipermeable. This permeability facilitates the delivery of oxygen and nutrients to tissue cells and the retrieval of carbon dioxide. Blood low in oxygen and high in carbon dioxide leaves the capillaries and enters tiny veins, called venules. Venous blood continues flowing through larger and larger veins until it returns to the heart via the superior and inferior venae cavae. It then returns to the lungs, which facilitate the release of carbon dioxide.

Flashpoint

Capillaries are the tiniest vessels in the body and are where the exchange of gases and nutrients occurs.

Venous blood travels under much less pressure than arterial blood. Because of this lack of pressure, venous blood cannot easily flow against gravity to ascend the legs and return to the heart. Veins thus contain one-way valves that facilitate circulation by preventing the backflow of blood. The pumping action created by the contraction and relaxation of leg muscles also helps to propel the blood forward.

Cardiovascular System Diseases and Disorders

There are many diseases and disorders of the cardiovascular system. The ones discussed in this chapter are hypertension, malignant hypertension, coronary artery disease, angina pectoris, myocardial infarction, heart failure, cor pulmonale, atrial fibrillation, cardiac tamponade, cardiomyopathy, shock, a variety of blood disorders, two common heart-valve disorders, several vascular disorders, and a number of inflammatory heart conditions.

Hypertension

ICD-9-CM: 401 (add fourth and fifth digit by type)   [ICD-10: I10-I15 (code by type)]

Hypertension, commonly known as *high blood pressure,* is a condition in which three separate blood-pressure readings over several weeks measure a systolic pressure above 140, a diastolic pressure above 90, or both. It is further categorized as stage 1 (systolic of 140 to 159 or diastolic of 90 to 99) and stage 2 (systolic 160 or above or diastolic 100 or above).

With the goal of identifying and treating hypertension earlier, experts have now defined **prehypertension** as systolic readings between 120 and 140 or diastolic readings between 80 and 90.

Flashpoint

If your systolic pressure is between 120 and 140 or your diastolic pressure is between 80 and 90, you have prehypertension.

Incidence

One-third of American adults over age 35 have hypertension, and a third of those do not know it. Incidence of hypertension increases with age and is higher in the African American population than other ethnic groups.

Etiology

Hypertension is classified as primary (also called *essential hypertension),* meaning the specific cause is unclear, or secondary, which means that it is caused by an underlying disorder. Primary hypertension makes up 90% to 95% of cases; secondary hypertension makes up the other 5% to 10%. Risk factors for primary hypertension include pregnancy, obesity, tobacco use, family history of hypertension, and endocrine disorders, such as diabetes. Causes of secondary hypertension include kidney disease, congenital abnormalities (present at birth) of the aorta, and narrowing of certain arteries.

Signs and Symptoms

Hypertension is known as a silent killer because most people are asymptomatic (symptom free) until complications arise due to advanced disease. In some cases, individuals may complain of headache; but unless high blood pressure is noted through the course of routine health screening or when individuals seek care for other problems, the first indicator may be a complication such as a stroke or heart attack.

Diagnosis

Diagnosis of hypertension is easily made based on repeated high blood-pressure readings over several weeks.

Flashpoint

Hypertension is known as a silent killer because most people don't know they have it until damage has occurred.

Treatment

Treatment of hypertension depends on the severity. In most cases, care providers try to employ conservative measures first, including modification of identified risk factors, such as weight loss, elimination of tobacco use, dietary changes, restriction of alcohol intake (one or two drinks per day), and regular exercise. If these measures fail to achieve the desired result, or hypertension is extreme, the provider will prescribe medication. The most commonly used medications include diuretics and antihypertensives. Because of the large list of medications to choose from and the variation in individual response, the provider must personalize the treatment plan for each individual patient.

Prognosis

Hypertension is a major contributor to the development of several serious conditions, including coronary artery disease, heart failure, myocardial infarction (heart attack), kidney failure, stroke, and vision loss. Therefore, it should be considered a serious disorder and should be treated aggressively, whether or not the patient is symptomatic.

Flashpoint

Hypertension contributes to many serious disorders like heart failure and heart attack.

Malignant Hypertension

ICD-9-CM: 401.0   [ICD-10: I13.0–I13.9 (hypertensive heart and renal disease; code by type)]

Malignant hypertension, also called *accelerated hypertension, nephrosclerosis,* and *arteriolar nephrosclerosis,* is a rare, life-threatening type of high blood pressure evidenced by papilledema (swelling of the optic nerve) and extremely high systolic and diastolic blood pressure.

Incidence

Malignant hypertension is rare, affecting only about 1% of those with hypertension. Unlike primary hypertension, it is more common in younger people (average age of 40), rather than older. Although it is more common in men, certain complications of pregnancy increase the risk in women. Other risk factors include African descent, history of kidney failure, and cigarette smoking.

Flashpoint

Malignant hypertension is life-threatening.

Etiology

The cause of malignant hypertension is not well understood. Constant high blood pressure causes thickening of the walls and dilation of small arteries, which results in damage to vascular organs. In some cases, certain drugs may contribute to the hypertensive state. Examples include oral contraceptives, cocaine, and monoamine oxidase inhibitors. Withdrawal from alcohol, beta blockers, and other substances may also trigger a hypertensive crisis.

Flashpoint

Malignant hypertension is an uncommon form of hypertension that occurs in young people.

Signs and Symptoms

Signs and symptoms of malignant hypertension include neurological changes such as headache, blurred vision, anxiety, confusion, lethargy, numbness, tingling or weakness in the extremities, and seizures. Other possible symptoms include chest pain, dyspnea, nausea, vomiting, and decreased urine production.

Diagnosis

In addition to significantly elevated blood pressure, generally greater than 220/120, other physical changes will be apparent. Upon examination of the patient's retina, the physician may note papilledema, soft exudates, and flame-shaped retinal hemorrhages. Cardiac examination may reveal an abnormal fourth heart sound. Echocardiogram may indicate enlargement of the left atrium and ventricle. Chest x-ray may reveal lung congestion, consistent with heart failure. Examination of the kidneys and results of kidney function tests such as blood urea nitrogen, creatinine, and urinalysis may indicate renal failure.

Treatment

Immediate treatment for malignant hypertension is needed, and hospitalization may be necessary. IV vasodilators (medications that relax and open blood vessels) may be used initially to bring the blood pressure down. This is usually followed by a regular schedule of oral antihypertensive medication, such as angiotensin converting enzyme (ACE) inhibitors or beta blockers.

Prognosis

While malignant hypertension can be a life-threatening emergency, prognosis is good when diagnosis and treatment are timely. Life expectancy was once poor, with a 5-year survival rate of less than 1%. Death was usually caused by heart failure, kidney failure, or stroke. However, current treatment has changed the prognosis dramatically; the 5-year survival rate is now 80%. Untreated hypertension can still cause kidney, brain, heart, and eye damage. Therefore, individuals with hypertension should see their health-care provider regularly.

Coronary Artery Disease

ICD-9-CM: 414.0   [ICD-10: I25.1]

Coronary artery disease (CAD) is defined as narrowing of the lumen (space within a vessel or other tubelike structure) of coronary (heart) arteries due to *arteriosclerosis* and *atherosclerosis*. Arteriosclerosis, commonly called *hardening of the arteries,* is the thickening and loss of elasticity and contractility of arterial walls. Atherosclerosis is a common form of arteriosclerosis marked by deposits of cholesterol, lipids, and calcium on the walls of arteries, which may restrict blood flow. CAD is the most common type of heart disease and is the leading cause of death in men and women in industrialized nations.

Flashpoint

CAD is caused by arteriosclerosis and atherosclerosis.

Incidence

Approximately 13 million Americans currently suffer from CAD; nearly half a million die from the disease each year. It develops slightly more often in men than in women.

Etiology

CAD results from the development of atherosclerosis and arteriosclerosis, which impede blood flow to heart muscle (see Fig. 10-4). Risk factors include hypertension, tobacco use, sedentary lifestyle, obesity, diabetes, advanced age, and family history of CAD.

Signs and Symptoms

Individuals with CAD are asymptomatic until the disease has advanced enough to cause angina (chest pain or pressure from insufficient delivery of blood and oxygen to heart muscle) or heart attack. Symptoms of angina include chest pain or discomfort that may radiate (spread) to the neck, jaw, back, shoulders, or arms.

Diagnosis

Diagnosis of CAD is based on presenting signs and symptoms and the results of diagnostic tests. A 12-lead electrocardiography (ECG) is done to check for **arrhythmias** (irregularities or loss of rhythm of the heartbeat; also called *dysrhythmias*) and ischemia (see Box 10-1). ECG is non-invasive and one of the most commonly performed heart tests. Cardiac catheterization and

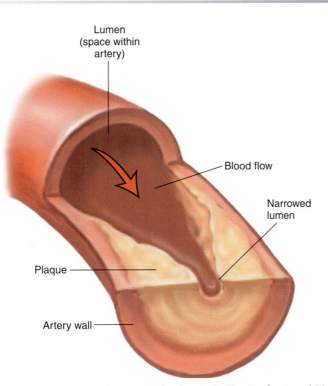

Lumen
(space within
artery)

Blood flow

Narrowed
lumen

Plaque

Artery wall

FIGURE 10-4 Coronary artery disease (From Eagle, S, et al. *The Professional Medical Assistant: An Integrative Teamwork-Based Approach.* 2009. Philadelphia: F.A. Davis Company, with permission.)

echocardiogram are two different tests that allow the physician to visualize the chambers, valves, and arteries of the heart as it pumps so that any areas of vessel narrowing or other structural problems can be seen. A cardiac stress test provides a carefully monitored environment in which the patient is challenged with physical exercise to see if it produces angina, dyspnea, or other symptoms. The patient is also encouraged to decrease their risk of CAD by changing poor diet and exercise habits (see Box 10-2).

Treatment

Treatment of CAD depends on the severity of the disease and the presence of symptoms. In most cases, health-care providers will employ conservative measures first, including lifestyle modifications such as weight loss, elimination of tobacco use, low-fat diet, alcohol restriction, and regular aerobic exercise. If these measures fail to achieve the desired results, or lipid levels are extremely high, the provider will prescribe medication to reduce cholesterol and triglyceride levels. If the disease is limited to one or two areas within cardiac arteries, the patient may undergo coronary **angioplasty.** In this procedure, the surgeon will place a stent or inflate a tiny balloon to open narrowed vessels. When disease is more extensive, the patient may undergo open heart surgery to place coronary artery bypass grafts to divert blood around areas of narrowing or blockage.

Prognosis

Prognosis for CAD varies depending on the extent and severity of disease and the patient's underlying health status. Health-care providers must take the condition seriously, because disease progression increases the risk of death from heart attack or other complications. Early diagnosis and aggressive management usually result in significantly increased length and quality of life.

> **Flashpoint**
> ECG is one of the most commonly performed heart tests.

> **Flashpoint**
> Angioplasty is the surgical repair of a vessel.

Angina Pectoris

ICD-9-CM: 413.9   [ICD-10: I20.9]

Angina pectoris is not a disease itself but is a symptom of heart disease, usually coronary artery disease. It is pain, pressure, or other discomfort felt in the chest, shoulders, arms, jaw,

Box 10-1 Diagnostic Spotlight

ELECTROCARDIOGRAPHY

Electrocardiography is a common, painless, noninvasive procedure that can be done in the physician's office during a routine physical examination. The electrocardiogram (ECG) is the written record that is produced in this procedure by an electrocardiograph machine. The electrocardiograph machine is connected to the patient with wires and electrodes that are sensitive to the electrical impulses generated by the patient's heart. This electrical activity is represented on electrocardiograph paper by specific waveforms, which the physician reviews and analyzes. The information obtained in this way aids in the diagnosis and treatment of cardiac problems. ECGs are also commonly done prior to major surgical procedures, to establish baseline health information about a patient and identify potential cardiac disorders.

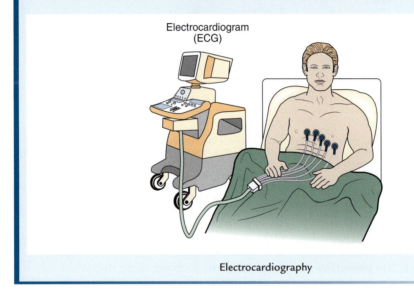

Electrocardiography

Box 10-2 Wellness Promotion

BE KIND TO YOUR HEART

Modifiable risk factors for heart disease include hypertension, tobacco use, alcohol abuse, sedentary lifestyle, poorly controlled diabetes, obesity, low levels of high-density lipoprotein (HDL), and high levels of cholesterol, triglycerides, low-density lipoprotein (LDL), and very low-density lipoprotein (VLDL). To reduce your risk for heart disease, follow these recommendations:

- Stop or reduce the use of tobacco products.
- Limit alcohol intake to two drinks (1 ounce of alcohol each) or less per day.
- Participate in aerobic exercise several times per week.
- Maintain blood pressure within recommended ranges.
- For diabetics, maintain blood glucose level within the recommended range.
- Keep cholesterol, LDL, VLDL, HDL, and triglycerides within the recommended ranges.
- Schedule a screening examination to find out what your cholesterol levels are.
- Eat a diet low in cholesterol and saturated fat.
- Attain and maintain a healthy weight.

or neck that is caused by insufficient blood and oxygen to the heart. Angina is often classified as stable, unstable, or variant (Prinzmetal's).

Incidence

Approximately 400,000 new patients are seen for angina each year, and nearly six million people suffer from the condition. Women are affected slightly more than men.

Etiology

Symptoms of all kinds of angina are caused by myocardial ischemia, or an inadequate supply of blood and oxygen to the heart muscle. Stable angina has a fairly predictable pattern of symptoms brought on by exertion that are relieved by rest or medication. Unstable angina doesn't follow this typical pattern and is therefore less predictable. It may occur with exertion or at rest and does not consistently respond to rest or medication. It increases in frequency, duration, and severity over time and is a signal of worsening heart disease. The uncertain nature of unstable angina makes it more dangerous than stable angina. Variant angina is rare, typically occurs at rest (often in the middle of the night), and is usually relieved by medication. It is thought to be caused by temporary coronary artery spasm. Risk factors for angina are the same as those for CAD.

Signs and Symptoms

Patients with angina complain of uncomfortable sensations in the chest, shoulders, arms, neck, or jaw. Common descriptors include pain, pressure, tightness, squeezing, and burning. Other symptoms may include dyspnea, nausea, vomiting, diaphoresis, anxiety, or fear. Symptoms are often brought on or worsened by physical exertion, large meals, emotional stress, or a cold environment. They are temporary, lasting for several minutes, and are relieved by rest or nitroglycerine medication.

Diagnosis

Angina is diagnosed through a careful history and the patient's description of symptoms. Blood may be tested to check cardiac enzymes such as troponin, to rule out heart attack, and to check blood lipid levels. ECG is done to identify any cardiac rhythm problems and to help rule out heart attack. Cardiac catheterization may be done so the physician can visualize the heart structures, particularly the coronary vessels, to identify any areas of narrowing. A stress test may be ordered to evaluate the heart's response to activity and to see if the symptoms are reproduced (see Box 10-3).

Treatment

Treatment for patients with angina is tailored to the specific type and severity. For many people with chronic stable angina or variant angina, medications such as beta blockers, nitrates,

> **Flashpoint**
> Angina is a warning sign that CAD may be present.

> **Flashpoint**
> Angina is relieved by resting or taking medication like nitroglycerine.

Box 10-3 Diagnostic Spotlight

CARDIAC STRESS TEST

A cardiac stress test has numerous other names, including *exercise stress test, exercise treadmill test, exercise tolerance test, stress test, exercise ECG test,* and—if radioactive isotopes are used—*nuclear stress test.* It is used to evaluate the heart's response to physical exercise. The patient walks on a treadmill or is given IV medication that causes a response similar to the body's response to exercise. The patient's heart rate, blood pressure, and symptoms are monitored by health-care providers who are familiar with emergency protocols and prepared to respond if the patient develops arrhythmias, dyspnea, chest pain, or other problems.

The American Heart Association recommends a cardiac stress test for patients with a medium risk of coronary artery disease based on smoking, hypertension, family history of heart disease, high cholesterol, or diabetes. However, patients who have had an MI within the previous 48 hours and those with unstable angina, uncontrolled arrhythmias, or certain other unstable conditions should not undergo stress testing.

calcium channel blockers, and angiotensin-converting enzyme inhibitors are effective in relieving or minimizing symptoms. Unstable angina, however, requires more aggressive treatment; in addition to medication, patients may need angioplasty or even heart bypass surgery.

Prognosis

Prognosis for patients with angina is generally good, with timely diagnosis and treatment. However, angina—especially unstable angina—usually indicates underlying coronary artery disease, which may be progressive and can lead to heart attack and possibly death.

Myocardial Infarction

ICD-9-CM: 410.00–410.92   **[ICD-10: I21.0–I22.9] (code by location and as initial or subsequent for both codes)**

Myocardial infarction (MI), commonly called *heart attack*, is defined as the death of heart muscle related to coronary artery occlusion (blockage), which cuts off the supply of blood, oxygen, and nutrients (see Fig. 10-5).

Incidence

More than one million individuals in the United States suffer from an MI each year, and about 350,000 of them die.

Etiology

Risk factors for MI are the same as for CAD: atherosclerosis and arteriosclerosis, hypertension, tobacco use, sedentary lifestyle, obesity, diabetes, advanced age, and family history of heart disease.

Signs and Symptoms

Symptoms of MI include pain, pressure, fullness, heaviness, or a squeezing sensation in the chest, arms, neck, jaw, back, or epigastric area; dyspnea; nausea; diaphoresis; and light-headedness. MI

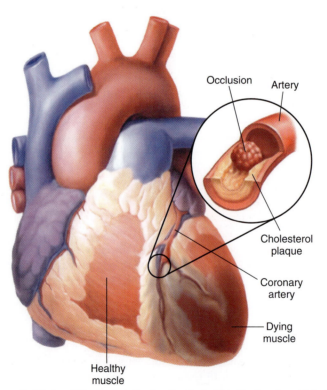

FIGURE 10-5 Myocardial infarction (From Eagle, S, et al. *The Professional Medical Assistant: An Integrative Teamwork-Based Approach.* 2009. Philadelphia: F.A. Davis Company, with permission.)

commonly causes heart arrhythmias. Half of those who experience an MI die within the first hour of symptom onset.

Diagnosis

Diagnosis of MI is based on presenting signs and symptoms and results of diagnostic tests. A 12-lead ECG detects cardiac ischemia and any abnormal heart rhythms. Blood is drawn to test for elevated cardiac enzymes. The most reliable indicator to confirm MI is an elevated troponin level, which shows how much heart-muscle damage has occurred. When the patient's condition is stable, testing may be done to determine the extent of CAD and necessity of surgical intervention. Such testing may include a nuclear heart scan, cardiac catheterization, and coronary angiography. These tests allow close inspection of heart chambers, valves, and coronary arteries.

Treatment

An MI is a life-threatening emergency; effective treatment must be early and aggressive. Unfortunately, many individuals delay seeking medical attention for 2 to 12 hours (see Box 10-4). Initial medications include aspirin, nitroglycerine, thrombolytics, beta blockers, and morphine. These drugs are usually followed by anticoagulants and, if needed, antihypertensives to manage

Flashpoint
Fifty percent of heart-attack victims die within an hour.

Box 10-4 Wellness Promotion

MI WARNING SIGNS

Unlike in the movies, it is not always clear in real life when someone is having a heart attack. Consequently, a person sometimes waits too long to summon help. Health-care workers should provide the following guidelines to patients at risk for a myocardial infarction (MI).

Major Signs of MI

Major signs of an MI include:

- mild or severe chest pain, pressure, fullness, heaviness, or squeezing that is constant and lasts for more than a few minutes, or goes away and then returns
- discomfort in other areas of the upper body, such as one or both arms, the back, neck, jaw, or upper stomach
- shortness of breath with or without chest discomfort
- nausea
- breaking out in a cold sweat
- dizziness or light-headedness

Different in Women

A woman's symptoms may vary from the major symptoms above and may include:

- nausea
- shortness of breath
- back or jaw pain
- chest discomfort (not as common)

What to Do?

If you suspect that you or a companion may be experiencing an MI, take these measures:

- Call 911.
- If you are the person experiencing symptoms, do **not** drive yourself to the hospital.
- While waiting for an ambulance, rest in a position of comfort to decrease oxygen demands on your heart.
- Take one aspirin.
- Take nitroglycerine if it has been prescribed.

blood pressure and other medications to lower triglyceride and cholesterol levels. Other supportive care includes treatment of arrhythmias and administration of IV fluids and oxygen. In some cases, emergency angioplasty is done to treat severely narrowed coronary arteries. Rehabilitation focuses on two areas: exercise and education. An individualized exercise plan supports each patient in gaining strength and endurance. The plan is designed around the patient's abilities, energy level, and personal interests. Education addresses risk reduction through lifestyle modifications and newly prescribed medications.

Prognosis

Flashpoint

For those who survive the first post-MI hour, prognosis is quite good.

The odds of dying from an MI are related to the patient's underlying health status, the possible development of life-threatening arrhythmias, and the timeliness of diagnosis and treatment. For those who survive the first post-MI hour, prognosis is good, with a 95% survival rate. Recovery and rehabilitation may take several weeks or months.

Heart Failure

ICD-9-CM: 428.0   [ICD-10: I50]

Heart failure, formerly called *congestive heart failure,* is the inability of the heart to pump enough blood to meet the needs of the body. The left ventricle is the part of the heart most affected in this condition, in which case the condition is referred to as *left-sided heart failure* and results in decreased effectiveness in pumping oxygen-rich blood to all parts of the body. Failure of the right ventricle, called *right-sided heart failure* or *cor pulmonale,* is less common. This condition impedes effective pumping of blood that returns to the lungs via the right side of the heart. As heart failure progresses, both sides become affected.

Flashpoint

Heart failure primarily affects the left ventricle.

Incidence

Approximately five million Americans suffer from heart failure, and the incidence is increasing. More than half a million individuals are newly diagnosed each year, and about 300,000 people die annually from causes related to heart failure. Those at greatest risk of developing heart failure include African Americans and the elderly.

Etiology

Heart failure is caused by ineffective pumping of the ventricles. The ventricles may lose effectiveness after heart muscle is lost due to MI or the heart is weakened by cardiomyopathy or other disorders, such as diseased heart valves, congenital heart defects, arrhythmias, CAD, diabetes, or hypertension. Damage from disorders such as kidney failure, sepsis (systemic infection), and other illnesses also contributes to heart failure.

Signs and Symptoms

Because left-sided heart failure results in fluid buildup in the lungs, the most common signs and symptoms are related to respiratory problems. Individuals commonly complain of dyspnea, especially with exertion, and general fatigue. Some individuals may experience orthopnea or **paroxysmal-nocturnal dyspnea** (episodes of dyspnea at night that occur repeatedly and without warning). Other symptoms include lower-extremity edema, decreased oxygen saturation, and the presence of **crackles** (abnormal lung sound heard on auscultation that indicates fluid in the alveoli).

Diagnosis

Diagnosis of heart failure is based on signs and symptoms, medical history, and diagnostic testing. Echocardiogram, which creates a moving picture of the heart using sound waves, is one of the most useful tests. It reveals data about the heart's size, shape, and valve function. It also reveals where blood flow is poor and whether all parts of the heart are working normally. Chest x-ray reveals pulmonary edema (fluid in the interstitium and alveoli of the lungs) and **cardiomegaly** (enlargement of the heart). A blood test for B-type natriuretic peptide will be elevated.

Flashpoint

Cardiomegaly is enlargement of the heart.

Treatment

Treatment of heart failure includes the administration of diuretics, antihypertensives, and inotropics such as digoxin (Lanoxin). Diuretics stimulate filtration and excretion of urine; excretion of urine reduces intravascular fluid and allows fluid to shift from the lungs back into blood vessels, thereby relieving dyspnea. Antihypertensives decrease the workload of the heart. Inotropics increase cardiac muscle contractility, thereby strengthening the pumping force of the heart. In cases of valvular disease, heart-valve replacement may be considered. Heart transplantation is considered only in extreme cases.

Prognosis

Of those with heart failure, approximately 10% to 20% die each year. However, early diagnosis and medical management can prolong life and increase its quality for most people.

Cor Pulmonale

ICD-9-CM: 415.0　　[ICD-10: I26.0]

Cor pulmonale, also called *right-sided heart failure*, is a condition of enlargement of the right ventricle or dilation from increased pressure of the right ventricle (see Fig. 10-6). Usually, pressure is greater in the left ventricle than the right because of the force needed to pump blood to the body. However, when certain disorders cause pressure to increase within vessels of the lungs, pulmonary hypertension develops. This, in turn, causes pressure to increase within the right ventricle, and cor pulmonale is the result.

Incidence

The exact incidence of cor pulmonale is unknown. However, the condition is thought to be a significant contributor in 7% of all heart disease among adults in the United States. It is known to be associated with chronic lung disease.

Etiology

Chronic cor pulmonale is usually caused by chronic obstructive pulmonary disease, but any condition leading to chronically low blood oxygen can be a cause. Examples include sleep apnea and blood disorders that increase blood viscosity. Other causes include disorders that result in fibrosis (scarlike changes), such as scleroderma, cystic fibrosis, and interstitial lung disease. These conditions result in a gradual increase of pulmonary vessels' resistance to blood flow. Muscle cells of the right ventricle respond by increasing in size to increase pumping force. This produces hypertrophy (increased tissue growth) of the ventricle.

Acute cor pulmonale is usually caused by massive pulmonary emboli (numerous blood clots lodging in the lungs) or injury from acute respiratory distress syndrome and mechanical ventilation. In the case of acute respiratory distress syndrome, lung tissue becomes stiff and less elastic because of alveolar injury and fluid accumulation. Patients are placed on a

> **Flashpoint**
> Cor pulmonale affects the right side of the heart.

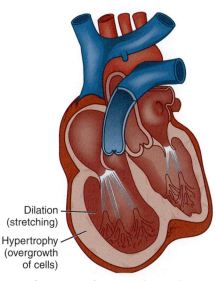

Dilation (stretching)

Hypertrophy (overgrowth of cells)

FIGURE 10-6 Right-sided heart enlargement in cor pulmonale

mechanical ventilator to help them breathe. The ventilator settings required to treat the syndrome exert increased pressure against lung tissues. The sudden increase in resistance to blood flow causes the right ventricle to become overloaded. As a result, it becomes dilated (stretched) and begins to fail.

Signs and Symptoms

Individuals with mild cor pulmonale usually have no specific symptoms associated with it, although they will very likely have symptoms associated with their chronic lung disorder. As dilation or hypertrophy of the right ventricle increases, they will begin to exhibit jugular-vein distention, edema of the feet and legs, fatigue, dyspnea, cough with or without hemoptysis (bloody sputum), chest pain or discomfort, exercise intolerance, and hepatomegaly (enlargement of the liver).

Diagnosis

Diagnosis is based upon the patient's medical history, physical-examination findings, and data from diagnostic tests. The physician may note abnormal heart sounds, such as murmurs, S_3, and S_4. Chest x-ray reveals enlargement of the right ventricle and proximal pulmonary artery. Echocardiography is likely to show dilation or hypertrophy of the right ventricle and possible pulmonary-valve dysfunction. ECG may indicate waveform deviations. Pulmonary function tests may identify underlying lung disorders. Heart catheterization allows measurement of pressures within the heart and provides the most accurate data for diagnosis; however, it is also more invasive than other tests.

Treatment

Treatment of cor pulmonale is aimed at relieving hypoxia (low oxygen level) and resolving the underlying cause. Depending upon the degree of heart failure, patients may respond to careful administration of medications such as diuretics, nitrates, phosphodiesterase inhibitors, and inotropics. Anticoagulants may be given to those with chronic cor pulmonale to reduce the risk of clot formation. Those with chronic obstructive pulmonary disease may benefit from oxygen therapy.

Prognosis

The prognosis for patients with cor pulmonale depends upon the underlying cause and the timeliness of diagnosis and treatment. Those with underlying chronic lung disease generally have a poorer prognosis than those with an acute condition, and they have a 5-year survival rate of just 30%. Liver damage may be a complication. Untreated cor pulmonale may be fatal. In severe cases, heart-lung transplantation may be considered.

Atrial Fibrillation

ICD-9-CM: 427.31   [ICD-10: I48]

There are many types of heart arrhythmias (see Box 10-5). One of the most common by far is atrial fibrillation, which occurs when irritable myocardial cells in the atrium that are not the SA node fire chaotically. As a result, the atria quiver uncontrollably rather than contracting normally. The ventricles, in turn, contract irregularly at a faster rate than normal, which results in a rapid, irregular heartbeat. Because of their chaotic quivering, the atria are ineffective in emptying. Sluggish blood flow may result in the formation of blood clots.

Incidence

Atrial fibrillation affects 5% to 10% of all individuals over the age of 70, which amounts to about 2.2 million Americans.

Etiology

The underlying cause of atrial fibrillation is not always clear. What is known is that depolarization of the atria is not triggered by signals from the SA node as normally occurs; instead, rapid, irregular electrical activity occurs in muscle cells throughout the atria (see Fig. 10-7). As a result, the atria fail to contract in an organized fashion and instead fibrillate, or quiver in a disorganized and ineffective manner. Impulses are sent along the conduction pathway to the AV node, where some of them are blocked. Ventricles continue to function normally but tend to contract with an irregular rhythm and a more rapid rate than normal. Known triggers for atrial fibrillation are many and

(text continues on page 292)

Box 10-5 Common ECG Rhythms

This table describes the features of some of the most common electrocardiograph (ECG) rhythms. Some are considered normal while others may be life-threatening.

Rhythm *Sinus Rhythms*	Characteristics	Signs and Symptoms	Required Response
Normal sinus rhythm (NSR) 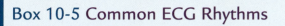 ECG of normal sinus rhythm (From Jones, SA. *ECG Success: Exercises in ECG Interpretation.* 2008. Philadelphia: F.A. Davis Company, with permission.)	• Rate: 60–100 beats/min • Rhythm: regular • P-R interval: 0.12–0.20 sec • QRS complex: less than 0.12 sec	None	No special action is required
Sinus bradycardia ECG of sinus bradycardia (From Jones, SA. *ECG Success: Exercises in ECG Interpretation.* 2008. Philadelphia: F.A. Davis Company, with permission.)	• Rate: less than 60 beats/min • Rhythm: regular • P-R interval: 0.12–0.20 sec • QRS complex: less than 0.12 sec	Usually none	The physician should be notified if the patient is symptomatic
Sinus tachycardia ECG of sinus tachycardia (From Jones, SA. *ECG Success: Exercises in ECG Interpretation.* 2008. Philadelphia: F.A. Davis Company, with permission.)	• Rate: greater than 100 beats/min • Rhythm: regular • P-R interval: 0.12–0.20 sec • QRS complex: less than 0.12 sec	Usually none	The physician should be notified if the patient is symptomatic
Sinus arrhythmia ECG of sinus arrhythmia (From Jones, SA. *ECG Success: Exercises in ECG Interpretation.* 2008. Philadelphia: F.A. Davis Company, with permission.)	• Rate: fluctuates with respiratory pattern • Rhythm: regular • P-R interval: 0.12–0.20 sec • QRS complex: less than 0.12 sec	None	No special action is required

Continued

Box 10-5 Common ECG Rhythms—cont'd

Rhythm *Atrial Arrhythmias*	Characteristics	Signs and Symptoms	Required Response
Sinus rhythm with premature atrial contractions (PACs) 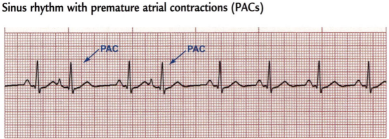 ECG of sinus rhythm with premature atrial contractions (From Jones, SA. *ECG Success: Exercises in ECG Interpretation.* 2008. Philadelphia: F.A. Davis Company, with permission.)	• Rate: 60–100 beats/min • Rhythm: regular, except when PACs occur • P-R interval: 0.12–0.20 sec; may vary in the PACs • QRS complex: less than 0.12 sec	Usually none, although palpitations are possible	No special action is required
Atrial fibrillation 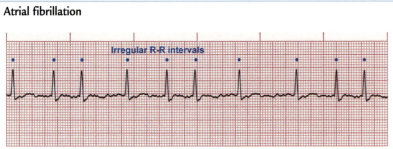 ECG of atrial fibrillation (From Jones, SA. *ECG Success: Exercises in ECG Interpretation.* 2008. Philadelphia: F.A. Davis Company, with permission.)	• Rate: possibly rapid • Rhythm: irregular • P waves: none • P-R interval: none • QRS complex: less than 0.12 sec	Possibly none, with controlled rate; with rapid, uncontrolled rate, possible palpitations, dyspnea, and dizziness	The physician should be notified if the patient is symptomatic
Atrial flutter 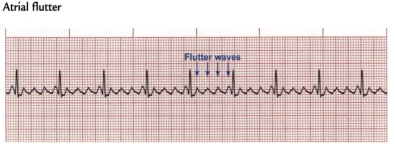 ECG of atrial flutter (From Jones, SA. *ECG Success: Exercises in ECG Interpretation.* 2008. Philadelphia: F.A. Davis Company, with permission.)	• Rate: atrial, rapid (250–350 beats/min); ventricular, variable (125–75 beats/min) • Rhythm: usually regular • P waves: none identifiable; sawtooth-patterned flutter waves present instead • QRS complex: less than 0.12 sec	Possible palpitations, shortness of breath, and dizziness	The physician should be notified immediately

Box 10-5 Common ECG Rhythms—cont'd

Rhythm *Ventricular Arrhythmias*	Characteristics	Signs and Symptoms	Required Response
Sinus rhythm with premature ventricular contractions (PVCs) ECG of sinus rhythm with premature ventricular contractions (From Jones, SA. *ECG Success: Exercises in ECG Interpretation.* 2008. Philadelphia: F.A. Davis Company, with permission.)	• Rate: 60–100 beats/min • Rhythm: regular except when PVCs occur • P-R interval: 0.12–0.20 sec; none when PVCs occur • QRS complex: less than 0.12 sec except in PVCs, which show up as bizarrely shaped, wide QRS complexes with no preceding P wave	Usually none, unless PVCs are frequent; possible palpitations	No special action is required unless the patient is symptomatic
Ventricular tachycardia ECG of ventricular tachycardia (From Jones, SA. *ECG Success: Exercises in ECG Interpretation.* 2008. Philadelphia: F.A. Davis Company, with permission.)	• Rate: rapid, usually 100–220 beats/min • Rhythm: usually regular • P waves: none • QRS complex: wide, oddly shaped, and greater than 0.12 sec	Dramatic hypotension, loss of consciousness	This is a life-threatening emergency that requires immediate notification of the physician. If the patient is pulseless and breathless, initiate cardiopulmonary resuscitation (CPR)
Ventricular fibrillation ECG of ventricular fibrillation (From Jones, SA. *ECG Success: Exercises in ECG Interpretation.* 2008. Philadelphia: F.A. Davis Company, with permission.)	• Rate: rapid (350–450 beats/min) • Rhythm: irregular, chaotic • P waves: none • QRS complex: none	Loss of consciousness, loss of pulse, imminent death	This is a life-threatening emergency that requires immediate notification of the physician. If the patient is pulseless and breathless, initiate CPR

Continued

Box 10-5 Common ECG Rhythms—cont'd

Rhythm	Characteristics	Signs and Symptoms	Required Response
Ventricular Arrhythmias			
Asystole 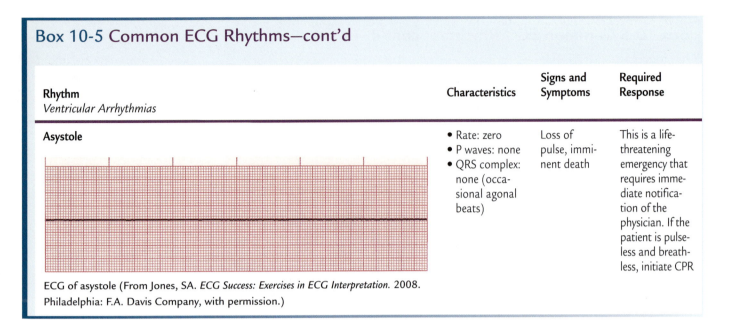	• Rate: zero • P waves: none • QRS complex: none (occasional agonal beats)	Loss of pulse, imminent death	This is a life-threatening emergency that requires immediate notification of the physician. If the patient is pulseless and breathless, initiate CPR

ECG of asystole (From Jones, SA. *ECG Success: Exercises in ECG Interpretation.* 2008. Philadelphia: F.A. Davis Company, with permission.)

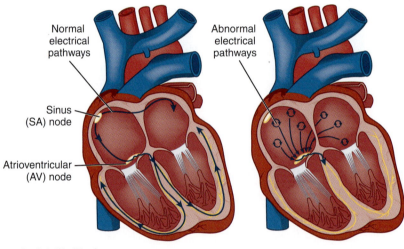

FIGURE 10-7 **Atrial fibrillation**

> ### Flashpoint
> During atrial fibrillation, the atria quiver chaotically instead of contracting normally.

include stress, exercise, alcohol withdrawal, cardiac surgery, cocaine intoxication, hypoxia, MI, and ***pulmonary embolism*** (obstruction by a blood clot of vessels in the lungs). Chronic atrial fibrillation also occurs in those with chronic forms of heart disease.

Signs and Symptoms

Individuals with atrial fibrillation are sometimes asymptomatic; however, most experience rapid, irregular heartbeat, hypotension, and chest ***palpitations*** (sensation of rapid or irregular beating of the heart). Other symptoms include dyspnea, dizziness, and exercise intolerance.

Diagnosis

Atrial fibrillation is diagnosed using a 12-lead ECG. However, atrial fibrillation is sometimes intermittent in nature and may be missed by an ECG, which only detects arrhythmias occurring at the moment it is performed. Therefore, accurate diagnosis may require that the patient wear a Holter monitor or an event recorder (see Box 10-6). These devices allow the detection of abnormal heartbeats as the individual goes about a daily routine. Other diagnostic techniques may include echocardiography and transesophageal echocardiography, which allow visualization of the heart as it beats.

Treatment

Conservative treatment of atrial fibrillation includes antiarrhythmic medication such as digoxin (Lanoxin), which slows the heart rate and often restores normal sinus rhythm. If medication is not successful, the patient will undergo *cardioversion,* which is a

Box 10-6 Diagnostic Spotlight

HOLTER MONITOR

A Holter monitor is a portable device that records the patient's cardiac rhythm over a 24- or 48-hour period. This type of testing is useful for patients with an irregular heartbeat or other symptoms that may be intermittent. Electrodes are applied to the patient, and the monitor is carried in a small pouch. The patient wears the monitor continuously for the prescribed period of time and records in a journal any symptoms, such as heart palpitations and dizziness, and any heavy physical activity. The patient may not shower or bathe while wearing the monitor but may take a sponge bath. After wearing the monitor for the designated period of time, the patient returns it to the medical office, where the data is downloaded. A cardiologist reviews and interprets the data and then discusses the results with the patient.

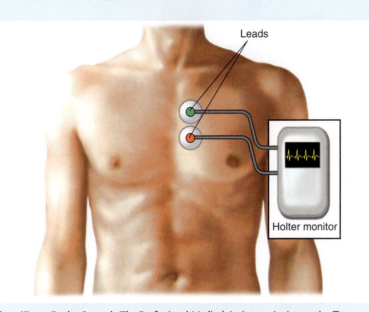

Holter monitor (From Eagle, S, et al. *The Professional Medical Assistant: An Integrative Teamwork-Based Approach.* 2009. Philadelphia: F.A. Davis Company, with permission.)

EVENT RECORDER

An event recorder is a small, portable monitor that the patient can wear around the neck like a pendant or clip onto a belt. It is attached to two electrodes on the patient's chest; the patient may activate it upon such symptoms as chest pain, dizziness, and palpitations. The data is then sent to the cardiology clinic via telephone for analysis. (Most event recorders allow telephone transmission of recordings.) This type of device is most ideal for patients whose symptoms are intermittent and unpredictable, and are therefore unlikely to manifest during an ECG test. Event recorders may be worn for as long as 30 days to capture events likely to be missed by an ECG or even a Holter monitor.

Continued

Box 10-6 Diagnostic Spotlight—cont'd

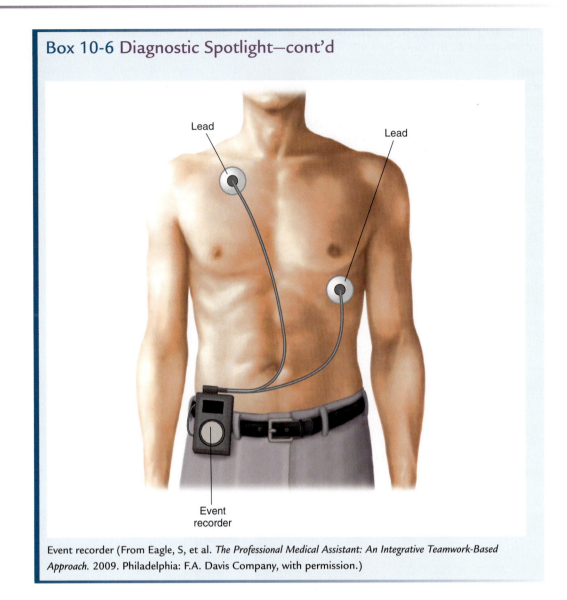

Lead

Lead

Event recorder

Event recorder (From Eagle, S, et al. *The Professional Medical Assistant: An Integrative Teamwork-Based Approach.* 2009. Philadelphia: F.A. Davis Company, with permission.)

synchronized shock of electrical current delivered to the chest wall while the patient is under sedation and analgesia. If these measures are unsuccessful, the patient may undergo **abla-tion** (destruction of electrical conduction pathways of the AV node). Subsequent placement of a pacemaker may prevent the chaotic atrial impulses from affecting the ventricles and ensure a stable heart rate.

> *Flashpoint*
>
> Cardioversion is a procedure in which an electrical shock is delivered to the sedated patient's heart.

Prognosis

Prognosis for those with atrial fibrillation is good, with accurate diagnosis and treatment. Even when restoration of normal sinus rhythm is not achieved, patients often lead productive lives for many years with atrial fibrillation at a controlled rate. Potential complications include formation of blood clots in the atria that may embolize to the brain and other vital organs and cause life-threatening complications, such as stroke or pulmonary embolism.

Cardiac Tamponade

ICD-9-CM: 423.3   [ICD-10: I31.9]

Cardiac tamponade, also called *pericardial tamponade,* is a serious condition in which the heart becomes compressed from an excessive collection of fluid or blood between the pericardial membrane and the heart. Compression restricts movement of the heart wall and prevents the heart chambers from adequately filling with blood.

Incidence
Cardiac tamponade is estimated to affect approximately two in 10,000 individuals.

Etiology
Cardiac tamponade develops when fluid or blood collects between the heart and pericardium, preventing the ventricles of the heart from fully expanding to fill with and pump blood (see Fig. 10-8). Causes can include a dissecting (tearing or rupturing) aortic aneurysm, advanced lung cancer, heart attack, pericarditis, heart surgery or other heart trauma, tumors on the heart, radiation therapy, systemic lupus erythematosus, kidney failure, or hypothyroidism.

Signs and Symptoms
Signs and symptoms associated with cardiac tamponade are related to reduced **cardiac output** (volume of blood pumped by the heart each minute) and increased pressure within the heart. They include anxiety, chest pain, dyspnea, palpitations, weak or absent pulse, fainting, and skin that is pale or dusky from low blood pressure and poor oxygen supply.

Diagnosis
Upon auscultation, the health-care provider notes heart sounds that are faint or distant sounding. Jugular veins may be distended in spite of low blood pressure. Other signs and symptoms include tachycardia, weight gain, and fluid retention. Echocardiogram reveals fluid collected in the pericardial space. Other tests may include ECG, chest x-ray, magnetic resonance imaging (MRI), computerized tomography (CT), and coronary angiography.

Treatment
Cardiac tamponade is a life-threatening emergency that requires immediate intervention. In addition to addressing the underlying cause, one of two procedures is done to drain the fluid and relieve pressure. Pericardiocentesis involves the insertion of a needle through the chest and into the pericardial sac. In some cases a catheter may be left in place for a time, to allow fluid to continue to drain and to prevent recurrence. A pericardial window is the other procedure, in which a portion of the pericardium is removed. This also allows the fluid to drain and prevents recurrence.

Prognosis
Cardiac tamponade is a medical emergency and may result in death if not treated promptly. However, prognosis is reasonably good with timely diagnosis and treatment. The condition may recur; potential complications include pulmonary edema, heart failure, and death.

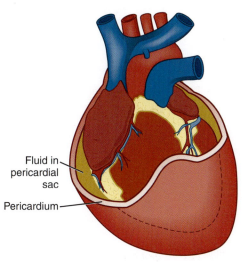

Fluid in pericardial sac

Pericardium

FIGURE 10-8 Cardiac tamponade

Cardiomyopathy

ICD-9-CM: 425 (add fourth digit by type)   [ICD-10: I42.0-I42.9 (code by type)]

Cardiomyopathy is a condition of the heart in which the heart muscle has deteriorated and functions less effectively. Common types include dilated, hypertrophic, and restrictive.

Incidence

Estimates of the incidence of cardiomyopathy vary widely, from 50,000 to 400,000 people diagnosed with some type of cardiomyopathy each year. Dilated cardiomyopathy, the most common type, usually affects middle-aged men. Hypertrophic cardiomyopathy is most common in young adults. Restrictive cardiomyopathy is the least common type. It can develop at any age but most commonly affects older people.

Etiology

In dilated cardiomyopathy, the left ventricle becomes enlarged, stretched, and weakened (see Fig. 10-9). This decreases its strength and effectiveness and increases risk of blood clot formation within the ventricle. Genetics may play a role since approximately 40% of cases are familial. However, other cases are related to pregnancy, alcoholism, or autoimmune responses.

Flashpoint

Cardiomyopathy results in a pump that is enlarged but weak.

In hypertrophic cardiomyopathy, the heart wall—especially the left ventricle—becomes thickened and stiffened, and the capacity of the chamber shrinks. As a result, less blood is pumped effectively. This type of cardiomyopathy is often linked to genetic disorders.

Restrictive cardiomyopathy is often idiopathic, which means the cause is not known. In some cases it is related to other disease processes. In this type of cardiomyopathy, the heart muscle loses elasticity and flexibility. As a result, it is not able to expand and fill with an adequate amount of blood.

Signs and Symptoms

Patients with mild cardiomyopathy are usually asymptomatic. However, as the condition progresses, individuals may experience fatigue, headaches, dizziness, blurred vision, dyspnea, chest pain or discomfort, edema of the feet and legs, *ascites* (abnormal fluid accumulation in the abdominal space between organs), heart murmur, and heart palpitations.

Diagnosis

Diagnosis of cardiomyopathy is based on information collected through history-taking, physical examination, and diagnostic testing. Chest x-ray indicates an enlarged heart. Echocardiogram produces images of the heart which provide information about increased size and dysfunction. ECG may indicate rhythm disturbances. Cardiac catheterization allows visualization of the heart

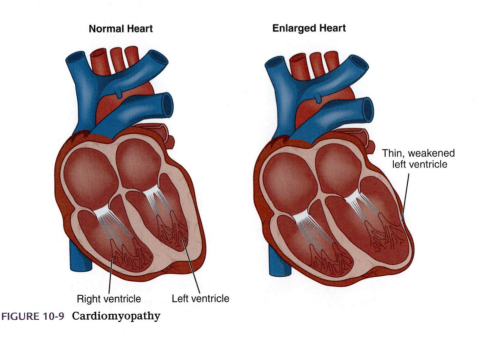

Normal Heart   **Enlarged Heart**

Thin, weakened left ventricle

Right ventricle   Left ventricle

FIGURE 10-9 Cardiomyopathy

as it pumps, measurement of pressure within the heart, and biopsy of heart tissue. Blood tests may be done to rule out or confirm causes. Elevated levels of B-type natriuretic peptide, a protein produced by the heart, indicate heart failure.

Treatment

Treatment for cardiomyopathy depends upon type and cause. A number of different medications may be used for all types: Anticoagulants decrease the risk of clot formation. Antiarrhythmics treat or minimize abnormal heart rhythms. Certain antihypertensives may be used to control blood pressure and maximize heart function. Vasodilators relax and open arteries, lowering blood pressure, decreasing the heart's workload, and improving blood flow to the heart. Diuretics are used to minimize lung congestion and edema in the extremities. Inotropics increase the heart's pumping strength and maximize cardiac output. Individuals with advanced disease may benefit from implantation of a pacemaker or cardioverter defibrillator. This device not only paces the heart but delivers an electrical shock, if needed, to correct abnormal rhythms. In some cases heart transplantation is considered.

The focus of treatment for dilated cardiomyopathy is controlling or minimizing heart failure. Therefore, most of the same measures are used as with heart failure.

Treatment of hypertrophic cardiomyopathy may include a procedure called septal myotomy-myectomy, in which some of the thickened heart muscle is surgically removed. A newer, less invasive procedure called alcohol ablation may also be used, in which alcohol is injected into one of the small arteries of the heart. This destroys extra heart muscle fed by that artery.

Treatment of restrictive cardiomyopathy may involve careful monitoring of water and salt intake, and daily weight measurement.

Prognosis

Prognosis for those with cardiomyopathy is variable and depends upon the type and severity. Complications include heart failure, stroke or heart attack related to clot formation, abnormal heart rhythms, and death.

> **Flashpoint**
> An elevated level of B-type natriuretic peptide indicates heart failure.

> **Flashpoint**
> Treatment for dilated cardiomyopathy is the same as for heart failure.

Shock

ICD-9-CM: 785.50 (unspecified; failure of peripheral circulation), 785.51 (cardiogenic), 785.59 (other)	[ICD-10: R57.9 (unspecified; failure of peripheral circulation), R57.0 (cardiogenic), R57.8 (other)]

Shock is a syndrome of inadequate *perfusion* (circulation of blood, nutrients, and oxygen through tissues and organs) as a result of low blood pressure. It is classified according to the underlying cause.

Incidence

Incidence varies with the type of shock involved.

Etiology

Types of shock include cardiogenic (caused by cardiac failure), hemorrhagic (caused by blood loss), septic (caused by massive infection), and anaphylactic (caused by an allergic reaction). Regardless of the cause, all forms of shock, if severe enough, ultimately lead to severe hypotension. Vital organs of the body are not adequately perfused, resulting in organ-system dysfunction and possible death.

Signs and Symptoms

Early symptoms of shock are variable, depending on the underlying cause; however, they always include anxiety and a decreased level of consciousness. Late signs of shock include tachycardia, profound hypotension, diaphoresis, confusion, pallor, a dramatic drop in oxygen saturation levels, a dramatic decrease in urinary output, and eventually death.

> **Flashpoint**
> There are many types of shock, but they all lead to severe hypotension.

Diagnosis

Diagnosis is based on recent medical history, the patient's presenting signs and symptoms, and physical-examination findings. Cardiogenic shock is diagnosed with measures to confirm MI or heart failure. Hemorrhagic shock is diagnosed by physical evidence of bleeding and a dramatic drop in red blood cells (RBCs), hematocrit, and hemoglobin. Septic shock is diagnosed by confirmation of the presence of infection through wound and blood cultures. Anaphylactic shock is generally easy to identify, as the patient exhibits obvious signs of a severe allergic reaction.

Treatment

Because shock may be life-threatening, timely diagnosis is important, as is aggressive treatment tailored to the specific cause. Hypotension is treated by blood transfusion or IV administration of fluids and vasoactive medications. The patient may be admitted to an intensive care unit, placed on cardiac monitors, and provided with respiratory support.

Prognosis

Flashpoint

The prognosis for late-stage shock is very poor.

Prognosis for the individual experiencing shock depends on the underlying cause and the speed of diagnosis and treatment. The outcome for a patient suffering from mild shock is good if appropriate treatment is initiated. However, survival for those suffering from severe, late-stage shock is very poor.

Blood Diseases and Disorders

There are many different types of blood disorders. Among the most common are the anemias, polycythemia vera, agranulocytosis, and disseminated intravascular coagulation.

Anemia

ICD-9-CM: 280-289   [ICD-10: D50.0-D53.9] (depends on specific type for both codes)

Anemia is generally defined as a reduction in the mass of circulating red blood cells. An individual is considered anemic when his or her hemoglobin level drops below a specified point; however, normal values vary depending on gender, pregnancy, age, race, and living altitude.

Incidence

Approximately 3.4 million Americans suffer from some form of anemia. Women and those with chronic disease are most commonly affected. Some of the numerous causes of anemia include blood loss, vitamin or mineral deficiencies, drop in RBC production as a result of kidney or bone-marrow failure, and disorders that cause excessive RBC destruction.

Flashpoint

Those most likely to suffer from anemia are women and people with chronic disease.

Etiology

Anemias are classified according to the color and size of the RBCs: those that cause RBCs to become pale are called hypochromic; those that cause them to become darker red are hyperchromic; and those that cause no color change are normochromic. Anemias are also classified according to RBC size. Those with small RBCs are labeled microcytic, those with large RBCs are macrocytic, and those with normal-size RBCs are normocytic. Anemias are also classified according to their cause, as follows:

- Autoimmune hemolytic anemia is caused by a defective response of the immune system in which it creates antibodies that destroy RBCs.
- Hemorrhagic anemia results from the loss of large volumes of blood.
- Iron-deficiency anemia comes from inadequate intake of iron in the diet.
- Folic acid deficiency anemia is the result of inadequate ingestion of folic acid in the diet.
- Pernicious anemia is caused by a defective response of the immune system in which the parietal cells of the stomach lining fail to secrete enough intrinsic factor to ensure intestinal absorption of vitamin B_{12} (see Chapter 9).

Flashpoint

There are many different types of anemia.

- Aplastic anemia is usually idiopathic, but some types are caused by exposure to chemical and antineoplastic (cancer-fighting) agents or ionizing radiation.
- Sickle cell anemia is the result of an inherited abnormality of the globin genes in hemoglobin.

Signs and Symptoms

Signs and symptoms of anemia vary with the specific type. Acute anemia generally causes weakness, fatigue, light-headedness, tachycardia, tachypnea, dyspnea, heart palpitations, angina, and headache. Chronic anemia may cause pallor and fissures at the corners of the mouth.

Diagnosis

In general, an individual has symptomatic anemia when the hemoglobin content of the blood is less than that required to meet the oxygen-carrying demands of the body. Diagnosis of a specific type of anemia is usually done by examining RBCs and other blood components under a microscope to determine their shape, size, and color.

Treatment

Treatment of anemia depends on the underlying cause. For example, iron-deficiency anemia is treated with iron and vitamin C supplements, while pernicious anemia is treated with vitamin B_{12} supplements, and sickle cell anemia with supplemental iron and blood transfusions.

Prognosis

Prognosis for individuals suffering from anemia depends on the specific type, the underlying cause, and the individual's response to therapy.

Polycythemia Vera
ICD-9-CM: 238.4   [ICD-10: D45]

Polycythemia vera has a number of other names, including *primary polycythemia, polycythemia rubra vera, myeloproliferative disorder, erythremia, splenomegalic polycythemia, Vaquez disease,* and *Osler disease.* It is a chronic disorder marked by increased production of all bone marrow cells, especially red blood cells. There is also an increase in RBC mass and hemoglobin concentration. As a result, individuals suffer problems related to increased blood volume and viscosity and an increased tendency to form blood clots.

Incidence

Approximately 6,000 Americans are affected by polycythemia vera, most between the ages of 40 and 60. It affects men more than women, especially those of Jewish ancestry.

Etiology

The exact cause of polycythemia vera is not known. However, it is thought to be associated with DNA mutation in bone-marrow cells responsible for blood-cell production.

Signs and Symptoms

The symptoms associated with polycythemia vera are related to increased blood volume and viscosity. They include orthopnea, headache, dizziness, dyspnea, abdominal "fullness" due to splenomegaly and hepatomegaly, chest discomfort, fatigue, red or bluish skin color, phlebitis, and vision changes. The skin may itch or burn, especially after a warm bath or shower.

Diagnosis

In the early stages of polycythemia vera, some people have no symptoms. The disease may be identified when testing is done for other reasons and abnormally high levels of RBCs, hematocrit, and hemoglobin are noted with low levels of oxygen. When suspicion is raised about polycythemia vera, further testing may be done. Bone marrow biopsy allows for the study of bone marrow cells. A complete blood count will reveal increased levels of red blood cells, white blood cells (WBCs), platelets, and other blood components. RBC mass may be abnormally high. Erythropoietin level will be very low. Because erythropoietin is a hormone responsible for stimulating RBC production in the bone marrow, the high number of RBCs causes its production to be reduced. In contrast, other types of polycythemia will often cause an increased erythropoietin level. This helps the physician identify which type of polycythemia the patient has.

Treatment

There is no cure for polycythemia vera. However, there are forms of treatment that help to minimize complications and improve quality and length of life. Weekly phlebotomy (blood drawing) may be done to reduce blood volume until the patient's hematocrit level falls below 45; thereafter, it may be repeated as needed. Certain types of chemotherapy may be used to decrease blood-cell production by bone marrow. Low-dose aspirin therapy may be used to reduce the risk of blood clotting and to help relieve the burning sensation in the hands and feet. Itching may be treated with antihistamines or UV light.

Prognosis

Prognosis varies depending on individual factors and the timeliness of diagnosis and treatment. Some people are relatively symptom free for many years, while the disease develops slowly. Others, without treatment, experience potentially life-threatening complications related to blood-clot formation, such as heart attack, stroke, deep vein thrombosis, and pulmonary embolism. They may also experience complications related to blood abnormalities, such as gastrointestinal bleeding, leukemia, and other cancers of the bone marrow or blood. Other complications include

Flashpoint
RBCs are studied to determine the specific type of anemia.

Flashpoint
Polycythemia vera causes the blood to be thicker than normal.

Flashpoint
Erythropoietin is a hormone that stimulates RBC production.

splenomegaly, peptic ulcers, joint inflammation, and kidney stones. Those who undergo treatment, however, can experience a relatively good quality of life for up to 20 years from diagnosis.

Agranulocytosis
ICD-9-CM: 288.0   [ICD-10: D70]

Agranulocytosis, also called *granulocytopenia, granulopenia,* and *neutropenia,* is a condition in which production of neutrophils, basophils, and eosinophils (types of WBCs) is dramatically decreased.

Incidence

The incidence of agranulocytosis in the United States is unclear. International estimates are 6,000 to 21,000 cases annually. The disorder affects individuals of all races and all ages, women slightly more often than men. Congenital forms are more common among children, while acquired forms are more common among the elderly.

Etiology

Agranulocytosis may be due to genetic conditions in which the bone marrow fails to produce adequate numbers of WBCs. More commonly, however, it is acquired. This means it is caused by other conditions or exposures that either destroy WBCs or decrease the bone marrow's ability to produce adequate numbers of WBCs, or both. Among the most common causes is exposure to chemicals and certain drugs that suppress bone marrow function. The list of drugs that can suppress the bone marrow is quite lengthy. The many classifications include analgesics, antibiotics, sulfonamides, cardiovascular drugs, diuretics, anticonvulsants, antihistamines, anti-inflammatory drugs, antithyroid drugs, hypoglycemics, antimalarials, phenothiazines, and neurological drugs. Certain viruses can also lead to agranulocytosis, including Epstein-Barr, influenza, cytomegalovirus, hepatitis B, and yellow fever. In some cases, an autoimmune reaction may also be the cause.

Flashpoint
Many medications, including antimicrobials, can cause agranulocytosis.

Signs and Symptoms

Individuals with agranulocytosis usually present with symptoms of infection, including fever, chills, sore throat, malaise, and weakness. They may have stomatitis (inflammation in the mouth) from fungal infection; painful aphthous ulcers in the mouth; tender, swollen gums; ulcers in the stomach; or bowel and skin infections. In severe cases septicemia may develop and progress quickly, as evidenced by tachycardia, hypotension, and shock.

Diagnosis

Diagnosis is based upon the patient's report of symptoms, physical-examination findings, and laboratory data. A careful history is needed to identify whether the patient has recently taken new medications, been exposed to chemicals or ionizing radiation, or had any recent viral or bacterial infections, and whether the patient has any autoimmune disorders. A complete blood count (CBC) with a differential analysis will reveal information about the various types of WBCs. Agranulocytosis is indicated by low numbers of neutrophils, basophils, and eosinophils. A neutrophil count of less than 500 is typically referred to as neutropenia; less than 100 is referred to as agranulocytosis. Culture of wounds or blood may reveal current infections and aid in selecting the most appropriate antimicrobial medication. A myelogram and bone marrow study may be done to exclude other diagnoses. If a genetic cause is suspected, genetic testing may also be done.

Flashpoint
Agranulocytosis is a neutrophil count of less than 100.

Treatment

Patients who are symptom free are monitored closely with frequent blood counts and are counseled on avoiding causative agents when possible. They are also counseled about avoiding infectious individuals, watching for signs and symptoms of infection, and calling their physician at the appropriate times. Infections are treated aggressively, with broad-spectrum antimicrobial agents. In some cases, granulocyte colony-stimulating factor may be given. As the name suggests, this substance stimulates production of granulocytes. Patients may also be considered for bone marrow transplantation if they have been otherwise in good health, are under the age of 40, and have a matched donor available.

Prognosis

Agranulocytosis puts individuals at high risk of infection. Should infection occur, it can progress rapidly to life-threatening septicemia. Chronic or repeated infections can sometimes lead to scarring and organ damage.

Disseminated Intravascular Coagulation
ICD-9-CM: 286.6   [ICD-10: D65]

Disseminated intravascular coagulation (DIC), sometimes called *consumption coagulopathy*, is a serious condition, arising as a complication of another disorder, in which widespread, unrestricted microvascular blood clotting occurs. This consumes platelets and clotting factors, putting the individual at risk of hemorrhaging. It also causes damage to tiny vessels and can produce organ dysfunction. DIC may be acute or chronic. The acute form tends to be more severe and more likely to cause organ failure than the chronic form.

Incidence

Incidence of DIC is estimated at 15,000 to 20,000 cases annually in the United States, or up to 1% of hospitalized patients. It occurs equally in men and women, in individuals of all ages. It is frequently associated with septicemia.

Etiology

DIC develops as a complication of other disorders that involve systemic inflammation. Key features include intravascular coagulation, which impairs circulation; clotting-factor depletion, which increases risk of hemorrhage; and end-organ damage. Numerous conditions are associated with DIC, including sepsis, surgery, severe head injuries, snakebites, obstetric complications, severe liver disease, malignancy, and serious burns.

Signs and Symptoms

The most common symptoms of DIC are bruising and bleeding from surgical or invasive-procedure sites and from the mucous membranes or gastrointestinal tract. Signs and symptoms of blood clots may also develop in limbs. Examples of this are deep vein thrombosis in the limbs and organ dysfunction such as kidney failure. Other indications may include hypotension, tachycardia, and altered consciousness.

Diagnosis

Diagnosis of DIC is suspected based upon signs and symptoms. Blood tests confirm diagnosis with results that may include a very low platelet count, a high value for fibrin degradation products, high partial thromboplastin time, high prothrombin time, and low serum fibrinogen.

Treatment

Treatment is aimed at correcting the underlying cause, minimizing the risk of clotting, and replacing blood components as needed. In some cases, heparin—an anticoagulant medication—is given to stop microvascular clotting. Plasma and platelets may be transfused to help replace clotting factors and stop bleeding.

Prognosis

Prognosis depends upon the underlying cause and the timeliness of diagnosis and treatment. The mortality rate of DIC is difficult to estimate, but DIC is known to significantly increase the mortality rate of many of the disorders that trigger it. Potential complications of DIC include severe hemorrhage, stroke, tissue necrosis in limbs affected by clotting, and possible organ damage leading to complications such as kidney failure.

Flashpoint
Patients with DIC are at risk of hemorrhaging.

Flashpoint
The most common symptoms of DIC are bruising and bleeding.

Heart-Valve Diseases and Disorders

Valvular heart disease can affect any of the four heart valves. Some valvular diseases are congenital and others are acquired secondary to damage from MI, heart failure, or other disorders. The mitral valve is the most commonly affected, because it is located between the left atrium and left ventricle, where the majority of the work of the heart occurs. The two most common disorders are mitral stenosis and mitral regurgitation.

Mitral Stenosis
ICD-9-CM: 394.0   [ICD-10: I05.0]

Mitral stenosis is a condition in which the mitral valve fails to open properly. This impedes normal blood flow and increases pressure within the left atrium and lungs (see Fig. 10-10).

Flashpoint
The mitral valve is the one most commonly affected by valvular heart disease.

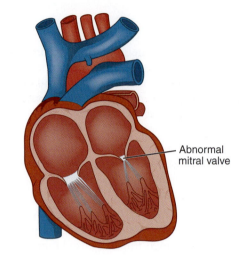

Abnormal mitral valve

FIGURE 10-10 **Mitral stenosis**

Incidence

Rheumatic fever is a common cause of mitral stenosis; as the rate of rheumatic fever in the United States has declined, so has the rate of mitral stenosis. In countries without ready access to antibiotics, untreated rheumatic fever is still a common cause.

Etiology

The most common cause of mitral stenosis is rheumatic fever, which is a potential complication of untreated strep throat. Rheumatic fever causes damage to the valve in the form of inflammation, thickening, and possible fusing. This leaves the valve narrowed, hardened, and less efficient. Mitral stenosis may also be caused by congenital defects, which may be familial. In these cases, infants are born with a narrowed, malformed valve.

Signs and Symptoms

Adults with mitral stenosis may be asymptomatic. As the condition worsens, they report exercise intolerance, hemoptysis, dyspnea, episodes of faintness, fatigue, palpitations, edema of the feet or ankles, orthopnea, and rarely, chest discomfort.

Diagnosis

Physical examination may reveal a heart murmur or snapping sound, irregular heartbeat, and lung congestion. Diagnostic tests that confirm diagnosis include cardiac catheterization, electrocardiogram, and transesophageal echocardiogram. Chest x-ray confirms lung congestion. Other studies may include MRI and Doppler ultrasound.

Flashpoint

Patients with mitral stenosis may have a heart murmur or other abnormal heart sound.

Treatment

Patients with mild mitral stenosis may not require treatment. Others may benefit from diuretic medication to reduce lung congestion and edema, inotropics such as digoxin to increase cardiac output and treat atrial fibrillation, and anticoagulants to prevent clot formation. Beta blockers or calcium channel blockers may also help control abnormal heart rhythms. Those with severe disease may undergo surgery to repair or replace the valve. A less invasive procedure called valvuloplasty or valvotomy may also be done. In this procedure, a catheter with a tiny balloon is inserted into the heart via a large vein. Once in place, the balloon is briefly inflated to widen the valve and separate the fused cusps.

Prognosis

The prognosis for individuals with mitral stenosis is variable. Life expectancy for infants born with the condition is very poor unless they undergo surgery. Older patients may require no treatment if they are asymptomatic; others may experience life-threatening heart failure without treatment. With timely diagnosis and treatment, prognosis is good. Potential complications include atrial fibrillation, pulmonary hypertension, pulmonary edema, heart failure, and thrombus formation leading to possible stroke or infarct of organs such as the intestines or kidneys.

Flashpoint

Prognosis for infants with mitral stenosis is very poor without surgery.

Mitral Regurgitation

ICD-9-CM: 394.1 (rheumatic insufficiency), 394.2 (mitral stenosis with insufficiency)   **[ICD-10: I05.1 (rheumatic insufficiency), I34.0 (mitral stenosis with insufficiency)]**

Mitral regurgitation, also called *mitral insufficiency* or *mitral incompetence,* is a condition in which the mitral valve does not close tightly and allows blood to flow backward into the left atrium (see Fig. 10-11).

Incidence

Estimates of the incidence of mitral regurgitation vary widely, from 2% to 20% of the population. Incidence is generally low among young individuals and rises with age.

Etiology

Mitral regurgitation occurs when the mitral valve fails to close properly. Faulty valve closure is usually from damage or weakness of the valve or the cords that connect the valve flaps to the heart wall. Rheumatic heart disease may damage the valve by causing stenosis or scarring. Other causes of damage include MI, endocarditis, trauma, and fibrosis. Approximately half of all cases are caused by myxomatous degeneration, a genetic condition in which the valve leaflets become stretched. This causes **mitral valve prolapse,** which is the abnormal displacement of the valve into the atrium each time it attempts to close.

Signs and Symptoms

Signs and symptoms of mitral regurgitation are variable and depend upon the severity of the problem. It usually develops slowly, and patients with chronic compensated mitral regurgitation may be symptom free unless they become overloaded with fluid. In this case, they are likely to develop signs and symptoms of heart failure. Those with acute mitral regurgitation will experience more sudden and pronounced evidence of heart failure, including dyspnea, orthopnea, exercise intolerance, chest pain, palpitations, cough, lower-extremity edema, and possible shock.

Diagnosis

Physical examination usually reveals a new or worsened heart murmur caused by the backflow of blood through the mitral valve. Other abnormal heart sounds may also be heard. Crackles may be heard in the lungs, indicating the presence of fluid related to heart failure. A variety of diagnostic tests may be done. Echocardiogram and transesophageal echocardiography produce moving images of the heart which reveal motion of the heart wall and valve, and blood backflow through the valve. Heart catheterization also allows

Flashpoint

Patients with mitral regurgitation are vulnerable to heart failure from fluid overload.

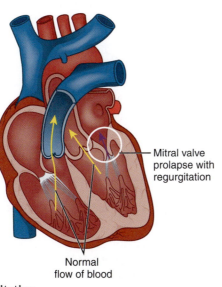

Normal flow of blood

Mitral valve prolapse with regurgitation

FIGURE 10-11 Mitral regurgitation

visualization of the heart in motion. ECG and Holter monitors may reflect abnormal heart rhythm. Chest x-ray helps the physician to examine the size and shape of the heart and to identify lung congestion. A cardiac stress test may be done to determine the patient's response to physical activity. Other possible tests include a color-flow Doppler, chest MRI, and CT scan of the chest.

Treatment

Treatment for mild mitral regurgitation may not be necessary. However, patients should be monitored by their health-care provider in case the condition worsens. Symptoms of moderate mitral regurgitation may be adequately relieved with medications, including diuretics to relieve lung congestion and leg edema, inotropics to strengthen the heart, antiarrhythmics to eliminate or control heart arrhythmias, anticoagulants to prevent clot formation, vasodilators to increase blood flow to the heart and reduce its workload, antihypertensives to control high blood pressure, and antibiotics if necessary to treat infection. In addition, a low-sodium diet may be advised to minimize fluid retention and edema. Severe symptoms may require valve repair or replacement.

Prognosis

Prognosis for patients with mitral regurgitation is variable and depends upon the severity and cause of the condition. Potential complications include arrhythmias, pulmonary edema, heart failure, and valve infection. Blood clots may also develop, leading to stroke.

Vascular Diseases and Disorders

There are numerous diseases and disorders that affect the veins and arteries of the body. Some of the more common ones are Raynaud disease, thromboangiitis obliterans, peripheral artery disease, aneurysm, varicose veins, and deep vein thrombosis.

Raynaud Disease
ICD-9-CM: 443.0　　[ICD-10: I73.0]

Raynaud disorders are categorized as either Raynaud disease or Raynaud phenomenon. Raynaud disease, or *primary Raynaud,* is diagnosed if there is no known underlying disorder that is triggering the Raynaud symptoms. It is a disorder that affects blood vessels in the fingers, toes, ears, and nose. In response to certain triggers, such as cold temperature, vessels constrict and blood flow diminishes. This form is usually mild to moderate.

Flashpoint

Symptoms of Raynaud occur when vessels spasm in response to certain triggers.

Raynaud phenomenon, sometimes called secondary Raynaud, develops secondary to other conditions. In extreme cases, this type of Raynaud can result in necrosis of the fingertips (see Fig. 10-12).

Incidence

It is estimated that 5% of Americans have Raynaud disease and that 80% of those are women. Primary Raynaud commonly develops in teens or young adults, while secondary Raynaud often develops later in life, around age 40. Genetics may play a role, although this has not been confirmed.

Flashpoint

The majority of patients with Raynaud are women.

Etiology

The physiology of both types of Raynaud is similar: An extreme vasomotor response to a trigger (usually cold or stress) results in vasoconstriction and diminished circulation in the affected body part. Tissue hypoxia may be mild or extreme. Secondary Raynaud may develop as a complication of disorders like systemic lupus erythematosus, arthritis, scleroderma, rheumatoid arthritis, Sjögren syndrome, carpal tunnel syndrome, obstructive arterial disease, and thyroid disorders, or of smoking, injuries to the extremities, and exposure to some chemicals and certain medications.

Signs and Symptoms

In response to a triggering event, vessels spasm; tissue in the affected body part becomes pale and may then turn bluish from lack of circulation. After the spasms end and blood flow returns, the area may turn red before it returns to a normal color. In addition to these color changes, the tissue often becomes cold and numb during vasospasm and then may tingle, sting, throb, or

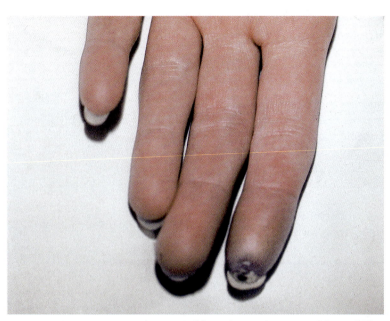

FIGURE 10-12 Raynaud phenomenon (From Goldsmith, LA, Lazarus, GS, and Tharp, MD. *Adult and Pediatric Dermatology: A Color Guide to Diagnosis and Treatment.* 1997. Philadelphia: F.A. Davis Company, with permission.)

ache after color returns. Swelling may also occur. Episodes can last anywhere from a minute to several hours.

Diagnosis

Diagnosis is suspected based upon the patient's description of signs and symptoms. The physician may investigate the possibility of underlying disorders. A cold-simulation test may be performed, in which the patient's hands are placed into cold water to trigger an episode. Other diagnostic testing may include noninvasive blood-flow studies and a nail-fold capillaroscopy. In this procedure, the skin at the base of the fingernail is examined under a microscope for changes to the blood vessels. Testing for antinuclear antibodies may detect the presence of antibodies indicating an autoimmune disorder. An elevated erythrocyte sedimentation rate (ESR) indicates an inflammatory or autoimmune disorder.

Treatment

Treatment may be unnecessary for those with mild Raynaud. Those with moderate to severe symptoms should seek treatment and practice good self-care to prevent or minimize symptoms (see Box 10-7). Medications such as calcium channel blockers may be used to dilate blood vessels. Some serotonin reuptake inhibitors and antidepressant medication may help to reduce the severity and frequency of symptoms. Other treatment options include biofeedback for mild symptoms and surgery for severe cases. Surgery may involve cutting nerves that send signals to the blood vessels of the fingertips.

Prognosis

Prognosis for patients with Raynaud depends upon the type, the severity of symptoms, and the timeliness of diagnosis and treatment. Mild cases may be a nuisance but pose no threat. Severe cases, by contrast, can result in tissue death, gangrene, and the need for amputation. Chronic, recurrent episodes may result in tissue changes such as atrophy and ulcerations that heal poorly.

Thromboangiitis Obliterans
ICD-9-CM: 443.1   [ICD-10: I73.1]

Thromboangiitis obliterans, sometimes called *Buerger disease,* is a type of vascular disease associated with tobacco use but not related to atherosclerosis. It is marked by inflammation and clot formation within small vessels of the hands and feet, which may lead to gangrene and the need for amputation (see Fig. 10-13).

Flashpoint
People with mild cases of Raynaud may not need treatment.

Flashpoint
There is a very strong connection between smoking and thromboangiitis obliterans.

Box 10-7 Wellness Promotion

REDUCING RAYNAUD TRIGGERS

The following self-care habits will help reduce the risk of triggering Raynaud symptoms:

- Avoid directly touching cold objects.
- Keep gloves or mittens next to the refrigerator and freezer and put them on before handling frozen or cold food.
- Always wear socks and shoes or warm house slippers.
- Dress warmly for cold environments, including overly air-conditioned areas.
- When possible, avoid medications or other substances that cause vasoconstriction, such as decongestants, oral contraceptives, caffeine, and nicotine.
- Keep hand warmers inside of coat pockets or even slip them inside gloves.
- Avoid using vibrating tools such as electric saws or sanders.
- Avoid excess stress.

Incidence

It is estimated that 60,000 to 180,000 Americans are affected by thromboangiitis obliterans. The most common age group affected is 20 to 40 years; men are affected three times more often than women. Among ethnic groups, the disease is most common in those of Jewish, Asian, and Far and Middle Eastern descent.

Etiology

The cause of thromboangiitis obliterans is not fully understood. It is clear, however, that a strong connection exists between this disease and the use of tobacco, especially heavy smoking. It is suspected that tobacco use triggers an immune reaction in which veins and arteries in the extremities become inflamed and develop clots. It is also believed that genetics plays a role and makes some individuals more likely than others to develop this disease.

Signs and Symptoms

This disease is characterized by chronic or recurrent inflammation and thrombosis in the vessels of the extremities, particularly the feet and hands. As a result, patients experience hand or foot pain with activity or at rest and ulcerations that frequently do not heal. Pain is especially common in the arch of the foot. Other symptoms may include burning, numbness, tingling, coldness, and cyanosis in the affected body part. Intermittent *claudication* may also occur. This is a sensation of tiredness, aching, cramping, pain, tightness, heaviness, or weakness in the leg (usually the calf) with exercise that is relieved with rest. The ulcerations may develop gangrene and require surgical amputation. Most patients experience symptoms in several limbs.

Flashpoint

Ulcerations that do not heal may require limb amputation.

Diagnosis

Diagnosis is made in part by excluding other causes, such as atherosclerosis, endocarditis, Raynaud disease, and clotting disorders. Physical examination of patients with thromboangiitis obliterans reveals absent or diminished pedal (foot) or radial (wrist) pulses. Many patients will have ulcerations on their fingers, toes, or feet and will complain of claudication when walking and pain at rest. A points system has been developed to aid in diagnosis. It includes criteria such as age of onset below 45, current or recent tobacco use, distal-extremity ischemia, involvement of arteries in fingers or toes, and exclusion of atherosclerosis, autoimmune disorders, diabetes, and other possible causes. An abnormally low ankle-brachial index indicates ischemia. This test is used to identify the severity of peripheral artery disease through measuring blood pressure in the lower leg and in the arm.

Diagnosis is confirmed by an angiogram of the lower and upper extremities, which indicates a "corkscrew" appearance caused by vessel damage, as well as blockages or areas of narrowing.

Treatment

Patients with thromboangiitis obliterans are treated symptomatically, because there is no cure. Discontinuation of tobacco use is strongly recommended and may slow further disease progression. Vascular surgery is sometimes helpful in restoring or improving circulation. Other recommendations include avoiding cold and avoiding medications that cause vasoconstriction.

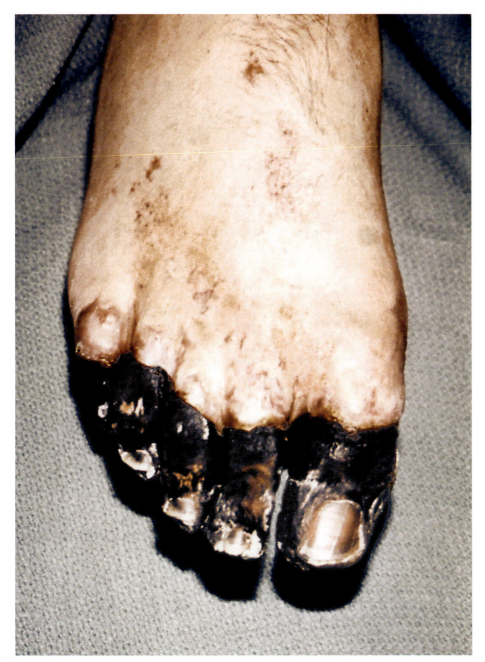

FIGURE 10-13 Thromboangiitis obliterans (Courtesy of the Centers for Disease Control and Prevention and William Archibald.)

Feet and hands should be protected as much as possible by wearing good-fitting shoes and socks, and gloves when appropriate.

Prognosis

Prognosis is good if the disorder is diagnosed early and tobacco use is stopped. Continued tobacco use will very likely lead to disease progression and the eventual need for limb amputation.

Peripheral Artery Disease

ICD-9-CM: 443.9   [ICD-10: I73.9]

Peripheral artery disease (PAD) is a condition of partial or complete obstruction of the arteries of the periphery (arms and legs). The term has gained preference over the term *peripheral vascular disease (PVD)*, which has a very similar meaning but refers to any

Flashpoint

Because there is no cure for this disorder, smoking cessation is strongly recommended.

condition that causes partial or complete obstruction of blood flow through both arteries and veins.

Incidence

PAD is known to affect more than eight million Americans and is most common among those over age 65. It is more common among men and smokers.

Etiology

PAD is caused by arteriosclerosis and atherosclerosis. It most commonly develops in the legs, in the femoral, popliteal, tibial, and peroneal arteries (see Fig. 10-14). Less often, it develops in the arteries of the arms, shoulders, or lower abdomen. Risk factors for the development of PAD include smoking, diabetes, hypertension, high cholesterol, obesity, and family history of heart disease, stroke, or PAD.

Signs and Symptoms

Signs and symptoms of PAD vary depending upon the specific arteries affected and the suddenness of the blockage. Sudden blockage occurs when a clot forms or lodges in an already narrowed vessel. Total blockage of an arm or leg artery may cause the extremity to become pale, cyanotic, cold, pulseless, painful, or numb. Gradual narrowing of a leg artery may result in intermittent claudication. Symptoms of PAD in the arms are rare and include pain, cramping, and a sensation of fatigue. Over time, skin changes may also occur, leaving the skin shiny and scaly or cracked. Hair and nails may not grow normally, and wounds may heal slowly or not at all.

Diagnosis

Diagnosis is based upon physical-examination findings, the patient's description of symptoms, and results of diagnostic tests. The physician may note a **bruit** (abnormal swooshing sound) over narrowed arteries. The ankle-brachial index will be abnormally low. A variety of radiological tests will reveal vessel narrowing or blockage. Examples include Doppler ultrasonography, angiography, magnetic resonance angiography, and computed tomographic angiography. Blood may be tested for elevated cholesterol and glucose, both of which increase the risk of PAD (see Box 10-8).

Treatment

Treatment for PAD is aimed at treating symptoms and stopping disease progression. Options include medication, exercise, risk modification, and surgery. Medications include antihypertensives

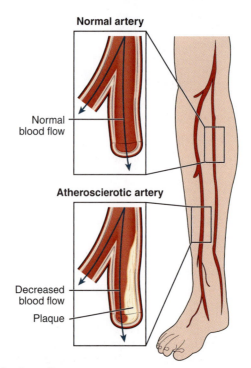

Normal artery

Normal blood flow

Atherosclerotic artery

Decreased blood flow

Plaque

FIGURE 10-14 **Peripheral artery disease**

Box 10-8 Diagnostic Spotlight

NORMAL LIPID LEVELS

Blood lipids are studied to determine a patient's risk of many forms of cardiovascular disease. Experts vary somewhat in their recommendations about what values are considered "normal." The ratio of "good" to "bad" fats is a factor. To some extent, having a very high level of HDL (high-density lipoproteins) offsets the risk posed by a high level of LDL (low-density lipoproteins). Individual patients should always consult with their physician to determine reasonable goals and treatment plans. In general, normal values are:

Total cholesterol: less than 200 mg/dL
Low-density lipoprotein (LDL—the "bad" cholesterol): less than 100 mg/dL
High-density lipoprotein (HDL—the "good" cholesterol): 40-60 mg/dL (higher is better)
Triglycerides: less than 150 mg/dL

to lower blood pressure, cholesterol-lowering agents to minimize or slow the worsening of PAD, and anticoagulants or antiplatelet medications to reduce the risk of clot formation. In some cases, thrombolytics may be used to dissolve blood clots within the vessel. Also useful may be cilostazol (Pletal), a medication that both prevents blood clots and dilates vessels. It helps relieve symptoms of claudication. Regular exercise with a physician's approval, such as walking for 30 minutes several times each week, may help improve symptoms. Risk modification includes exercise, smoking cessation, careful management of diabetes, weight loss, and a low-fat, low-cholesterol diet. One surgical option is balloon angioplasty with or without stent placement to open up the vessel. Another is bypass surgery to create an alternate route for blood flow. Yet another option is endarterectomy, a procedure in which the physician removes plaque from the artery. In severe cases where the limb cannot be salvaged, amputation may be necessary.

Flashpoint
Risk modification for PAD is the same as for CAD.

Prognosis

Prognosis depends upon the vessels involved and the timeliness of diagnosis and treatment. Ischemia can lead to tissue necrosis and gangrene formation, necessitating amputation. Other potential complications include stroke or heart attack as a result of vessel narrowing and clot formation.

Aneurysm

ICD-9-CM: 442.0-442.89   [ICD-10: I72.0-I72.9] (code by site for both codes)

An aneurysm is an abnormal dilation, of more than 50%, in the wall of a blood vessel (usually an artery) due to weakness in the vessel wall. Brain aneurysm is the most common type, followed by abdominal aortic aneurysm (AAA—see Fig. 10-15).

Incidence

One in 15 Americans has a brain aneurysm, although most will not realize it unless they become symptomatic. Every year, approximately 30,000 suffer from bleeding. Brain aneurysms are most common in adult women between the ages of 35 and 60. AAA, however, is most common among white males over the age of 60; approximately 15,000 Americans die from a ruptured AAA each year.

Flashpoint
Most aneurysms occur in vessels of the brain or in the aorta.

Etiology

AAA is caused by atherosclerosis and weakness in the vessel wall. Brain aneurysms are usually congenital. General risk factors that compound vessel injury and increase aneurysm expansion and risk of rupture are diabetes, hypertension, tobacco use, alcohol abuse, and insomnia.

Signs and Symptoms

Patients with brain aneurysm or AAA are usually asymptomatic unless the aneurysm ruptures. Rupture of a brain aneurysm causes sudden, severe headache and hemorrhagic stroke. AAA rupture causes pain in the abdomen or back that may radiate into the groin or flank. The patient may also complain of a feeling of fullness. Without immediate medical attention, severe hypotension, shock, and death quickly follow.

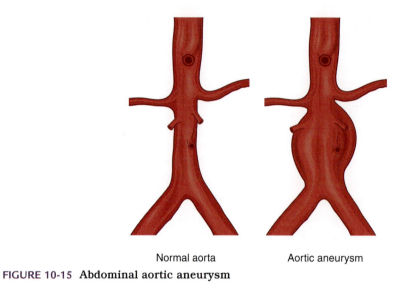

Normal aorta   Aortic aneurysm

FIGURE 10-15 Abdominal aortic aneurysm

Diagnosis

Abdominal aortic aneurysm may be discovered upon examination, when a pulsating mass is noted in the mid-abdomen. A bruit may be heard upon auscultation. Radiological studies, such as MRI, CT scan, and ultrasound, confirm the diagnosis for all types of aneurysm. In some cases, aneurysm is noted when patients undergo examination or radiological testing for other purposes.

Treatment

When an aneurysm is found, it is usually examined repeatedly over time to determine whether it is increasing in size. This approach is sometimes called *watchful waiting.* Traditional treatment of unstable aneurysms includes surgery to insert a graft or clip to stabilize the area. In the late 1990s, a treatment method known as coil *embolization* was developed to treat brain aneurysms. In this procedure, a microcatheter is inserted through a large vessel near the groin and threaded to the aneurysm. Coils are inserted into the aneurysm to fill it from within, thus plugging it and preventing blood from entering. When a patient is identified as having a dissecting (tearing) or ruptured aneurysm, emergency measures are initiated, including surgery, blood and fluid replacement, and respiratory support.

Prognosis

Prognosis depends on the type and location of the aneurysm and whether or not it is identified prior to rupture. When intervention occurs prior to rupture, chances of survival are good; however, once an aneurysm ruptures, the survival rate is low. Among those who suffer a ruptured brain aneurysm, 10% to 15% will die before reaching a hospital. Of those who survive the initial event, 50% will die within 30 days. Of those who survive long-term, approximately 50% will have some type of permanent neurological deficit.

Flashpoint

The survival rate for patients with a ruptured aneurysm is very low.

Varicose Veins
ICD-9-CM: 454.0-454.9   [ICD-10: I83.0-I83.9] (code by complications for both codes)

Varicose veins are enlarged, dilated superficial veins, which most commonly develop in the legs.

Incidence

An estimated 12 million Americans suffer from varicose veins. Women suffer from varicose veins more than men, with over 40% of all women over age 50 affected.

Etiology

Varicosities develop in veins rather than arteries because venous blood travels under low pressure and must flow against gravity to return to the heart. Blood flow is helped along by the presence of one-way valves in veins as well as the pumping action of surrounding leg muscles. When valves become incompetent and fail to close properly, blood movement becomes sluggish. This sluggishness results in vein engorgement, which further worsens valvular incompetence. It is unclear why this problem develops in some individuals and not in others; however, family history of varicose veins is a known risk factor. Others risk factors include obesity, pregnancy, and prolonged sitting or standing.

Signs and Symptoms

Signs and symptoms of varicose veins include the appearance of distended, knotted-looking superficial veins of the legs and feelings in the legs of pain, aching, and fatigue (see Fig. 10-16). Symptoms worsen with prolonged standing and are temporarily relieved by elevating the legs.

Diagnosis

Diagnosis is based on the appearance of the veins and a description of symptoms from the patient.

Treatment

Conservative treatment aims at relieving symptoms and promoting the return of venous blood to the heart. It includes taking rest periods during which legs are elevated above the heart, wearing support hose, and performing ambulation or leg exercises every hour throughout the day. Patients should avoid activities that impede circulation, including wearing hose with tight leg bands, wearing girdles, crossing the legs, and sitting or standing for a prolonged time. Weight loss is encouraged if obesity is a factor. More aggressive treatment includes stripping (surgical procedures to remove the affected veins) and ligation (suturing), or injection of a sclerosing solution that causes the vein to collapse, harden, and eventually atrophy.

Prognosis

In most cases, varicose veins pose no significant health risk other than discomfort and embarrassment related to their appearance. However, severe varicose veins do contribute to the development of deep vein thrombosis, which can be serious.

Flashpoint

Risk factors for varicose veins include family history, obesity, pregnancy, prolonged sitting or standing, and being female.

Flashpoint

Severe varicose veins increase the risk of deep vein thrombosis.

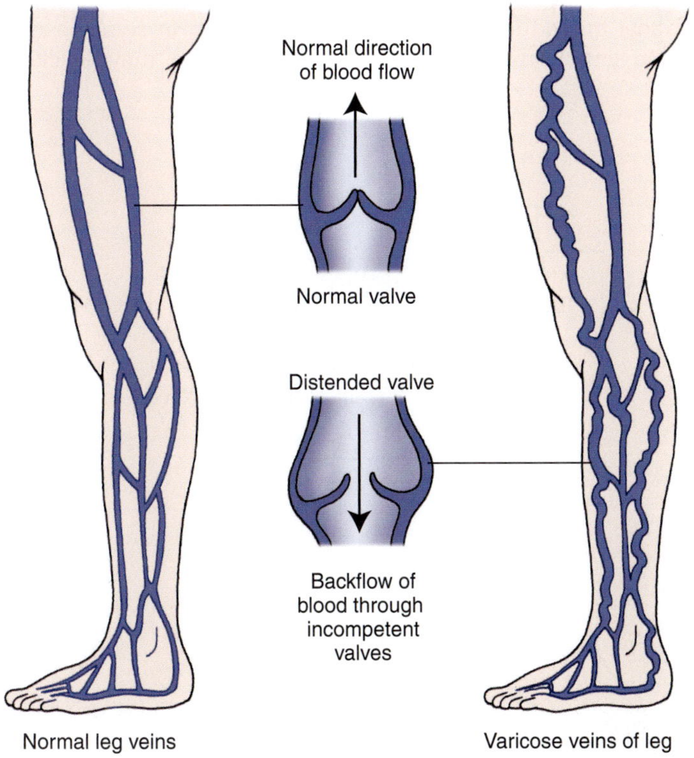

FIGURE 10-16 **Varicose veins** (From Eagle, S. *Medical Terminology in a Flash! An Interactive, Flash-Card Approach.* 2006. Philadelphia: F.A. Davis Company, with permission.)

Deep Vein Thrombosis
ICD-9-CM: 453.40   [ICD-10: I80.2]

Deep vein thrombosis (DVT), also known as *thrombophlebitis* and *venous thromboembolism* (VTE), occurs when a blood clot develops in a deep vein, usually in the legs.

Incidence

The condition most commonly develops in adults over the age of 60 and those with impaired mobility, such as those who are bedridden or paralyzed.

Etiology

DVT usually occurs secondary to vessel injury and blood **stasis** (sluggish blood flow) caused by poor circulation and immobility. Platelets begin to gather and fibrin formation occurs in areas of injury, creating a blood clot, and then inflammation ensues (see Fig. 10-17). Other contributing factors include clotting disorders, heart failure, estrogen use, malignancy, obesity, and pregnancy.

Signs and Symptoms

Common symptoms of DVT include a dull ache in the area of the clot, a feeling of heaviness, and localized edema, redness, and heat.

Diagnosis

A tentative diagnosis is based on physical-examination findings, the patient's description of symptoms, and tenderness on palpation. Blood may be drawn to check D-dimer; a low value rules out DVT, and a high value (greater than 300) indicates possible DVT. Diagnosis is confirmed with compression ultrasonography, which reveals the failure of a vein to compress where a clot is located. Radiographic venography may also help confirm the diagnosis.

Flashpoint

Compression ultrasonography may be done to confirm diagnosis.

Treatment

DVT is treated with anticoagulant medication. The patient should rest and refrain from vigorous exercise until the condition resolves. The health-care provider may also advise the patient to elevate the limb and apply warm compresses.

Flashpoint

A serious complication of DVT is pulmonary embolism.

Prognosis

A potential complication of DVT is embolization of the clot to the lungs, resulting in pulmonary embolism, which may be a life-threatening event. However, with timely diagnosis and intervention, most individuals recover without incident. In some cases, **postphlebitic syndrome,** a chronic condition marked by edema and aching, may develop.

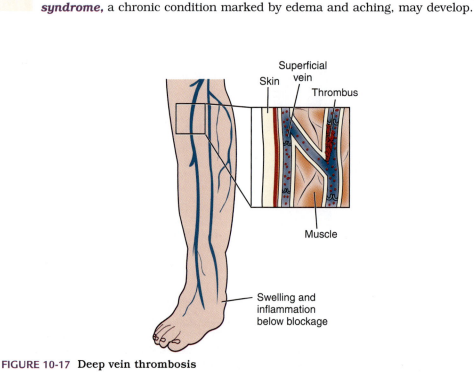

FIGURE 10-17 Deep vein thrombosis

Inflammatory Heart Diseases and Disorders

Several heart conditions have inflammation as a central part of the pathology. They include rheumatic heart disease, pericarditis, myocarditis, and endocarditis.

Rheumatic Heart Disease

ICD-9-CM: 392.0   [ICD-10: I01.0-I01.9 (code by site of heart damage)]

Rheumatic heart disease is a complication of rheumatic fever in which inflammation and damage occur to parts of the heart, most commonly the valves.

Incidence

At one time, rheumatic heart disease was the most common cause of death in young people between the ages of 5 and 20. Since the 1960s, incidence and mortality have dropped to nearly zero in developed countries; however, it continues to be a major health problem in less-developed countries, affecting as many as 30 million young people and accounting for more than 200,000 deaths each year.

Etiology

As many as 3% of individuals who develop pharyngitis caused by group A beta-hemolytic streptococci—strep throat—will develop rheumatic fever several weeks later. In some, inflammation and damage to various heart structures occurs from an autoimmune reaction in which the body forms antibodies that then migrate to structures such as heart valves, especially the mitral valve. There, the antibodies grow and cause scarring or stenosis. This damage may result in muscle and valve dysfunction that causes heart failure and arrhythmias.

Streptococcal infections are spread by direct contact with secretions from the mouth or respiratory tract. Patients may continue to be infected for weeks after symptoms have resolved. Crowded living conditions increase the likelihood of spreading.

Signs and Symptoms

Common signs and symptoms of rheumatic heart disease are those of heart failure, including dyspnea, edema, tachycardia, and new or worsened heart murmurs.

Diagnosis

Diagnosis of rheumatic heart disease is based on several criteria. These include recent evidence of group A streptococcal pharyngitis, the presence of rheumatic fever, and symptoms of heart failure such as dyspnea, activity intolerance, and rapid heart rate. (See Chapter 11 for further information about streptococcal pharyngitis.)

Treatment

Treatment of rheumatic heart disease is aimed at preventing or reducing inflammation and the damage it causes. This is done with anti-inflammatory medication, such as corticosteroids, and NSAIDS, such as high-dose aspirin. Antibiotics (e.g., penicillin) are used to treat streptococcal infections. Chronic administration of low-dose antibiotics may be used to prevent recurrence. Individuals with evidence of heart failure may require diuretics and digoxin therapy.

Prognosis

Prognosis is generally good for patients with rheumatic heart disease, depending upon how early it is diagnosed and treated. Approximately 60% to 80% of those who complete antibiotic therapy will experience resolution of valvular disease. Response to anti-inflammatory therapy is also very good. Prognosis is not quite as good for those with chronic disease. Complications include permanent damage to heart structures, leading to arrhythmias, heart failure, and death. Chronic disease is the most common reason for mitral valve stenosis and heart-valve replacement surgery in the United States. The best way to prevent rheumatic heart disease is early diagnosis and treatment of strep throat (see Box 10-9).

Pericarditis

ICD-9-CM: 420.90   [ICD-10: I30.9] (unspecified for both codes)

Pericarditis is a condition in which the pericardium becomes inflamed (see Fig. 10-18). It may be acute or chronic, may have a variety of causes, and in some cases may be life-threatening. Acute pericarditis lasts 2 or 3 weeks, with a recurrence possible during the following year. Chronic pericarditis lasts 6 to 12 months after the acute episode.

Flashpoint

Rheumatic heart disease continues to be a serious global health problem.

Flashpoint

Chronic rheumatic disease is the most common reason for heart-valve replacement in the United States.

Box 10-9 Wellness Promotion

PREVENTING RHEUMATIC HEART DISEASE

Taking active steps to prevent rheumatic fever will prevent some forms of heart disease. Measures include:

- timely and accurate diagnosis and treatment of pharyngitis (sore throat) caused by streptococci.
- timely and accurate diagnosis and treatment of rheumatic fever—symptoms appear about 3 weeks after an episode of strep throat and include fever; chest pain; heart palpitations; dyspnea; fatigue; skin rash; small, painless skin nodules; and red, painful, swollen joints.
- identification of individuals with a history of rheumatic fever—they are much more vulnerable to repeated episodes of rheumatic fever and to heart damage, and they may need to be on continuous antibiotic therapy.

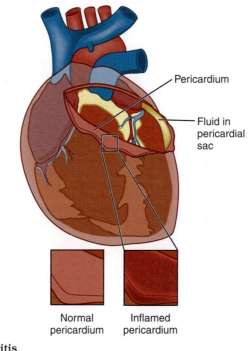

Pericardium

Fluid in pericardial sac

Normal pericardium

Inflamed pericardium

FIGURE 10-18 **Pericarditis**

Incidence

Accurate incidence of pericarditis is difficult to estimate because of the many undiagnosed cases. However, it has been estimated that pericarditis accounts for one in every 1,000 hospital admissions.

Etiology

Causes of pericarditis are numerous; the most common is some type of viral, bacterial, or fungal infection. The condition can also develop as a complication of certain medications, heart attack, or some diseases, such as rheumatic fever, cancer, rheumatoid arthritis, systemic lupus erythematosus, tuberculosis, and scleroderma. Other causes include injury from radiation therapy, trauma, and surgery.

Signs and Symptoms

Some individuals with pericarditis are asymptomatic. In those who have symptoms, the most common complaint is substernal chest pain that may radiate to the neck, arms, or upper back and is worse with certain activities, such as swallowing, coughing, or lying down. It is usually relieved or lessened by sitting upright and leaning forward. Other symptoms may include tachycardia, mild fever, chills, dyspnea, and diaphoresis.

Diagnosis

Diagnosis of pericarditis is based on medical history, physical-examination findings, and a variety of diagnostic tests. Upon auscultation, the physician may note a pericardial rub, which is an odd creaking, scratching sound produced by the heart muscle moving against the inflamed pericardium. Other examination findings might include distended jugular veins and edema in the feet and ankles. An ECG may reveal an elevated ST segment. Tests such as echocardiogram, CT, and MRI may reveal thickening of the pericardium or **pericardial effusion** (increased fluid collection between the heart and pericardium).

Treatment

Treatment of pericarditis is aimed at the underlying cause but most commonly includes analgesics and NSAIDs. Severe cases may require corticosteroid medication and possible hospitalization. Pericardiocentesis may be done in such cases. This is a procedure in which a sterile catheter is placed to drain fluid from the pericardium, to eliminate or reduce effusion.

Prognosis

The prognosis for pericarditis is generally good, depending upon the underlying cause and the timeliness of appropriate treatment. A potential complication is the development of constrictive pericarditis, in which extensive scarring and thickening of the pericardium results in loss of elasticity. This causes compression of the heart, restricting its ability to fill with and pump blood effectively. This can lead to heart failure and kidney disease.

Myocarditis

ICD-9-CM: 429.0   [ICD-10: I51.4]

Myocarditis is a condition in which the middle layer of the heart wall becomes inflamed.

Incidence

Incidence of myocarditis is difficult to determine, since many cases go unreported. It is estimated that approximately 24,000 individuals in the United States experience this disorder each year.

Etiology

There are many causes of myocarditis, but most are bacterial, viral, fungal, or parasitic infections. Viral causes include coxsackie (most common), cytomegalovirus, hepatitis C, herpes, HIV, Epstein-Barr, influenza, rubella, and parvovirus. Bacterial causes include *Chlamydia*, *Mycoplasma*, streptococci, *Staphylococcus aureus*, and *Treponema*. Fungal causes include *Aspergillus*, *Candida*, *Coccidioides*, *Cryptococcus*, *Histoplasma*, and *Schistosoma* (the parasitic blood fluke) causing the infection. Parasitic causes are uncommon in the United States but are a primary global cause of myocarditis. Offenders include *Trypanosoma cruzi*, *Toxoplasma*, and Chagas disease. Other possible causes include toxins and drugs (legal and illegal), chemical exposure, and diseases like rheumatic fever, sarcoidosis, systemic lupus erythematosus, and rheumatoid arthritis. Regardless of cause, the process of inflammation and healing within heart muscle leaves scar tissue in the place of healthy muscle. As a result, the myocardium is left thickened, weakened, and less elastic. This often leads to heart failure.

Signs and Symptoms

Some individuals with myocarditis are symptom free. Others may complain of chest pain or aching, fatigue, palpitations, faintness, mild dyspnea, and joint pain. Other signs include abnormal heart rhythm, edema of the joints or legs, and fever.

Diagnosis

Notable examination findings may include a new heart murmur or other abnormal heart sounds, tachycardia, fluid in the lungs, and edema in the legs. Chest x-ray confirms lung congestion, and ECG confirms tachycardia or other rhythm abnormalities. An elevated WBC count and positive blood culture indicate infection. Elevated cardiac enzymes in the blood indicate heart-muscle damage. Antibody testing may reveal an autoimmune process. Echocardiogram produces moving images of the heart as it beats

Flashpoint

Unlike pain from an MI, pericarditis pain is relieved or lessened by sitting upright and leaning forward.

Flashpoint

Pericarditis usually responds to analgesic and anti-inflammatory medication.

Flashpoint

Many different organisms can cause myocarditis.

Flashpoint

Patients with myocarditis may complain of chest pain, fatigue, palpitations, faintness, dyspnea, and joint pain.

and provides information about motion of the heart wall, heart size, and presence of fluid surrounding the heart. Heart-muscle tissue may be biopsied to confirm the cause.

Treatment

Treatment of myocarditis is aimed at the cause and usually includes anti-inflammatory medication to reduce inflammation and edema, analgesics for pain, antibiotics if infection is indicated, and diuretics to treat edema and lung congestion. Cardiac medications are also given if needed, including angiotensin-converting enzyme inhibitors to increase blood flow to the heart, antiarrhythmics to treat rhythm problems, and inotropics to increase muscle strength. Rest and a low-sodium diet may also be advised. In cases of extreme heart damage, transplantation may be considered.

Prognosis

Prognosis for patients with myocarditis is variable. Many recover fully; others suffer varying degrees of heart failure, which may become chronic. Other potential complications include arrhythmias, pericarditis, and cardiomyopathy. The mortality rate for acute myocarditis is 20% to 30%.

Endocarditis
ICD-9-CM: 421.9   [ICD-10: I33.9] (unspecified for both codes)

Endocarditis is an infection of the inner lining of the heart. It may affect the inside of one or more chambers and any of the valves.

Flashpoint

Endocarditis is an infection of the inner lining of the heart.

Incidence

Endocarditis is more common in men than in women, and half of all cases occur in patients over age 50. Among younger individuals it develops most commonly in those with congenital heart defects.

Etiology

Endocarditis is usually caused when bacterial infection from organisms that originated in other parts of the body, such as the skin, intestinal tract, or respiratory tract, travels to the heart via the bloodstream. Rarely, fungi may also be a cause. Pathogens can enter the bloodstream in any number of ways: injection drug use; central venous access lines; prior heart-valve surgery; tonsillectomy; endoscopic examination or surgery of the intestinal, urinary, or respiratory tract; and recent dental surgery. Individuals at greatest risk are those with some type of already present heart defect, such as atrial septal defect, ventricle defect, a prosthetic heart valve, or damage from a previous episode of endocarditis. The defect provides a roughened area where bacteria can attach and grow. These growths are often referred to as *vegetations* (see Fig. 10-19).

Flashpoint

Bacterial growths on infected heart valves are often called vegetations.

Signs and Symptoms

Symptoms may develop slowly or suddenly. Endocarditis may be difficult to identify because of the vagueness of early symptoms, which include fever, chills, fatigue,

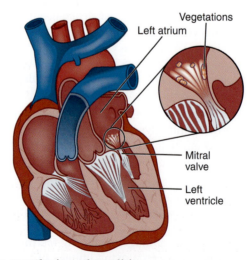

FIGURE 10-19 **Vegetative growths in endocarditis**

weakness, pallor, anorexia, weight loss, muscle and joint aches, cough, and night sweats. As the condition becomes more advanced, the individual may develop a new heart murmur, dyspnea with activity, and edema in the feet and legs. Other signs and symptoms include hematuria; spleen tenderness; red, tender nodes in the pads of toes and fingers; red, painless spots on the palms and soles; and splinter hemorrhages under the fingernails.

Diagnosis

Diagnosis may be suspected based on examination findings and patient symptoms. A variety of tests may be done; the most conclusive is transesophageal echocardiogram, which may reveal vegetations. Other tests might include erythrocyte sedimentation rate (ESR), CBC, ECG, and blood culture. An elevated ESR indicates an inflammatory condition. The CBC may reveal elevated WBC count, which indicates infection. An ECG will reveal any heart-rhythm disturbances. A positive blood culture may help to identify the causative pathogen and aid the physician in antibiotic selection.

Treatment

Individuals with endocarditis will be given IV antibiotics for as long as 6 weeks. Valve damage may require replacement surgery.

Prognosis

Prognosis is generally good, with timely diagnosis and treatment. Potential complications include arrhythmias, heart failure, pericarditis, and MI. Pieces of the vegetation may break off and travel to the brain, causing stroke; to the lungs, causing pulmonary embolism; or to other organs, such as the kidneys, causing tissue damage. Untreated endocarditis can result in damage or destruction of the heart lining, leading to heart failure. Untreated infection can be fatal.

Flashpoint

Patients may need antibiotic treatment for up to 6 weeks.

STOP HERE.
Select the flash cards for this chapter and run through them at least three times before moving on to the next chapter.

Student Resources

American Heart Association: http://www.heart.org
The Cardiomyopathy Association: http://www.cardiomyopathy.org
Healthcommunities.com Cardiology Channel: http://www.cardiologychannel.com
Texas Heart Institute: http://www.texasheartinstitute.org
Vascular Disease Foundation: http://www.vdf.org

Chapter Activities

Learning Style Study Strategies

Try any or all of the following strategies as you study the content of this chapter:

Visual and auditory learners: At your college or city library, check out and watch any videos on specific diseases you need to learn about.

Kinesthetic and verbal learners: Join a study buddy or group and use sidewalk chalk to draw a huge, anatomically correct illustration of the heart on an area of pavement. Label all parts with anatomical names and combining forms. Take turns walking along the path of blood flow, verbally naming the parts as you walk over them.

Practice Exercises

Answers to Practice Exercises can be found in Appendix D.

Case Studies

CASE STUDY 1

May Seibert is a 72-year-old woman who presented to her family doctor with complaints of a recent onset of chest palpitations, occasional shortness of breath, and fatigue. She notes that her symptoms are interfering with her usually daily walk and are worse when she climbs stairs. When reviewing Mrs. Seibert's ECG, the physician notes that her rhythm is rapid and irregular, with no identifiable P waves, and concludes that she is in a rhythm known as atrial fibrillation.

1. Is Mrs. Seibert typical of those who commonly develop atrial fibrillation? Explain why or why not.

2. Describe the activity of her atria during this rhythm.

3. If Mrs. Seibert's ECG had been normal, the physician might have decided to have her wear one of two devices available that collect data about her heart activity. Describe these devices and how they work.

4. What medication will the physician likely order for Mrs. Seibert to try to slow her heart rate and restore normal sinus rhythm?

5. If the medication is not successful, what other treatment options might be considered?

CASE STUDY 2

Rebecca Han is a 22-year-old woman who has just been diagnosed with Raynaud disease. The physician has asked the medical assistant to provide some general education for Rebecca and answer questions she may have related to self-care. How should the medical assistant answer Ms. Han's questions?

1. The physician told me what this condition is, but I can't remember everything she said. Could you explain it to me again?

2. How did I catch this?

3. Why do my fingers change color and hurt so much when they get cold?

4. What can I do to keep from triggering my symptoms?

CASE STUDY 3

Del Pruitt is a 62-year-old man who came to see his primary care provider today with complaints about his leg. After evaluating Mr. Pruitt, the physician diagnoses him with thrombophlebitis.

1. What is the other common name for this disorder?

2. Given Mr. Pruitt's diagnosis, what presenting signs and symptoms did he probably have?

3. Is Mr. Pruitt typical of someone who develops this disorder?

4. What are the usual cause and risk factors for this disorder?

5. What type of diagnostic tests may have been done to confirm Mr. Pruitt's diagnosis?

6. What class of medication is the physician likely to prescribe for Mr. Pruitt?

7. List two specific medications, by name, that might be prescribed. (Hint: See Appendix C.)

8. What other self-care advice might the physician give Mr. Pruitt?

9. What potentially life-threatening complication are Mr. Pruitt and his physician hoping to avoid?

Multiple Choice

1. Which of the following terms is **not** matched with the correct definition?

   a. Ablation: destruction of electrical conduction pathways of the AV node

   b. Cardioversion: synchronized shock of electrical current delivered to the chest wall while the patient is under sedation and analgesia

   c. Claudication: abnormal fluid accumulation in the abdominal space between organs

   d. Depolarization: electrical change in cardiac muscle cells that causes them to contract

2. The term *bruit* is defined as:

   a. Abnormal lung sound heard on auscultation that indicates fluid in the alveoli

   b. Sensation of rapid or irregular beating of the heart

   c. Sluggish blood flow

   d. Abnormal swooshing sound

3. A term which refers to contraction and relaxation of all chambers of the heart is:

   a. Cardiac cycle

   b. Cardiac output

   c. Perfusion

   d. Blood pressure

4. In which of the following disorders is the patient at greatest risk of acquiring an infection?

   a. Anemia

   b. Raynaud disease

   c. Agranulocytosis

   d. Disseminated intravascular coagulation

5. Which of the following disorders is most closely associated with smoking?

   a. Anemia

   b. Thromboangiitis obliterans

   c. Varicose veins

   d. Cardiomyopathy

Short Answer

1. **Describe the similarities and differences between angina and MI.**

2. **Define the two primary contributors to the development of coronary artery disease.**

3. **List nine steps to reduce risk of heart disease.**

RESPIRATORY SYSTEM DISEASES AND DISORDERS

11

Learning Outcomes

Upon completion of this chapter, the student will be able to:

- Define and spell terms related to the respiratory system
- Identify key structures of the respiratory system
- Discuss the roles of the upper airway, lower airway, and lungs as part of the respiratory system

- Identify characteristics of common respiratory system diseases and disorders, including:
  - description
  - incidence
  - etiology
  - signs and symptoms
  - diagnosis
  - treatment
  - prognosis

KEY TERMS	
asbestosis	form of pneumoconiosis caused by inhalation of asbestos fibers
atelectasis	condition of collapse or airlessness in parts of the lung
berylliosis	form of pneumoconiosis caused by inhalation of or exposure to beryllium
chronic hypoxia	chronic lack of oxygen
coal worker's pneumoconiosis	form of pneumoconiosis caused by inhalation of coal dust; also called *anthracosis* or *black lung*
crackles	abnormal lung sound heard on auscultation that indicates fluid in the alveoli
decortication	procedure done under general anesthesia in which scar tissue, pus, or other debris is removed from the pleurae and pleural space
empyema	collection of fluid in the pleural space containing infectious matter, such as bacteria and white blood cells
flail chest	injury in which three or more ribs are fractured in two or more places, creating a free-floating segment
hemoptysis	spitting or coughing up blood from the respiratory tract
hypercapnea	chronic retention of carbon dioxide, leading to symptoms of mental cloudiness and lethargy
hypoxemia	condition of low blood oxygen
orthopnea	difficulty breathing that is eased by sitting, rather than lying down
paradoxical motion	motion of a free-floating fractured rib segment in the opposite direction from the rest of the chest as the patient breathes
pH scale	tool for measuring the acidity or alkalinity of a substance

Continued

KEY TERMS—cont'd	
pleural friction rub	low-pitched scratching, creaking, grating sound made by the pleurae as they rub against one another
pleurodesis	procedure in which a sterile, irritating substance is infused into the pleural space, causing the pleural linings to develop scar tissue and fuse to one another
silicosis	form of pneumoconiosis caused by inhalation of silica (quartz) dust; also called *grinder's disease, progressive massive fibrosis,* and *potter's rot*
wheezes	musical sound caused by narrowed air passages

Abbreviations

Table 11-1 lists some of the most common abbreviations related to the respiratory system.

Structures and Functions of the Respiratory System

The respiratory system, also called the *pulmonary system,* is made up of the upper airway, lower airway, and lungs. The respiratory system facilitates breathing and the exchange of gases—especially oxygen and carbon dioxide, which are vital to life and health.

Structures of the Respiratory System

The respiratory system is divided into the upper and lower airways and the lungs (see Fig. 11-1).

TABLE 11-1

ABBREVIATIONS

Abbreviation	Meaning	Abbreviation	Meaning
ABG, ABGs	arterial blood gases	O_2	oxygen
ARDS	acute respiratory distress syndrome	PE	pulmonary embolism
CBC	complete blood count	PFTs	pulmonary function tests
CO_2	carbon dioxide	pH	potential of hydrogen
COPD	chronic obstructive pulmonary disease	PPD	purified protein derivative (TB test)
CPAP	continuous positive airway pressure	SOB	short of breath
CWP	coal worker's pneumoconiosis	TB	tuberculosis
ENT	ears, nose, and throat	URI	upper respiratory infection
NPC	nasopharyngeal carcinoma, nonproductive cough	VC	vital capacity

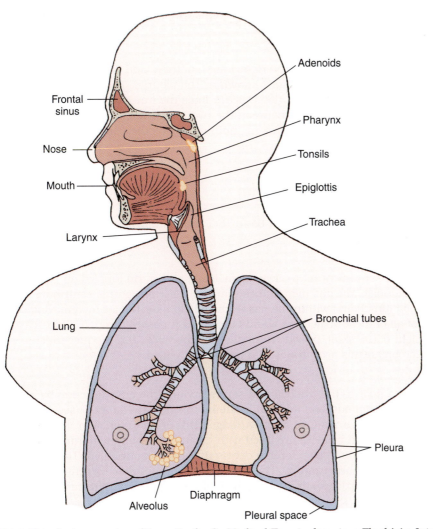

FIGURE 11-1 Respiratory system (From Eagle, S. *Medical Terminology in a Flash! An Interactive, Flash-Card Approach.* 2006. Philadelphia: F.A. Davis Company, with permission.)

Upper Airway

The main structures of the upper airway consist of the mouth, nose, sinuses, and pharynx (throat). The pharynx is further divided into the nasopharynx (back of the nose) and oropharynx (back of the mouth). The nose begins with the nares (nostrils) and extends back to the nasopharynx. The nasal passages are divided into right and left sides by the nasal septum. The hard palate divides the nasal cavity from the mouth, which sits beneath it. The sinus cavities—maxillary, frontal, ethmoidal, and sphenoidal—are air-filled spaces named for the facial bones within which they are located. Many of the upper-airway structures, like the mouth and oropharynx, are shared by the gastrointestinal and respiratory systems.

Lower Airway

The lower airways consist of the epiglottis, trachea, bronchial tubes, and lungs. The trachea (sometimes called the *windpipe*) begins superiorly with the larynx (sometimes called the *voice box*) and extends inferiorly to the middle of the chest. It is approximately 5 inches long and gets its shape and strength from numerous rings of cartilage. In the center of the chest, the trachea divides into the two primary bronchi, each of which leads to smaller and smaller bronchi and, eventually, to tiny bronchioles. The structure of the bronchi changes to less cartilage and more smooth muscle as they become smaller. The bronchioles end at the alveoli, which are microscopic air sacs within the lungs. There are approximately 300 million

Flashpoint

Many structures, like the mouth and oropharynx, are shared by gastrointestinal and respiratory systems.

alveoli in each lung, covered with a delicate capillary bed (microscopic blood vessels) that provides them with a rich blood supply.

Lungs

The lungs are divided into lobes; the right lung has three and the left lung, two. The lungs are covered with two thin membranes known as the pleurae. The visceral pleura lies directly on the lungs, while the parietal pleura lines the inner wall of the thorax. A small amount of pleural fluid lies in the space between the two membranes. This space is sometimes referred to as a *potential space,* because there is nothing there other than a small amount of this fluid.

Functions of the Respiratory System

The functions of the respiratory system can be further broken down by the upper and lower airways and the lungs.

Upper Airway

The structures of the upper airway act to cleanse, moisten, and warm inhaled air before it continues its journey to the lungs. Mucous membranes that line these structures contribute moisture to humidify the air. Cilia (tiny hairs) within the nasal cavity help filter the air by removing debris. The rich blood supply of all of these structures warms the air as it passes through. Sinus cavities serve to decrease the weight of the skull, provide resonance for the voice, and produce mucus, which helps eliminate microorganisms as it drains into the nasal cavities.

Lower Airway

The epiglottis acts as a door to the trachea and serves a vital protective function by opening to let in air and closing to keep out food and fluid. The larynx vibrates as air passes through it, creating vocal sounds. The numerous C-shaped cartilage rings of the trachea provide strength and keep it open. The trachea and bronchi are lined with ciliated mucous membranes which further moisten air and secrete mucus to trap foreign debris that has been inhaled. The cilia move in a wavelike fashion to propel debris upward. The trachea and bronchi are extremely sensitive; the presence of foreign particles stimulates a powerful cough reflex that further helps to expel foreign debris.

Lungs

The lungs expand and contract with each breath in and out. The elastic quality that allows them to do this is sometimes called *recoil.* The pleural fluid between the visceral and parietal pleurae acts as a sort of lubricant, which helps the process along as the lungs continually expand and contract.

A person takes oxygen (O_2) into the lungs by inhaling, or breathing in, which is usually an unconscious act. A person may, however, exert conscious control to take extra-large breaths or even hold the breath for a short time. At some point, however, the person will have an overwhelming urge to breathe, which is triggered by a buildup of carbon dioxide (CO_2) in the blood. This buildup causes the blood to become more acidic. To be healthy, a person's blood must remain slightly alkaline—within the narrow range of 7.35 to 7.45 on the **pH scale.** This scale, whose name stands for *potential of hydrogen,* is a tool for measuring the acidity or alkalinity of a substance—the blood, in this case. As the blood becomes more acidic and the pH level drops, the urge to breathe is triggered. The act of inhalation brings fresh, oxygen-rich air into the person's lungs so that the oxygen can be absorbed into the blood. By exhaling, or breathing out, the body eliminates excess CO_2, thus restoring a normal blood pH level. Contrary to what most people think, the stimulus to breathe is not lower O_2 levels in the blood but the lowered pH level caused by CO_2 buildup.

Gas exchange, so vital to life, takes place within the millions of tiny alveoli contained within each lung. They expand somewhat like tiny balloons during inhalation, as air enters and fills them. They contract and partially deflate during exhalation, as much of the air moves out of the lungs. Because the walls of the alveoli and the capillary beds are each just one cell thick, gases move easily back and forth. Excess CO_2 leaves the capillaries, moves into the air space in the alveoli, and is then exhaled. Oxygen moves from the air space in the alveoli into the capillary blood and is then distributed to various parts of the body by the circulatory system.

Common Upper Respiratory System Diseases and Disorders

There are many diseases and disorders of the upper respiratory system. Some are structural in nature, like sleep apnea, deviated septum, and nasal polyps, or caused by injury, such as epistaxis. Others are infectious or inflammatory illness, such as upper respiratory infection, sinusitis, pharyngitis, allergic rhinitis, and laryngitis.

Sleep Apnea

ICD-9-CM: 780.57   [ICD-10: G47.3] (unspecified for both codes)

Sleep apnea, sometimes called *sleep-disordered breathing,* is a common condition in which individuals stop breathing, possibly hundreds of times, during sleep. It is classified as obstructive, the most common form; central, a less common form; or complex, a mix of the two.

Incidence

Sleep apnea is estimated to affect between 12 and 18 million Americans. It affects approximately 10% of all middle-aged men and 5% of all middle-aged women, but it can also affect children. It is more common among African Americans than Caucasians. Incidence is higher among obese individuals.

> **Flashpoint**
> A person with sleep apnea can awaken hundreds of times during the night without even knowing it!

Etiology

In obstructive sleep apnea, air flow is blocked by upper-airway tissue but respiratory efforts continue (see Fig. 11-2A). This results in a repetitive pattern of snoring, snorting, and gasping as the individual rouses from sleep just enough to finally take several effective breaths. As carbon dioxide is eliminated and the need for oxygen is satisfied, the person slips back into a deeper sleep. Then muscles in the throat relax and the airway becomes obstructed once again. Because this pattern repeats itself hundreds of times during the night, normal sleep patterns are disrupted, interfering with truly restful sleep. Risk factors that contribute to airway obstruction during sleep include obesity, age of at least 40, neck circumference greater than 44 centimeters (17.5 inches), narrowed airway, family history of sleep apnea, smoking, use of alcohol or sleeping medication, and being male.

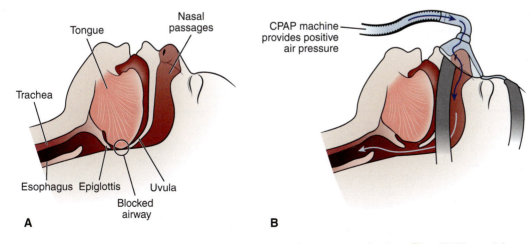

FIGURE 11-2 Sleep apnea: (A) the airway closes during apnea episodes; (B) a CPAP machine provides positive air pressure to keep the airway open

In central sleep apnea, breathing stops because of a failure of the brain to send signals to muscles that control breathing, not because of airway obstruction. Risk factors for central sleep apnea include history of brain tumor or stroke, certain heart disorders, such as heart failure, certain arrhythmias, and being male. Mixed sleep apnea is a combination of both mechanisms. Risk factors for mixed sleep apnea are the same as for the other two.

Signs and Symptoms

People with sleep apnea are often unaware that they have it, thinking they are sleeping well through the night. However, they rarely feel rested in the morning and often struggle with day-time drowsiness. In addition, they may note morning headache, dry mouth, and sore throat.

More often than not, it is the patient's spouse or significant other who notices the snoring and observes the apnea periods.

Flashpoint

Sleep apnea is often noticed by a spouse or other person, who hears the snoring and sees the person stop breathing.

Diagnosis

Sleep apnea is diagnosed by history, physical examination, and sleep studies. During sleep studies the patient stays overnight in a sleep lab, where several types of tests are done. Continuous pulse oximetry is a test in which a small sensor is placed on the patient's finger to detect abnormal drops in oxygen level during sleep. This test can also be done at home. During nocturnal polysomnography, the patient has sensors applied that detect heart, lung, and brain activity in addition to body movements, breathing patterns, and oxygen levels. The information gathered in a sleep study identifies the number, frequency, and severity of apnea periods as well as the number of nighttime awakenings. Patients are sometimes surprised to learn that they awaken hundreds of times during the night without knowing it.

Some patients are referred to other specialists, such as ear, nose, and throat (ENT) doctors, neurologists, and cardiologists, who may further evaluate them for potential causes of obstructive and central sleep apnea. These specialists may also aid in the design of a treatment plan.

Treatment

For many patients, conservative measures and good self-care are all that is needed to reduce or eliminate sleep apnea. Measures include weight loss, smoking cessation, avoidance of sleep medications and alcohol, sleeping on the side rather than the back, and use of a saline nasal spray before bed to help keep nasal passages open. Individuals with more severe sleep apnea may benefit from using an oral device fitted by their dentist, or may need to use a continuous positive airway pressure (CPAP) breathing machine (see Fig. 11-2B). Those with severe obstructive sleep apnea may also benefit from surgery to remove nasal polyps, tonsils, adenoids, or other airway tissues, and to correct structural defects.

Flashpoint

A CPAP machine can eliminate sleep apnea and help the patient sleep well.

Prognosis

Prognosis is very good for individuals whose sleep apnea is identified and appropriately treated. On the other hand, untreated sleep apnea can lead to a variety of problems. It is known to contribute to hypertension and cardiovascular disease, and increases risk of heart attack and stroke. It contributes to obesity, memory impairment, impotence, headaches, irritability, depression, daytime sleepiness, and impaired mental functioning. This can result in accidents, injury, and death on the job or on the road. In children it can lead to hyperactivity, inattentiveness, and other behavior problems at school.

Deviated Septum

ICD-9-CM: 470   [ICD-10: J34.2]

The nasal septum is the wall that divides the right and left sides of the nose. Ideally, it is straight and located in the center so that each naris is equal in size. When it is displaced to the side, causing the two nares to be unequal, it is said to be deviated (see Fig. 11-3). If the deviation is severe enough, it can impede normal air flow, leading to breathing difficulty and frequent episodes of sinusitis.

Flashpoint

Approximately 80% of the population has some degree of septal deviation.

Incidence

The exact incidence of deviated septum is unknown, since many people do not seek treatment for it and may not even realize they have it. However, it is estimated that 80% of the population has some degree of septal deviation.

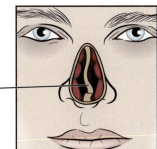

FIGURE 11-3 **Deviated septum**

Deviated or irregular nasal septum

Etiology

Many people are born with a deviated septum. Others develop the problem due to nasal trauma from accidents, sports injury, and other activities.

Signs and Symptoms

Some individuals complain of frequent sinusitis, especially if the sinus cavities are unable to drain properly. Others may complain of nasal stuffiness, nosebleeds, facial pain, headaches, or noisy breathing sounds during sleep. However, many people don't know that they have a deviated septum unless it is noted upon examination for some other reason.

Diagnosis

Deviated septum is easily diagnosed with physical examination. The physician examines the nasal passages using a nasal speculum and a light.

Treatment

Patients with a mildly deviated septum may require no treatment. Those with moderate deviation may benefit from medications such as decongestants, antihistamines, and nasally administered corticosteroids. These medications help to temporarily reduce nasal-membrane inflammation and edema and to open nasal passages. For a permanent solution, surgery may be necessary. Septoplasty is surgical repair of the septum to straighten and reposition it.

Prognosis

A deviated septum may be a minor nuisance for some people. For others it may have a significant impact on quality of life, contributing to frequent sinus infections, snoring, and sleep apnea. Prognosis for those who undergo appropriate treatment is very good.

Flashpoint
Septoplasty is a procedure to repair and straighten the septum.

Upper Respiratory Infection

ICD-9-CM: 465.9   [ICD-10: J06.9] (unspecified for both codes)

Incidence

Upper respiratory infections (URIs) are so common that they are often called the *common cold.*

It is estimated that there are more than one billion cases of URI in the United States each year. Often affected are children, who average three to eight colds each year.

Etiology

More than 200 viruses are known to cause the common cold. It is the most common reason people miss school and work. Upper respiratory infections are very contagious and are spread via the virus contained in the fluid from nasal secretions (see Box 11-1). Virus particles can become airborne when someone sneezes and may also be spread by hand-to-face contact. People are most contagious within the first 2 or 3 days of a cold.

Flashpoint
No wonder it's called the common cold: There are over a billion cases each year!

Signs and Symptoms

Common signs and symptoms of URI vary with the specific virus but generally include rhinitis (nasal inflammation), nasal congestion, sneezing, sore throat, cough, headache, muscle aches, decreased appetite, and malaise. Small children may run a fever up to 102°F, but older children

Box 11-1 Wellness Promotion

DON'T CATCH THE COMMON COLD
Follow these measures to protect yourself from catching the cold virus and help make the common cold less common.

Avoid
- Being in crowds during cold and flu season
- Sharing towels with others
- Inhaling secondhand smoke

Be Sure To
- Wash your hands frequently—after wiping your nose and toileting and before eating and preparing food.
- Use instant hand sanitizers when you can't wash.
- Clean commonly touched surfaces (doorknobs, shopping-cart handles, counter-tops, etc.) with disinfectants.
- Shop for a day care with six or fewer children, to reduce your child's exposure.
- Get enough sleep.
- Take a multivitamin.

Self-Care
- Drink plenty of water (at least eight glasses per day).
- Eat a balanced diet.
- Get regular exercise.
- Eat yogurt (bacteria in some active yogurts help prevent colds).
- Breastfeed infants.

and adults are usually afebrile. Symptoms occur within 2 or 3 days of exposure and usually last 7 to 10 days.

Diagnosis
Diagnosis is based upon a description of symptoms and physical-examination findings.

Treatment
Treatment of the common cold includes caffeine- and alcohol-free fluids and rest. Over-the-counter cold remedies may lessen some symptoms, and analgesics may relieve muscle aches and fever. Antibiotics are not appropriate, because they have no effect on viruses.

Flashpoint

To effectively rehydrate, fluids must be free of caffeine and alcohol.

Prognosis
Prognosis for those afflicted by URI is generally excellent. Complications may include secondary ear infection, sinus infection, bronchitis, pneumonia, and worsening of asthma in those with asthmatic conditions.

Sinusitis

| ICD-9-CM: 461.0–461.9 (acute, code by site), 473.0–473.9 (chronic, code by site) | [ICD-10: J01.0–J01.9 (acute, code by site), J32.0–J32.9 (chronic, code by site)] |

Sinusitis is a condition in which the lining of the sinus cavities becomes inflamed (see Fig. 11-4).

Incidence
An estimated 30 million people in the United States have sinusitis. Over $65 billion is spent each year on medical care and surgical treatments for sinus disease.

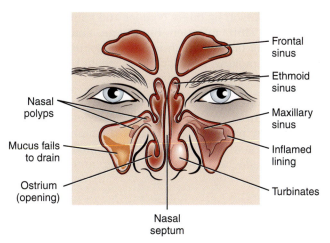

FIGURE 11-4 Sinusitis

Etiology

Sinusitis is caused when the sinus cavities become blocked due to swelling or growth of polyps. Primary contributors include bacterial and viral infections; other contributors include overuse of decongestant nasal sprays and smoking.

Signs and Symptoms

A common sign of acute sinusitis is when a cold seems to improve and then worsens again. Pressure or pain is often felt in the face, including the cheeks and forehead, between the eyes, and even in the teeth. Other symptoms may include nasal congestion, fever, malaise, and a cough and sore throat (due to postnasal drainage) that are worse in the mornings.

Diagnosis

Diagnosis is usually based upon a description of symptoms and physical-examination findings. In some cases sinus films may be done, including standard x-rays, computed tomography (CT), or magnetic resonance imaging (MRI).

Flashpoint

Pain from sinusitis can be felt in the cheeks and forehead, between the eyes, and even in the teeth.

Treatment

Antibiotics are prescribed for 10 to 14 days and should be taken until gone, even if symptoms begin to improve after a few days. Decongestants may also be prescribed. Other treatment includes rest, fluids, moist heat compresses, humidifiers, and hot showers (breathing in the steam).

Prognosis

Most people recover fully, with appropriate diagnosis and treatment. Potential complications include chronic sinusitis, osteomyelitis (bone infection), and orbital cellulitis (bacterial skin infection around the eyes).

Pharyngitis

ICD-9-CM: 462 (acute), 427.1 (chronic)   [ICD-10: J02 (acute), J31.2 (chronic)]
Pharyngitis, commonly called a *sore throat,* is inflammation of the pharynx.

Incidence

In the United States, children have an average of five cases and adults an average of two cases of pharyngitis per year.

Etiology

The usual causes of pharyngitis are a viral URI or seasonal allergies which cause postnasal drip, irritating the throat. Organisms that may be responsible for bacterial pharyngitis include streptococci, *Mycoplasma pneumoniae, Chlamydophila pneumoniae,* and *Neisseria gonorrhoeae.*

Infection is spread from person to person by direct contact and contact with oral secretions. Other causes of pharyngitis include sinus infection, diphtheria, and mononucleosis caused by Epstein-Barr virus (EBV). Risk factors which make people more vulnerable to pharyngitis include inhaling pollutants, smoking, and breathing secondhand smoke.

Signs and Symptoms

The throat is described as scratchy and sore, which makes swallowing painful and difficult. Upon examination, the throat appears red and edematous. Tonsils may be swollen and covered with white or gray patches. Cervical (neck) lymph nodes are usually tender and swollen. Individuals with a strep infection will have similar, but more severe, symptoms. They may also complain of headache and abdominal pain and may have a fever as high as 104°F.

Diagnosis

Diagnosis is based upon a description of symptoms and physical-examination findings. In some cases a throat culture may be used to differentiate viral from bacterial pharyngitis. A rapid strep test, which provides results within 15 minutes, may be done to identify whether the patient has a strep infection. However, a negative result must be confirmed by culture, since the test is not 100% accurate.

Treatment

Viral pharyngitis usually resolves without medication and responds well to conservative treatment, including analgesics and warm saline gargles. Antibiotics are prescribed for bacterial pharyngitis. Those who suffer from chronic infections may benefit from a tonsillectomy.

Prognosis

Most people recover fully with conservative treatment. However, potential complications include rheumatic fever, scarlet fever (with streptococcal infections), tonsil abscess, and glomerulonephritis.

Allergic Rhinitis

ICD-9-CM: 477.0–477.9   [ICD-10: J30.1–J30.4] (code by allergen for both codes)
Rhinitis is inflammation of the nasal membranes. The most common cause is allergies.

Incidence

Allergic rhinitis affects approximately 20% of the population in the United States. Costs associated with treating allergic rhinitis and its complications are estimated at over $5 billion per year.

Etiology

The primary risk factor for allergic rhinitis is a genetic predisposition. Susceptible people develop a sensitivity to certain allergens and then experience allergic reactions when subsequently reexposed. Common triggers include pollen, dust, mold, and pet dander.

Signs and Symptoms

Common signs and symptoms of allergic rhinitis include sneezing, nasal congestion, itching, redness, postnasal drip, rhinorrhea (runny nose), and sinus congestion. Systemic symptoms may include malaise, fatigue, and sleepiness. Symptoms may last for hours or days.

Diagnosis

Diagnosis of allergic rhinitis is based upon description of symptoms and physical-examination findings.

Treatment

Patients with allergic rhinitis may be treated with medications such as antihistamines, decongestants, and nasal steroids. They may decrease their exposure to allergens by using air filters in the home and workplace. They may also discuss allergy desensitization with an allergy specialist. This is accomplished through a series of injections.

Prognosis

Allergies are generally chronic but can usually be managed reasonably well with medications. Complications may include otitis media (middle ear infection) and acute or chronic sinusitis.

Laryngitis

ICD-9-CM: 464.0 (acute), 476.0 (chronic)   **[ICD-10: J04.0 (acute), J37.0 (chronic)]**

Laryngitis is a condition of inflammation of the larynx (voice box). It is usually evidenced by a temporary loss of the voice (hoarseness).

Incidence

The exact incidence of laryngitis is not clear, since people often treat themselves and do not see a physician unless complications arise. However, it is known to be very common.

Etiology

Any condition that causes inflammation and swelling of the larynx can cause laryngitis. Acute cases last less than 3 weeks and chronic cases last longer than 3 weeks. Among the most common causes of acute laryngitis are the many strains of cold viruses and influenza viruses. Other types of viral and bacterial infection may be responsible as well. Examples include measles, pertussis, bronchitis, and EBV. Overuse of the voice and exacerbation of allergies may also be responsible. Chronic laryngitis may be caused by asthma inhalers, cigarette smoke, and pollution. Individuals with chronic laryngitis should be evaluated by their health-care provider, since it can also be a sign of throat cancer.

Signs and Symptoms

The primary symptom of laryngitis is partial or complete loss of the voice. Other symptoms may be those associated with the underlying disorder that triggered the laryngitis, including sore throat, tender or swollen lymph nodes, congestion, rhinorrhea, cough, dyspnea, fatigue, fever, and malaise.

Flashpoint
Chronic laryngitis should be evaluated, because it could be a sign of throat cancer.

Diagnosis

Diagnosis is usually based upon the patient's complaints of symptoms and physical examination. Upon examination, the oropharynx may appear reddened and tonsils may be enlarged and inflamed. Examination of the larynx with a tiny mirror or nasolaryngoscope will help the physician identify redness and swelling. The physician may also examine the patient's eyes, ears, nose, and lungs for other evidence of a respiratory infection. Individuals with chronic hoarseness may be referred to an ENT specialist for further evaluation.

Treatment

Most individuals with acute laryngitis respond well to self-care measures such as rest, analgesics, fluids, avoidance of smoke, and use of a humidifier. More severe cases may require treatment with corticosteroids. Antibiotics are not helpful unless a bacterial infection is the cause.

Prognosis

Prognosis is excellent for most individuals with acute laryngitis, with recovery in 7 days or so. In rare cases, airway obstruction could be a complication of related infections, such as epiglottitis or croup. Prognosis for those with chronic laryngitis is generally good but depends upon the underlying cause and the timeliness of diagnosis and treatment.

Nasal Polyps

ICD-9-CM: 471.9   [ICD-10: J33.9] (unspecified for both codes)

Nasal polyps are rounded tissue growths on the nasal or sinus mucosa (see Fig. 11-5). They may be very small or large enough to block the passageway and impede breathing. They are usually not cancerous.

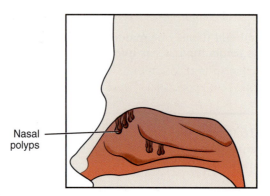

FIGURE 11-5 Nasal polyps

Incidence

Nasal polyps are most common in people who have asthma, allergies, or frequent sinus infections. They are most common in adults, although children with cystic fibrosis also often develop them.

Etiology

The reason that nasal polyps form is not well understood. However, it is known that they develop in response to tissue inflammation caused by allergies, asthma, and infections, and in response to the presence of foreign bodies. They are also more common in those with cystic fibrosis and those who are allergic to aspirin. In some cases nasal polyps disappear after infection clears, but in other cases they persist.

Signs and Symptoms

People are often unaware that they have nasal polyps until they are examined by a physician. Common complaints include nasal congestion, runny nose, postnasal drip, sneezing, reduced sense of smell and taste, snoring, facial pain and headaches, itching around the eyes, and chronic infections.

Diagnosis

The physician is usually able to detect some of the polyps on physical examination. More detailed examination may be done by nasal endoscopy, in which an instrument with a tiny camera or magnifying lens is used to examine the inner nasal passages. CT scan may also be done. The sweat test may be done on children to rule out cystic fibrosis. It is a noninvasive test that measures the amount of salt in perspiration. Allergy tests may also be done to identify specific allergies that contribute to the problem.

Treatment

Corticosteroid medication may be used to reduce the size of nasal polyps; however, surgery is often needed to eliminate them. Antibiotics may be used if infection is a contributing factor. Underlying disorders such as allergies may be treated with antihistamines.

Prognosis

Polyps often prevent sinuses from properly draining and therefore contribute to frequent sinus infections. They may also contribute to obstructive sleep apnea. Results of surgery are generally good. However, polyps sometimes grow back, especially if the underlying disorder (such as allergies) continues.

Epistaxis

ICD-9-CM: 784.7   [ICD-10: R04.0]

Epistaxis, commonly known as a *nosebleed*, is an episode of bleeding from the nose. Blood loss is usually minor, although major hemorrhage is possible. Epistaxis is classified as anterior or posterior depending on the location of the bleeding. Anterior epistaxis is the more common, less serious form; posterior epistaxis is less common but is likely to be more serious.

Incidence
Epistaxis is very common, occurring in both genders in one in every seven people. Incidence is greatest among young people between 2 and 10 years old and those over age 50.

Etiology
The mucous-membrane lining of the nasal passages is very vascular. Therefore, simple forms of traumatic injury can cause bleeding. Examples include blowing the nose, repeated sneezing, injuries to the nose, picking the nose, and foreign bodies. Risk increases with use of nasal sprays, cold or dry air, use of nonhumidified oxygen, hypertension, alcohol consumption, allergies, sinusitis, pregnancy, clotting disorders, and use of aspirin or anticoagulant medication.

Signs and Symptoms
The primary sign of epistaxis is bleeding from the nose. Physical discomfort may or may not be present. Swallowing blood typically causes nausea.

Diagnosis
Diagnosis is based upon presenting signs and symptoms. For mild to moderate epistaxis, no diagnostic tests are needed. If bleeding is severe or prolonged, testing might include nasal endoscopy, skull x-rays, CT scan, and complete blood count (CBC). Coagulation tests may also be done, including prothrombin time, international normalized ratio, and partial thromboplastin time.

Treatment
In most cases, simple first-aid measures are sufficient to stop epistaxis. This includes applying direct pressure to the soft part of the nose for at least 10 minutes. To prevent nausea, the individual should lean forward and spit blood out rather than swallow it. More severe epistaxis may require treatment by a medical professional. Measures include cauterization with silver nitrate sticks, application of vasoconstricting decongestant nasal sprays, and nasal packing. A calcium alginate mesh called NasalCEASE may be placed to speed coagulation. In rare cases endoscopic surgery is needed to stop the bleeding.

Prognosis
Prognosis is excellent with proper intervention. Potential complications include hypovolemia (state of decreased blood volume), anemia, infection, sinusitis, and aspiration.

Common Lower Respiratory System Diseases and Disorders

There are numerous lower respiratory diseases and disorders. Some infectious illness are pneumonia, legionellosis, histoplasmosis, influenza, pulmonary tuberculosis, and Epstein-Barr virus. Obstructive disorders of the lower respiratory system include bronchitis, bronchiectasis, pulmonary emphysema, asthma, and pneumoconiosis. Yet other conditions include pulmonary embolism, pleurisy, pulmonary edema, pleural effusion, pneumothorax, hemothorax, and acute respiratory distress syndrome (ARDS).

Pulmonary Embolism

ICD-9-CM: 415.19　　　[ICD-10: I26.9] (unspecified for both codes)
Pulmonary embolism (PE) is a common, life-threatening condition that occurs when a blood clot or other matter becomes lodged in an artery in the lungs (see Fig. 11-6).

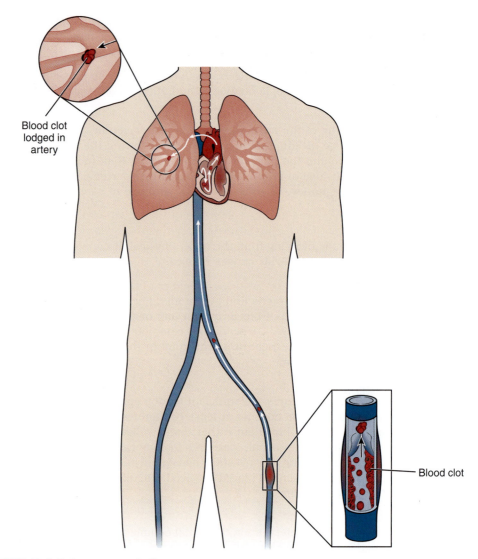

FIGURE 11-6 Pulmonary embolism

Incidence

More than 650,000 individuals die from PE each year in the United States, making it the third-most common cause of death. It is most common among hospitalized patients, although there are many other risk factors. It affects people from all racial groups and both genders, although incidence is increased among women taking oral contraceptives. PE affects all age groups, but risk does increase with advanced age.

Flashpoint

More than 650,000 people die from PE in the United States each year!

Etiology

PE most commonly is a complication of deep vein thrombosis (DVT), particularly in the veins of the lower legs. DVT develops in the veins as a result of venous stasis (congestion or sluggish blood flow), hypercoagulability (tendency to form blood clots), and inflammation in the vein wall. These three factors are sometimes called the *Virchow triad*. When all or part of the clot breaks free from the vessel wall, it travels with flowing blood until it reaches a vessel too small to let it pass, nearly always in the lungs. This not only disrupts blood flow through the lungs but also results in increased pressure as the heart pumps harder to try to push blood through the blocked pulmonary capillary bed. As a result, the patient may suffer from cor pulmonale, a type of heart failure. There are many risk factors for PE but the most common include a previous history of PE or DVT, pregnancy, lengthy immobilization, recent surgery, cancer, obesity, and smoking.

Signs and Symptoms

Symptoms of PE include dyspnea, anxiety, **hemoptysis** (spitting or coughing up blood from the respiratory tract), wheezing, cyanosis, diaphoresis, tachycardia, and chest pain, especially during inspiration. However, many patients do not present with these classic symptoms. Many have atypical symptoms such as syncope, abdominal pain, high fever, new onset of heart arrhythmia, or even hiccups.

Diagnosis

Diagnosis is based upon presenting signs and symptoms and diagnostic studies. The physician may choose from a variety of tests to confirm diagnosis; the most definitive is pulmonary angiography, although it is riskier than some of the others and therefore is not always done first. Chest x-ray may be done to rule out other lung disorders. Electrocardiography (ECG) will help to rule out myocardial infarction or arrhythmia problems. Blood will be drawn to check cardiac enzymes and D-dimer. The latter helps to identify whether DVT is a factor. Other studies may include lung scan, lung spiral CT, and duplex ultrasound of veins in the legs.

> **Flashpoint**
> Hemoptysis is coughing up blood from the respiratory tract.

Treatment

Patients with PE are treated with injections of anticoagulant medication, followed by oral anticoagulants for several months. A very large PE might be treated with thrombolytic medication, or in some cases, surgically removed by thrombectomy or embolectomy.

Prognosis

Prognosis for patients with PE is widely variable and depends upon the severity and on the timeliness of diagnosis and treatment. A massive PE may be immediately fatal. Approximately one-third of those who go undiagnosed and untreated do not survive. On the other hand, those with minor PEs may be completely unaware of the problem. Individuals who suffer one PE are at risk for another and for cor pulmonale in the future.

Pneumonia

ICD-9-CM: 480.0–480.9 (viral, by organism), 482.0–482.9 (bacterial, by organism)   **[ICD-10: J12.0–J12.9, J13, J14 (viral, by organism), J15.0–J15.9 (bacterial, by organism)]**

Pneumonia is an infection of the lungs, which may be mild or severe, and in some cases, is life-threatening.

Incidence

More than three million people in the United States develop pneumonia each year, and more than a half million of them are hospitalized. Most recover fully, but approximately 5% die.

> **Flashpoint**
> More than three million Americans develop pneumonia every year.

Etiology

Pneumonia may be caused by bacteria, viruses, or chemical irritants. In some cases, an infectious organism becomes airborne when an ill person coughs or sneezes. If it is inhaled by another person and grows in the lungs, then pneumonia may develop. Aspiration (inhalation) of chemical irritants, such as stomach fluids, food, or drink, might occur during CPR or a choking episode. Those at greatest risk of developing pneumonia include those with weakened immune systems, chronic lung disease, heart disease, alcoholism, seizure disorders, and swallowing disorders.

Signs and Symptoms

Those with pneumonia usually develop coldlike symptoms followed by a fever. Other symptoms include a productive cough, shaking chills, shortness of breath, chest pain with deep breaths, muscle aches, and malaise.

Diagnosis

Diagnosis is based upon a description of symptoms, physical-examination findings, and a chest x-ray. Lung sounds heard upon auscultation usually include **wheezes** (musical sound caused by narrowed air passages) and *crackles* (abnormal lung sound heard on auscultation that indicates fluid in the alveoli), which are caused by inflammation of the airways and fluid accumulation (see Fig. 11-7). A sputum (respiratory secretions) sample may be collected and examined in the laboratory to identify the causative microorganism. A culture and sensitivity test may be done to determine the most appropriate antimicrobial for treatment. Examination of a blood sample may reveal increased white blood cells (WBCs).

Treatment

Treatment is based on the cause. Bacterial pneumonia is treated with antibiotics; patients with other forms of pneumonia are usually treated with supportive care including oxygen, fluids, and respiratory support.

Prognosis

In past years, a third of those infected died from pneumonia; but since the advent of antimicrobial medications, most people recover. Therefore, prognosis and survival is generally good.

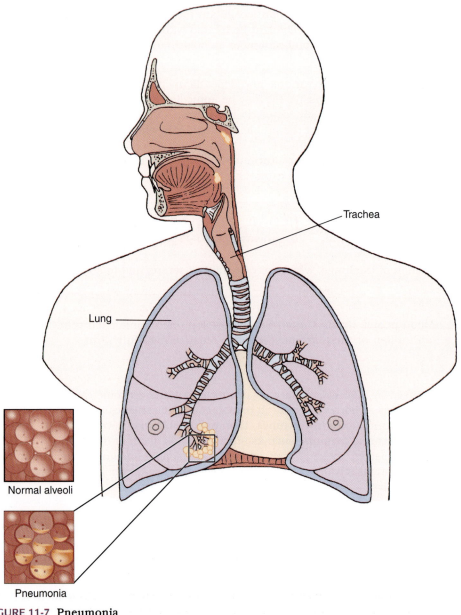

Trachea

Lung

Normal alveoli

Pneumonia

FIGURE 11-7 Pneumonia

However, there is a 5% mortality rate, usually affecting patients in a weakened state. Complications include pleural effusion and **empyema** (collection of fluid in the pleural space containing infectious matter, such as bacteria and white blood cells).

Legionellosis

ICD-9-CM: 482.84   [ICD-10: A48.1]

Legionellosis is a bacterial lung infection caused by *Legionella pneumophila*. It was identified and given its name after an outbreak among people at an American Legion convention in 1976. It was also identified as having two forms: the more serious Legionnaires' disease and the milder Pontiac fever.

Incidence

As many as 18,000 Americans develop Legionnaires' disease each year; an unknown number of people contract Pontiac fever. Outbreaks, which gain the most attention, usually occur in the summer or early fall. However, most patients contract the disease on an individual basis rather than as part of an outbreak. At greatest risk are those over age 65, those with weak immune systems, those who smoke, and those with chronic lung disease.

Flashpoint

There are two forms of legionellosis: Legionnaires' disease and the milder Pontiac fever.

Etiology

The *Legionella* bacteria thrive in warm (95°F to 115°F), stagnant water, like that found in hot-water tanks, cooling towers, large air-conditioning systems, and spas in public places like hotels, hospitals, and workplaces. People become infected by breathing in contaminated mist. The illness is not spread by person-to-person contact.

Signs and Symptoms

Flashpoint

Legionella bacteria thrive in warm, stagnant water.

Symptoms begin 2 to 14 days after exposure and include flu-like symptoms of fever, chills, fatigue, anorexia, muscle aches, and headaches. Legionnaires' disease may cause severe pneumonia, leading to respiratory failure. Pontiac fever causes a milder version of the same symptoms without pneumonia.

Diagnosis

Diagnosis of pneumonia may be suspected based upon history and physical examination, but Legionnaires' disease must be confirmed with laboratory tests. Chest x-ray will reveal areas of density indicating lung congestion consistent with pneumonia. A urinary antigen test can detect the *Legionella* bacteria in a urine sample. Confirmation may also be obtained by identifying the organism in a sputum specimen or biopsied lung tissue. Blood can also be checked for antibodies, but this takes several weeks and occurs after the fact.

Treatment

Legionellosis responds well to antibiotics if identified and treated early enough. Most commonly used are agents from the fluoroquinolone, macrolide, and tetracycline classes. Pontiac fever usually does not require antibiotic therapy.

Prognosis

Individuals with Pontiac fever experience a limited course of an influenza-like illness but do not develop pneumonia. They recover within 5 days without any special treatment. Those affected with Legionnaires' disease can become very ill with pneumonia. Healthy individuals usually recover, but those with a weakened immune system may not. The mortality rate is between 5% and 30%.

Histoplasmosis

ICD-9-CM: 115.05   [ICD-10:B39.2]

Histoplasmosis, also known as *Darling disease*, is a fungal disease caused by *Histoplasma capsulatum* (see Fig. 11-8). It most commonly affects the lungs but can affect other organs.

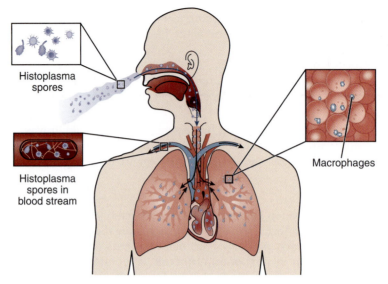

FIGURE 11-8 Histoplasmosis

Incidence

The histoplasmosis fungus is extremely common in many parts of the world. It is estimated that 80% of those living in such areas have been infected. But not everyone who becomes infected becomes ill; therefore, many people do not know they have it.

Etiology

H. capsulatum is present in soil contaminated with bird or bat droppings and can become airborne as dust is stirred into the air. People at greatest risk of infection are those who work with the soil, including landscapers, farmers, construction workers, gardeners, archeologists, and geologists. After being inhaled into the lungs, the microscopic spores settle in the alveoli, germinate, and grow. Macrophages trap some of them and carry them to lymph nodes in the chest, as well as to other parts of the body, via the bloodstream. In individuals with a weak immune system, this can cause systemic illness that can be fatal. This illness cannot be passed from one person to another. Those at greatest risk of becoming ill include the very young and the very old, those with HIV or AIDS, those receiving chemotherapy, and those taking immunosuppressive medications.

> **Flashpoint**
>
> *Histoplasma capsulatum* is very common in the soil, so farmers and others who work with soil are at risk.

Signs and Symptoms

Most people do not become ill and therefore may exhibit no signs or symptoms. However, those who do will begin to feel ill approximately 10 to 12 days after exposure. They will have flu-like symptoms of fever, chills, sweats, headache, dry cough, chest pains, and weight loss. Those with widespread disease exhibit a wide variety of symptoms, since most major organ systems become involved. They can develop pneumonia, anemia, meningitis, pericarditis, adrenal problems, and ulcerations in the mouth or intestinal system. They will very likely die without treatment.

> **Flashpoint**
>
> Many infected people do not become ill with histoplasmosis, but those who do may die without treatment.

Diagnosis

Diagnosis may or may not be suspected based upon the patient's presenting signs and symptoms. A good medical history should indicate whether exposure was likely and whether the patient may have a suppressed immune system. Laboratory tests on sputum, blood, or tissue samples are needed to confirm diagnosis. The most reliable test, a fungal culture, can take several weeks to grow. Therefore, serology (blood) tests are done to identify the presence of antigens and antibodies. Chest x-ray or CT may be done to identify inflammation, enlarged lymph nodes, or other complications. If tissue biopsy is required, a bronchoscopy may be done (see Box 11-2). This also allows the physician to visually examine the airways of the lungs.

Box 11-2 Diagnostic Spotlight

BRONCHOSCOPY

Bronchoscopy may be used for diagnostic or therapeutic purposes. It is a procedure in which the physician inserts a lighted scope with a tiny camera through the mouth or nose into the air passages to identify tumors, take tissue specimens, or remove foreign objects.

- A chest x-ray will likely be done beforehand to help the physician identify areas to examine during the procedure.
- The patient should not eat or drink for 8 to 10 hours before the procedure.
- The patient will be asked to empty his or her bladder just before the procedure and to remove dentures, eyeglasses or contacts, hearing aids, jewelry, etc.
- The patient will be given medication to help him or her relax, to numb the throat, and to dry up oral secretions.
- The patient must have someone available to drive him or her home.
- The patient's ability to breathe will be uninterrupted.
- The patient will be monitored throughout the procedure, which usually takes 1 hour or less.
- Results of a biopsy or culture will usually be available 2 to 7 days later.

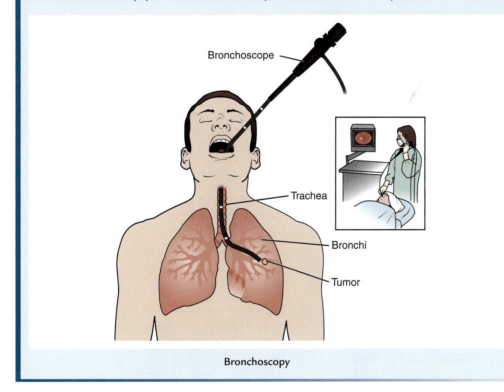

Bronchoscope

Trachea

Bronchi

Tumor

Bronchoscopy

Treatment

Individuals who are asymptomatic or have very mild cases do not require treatment. Those with severe or chronic illness are treated with antifungal medication. Occasionally, those with severe respiratory disease are also given corticosteroids.

Prognosis

Prognosis is excellent for those with mild infection but is more guarded for those with severe illness. People with disseminated disease will die without treatment. Potential serious complications for those with severe disease include lymph-node enlargement,

Flashpoint

There are many possible complications for patients with histoplasmosis.

pericarditis, arthritis, adrenal insufficiency, meningitis, hepatomegaly, splenomegaly, fibrosing mediastinitis (development of scar tissue that begins blocking the esophagus, large blood vessels, and other structures in the chest), and ocular (eye) involvement leading to vision loss.

Influenza

ICD-9-CM: 487.1   [ICD-10: J10.1]

Influenza, commonly called the *flu,* is a common, contagious, acute viral respiratory illness (see Fig. 11-9). Outbreaks can occur as often as every year.

Incidence

Approximately 20% of the U.S. population gets the flu each year, over 200,000 are hospitalized, and more than 35,000 die. Those at greatest risk are the very young and very old and those with chronic health disorders and weakened immune systems.

Flashpoint

More than 35,000 Americans die from influenza every year.

Etiology

There are a number of flu viruses, often categorized as types A, B, and C. Types A and B cause the flu that circulates almost every winter; occasionally, a stronger strain of these types causes a deadly pandemic or more serious local outbreak. Types A and B are constantly changing, with new strains appearing regularly, while type C is more stable. All three commonly spread from person to person in respiratory droplets and secretions through coughing, sneezing, and kissing. They may also be spread through contact with surfaces with viruses on them (doorknobs, etc.) followed by contact with the mouth or nose. A person may be infectious up to 1 day before symptoms develop and up to 5 days after.

Flashpoint

Influenza is easily spread through respiratory droplets and secretions.

Signs and Symptoms

The most common signs and symptoms of the flu include fever as high as 105ºF, chills, sweats, anorexia, headache, muscle aches, nasal congestion or rhinitis, fatigue, sore throat, and dry cough. Occasionally patients also complain of gastrointestinal symptoms such as nausea, vomiting, and diarrhea.

Diagnosis

Diagnosis of influenza is usually based upon physical-examination findings and description of symptoms. Confirmation of diagnosis may be made from a throat culture. If secondary bacterial pneumonia is suspected, a sputum specimen may be collected and cultured.

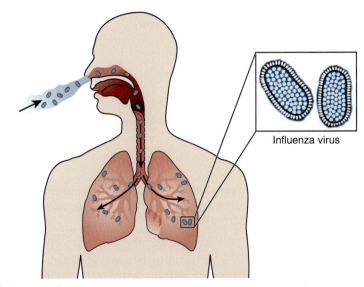

Influenza virus

FIGURE 11-9 Influenza virus

Treatment

Treatment of the flu is usually aimed as supportive care and includes fluids, rest, and antipyretic (fever-reducing) and analgesic medication. Sore throat may be soothed by warm saltwater gargles and throat lozenges. In some cases, antiviral medication may be helpful. Antibiotics are not effective against the flu virus but may be appropriate for secondary bacterial infections. Aspirin should not be given to children because of the risk of Reye syndrome. Education is aimed at prevention, with an emphasis on flu vaccination (see Box 11-3) and standard precautions such as hand washing. In severe cases, hospitalization may be needed.

Prognosis

Most people recover fully from influenza. However, complications may include dehydration, bacterial pneumonia, bronchitis, and sinus or ear infections.

> **Flashpoint**
> Antibiotics do not help patients who are ill with influenza, because it is caused by a virus.

Pulmonary Tuberculosis

ICD-9-CM: 011.90   [ICD-10: A15.9] (unspecified for both codes)

Pulmonary tuberculosis (TB) is a contagious lung infection caused by an organism called *Mycobacterium tuberculosis*. The infection can also spread to and affect other organ systems.

Incidence

It is estimated that between 10% and 30% of the population is affected by TB. However, this varies widely. Populations that experience poverty, crowding, unsanitary conditions, malnutrition, and poor access to health care suffer higher rates than others. Pulmonary TB is acquired most commonly by individuals whose immune systems are weakened and do not isolate the primary infection. This includes the very young, the very old, and the immunocompromised.

Etiology

Primary infection with *M. tuberculosis* usually begins in the lungs, after inhalation of the bacterium. In most cases the lungs successfully encapsulate the infection, and the individual recovers without further complications. Pulmonary TB develops several weeks after the primary infection or may develop or recur after lying dormant for a number of years. Those who are immunocompromised are more likely to experience such reactivation at a later time.

> **Flashpoint**
> TB is most common among those who experience poverty, crowding, unsanitary conditions, malnutrition, and poor access to health care.

Box 11-3 Wellness Promotion

INFLUENZA VACCINATION

Influenza vaccination helps prevent or minimize influenza outbreaks and the many complications caused by this illness. Guidelines for vaccination include:

- Vaccination is recommended for health-care providers and vulnerable individuals, such as the elderly, residents of long-term care facilities, those with cancer and lung disease, those with weakened immune systems, infants between 6 and 23 months old, and children on long-term aspirin therapy.
- Individuals should consult with their physician before being vaccinated.
- Influenza vaccination should **not** be given to individuals:
  - who have allergies to chicken or eggs
  - who have experienced a previous severe reaction to flu vaccine
  - who have a history of Guillain-Barré syndrome in the past 6 weeks
  - who are under 6 months old
  - who are currently ill with a febrile illness

Signs and Symptoms

Up to 20% of individuals may be asymptomatic. Others present with productive cough, hemoptysis, fever, night sweats, weight loss, anorexia, fatigue, chest pain, and dyspnea.

Diagnosis

Diagnosis of TB is based upon history, presenting symptoms, and physical-examination findings. Upon auscultation, the lungs may have crackles. Other findings include enlargement and tenderness of the cervical lymph nodes. Diagnostic testing may include chest x-ray, sputum cultures, bronchoscopy, and a tuberculin skin test. It is important to note that a positive TB skin test indicates exposure but does not confirm the presence of active disease. Furthermore, an individual who has tested positive will always test positive thereafter; therefore, skin testing is of no further use for that person. Other tests for tuberculosis may include a thoracentesis and chest CT.

Flashpoint

A positive TB skin test indicates that the individual has been exposed but does not confirm the presence of active disease.

Treatment

A course of treatment usually lasts 6 months or longer and includes multiple drugs. All anti-tubercular drugs have some toxicity; thorough patient education and careful monitoring are important. The importance of completing treatment should be stressed so that the patient can prevent relapse and reduce the risk of antibiotic resistance.

Prognosis

Symptoms generally resolve within 3 weeks, although chest x-ray will not reveal improvement until later. Prognosis is excellent if the disease is diagnosed and treated early. Delayed treatment can result in permanent lung damage. Incomplete treatment contributes to the emergence of drug-resistant strains of the disease.

Epstein-Barr Virus

ICD-9-CM: 075   [ICD-10: B27.0]

Infectious mononucleosis, often called *mono* and also known as *glandular fever*, is an infection caused by the Epstein-Barr virus (EBV), a member of the herpesvirus family that is a common human virus.

Incidence

The Epstein-Barr virus is extremely common—it has infected an estimated 95% of adults under age 40. When individuals are infected with the virus during their teen or young adult years, it causes infectious mononucleosis between 35% and 50% of the time. Younger children are often asymptomatic or have such mild cases that they are indistinguishable from other mild viruses. Adults older than age 35 rarely have an active infection.

Flashpoint

It is estimated that 95% of young adults have been infected with the Epstein-Barr virus.

Etiology

EBV is transmitted by intimate contact with saliva of an infected person. This is why it has often been called the "kissing disease" among young people. It is not usually transmitted via air like cold viruses are, and is not transmitted via blood. Because many healthy people have the virus and don't know it, most are not at significant risk of acquiring an active infection from anyone else. Therefore, no special precautions are recommended.

Signs and Symptoms

The active infection lasts about 4 weeks, with symptoms of fever, pharyngitis, cervical lymphadenopathy (swelling and tenderness of the lymph nodes), headaches, fatigue, and anorexia. Splenomegaly or hepatomegaly may develop. If symptoms last longer than 4 months, chronic EBV infection may be present; however, this may be confused with chronic fatigue syndrome and should be further investigated.

Flashpoint

Chronic EBV is sometimes confused with chronic fatigue syndrome.

Diagnosis

Diagnosis is based upon history, description of symptoms, and diagnostic tests. The most common test is the Monospot test, also called the *Paul-Bunnell test*, which identifies certain antibodies produced by infection with EBV. Other tests include antinuclear antibody and

CBC, which may reveal elevated WBC count generally and elevation in a specific type of WBC called lymphocytes.

Treatment

There is no cure for EBV; treatment is aimed at relieving symptoms and includes bedrest, fluids, and analgesics. Corticosteroids may be considered in some cases to help relieve pharyngitis and lymphadenopathy. Sports and demanding physical activities should be avoided, due to risk of splenic rupture, until the physician says it is safe to participate. Aspirin should not be given to young people. Because EBV is a virus, it does not respond to antibiotics.

Prognosis

Symptoms usually resolve within 4 weeks, and complete recovery occurs within 3 to 4 months. Once a person is infected, the virus often remains dormant in the body. In most cases it causes no further problems for the individual; however, in rare cases it can play a role in the development of Burkitt lymphoma and nasopharyngeal carcinoma. A rare but serious complication is splenic rupture, which can cause life-threatening hemorrhage.

Chronic Obstructive Pulmonary Disease

Chronic obstructive pulmonary disease (COPD), also known as *chronic obstructive lung disease (COLD)*, affects 11% of the American population. It refers to a variety of lung disorders that create obstructive changes in the bronchi and alveoli. These disorders include chronic bronchitis, bronchiectasis, pulmonary emphysema, asthma, and pneumoconiosis. The greatest risk factor for COPD is smoking, but others include air pollution, occupational exposure to dust and chemicals, and repeated lower respiratory infections (see Box 11-4). While the initial cause may be different in each case, the result is similar: severe lung damage and impaired air exchange. As the lungs become less functional, chronic air-trapping occurs and structural changes develop. Chest dimension becomes more barrel-like and the lungs flatten on the bottom and rob the diaphragm (an important respiratory muscle) of its effectiveness (see Fig. 11-10). Cilia in the airway normally move foreign debris upward to be coughed out, but when cigarette smoke is a contributing factor, they become clogged with tar and dysfunctional.

Flashpoint
The greatest risk factor for COPD is smoking.

Box 11-4 Wellness Promotion

SELF-CARE MEASURES FOR PATIENTS WITH COPD

Patients with COPD can improve immediate and long-term quality of life by following these guidelines:

- Stop or reduce smoking. Information on smoking-cessation programs is available from your health-care provider.
- Do not smoke or use flames around oxygen.
- Avoid secondhand smoke and other forms of air pollution.
- Avoid exposure to others with contagious respiratory disorders.
- Obtain an annual influenza vaccination.
- Pay attention to your nutritional needs:
  - Plan small, nutritious meals with between-meal snacks.
  - Consider drinking high-energy, nutritious supplements, such as Ensure.
  - Take a daily multivitamin.
- Take medication as prescribed.
- Keep emergency medication (such as an inhaler) handy.
- Pace your activities and take frequent rest breaks.
- Use pursed-lip breathing when you feel severely short of breath.
- Keep well-hydrated to help thin respiratory secretions.

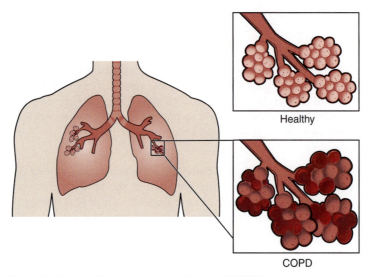

FIGURE 11-10 Chronic obstructive pulmonary disease (COPD)

The net result of all of these physical changes is that patients will begin to experience some or all of the following symptoms:

- **Orthopnea:** The need to remain upright in order to breathe effectively. Physicians often quantify the severity of orthopnea by referring to the number of pillows the patient must recline against while sleeping (e.g., three-pillow orthopnea).
- **Hypercapnea:** The chronic retention of CO_2, leading to symptoms of mental cloudiness and lethargy. In some cases, it also changes the way the person's body determines when to breathe. Breathing becomes triggered by the hypoxic drive, and the urge to breathe is based on too low an O_2 level. In individuals with healthy lungs, by contrast, the drive to breathe is normally stimulated by dropping pH levels as the blood becomes more acidic; this is directly related to the rising CO_2 level. The hypoxic drive becomes a problem when the person with COPD needs supplemental O_2. If health-care providers give too much, it could actually knock out the individual's drive to breathe, leading to respiratory arrest.
- **Chronic hypoxia:** A chronic lack of oxygen. As gas exchange becomes less effective, breathing becomes more and more difficult. Eventually the person becomes dependent on supplemental oxygen. Yet in the last stages of the disease, supplemental O_2 provides little relief, and the patient becomes severely dyspneic with even the slightest exertion.

No matter the cause of a patient's COPD, many important self-care measures are the same. The sooner patients begin these measures, the better their prognosis will be.

Flashpoint

Supplemental oxygen is of little help in the final stages of COPD.

Bronchitis
ICD-9-CM: 466.0 (acute), 491.0 (chronic)   **[ICD-10: J60.9 (acute), J42 (chronic)]**
Acute bronchitis is an infection of the bronchial passages and is usually caused by a virus (see Fig. 11-11). Chronic bronchitis is similar, but the condition persists for months or even years.

Incidence
Those most vulnerable to bronchitis are those who smoke and those who have chronic respiratory conditions.

Etiology
Bronchitis is usually caused by the same viruses that cause the common cold. Less commonly, the cause may be bacterial or—rarely—fungal. The infection is spread the same way the common cold is spread, by respiratory secretions from coughing or sneezing and by direct contact.

Flashpoint

Bronchitis is caused by the same viruses that cause the common cold.

Signs and Symptoms
The most common symptom of bronchitis is a persistent cough that is usually productive of thick sputum. Other symptoms include wheezing, shortness of breath, and mild

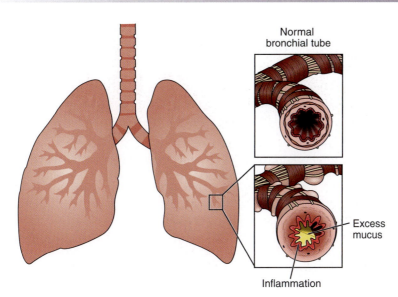

FIGURE 11-11 Bronchitis

fever. The acute phase usually lasts a week or so but the cough may continue for several weeks. Lungs are usually clear to auscultation, but occasional scattered wheezes and crackles may be heard. The primary symptom of chronic bronchitis is a productive, chronic cough that is generally worse in the mornings. Symptoms are worsened by respiratory infections.

Diagnosis

Diagnosis is usually based upon history and presenting symptoms. Testing may be done to rule out other disorders and may include chest x-ray, pulmonary function tests, blood and sputum analysis, and arterial blood gases (see Box 11-5).

Flashpoint
Chronic bronchitis causes a chronic productive cough that is usually worse in the mornings.

Treatment

Because the cause of acute bronchitis is usually viral, antibiotics will not help. Treatment is usually conservative and includes fluids, rest, humidifiers, and cough medication. A cough that is productive of thick secretions may be treated with expectorant medication, which helps loosen and liquefy secretions so they are more easily expelled. Coughs that are nonproductive may be suppressed with antitussive medication. In some cases, bronchodilator medication may be used to help open narrowed airways, and corticosteroids may be used to suppress inflammation. Those with chronic bronchitis may eventually need oxygen therapy and more aggressive pulmonary care, including percussion and drainage. Smokers are encouraged to stop or at least reduce the number of cigarettes smoked each day. If a secondary bacterial infection is suspected, antibiotics may be prescribed.

Prognosis

Those with acute bronchitis usually recover completely, although the cough may linger for several weeks. The prognosis for those with chronic bronchitis is more guarded because of the cumulative damage, which results in obstructive changes.

Flashpoint
Antibiotics may not help bronchitis, since the cause is usually viral.

Bronchiectasis
ICD-9-CM: 494.0   [ICD-10: J47]

Bronchiectasis is a condition of chronic, irreversible dilation (widening) of portions of the bronchi. It may be congenital (present at birth) or may develop from the damaging effects of a long-standing infection.

Incidence

It is unclear exactly how many people have bronchiectasis. Approximately 1,000 people die from it each year, and another 6,000 are hospitalized. Nearly half of all cases occur in patients with cystic fibrosis. Incidence has decreased with antibiotic treatment of acute infections.

Flashpoint
Nearly half of bronchiectasis cases occur in patients with cystic fibrosis.

Box 11-5 Diagnostic Spotlight

PULMONARY FUNCTION TESTS

Pulmonary function tests (PFTs), also called *spirometry,* are a group of tests used to evaluate the respiratory system and determine the degree of airway obstruction caused by obstructive disorders. The tests measure various aspects of expiratory flow and lung volume, including:

- Total lung capacity—the total volume of air in the lungs after a maximal inhalation. It is reduced in patients with restrictive lung disease and increased in those with obstructive lung disease.
- Tidal volume—the volume of air typically inhaled and exhaled with each normal breath. It is reduced in elderly patients and those with restrictive lung disease.
- Vital capacity—the volume of air that can be exhaled from the lungs after a maximal inspiration. It is reduced in elderly patients and those with **atelectasis** (condition of collapse or airlessness in parts of the lung) and pulmonary edema.
- Residual volume—the amount of air remaining in the lungs after a forced maximal exhalation. It is increased in elderly patients and those with COPD.
- Functional residual capacity—the amount of air remaining in the lungs after a normal exhalation. It is increased in elderly patients and those with COPD (see Fig. 11-10).
- Forced expiratory volume (FEV)—the amount of air that can be quickly exhaled.
- FEV1—the volume of air that can be forcibly exhaled in 1 second.
- Forced vital capacity (FVC or FEV6)—the amount of air that can be completely and forcibly exhaled after a maximal inhalation.

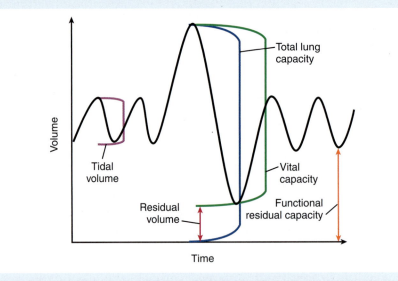

Pulmonary function test (From Eagle, S, et al. *The Professional Medical Assistant: An Integrative Teamwork-Based Approach.* 2009. Philadelphia: F.A. Davis Company, with permission.)

Etiology

Some cases of bronchiectasis are congenital; however, most develop as a result of obstruction or infection from bronchopneumonia, chronic bronchitis, tuberculosis, cystic fibrosis, or whooping cough. These infections damage the walls of the bronchi and cause chronic inflammation. Damaged cilia become less effective, making secretions and debris more likely to accumulate. This provides a rich medium for bacterial growth, which further worsens the problem. Walls of medium-sized airways lose elasticity and become widened. Smaller ones may be completely destroyed over time.

Signs and Symptoms

Signs and symptoms of bronchiectasis develop gradually and slowly worsen over many years. They include chronic productive cough, often with hemoptysis or foul-smelling sputum, and chest pain. Other symptoms include wheezing, dyspnea, fatigue, weight loss, pallor, and fingernail clubbing. Patients tend to have repeated bouts of pneumonia, and as the condition worsens they may develop cor pulmonale or respiratory failure and cyanosis.

Diagnosis

Physical examination may reveal abnormal lung sounds on auscultation. Chest x-rays are commonly done but may be normal with early disease. A chest CT scan is most accurate and helps to identify the severity of the disease. After diagnosis, further testing may be done to identify causative disorders. These include tests for HIV/AIDS and cystic fibrosis. Occasionally, bronchoscopy is done as well. This allows visualization of the air passages and collection of sputum and tissue samples.

Flashpoint

Bronchiectasis may cause chronic cough with hemoptysis or foul-smelling sputum.

Treatment

There is no cure for bronchiectasis. Therefore, treatment is aimed at reducing secretions, preventing or resolving infections, relieving obstruction, and preventing or minimizing complications. Antibiotics are given when bacterial infection is a factor. Bronchodilating medication and chest physiotherapy help promote drainage of secretions. Inhaled corticosteroids may be given to decrease inflammation. Mucolytic and expectorant medications and saline mist may be used to help thin secretions so they can be more easily coughed up. Cough suppressants are generally avoided, because they may worsen the condition. Bronchoscopy may be done to remove mucous plugs if bronchial obstruction occurs. Supplemental oxygen may be appropriate for severe disease. In severe cases, usually those associated with advanced cystic fibrosis, lung transplantation may be considered. All individuals are cautioned to avoid smoking and exposure to air pollution and people with infectious respiratory illness. Vaccinations, including the annual influenza vaccine, are recommended to reduce the risk of infectious illness.

Prognosis

Prognosis is guarded and depends upon the patient's self-care practices and access to health care, and upon whether complications arise. Many individuals are able to lead reasonably normal lives. Prognosis is poorer for those with other complicating lung disorders. Those who receive a heart-lung or double lung transplant have a 5-year survival rate of 65% to 75%.

Flashpoint

Cough suppressants are avoided because they may worsen the condition.

Pulmonary Emphysema
ICD-9-CM: 492.8   [ICD-10: J43.9]

Pulmonary emphysema is a lung disorder marked by the destruction of the alveolar walls and an abnormal increase in the size of air spaces distal to the terminal bronchiole. These changes result in the loss of normal elastic properties of the lungs and make exhaling air more difficult.

Incidence

Emphysema is a common chronic respiratory disorder, affecting as many as 30 million Americans and causing over 100,000 deaths each year.

Etiology

There are a number of contributors to the development of emphysema, including industrial exposure and repeated or chronic respiratory infections. However, the main risk factor is cigarette smoking. The average smoker smokes one or two packs of cigarettes each day, which means the lungs are subjected to chronic irritation caused by smoke, tar, and other toxins 20 to 40 times each day for years on end. As a result, the lung tissue becomes inflamed. Under normal circumstances, body tissue is able to repair itself; however, repetitive smoke exposure inflicts chronic damage and inflammation, and prevents healing. The walls of the delicate alveoli lose their elasticity and become permanently distended, like tiny balloons that have been inflated too many times. They also become thickened in some areas and eroded in others, resulting in an overall loss of function. Over time, these changes lead to chronic air-trapping and changes in chest dimension. The chest takes on a barrel-like shape that is characteristic of COPD and the diaphragm flattens out and loses much of its effectiveness. All of these things decrease the effectiveness of respiration and gas exchange.

Signs and Symptoms

Most patients are asymptomatic until they lose over half of their lung function. This lulls many into a false sense of security; they believe they still have time to quit smoking before any real damage is done. Initial signs of emphysema include dyspnea with exertion, which gradually worsens, and the development of a chronic productive cough. Characteristic changes in chest size and shape develop and lung sounds become chronically decreased. In later stages, weight loss occurs, and as heart failure develops, lower-leg edema may occur. Fingernail clubbing also develops (see Fig. 11-12). The patient experiences progressively worse orthopnea and chronic hypoxia, which may cause circumoral cyanosis. Other symptoms may include tachycardia and hypertension. During the last few years of life, the patient with emphysema has great difficulty performing basic self-care activities.

Diagnosis

Diagnosis of pulmonary emphysema is based upon history, physical-examination findings, chest x-ray, and pulmonary function tests. Tidal volume and residual volume are increased, while vital capacity and expiratory volume are decreased. Radiological studies reveal a flattened diaphragm and cardiomegaly. On good days, the lungs may sound clear but decreased; on bad days they will sound wheezy, with scattered crackles and rhonchi. Arterial blood gases (ABGs) may reveal chronically low oxygen saturation and carbon dioxide retention.

Treatment

The most critical intervention is avoiding exposure to the causative substances, such as tobacco smoke and other environmental irritants, and avoiding anyone with infectious respiratory illnesses. An annual influenza vaccine should be given. A variety of medications are used to manage the disease and treat acute exacerbations. These include bronchodilators to open airways, corticosteroids to reduce inflammation, expectorants to make a productive cough more effective, and antibiotics as needed for secondary bacterial infections. Eventually, supplemental oxygen will be needed, but patients must carefully follow physician recommendations, since too much oxygen can in some cases cause complications.

Prognosis

Prognosis is poor and depends largely on how early the patient receives diagnosis and treatment and whether further exposure to inhaled irritants is eliminated. Death from emphysema and other forms of COPD is very common in the United States.

Asthma

ICD-9-CM: 493.90 (acute), 493.20 (chronic)   **[ICD-10: J45.0 (acute), J44.8 (chronic)]**

Asthma, also called *reactive airway disease*, affects individuals who also suffer from allergies. It is a disorder in which the airways overreact to certain triggers with inflammation, narrowing,

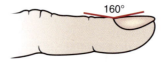

Normal finger

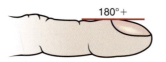

Clubbed finger

FIGURE 11-12 Fingernail clubbing

Normal bronchiole   **Asthmatic bronchiole**

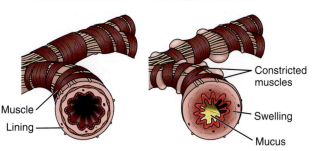

FIGURE 11-13 **Asthma**

and production of thick mucus (see Fig. 11-13). There are two types of asthma: allergic and non-allergic.

Incidence

Asthma affects approximately 20 million Americans and costs an estimated $18 billion each year in direct and indirect costs. It is estimated that each day in the United States, with regard to asthma, 30,000 people suffer an attack, 5,000 people visit the emergency room, 1,000 are admitted to the hospital, and 10 to 15 people die. Even more alarming is the fact that since 1980, asthma-related deaths have increased by more than 50% among all age groups and by 80% among children. In fact, asthma is the most common chronic disease suffered by children. African Americans and Latinos suffer higher rates of illness and death than other groups. These differences appear to be correlated with poverty, air quality, indoor allergens, and lack of access to adequate education and medical care.

Etiology

Asthma is caused by allergens, such as pollen, dust mites, pet dander, or other irritants, that are inhaled into the lungs and air passages and cause inflammation. Nonallergic asthma is triggered by nonallergy factors such as exercise, cold air, stress, anxiety, smoke, and viruses. Risk factors for asthma include having one or both parents with asthma.

Flashpoint
Asthma is the most common chronic disease suffered by children.

Signs and Symptoms

Signs and symptoms of both forms of asthma are similar and include coughing, wheezing, shortness of breath, and chest tightness. The increased respiratory effort and shortness of breath often result in anxiety and tachycardia. The individual prefers to sit upright for maximal lung expansion and may have difficulty speaking in complete sentences.

Diagnosis

In an emergent situation, diagnosis is usually based upon the patient's description of symptoms, physical-examination findings, oxygen saturation readings, and peak flow measurement (see Box 11-6). Auscultation reveals tight-sounding lungs with decreased breath sounds due to poor air exchange, as well as other abnormal sounds such as wheezes. Pulmonary function tests may be done but may be deferred for the critical patient. Chest x-ray may reveal changes related to hyperinflation of the lungs and mucous plugs. A CBC with differential may reveal an elevated level of eosinophils (a type of WBCs). Blood testing may indicate elevated immunoglobulin E levels. Allergy testing may also be done.

Flashpoint
The patient with asthma may have difficulty speaking in complete sentences.

Treatment

Patients suffering acute asthmatic episodes are treated with bronchodilating medications, which help open airways. Depending on the severity of the attack, corticosteroids may be used to decrease inflammation and airway reactivity. Long-term management includes identification of allergens, desensitization therapy, preventive use of medications such as steroid inhalers, and avoidance of known triggers.

Prognosis

Prognosis is variable, depending upon the type and extent of the asthma and the patient's access to health-care resources.

Box 11-6 Diagnostic Spotlight

PEAK FLOW METER

A peak flow meter is a handheld device used to measure how much air patients can blow out of their lungs in one breath, allowing them to establish a baseline measurement. When patients are experiencing episodes of dyspnea, such as during an asthma flare-up, they can then measure again and compare with their baseline. This allows them to better quantify just how well or how poorly they are breathing and take appropriate action according to the plan they have designed with their health-care provider. Patients are often encouraged to keep a journal of their peak flow readings and associated symptoms and bring it with them to their doctor's appointment.

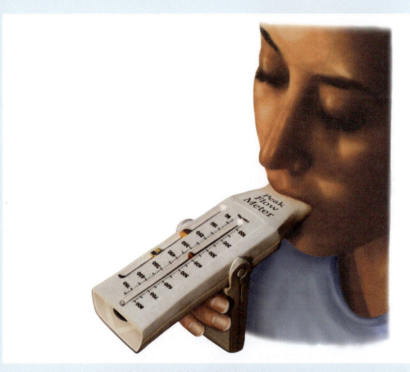

Peak flow meter. (From Eagle, S, et al. *The Professional Medical Assistant: An Integrative Teamwork-Based Approach.* 2009. Philadelphia: F.A. Davis Company, with permission.)

Pneumoconiosis

ICD-9-CM: 500–505   **[ICD-10: J63.0–J63.8] (code by type of causative agent for both codes)**

Pneumoconiosis is any disease of the respiratory tract caused by chronic or repetitive inhalation of dust particles. There are several variations:

> **Flashpoint**
>
> Pneumoconiosis is caused by chronic inhalation of dust particles.

- ***Coal worker's pneumoconiosis (CWP),*** also called *anthracosis* or *black lung:* caused by inhalation of coal dust
- ***Asbestosis:*** caused by inhalation of asbestos fibers
- ***Silicosis,*** also called *grinder's disease, progressive massive fibrosis,* and *potter's rot:* caused by inhalation of silica (quartz) dust
- ***Berylliosis:*** caused by inhalation of or exposure to beryllium

Incidence

All forms of pneumoconiosis can develop in individuals of all races, both genders, and any age; however, all are directly related to length and intensity of exposure. Therefore, individuals who have worked longer in an exposure environment are more likely to develop the disease. All types of pneumoconiosis were much more prevalent in past years, before industrial safety measures were instituted. In recent years, incidence has dropped dramatically. For example, since the year 2000, incidence of CWP has dropped by over 35%, and death from silicosis has dropped by 84% since 1999.

Etiology

All types of pneumoconiosis are caused by chronic inhalation of the offending substance. The exact pathology varies slightly with the type of substance, and the type and length of exposure, but in all cases tissue inflammation develops and the affected tissue becomes edematous (swollen). Macrophages (specialized WBCs) arrive to attempt to engulf and eliminate the offending substance. However, with chronic exposure, inflammation and damage continue. Immune defenses eventually become overwhelmed and permanent tissue damage occurs in the form of fibrosis (scarring). Variables that increase severity of the disorder include tobacco smoking, age at first exposure, and size and type of dust particles.

Signs and Symptoms

Most individuals with pneumoconiosis are asymptomatic for quite some time—as long as 20 years, in some cases. As the disease becomes more advanced, signs and symptoms (which are similar for all types) become noticeable. They include cough and dyspnea, especially with exertion. As the disease worsens, symptoms become more chronic and more pronounced. These include anorexia, weight loss, chest pain, fatigue, fever, night sweats, more pronounced episodes of dyspnea, and cor pulmonale.

Diagnosis

Diagnosis of pneumoconiosis is based upon the patient's signs and symptoms, physical-examination findings, and results of radiological testing. The health-care provider may note clubbing of the patient's fingernails and, upon auscultation, crackles in the lungs. These changes are especially likely in the patient with asbestosis. Chest x-ray may indicate fibrotic changes and nodules. Pulmonary function tests will reveal reduced vital capacity and tidal volume. In some cases CT scan may also be done. Bronchoscopy may be done, especially if cancer is suspected. The tuberculin skin test may be done for the patient who is suspected of having silicosis, because that condition increases susceptibility to tuberculosis.

Flashpoint

People with pneumoconiosis may be symptom free until the disease becomes quite advanced.

Treatment

There is no cure for any form of pneumoconiosis. The most effective treatment is early diagnosis and cessation of further exposure; otherwise, patients are treated symptomatically, with bronchodilators to help open air passages, corticosteroids to reduce inflammation, antibiotics if secondary bacterial infection is suspected, and supplemental oxygen as breathing becomes less effective.

Flashpoint

There is no cure for any form of pneumoconiosis.

Prognosis

Outcome may be good if the disease is identified early and exposure to the offending substance is discontinued. However, chronic exposure is likely to result in disabling lung disease. Individuals who suffer an initial episode of respiratory failure severe enough to require mechanical ventilation have been found to have a mortality rate of 40%. Asbestosis increases the patient's risk of developing a deadly form of lung cancer called mesothelioma by six times. If the patient also smokes, the risk of developing this type of lung cancer is 59 times higher than average. Other complications of pneumoconiosis include other forms of lung cancer, pulmonary hypertension, and cor pulmonale.

Flashpoint

Asbestosis and smoking dramatically increase the risk of a deadly form of lung cancer.

Pleurisy

ICD-9-CM: 511.0–511.9 (code by cause)   [ICD-10: R09.1, J90.0 (with effusion)]

Pleurisy, also called *pleuritis,* is a condition in which the pleurae become inflamed, causing sharp inspiratory pain in the chest.

Incidence

It is difficult to estimate the incidence of pleurisy, since it can be associated with any disease or disorder that causes inflammation of the pleurae. However, it is known to be very common.

Etiology

Normally the pleural membranes slide smoothly against one another as the lungs expand and contract. This is facilitated by a small amount of fluid between them. The cause of pleurisy isn't always known, but any condition that causes inflammation of either pleural membrane can result in pain as friction from movement occurs. Any number of disorders can cause inflammation. Viral infections such as influenza and pneumonia are the most common. Others include bacterial, fungal, or parasitic infection; trauma; cancer; sarcoidosis; connective-tissue diseases such as scleroderma, systemic lupus erythematosus, or rheumatoid arthritis; and reactions to some drugs.

Flashpoint

Pleuritic pain is caused by friction as the inflamed pleural membranes slide over one another.

Signs and Symptoms

The most prominent symptom of pleurisy is sharp, stabbing chest pain on breathing in. Pain may radiate into the back or shoulder, may be worsened by coughing or moving, and may be lessened by shallow breathing or lying on the painful side. Other symptoms depend upon the underlying cause and may include nonproductive cough, dyspnea, fever, chills, and sore throat.

Diagnosis

Upon auscultation, the physician may note a **pleural friction rub,** which is a low-pitched scratching, creaking, grating sound made by the pleurae as they rub against one another. Diagnostic tests may include chest x-ray, CBC, ECG, and sputum analysis. Imaging tests such as chest x-rays, CT scan, or ultrasound may be done to identify air or abnormal amounts of fluid between the pleurae, or to identify the presence of trauma or disease. Thoracentesis may be done to remove and study a sample of pleural fluid (see Box 11-7). If necessary, a thoracoscopy

Box 11-7 Diagnostic Spotlight

THORACENTESIS

Thoracentesis is a procedure in which fluid is removed from the pleural space to allow lung reexpansion (in the case of a collapsed lung) or diagnosis. By studying the fluid, the physician might note bacteria, cancer cells, or other abnormal findings. This information helps to diagnose illnesses like infection, cancer, and cirrhosis. The patient is positioned in a bed or chair, leaning forward with arms resting on a table, and instructed to hold very still. After applying antiseptic and numbing the area, the physician inserts a flexible catheter (tube) with the aid of a needle and withdraws the fluid. A chest x-ray may be done afterward to check for complications.

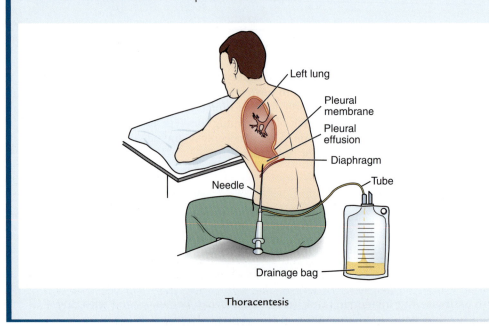

Thoracentesis

may also be done. In this procedure, the physician inserts a scope with a tiny camera though a small incision between two ribs to visually examine the inner chest and obtain tissue samples.

Treatment

Pleuritic pain is treated with analgesic and anti-inflammatory medication. If an excessive amount of pleural fluid has collected, it may be drained by thoracentesis or insertion of a chest tube. Antibiotics may be appropriate if bacterial infection is suspected. Severe cases may require **decortication.** This is a procedure done under general anesthesia in which scar tissue, pus, or other debris is removed from the pleurae and pleural space.

Prognosis

The prognosis for patients with pleurisy depends upon the underlying cause. Cases caused by viral infection are usually self-limiting and resolve within a week. More severe or complicated cases can lead to pleural effusion, pneumothorax, and hemothorax.

> **Flashpoint**
> Decortication is a procedure in which scar tissue, pus, or other debris is removed from the pleurae.

Pulmonary Edema

ICD-9-CM: 518.4 (acute), 428.1 (acute with mention of heart failure), 514 (chronic)   **[ICD-10: J81 (acute or chronic), I50.1 (acute with mention of heart failure)]**

Pulmonary edema is a serious condition in which fluid has accumulated in the tissues and alveoli of the lungs. Its presence hinders the exchange of oxygen and carbon dioxide and leads to respiratory failure. See Chapter 10 for a detailed description of heart failure.

Pleural Effusion

ICD-9-CM: 511.9   [ICD-10: J90]

A pleural effusion is an excess collection of fluid between the visceral and parietal pleurae that line the lungs.

Incidence

The general incidence of pleural effusion is not clear. However, it is known to be very common among patients admitted to the intensive care unit and among patients who have undergone open heart surgery.

Etiology

Normally there is a small amount of pleural fluid located between the two pleurae. It acts to lubricate the surfaces so they can slide smoothly against one another as the lungs expand and contract. An effusion develops when an abnormally large amount of fluid collects there. Effusions are classified as either transudative or exudative. Transudative effusions are caused by abnormal pressure, such as occurs with heart failure. Exudative effusions contain a large amount of protein and are caused by inflammation, cancer, and conditions like pneumonia, tuberculosis, asbestosis, and sarcoidosis. These conditions cause an effusion by increasing production of pleural fluid, creating conditions that inhibit lymphatic drainage of pleural fluid, or both. If the effusion contains infectious matter like bacteria and white blood cells, it is called empyema.

Signs and Symptoms

Signs and symptoms of pleural effusion include shortness of breath, pleuritic chest pain, and cough. If empyema is present, the patient may have a fever and a cough productive of foul-smelling sputum and may complain of anorexia and fatigue.

> **Flashpoint**
> Empyema is a condition in which the effusion fluid contains infectious matter.

Diagnosis

Pleural effusion is suspected based upon the patient's signs and symptoms and physical-examination findings. The physician may note decreased lung sounds and pleural friction rub upon auscultation. Diagnosis is confirmed with chest x-ray if more than 300 milliliters of fluid is present, or with a thoracic CT scan. Thoracentesis is often done as a diagnostic and treatment measure. Fluid analysis allows the physician to determine whether the effusion is transudative or exudative and to detect the presence of bacteria, cancer cells, or other abnormalities. This information helps identify the specific underlying cause and aids in the creation of a treatment plan.

Treatment

Treatment is aimed at resolving the underlying cause and removing the effusion fluid. Medications vary depending upon cause, including antibiotics for bacterial infection and chemotherapy for cancer. Effusion fluid is drained by thoracentesis or by insertion of a chest tube. Individuals who suffer chronic or repeated effusions may undergo *pleurodesis.* In this procedure, some form of sterile, irritating substance (such as talc) or chemical (such as bleomycin) is infused into the pleural space. This causes the pleural linings to develop scar tissue and fuse to one another, and inhibits further fluid accumulation. Complicated cases of empyema may require surgical decortication.

Prognosis

Prognosis for patients with pleural effusion depends upon the underlying cause and the patient's overall health status. Potential complications of the condition and its treatment include pneumothorax, infection, and bleeding.

Pneumothorax

ICD-9-CM: 512.0–512.8   [ICD-10: J93.0–J93.9] (code by cause for both codes)

Pneumothorax, commonly called a *collapsed lung,* is a condition in which air has collected in the chest cavity between the pleural membranes. Pneumothorax is categorized as open, closed, spontaneous, or tension.

Incidence

Flashpoint

Pneumothorax is often called a collapsed lung.

Incidence of pneumothorax varies by type. Spontaneous pneumothorax is most common in tall, thin men who smoke, between the ages of 20 and 40. Tension pneumothorax is associated with injuries caused by blunt-force trauma to the chest wall. It is estimated that three out of 1,000 people suffer spontaneous pneumothorax at some time in their lives. Incidence of tension pneumothorax is less certain but has been estimated at one per 14,000 men and one per 50,000 women.

Etiology

An open pneumothorax is one in which the pleural cavity has been disrupted and exposed to the atmosphere by some type of injury. A closed pneumothorax is one in which there is no open wound allowing air in from the external atmosphere; it may be caused by internal injuries such as rib fractures. In a spontaneous pneumothorax, a weak area on the lungs (sometimes called a *bleb*), something like an air blister, ruptures and begins leaking air into the pleural space. The reason this happens is not clear, although family history is thought to play a role. In other cases, the affected area of the lung has been weakened by disease such as tuberculosis or cancer. This type of pneumothorax is also sometimes called *secondary pneumothorax,* since it develops secondary to (because of) another disorder.

A tension pneumothorax can begin as any of the other types but progresses to a tension pneumothorax when continued air collection and pressure begin to compress great vessels and the heart, trachea, and remaining functional lung after having already fully collapsed the first one. This is a life-threatening emergency that requires immediate intervention. Risk factors for pneumothorax include smoking, lung disease, and a history of prior pneumothorax.

Signs and Symptoms

A minor pneumothorax, especially a spontaneous one, may cause no signs or symptoms. When the lung is more than 25% collapsed, patients may become symptomatic and begin to experience chest pain, dyspnea, tachycardia, and cyanosis. Other symptoms vary depending upon the underlying cause and severity. Individuals with tension pneumothorax will become severely dyspneic, hypoxemic, and hypotensive as their condition rapidly deteriorates.

Diagnosis

Diagnosis may be suspected based upon other injuries the patient has suffered, a description of the mechanism of injury (how the injury occurred), and presenting signs and symptoms. Upon auscultation, the physician will note diminished or absent lung sounds on the affected side and possibly unequal chest expansion. Arterial blood gases will reveal **hypoxemia** (condition of low blood oxygen) and possible respiratory acidosis (low blood pH). The diagnosis is confirmed with a chest x-ray.

Treatment

A minor pneumothorax may require no treatment other than follow-up evaluation to ensure that it resolves. More severe cases require treatment to reexpand the collapsed lung by removing trapped air from the pleural space. This is usually done by the insertion of a chest tube connected to a chest drainage unit (see Fig. 11-14), although a small pneumothorax may be treated with a smaller portable device called a Heimlich valve.

Prognosis

Prognosis for the patient with a pneumothorax depends upon the underlying cause, the severity of the condition, and the speed of intervention. The most common complication is a repeated pneumothorax at a later date. This occurs in about 50% of patients. Those most likely to experience a recurrence are smokers, those with HIV or AIDS, and those with lung disease. Tension pneumothorax has a high mortality rate.

Hemothorax

ICD-9-CM: 511.8   [ICD-10: J94.2]

Hemothorax is a condition in which blood or bloody fluid has collected in the chest cavity between the pleural linings, compressing the lung and causing respiratory distress.

Incidence

The exact incidence of hemothorax is unclear, since very minor cases may go undetected and untreated. However, it is estimated that around 300,000 cases occur each year as a result of traumatic injury.

Etiology

Hemothorax nearly always results from traumatic injury, such as that inflicted in motor vehicle accidents or violent crime. These types of injuries create a disruption in the pleurae and inflict injury to lung tissue and associated blood vessels. A severe form of injury that often results in life-threatening hemothorax is **flail chest.** This is an injury in which three or more ribs are fractured in two or more places. The resultant "island" rib segment moves in the opposite direction from the rest of the chest each time the patient attempts to breathe, which is referred to as **paradoxical motion.** This causes further tissue trauma and makes breathing extremely painful and difficult.

Regardless of the cause of injury, bleeding occurs into the intrapleural space and compresses lung tissue, causing lung collapse. Hemorrhage may be severe, depending upon the extent of injury. An adult's intrapleural space can hold up to 4 liters (over 4 quarts) of

Flashpoint
Pneumothorax can cause acidosis and hypoxemia.

Flashpoint
A minor pneumothorax may require no treatment at all, but a major one can be deadly.

Flashpoint
Hemothorax nearly always results from traumatic injury.

Flashpoint
Flail chest is often deadly because it causes severe respiratory distress.

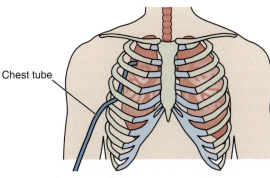

Chest tube

FIGURE 11-14 A chest tube to eliminate air from a pneumothorax

blood; therefore, life-threatening blood loss, not visible to the naked eye, can occur. In addition, life-threatening respiratory distress can occur.

Signs and Symptoms

Signs and symptoms associated with hemothorax are those related to respiratory compromise from the collapsed lung, shock from blood loss, and hypoxemia related to both of these problems. The patient experiences chest pain, dyspnea, tachycardia, hypotension, pallor, and cyanosis. During early stages the patient will be anxious and restless, but as the condition worsens the patient becomes exhausted and lethargic.

Diagnosis

Diagnosis of hemothorax must occur quickly so that life-saving interventions can be initiated in a timely fashion. Upon examination, the physician will note unequal chest expansion and, in the case of flail chest, paradoxical movement of the flail segment. Tracheal deviation may also occur as a hemothorax progresses into a tension hemothorax (similar to tension pneumothorax, but with blood instead of air collecting in the pleural space), as well as bruising or other visible signs of injury. Upon auscultation, the physician will observe decreased or absent breath sounds on the affected side. To confirm diagnosis and identify the severity of injury, a chest x-ray will be done. In some cases, chest CT scan is also done, but there may not be time for this procedure if the patient's condition is critical.

Treatment

Treatment of hemothorax is aimed at facilitating lung reexpansion and promoting circulatory stability and effective oxygenation. Blood is drained from the chest cavity with a chest tube connected to a drainage unit. This allows the lung to reexpand and also enables accurate measurement of intrapleural blood loss. Depending upon the severity of hemorrhage, blood transfusion may be given. Supplemental oxygen is administered, and if necessary the patient is placed on mechanical ventilation. In some cases surgery is done to repair internal injuries.

Flashpoint

The patient with hemothorax may need mechanical ventilation, especially in a case of flail chest.

Prognosis

Prognosis for patients suffering hemothorax is variable and depends on the severity of injury and the speed of treatment initiation. Potential immediate complications include shock and death; potential delayed complications include respiratory problems such as ARDS and empyema.

Acute Respiratory Distress Syndrome

ICD-9-CM: 518.5   [ICD-10: J80]

Acute respiratory distress syndrome (ARDS), also called *noncardiogenic pulmonary edema* and *shock lung*, is an acute, life-threatening condition of lung injury that is always secondary to some other lung trauma or disorder. It nearly always leads to respiratory failure and the need for mechanical ventilation.

Incidence

The exact incidence of ARDS is unclear, because of varying definitions. It is estimated that 200,000 Americans suffer from it each year.

Etiology

There are two general categories of causes of ARDS. One involves direct injury to lung tissue, such as with smoke inhalation, near drowning, or aspiration of stomach contents. The other is more common but less well understood; it involves indirect injury to the lungs from severe infection, hemorrhagic shock, conditions of inflammation such as pancreatitis, adverse drug reactions, or oxygen toxicity. Regardless of the cause, when lung tissue is injured it becomes edematous as fluid, proteins, and macrophages gather. This causes the lungs to become heavy and less compliant (stiffer). In addition, alveolar flooding occurs as fluid shifts from capillaries into the alveoli. The result of both of these processes is severely impaired gas exchange, leading to extreme dyspnea.

Flashpoint

The lungs in a patient with ARDS become heavy and noncompliant.

Signs and Symptoms

Signs and symptoms of ARDS include progressive dyspnea, cyanosis, anxiety, confusion, restlessness, and tachycardia. Without intervention, symptoms progress until the patient becomes severely exhausted, hypoxemic, and lethargic, and suffers complete respiratory failure.

Diagnosis

Diagnosis of ARDS may be suspected based upon signs and symptoms including hypoxemia, indicated by decreased oximeter readings and ABG results. Chest x-ray will reveal bilateral infiltrates and an eventual "whiteout" appearance. Sputum culture may reveal the offending organism when infection is a factor.

Treatment

Treatment of ARDS is aimed at resolving the underlying cause and providing ventilation support, including supplemental oxygen and, very likely, mechanical ventilation. This permits the patient to rest, usually with the aid of analgesics and sedatives. It also allows the administration of higher oxygen levels and a variety of ventilator settings that help to maximize the lungs' ability to exchange gases. Other supportive care is provided to aid the body with healing. Measures include IV fluids, enteral nutrition (liquid feedings through a tube), and careful monitoring.

Flashpoint

Patients with ARDS often require mechanical ventilation.

Prognosis

The prognosis for patients with ARDS is guarded and depends upon the underlying cause, the patient's age and underlying health status, and the earliness and aggressiveness of treatment. The mortality rate varies between 40% and 70%. Those who survive severe cases of ARDS usually have some degree of permanent lung fibrosis.

STOP HERE.
Select the flash cards for this chapter and run through them at least three times before moving on to the next chapter.

Student Resources

American Sleep Apnea Association: http://www.sleepapnea.org
ARDS Support Center: http://www.ards.org
Asthma and Allergy Foundation of America: http://www.aafa.org
Centers for Disease Control and Prevention Seasonal Influenza (Flu) page: http://www.cdc.gov/flu
FamilyDoctor.org: http://www.familydoctor.org
Healthcommunities.com Pulmonology Channel: http://www.pulmonologychannel.com
MedicineNet.com Pneumonia Index: http://www.medicinenet.com/pneumonia
MedlinePlus: http://www.nlm.nih.gov/medlineplus
National Emphysema Foundation: http://www.emphysemafoundation.org

Chapter Activities

Learning Style Study Strategies

Try any or all of the following strategies as you study the content of this chapter:

Visual and kinesthetic learners: Visual information is powerful for you and enables you to remember data better. Therefore, use one or more search engines (this also requires kinesthetic activity on your part) online to locate visual images associated with specific diseases and disorders as you study them.

Auditory learners: Ask your instructor to explain concepts you find confusing. Hearing this information can be very helpful for you.

Verbal learners: With a study buddy or study group, take turns "selling" a disease or diagnostic test by giving humorous sales pitches about its "benefits."

Practice Exercises

Answers to Practice Exercises can be found in Appendix D.

Case Studies

CASE STUDY 1

Mr. and Mrs. Reeves have come to the clinic for his annual checkup today. Mrs. Reeves states that her husband's snoring has gotten progressively worse and is keeping her awake at night. Furthermore, she has noted that he seems to actually stop breathing at times. The couple have some questions for the medical assistant.

1. Is this a problem that needs further investigation?

2. How could Mr. Reeves be evaluated for this problem?

3. What kind of information is obtained during this testing?

4. Is it true that this problem is very common and very serious? Could Mr. Reeves actually die in his sleep?

5. What symptoms would Mr. Reeves have if he really has sleep apnea?

6. Would it help if Mr. Reeves lost weight and stopped smoking? What else could he do?

CASE STUDY 2

Nicole Daniels is a 24-year-old woman who states that she went to the dentist because her teeth kept hurting. However, her dentist said that her teeth are all fine and suggested that she be evaluated for a possible sinus infection.

1. In addition to her teeth hurting, what other symptoms might Ms. Daniels have if she has sinusitis?

2. How might the physician determine whether Ms. Daniels actually has sinusitis?

3. What type of treatment might the physician recommend?

How should the medical assistant answer these questions that Ms. Daniels has?

4. How could a sinus infection make my teeth hurt?

5. Can these be spread between people?

CASE STUDY 3

Maya and Sayoko are medical assistants who work in a family practice office. Flu season is approaching, so their office manager has asked them to make some patient-education posters to put around the clinic.

1. What kind of statistics might they put on the poster to emphasize the extent of the influenza problem?

2. What should they say about what causes the flu?

3. What signs and symptoms should they warn people to watch out for in someone else who might have influenza?

4. What self-care measures might they describe that treat influenza?

5. What medication should be avoided when treating children who have influenza, and why?

6. Whom is influenza vaccination recommended for?

7. What are the possible complications of influenza?

Multiple Choice

1. Which of the following terms is **not** matched with the correct definition?

   a. Crackles: abnormal lung sound heard on auscultation that indicates fluid in the alveoli

   b. Hemoptysis: spitting or coughing up blood from the respiratory tract

   c. Wheezes: musical sound caused by narrowed air passage

   d. Pleural friction rub: motion of a free-floating fractured rib segment in the opposite direction from the rest of the chest as the patient breathes

2. The term *hypercapnea* means:

   a. Collection of fluid in the pleural space containing infectious matter, such as bacteria and white blood cells

   b. Chronic retention of carbon dioxide leading to symptoms of mental cloudiness and lethargy

   c. Need to remain upright in order to breathe effectively

   d. Chronic lack of oxygen

3. Decortication is:

   a. A procedure done under general anesthesia in which scar tissue, pus, or other debris is removed from the pleurae and pleural space

   b. Surgical removal of a lobe of the lung

   c. Surgical removal of an entire lung

   d. A tool for measuring the acidity or alkalinity of a substance

4. Which of the following is **not** a type of pneumoconiosis?

    a. Asbestosis

    b. Berylliosis

    c. Silicosis

    d. Histoplasmosis

5. Which of the following disorders are likely to be treated with the insertion of a chest tube?

    a. Pulmonary effusion

    b. Hemothorax

    c. Pneumothorax

    d. All of these

Short Answer

1. **Describe the path that oxygen takes to get from the external atmosphere into the bloodstream. Be sure to name all key structures.**

2. **Describe the mechanism that stimulates a healthy person to take a breath, to breathe faster and more deeply, and to breathe slower and more shallowly.**

3. **Describe first-aid measures and medical treatment for epistaxis.**

GASTROINTESTINAL SYSTEM DISEASES AND DISORDERS

12

Learning Outcomes

Upon completion of this chapter, the student will be able to:

- Define and spell terms related to the gastrointestinal system
- Identify key structures of the gastrointestinal system
- Discuss the roles of ingestion, digestion, and excretion played by the gastrointestinal system

- Identify characteristics of common gastrointestinal system diseases and disorders, including:
  - description
  - incidence
  - etiology
  - signs and symptoms
  - diagnosis
  - treatment
  - prognosis

KEY TERMS	
absorption	process by which nutrients move from the digestive tract into the bloodstream
bolus	rounded mass of chewed food that is ready for swallowing
cholecystectomy	surgical removal of the gallbladder
chyme	liquid mixture of stomach acids and partially digested food in the stomach and intestines
defecation	elimination of feces from the bowel; also called *bowel movement*
digestion	process by which food is broken down mechanically and chemically in the gastrointestinal tract and converted into absorbable forms
dysentery	group of disorders marked by intestinal inflammation and diarrhea
dysphagia	pain or difficulty with swallowing
excretion	process of eliminating bulk waste (feces) from the anus
flatulence	gassiness
hepatomegaly	enlargement of the liver
impaction	cavity that is tightly packed or overloaded
ingestion	oral consumption
intussusception	telescoping of the bowel into itself
jaundice	condition of increased bilirubin in the blood that results in yellow staining of the skin and mucous membranes
lavage	irrigation or rinsing out of a body cavity
lower endoscopy	visual examination of the lower digestive tract with a scope

Continued

KEY TERMS—cont'd	
peristalsis	rhythmic, wavelike muscular contractions of a tubular structure
portal hypertension	increased pressure in the vein entering the liver
proctoscopy	visual examination of the anus and rectum with a scope
steatorrhea	presence of fat in the stool
strangulated hernia	herniated tissue that has had the blood supply cut off, resulting in necrosis and possible septicemia
upper endoscopy	visual examination of the upper digestive tract with a scope
volvulus	twisting of the bowel on itself resulting in obstruction

Abbreviations

Table 12-1 lists some of the most common abbreviations related to the gastrointestinal system.

Structures and Functions of the Gastrointestinal System

The gastrointestinal (GI) system includes the alimentary canal and accessory organs of digestion. Together, these structures provide nutrients to all cells of the body.

Structures of the Gastrointestinal System

The structures of the GI system include the mouth, pharynx, esophagus, stomach, and intestines, as well as the accessory organs of digestion: the pancreas, liver, and gallbladder.

Alimentary Canal

The alimentary canal, also known as the *digestive tract* or *gastrointestinal tract,* is the route of digestion; it includes all structures from the mouth to the anus, excluding the accessory organs of digestion. At the beginning of the alimentary canal is the mouth, including the tongue, teeth, and gums. The uvula is a small, finger-shaped portion of soft tissue that hangs from the upper back part of the mouth. Contiguous with the mouth is the pharynx, which is shaped like a funnel. The pharynx begins at the back of the mouth and extends to the esophagus, a long,

TABLE 12-1			
ABBREVIATIONS			
Abbreviation	**Meaning**	**Abbreviation**	**Meaning**
ac	before meals	NPO, npo	nothing by mouth
BM	bowel movement	pc	after meals
EGD	esophagogastroduodenoscopy	PO, po	by mouth
GI	gastrointestinal	PR	per rectum
N&V	nausea and vomiting	supp	suppository
NG	nasogastric		

tubelike structure that passes through the diaphragm to connect the mouth to the stomach. At the beginning of the esophagus is a small, cartilaginous flap called the epiglottis, which hangs between the esophagus and the trachea. At the lower end of the esophagus is a muscular opening called the lower esophageal sphincter (LES), also called the *cardiac sphincter* because of its location near the heart. The LES separates the esophagus from the stomach.

The abdominal cavity holds the stomach, small intestine, large intestine, and rectum. This cavity is lined with a membrane called the peritoneum. The stomach, which is lined with folds called rugae, is composed of three major areas: the fundus (upper portion), body (middle portion), and pylorus (lower portion). The pyloric sphincter, another circular muscle, lies between the lowest portion of the stomach and the small intestine.

The small intestine is a coiled tube that measures about 20 feet long and consists of the duodenum (upper portion), jejunum (middle portion), and ileum (end portion). The small intestine is lined with villi, which are tiny, fingerlike projections surrounded by capillaries and lymph vessels. The ileocecal valve connects the ileum with the large intestine at the cecum. The large intestine includes the cecum and the colon. The cecum is a small pouch at the beginning of the large intestine. The appendix is a small, tubelike organ that hangs from the cecum in the right lower quadrant of the abdomen. The cecum connects to the colon, which consists of four portions: ascending colon, transverse colon, descending colon, and sigmoid colon. The last part of the alimentary canal, the rectum, begins at the sigmoid colon and ends at the anus (see Fig. 12-1.)

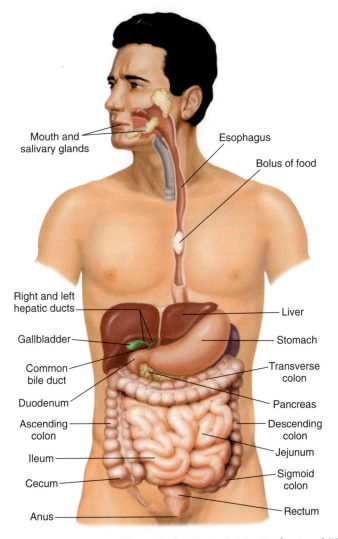

FIGURE 12-1 Gastrointestinal system (From Eagle, S, et al. *The Professional Medical Assistant: An Integrative Teamwork-Based Approach.* 2009. Philadelphia: F.A. Davis Company, with permission.)

Accessory Organs of Digestion

The accessory organs of digestion are the liver, gallbladder, and pancreas. While these organs serve other functions for other body systems, they are referred to as accessory organs of digestion when discussing the GI system because they serve important functions in the digestive process.

> **Flashpoint**
>
> Accessory organs like the pancreas and liver help you digest and utilize nutrients.

Liver

The liver consists of two large lobes and fills the upper right and center of the abdominal cavity, just below the diaphragm. It is the largest glandular organ of the body. The hepatic duct of the liver extends to the duodenum of the large intestine.

Gallbladder

The gallbladder is a 3- to 4-inch-long sac on the inferior surface of the liver. The gallbladder is connected to the common bile duct, which also connects to the duodenum.

Pancreas

The long, somewhat flat pancreas lies posterior and inferior to the stomach. Within the pancreas lie specialized cells called the islets of Langerhans. There are two types of these cells: alpha and beta. The pancreas also contains the pancreatic duct, which connects with the hepatic duct at the duodenum of the large intestine.

Functions of the Gastrointestinal System

The structures of the upper GI system aid in the process of **ingestion** (oral consumption) and **digestion** of food and fluids. Digestion is the process by which food is broken down mechanically and chemically in the gastrointestinal tract and converted into absorbable forms.

> **Flashpoint**
>
> Digestion turns the food you eat into usable nutrients.

The major products of digestion are proteins, fats, vitamins, minerals, water, and glucose. Digestive enzymes called proteases and lipases break down proteins and fats. As food is digested, vitamins and minerals move into the bloodstream, which delivers water-soluble vitamins to the tissues and fat-soluble vitamins to the liver and muscle tissue for storage. Insulin is essential for enabling glucose to leave the bloodstream and enter the tissues. These products of digestion are necessary for many biochemical reactions in cells of all parts of the body.

The GI system also performs **excretion,** the process of eliminating bulk waste (feces) from the anus. Digestion and excretion are carried out by the organs of the alimentary canal and the accessory organs of digestion.

Alimentary Canal

Digestion starts in the mouth, where teeth mechanically begin breaking down food. As food is chewed, the salivary glands of the mouth secrete saliva to mix with the food. Saliva moistens food and contains ptyalin, a chemical that starts to break down starches. The tongue helps to form the food into a **bolus,** which is a rounded mass of chewed food that is ready for swallowing. The tongue helps distinguish the taste of food. Specific areas on the tongue detect the different flavors of food, including sweet, salty, sour, and bitter (see Fig. 12-2.)

As a person swallows food, the uvula prevents the food from entering the nasal cavity. The epiglottis covers the trachea to prevent food from entering the respiratory tract. The bolus continues into the esophagus, where rhythmic involuntary muscular contractions called **peristalsis** move it downward into the stomach.

> **Flashpoint**
>
> The epiglottis covers the trachea when you swallow to keep you from choking.

The LES lets the bolus in and prevents backflow of gastric secretions up into the esophagus. The rugae allow the stomach to expand to accommodate large quantities of food. The fundus and body of the stomach are mostly holding areas for the food. The majority of digestion happens in the lowest portion, the pylorus. Gastric secretions within the stomach are highly acidic, with an average pH of 1.7. These secretions continue the breakdown of food to enable **absorption,** which is the process by which nutrients move from the digestive tract into the bloodstream. At this point in the digestive process the food is referred to as **chyme,** a liquid mixture of stomach acids and partially digested food in the stomach and intestines. The pyloric sphincter allows chyme to be released from the stomach into the small intestine a little at a time.

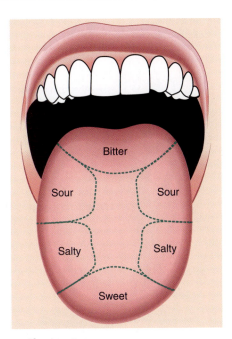

FIGURE 12-2 Areas of taste on the tongue

The villi of the small intestine increase its surface area, allowing greater absorption of water and nutrients into the blood. Most of this absorption occurs in the small intestine (see Fig. 12-3). All products of digestion that are not absorbed by the small intestine are deemed waste products. They continue into the large intestine, where water is absorbed and stool becomes more solid. For years the appendix has been thought to serve no useful function; more recently, however, researchers have found evidence that it may act to produce and store useful bacteria. This comes in handy if normal flora get cleared from the colon, as can happen with some types of illness. The appendix may then act to repopulate the colon with the right types of bacteria.

The large intestine secretes mucus to facilitate the passage of stool. No digestion occurs there, but water and some minerals are absorbed. This turns the stool from liquid into a semisolid mass ready to be expelled. The most distal part of the colon is the sigmoid colon. It acts along with the rectum and anus to expel stool in the process of ***defecation*** (elimination of feces from the bowel; also called *bowel movement*).

Flashpoint
Digestion largely takes place in the small intestine.

Accessory Organs of Digestion
Although the liver, gallbladder, and pancreas are not part of the alimentary canal, they play vital roles in the digestion, absorption, storage, and chemical conversion of vital nutrients.

Liver
The liver is involved in digestion, absorption, storage, and excretion. Its contributions to the digestive process include:

- manufacture of bile, a fat emulsifier, which it sends to the gallbladder for storage
- production and storage of glycogen, which can be converted to glucose when needed by cells
- detoxification of drugs and alcohol, making them water soluble so they can be excreted by the kidneys
- storage of fat-soluble vitamins A, D, E, and K for use when needed by cells
- manufacture of blood lipids, such as cholesterol and other lipoproteins, that protect arterial walls from damage and transport fat-soluble substances, such as vitamins, to various tissues via the bloodstream
- destruction of old erythrocytes, recycling the iron from those blood cells—and sending it to muscles and back to bone marrow to make new erythrocytes—and releasing bilirubin, which gets excreted in feces
- use of dietary protein sources to manufacture blood-clotting proteins, such as prothrombin and fibrinogen, which aid in repair of injured artery, vein, and capillary walls

Flashpoint
The liver detoxifies things like drugs and alcohol.

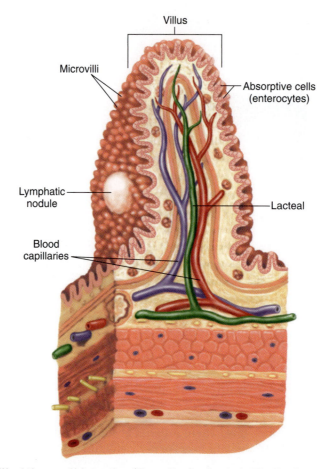

FIGURE 12-3 **Villi of the small intestine** (From Eagle, S, et al. *The Professional Medical Assistant: An Integrative Teamwork-Based Approach.* 2009. Philadelphia: F.A. Davis Company, with permission.)

Gallbladder

The gallbladder acts as a storage pouch for bile. Bile, produced in the liver, is sent to the gallbladder through the right and left hepatic ducts for storage. As fatty food passes into the duodenum, the gallbladder secretes the bile into the duodenum through the common bile duct to break down those fats.

Pancreas

The pancreas secretes substances into the duodenum through the pancreatic duct and directly into the bloodstream through capillaries of the islets of Langerhans. The pancreas secretes the pancreatic enzymes and sodium bicarbonate into the duodenum to neutralize stomach acid. These pancreatic enzymes include:

- trypsin to break down proteins
- lipase to break down fats
- amylase to break down carbohydrates

The specialized cells of the islets of Langerhans secrete insulin and glucagon, two hormones that regulate blood glucose levels. Insulin is secreted by the beta cells of the islets of Langerhans in response to increased blood glucose levels after eating. It binds to glucose molecules in the bloodstream, allowing them to diffuse into the tissues. Glucagon is secreted by the alpha cells of the islets of Langerhans in response to low blood glucose levels. It releases a storage form of glucose called glycogen from the liver. The release of glycogen occurs while the person is sleeping and fasting (see Fig. 12-4).

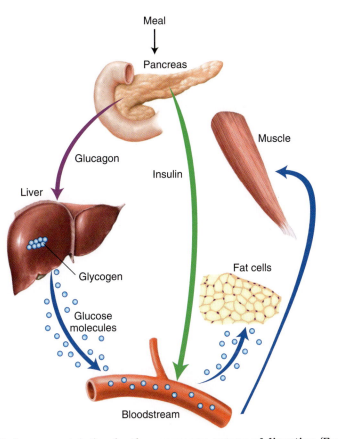

FIGURE 12-4 **Blood glucose regulation by the accessory organs of digestion** (From Eagle, S, et al. *The Professional Medical Assistant: An Integrative Teamwork-Based Approach.* 2009. Philadelphia: F.A. Davis Company, with permission.)

Because the pancreas secretes substances into the bloodstream (insulin and glucagon) and into the alimentary canal (sodium bicarbonate and pancreatic enzymes), it is considered an exocrine (outside of the bloodstream) and endocrine (into the bloodstream) gland. For more information on the endocrine functions of the pancreas, see Chapter 13.

Flashpoint

The pancreas secretes insulin, glucagon, and important digestive enzymes.

Gastrointestinal System Diseases and Disorders

There are innumerable diseases and disorders of the GI system. They are often categorized according to the part of the system they affect: the oral cavity, upper GI system, lower GI system, and accessory organs.

Diseases and Disorders of the Oral Cavity

Disorders of the oral cavity are quite common. Because the mouth is used so extensively in day-to-day activities like talking, eating, drinking, and kissing, such disorders can have a significant impact on quality of life. Therefore, prevention and early detection and treatment are important. The good news is that most of these disorders are self-limiting, heal without extensive treatment, and are easy to prevent or minimize—and some are curable. Common disorders of the oral cavity include aphthous ulcers, herpes simplex, dental caries, gingivitis, impacted third molars, and oral thrush. Notice that several of these disorders are easily prevented or treated with regular dental hygiene (see Box 12-1).

Flashpoint

Several disorders of the oral cavity are easily prevented or treated with regular dental hygiene.

> ## Box 12-1 Wellness Promotion
>
> ### BE KIND TO YOUR MOUTH
> Many oral disorders can be prevented or minimized through good self-care. Follow these measures to create and maintain good oral health:
>
> - Brush your teeth and floss after meals.
> - Get regular dental check-ups.
> - Avoid exposure to HSV-1.
> - Get enough sleep.
> - Take a multivitamin.
> - Avoid tobacco products.
> - Follow measures to protect and strengthen your immune system (see Box 9-6).

Aphthous Ulcers
ICD-9-CM: 528.2   [ICD-10: K12.0]

Aphthous ulcers, commonly known as *canker sores*, are ulcerations in the mouth and oropharynx. Recurrent aphthous stomatitis is a condition in which lesions recur within the mouth repeatedly.

Incidence

Estimates of the incidence of recurrent aphthous stomatitis vary widely, between 5% and 65% of the population. It typically begins in childhood or adolescence. Women are affected slightly more than men.

Etiology

The exact cause of aphthous ulcers is not understood. In many cases there seems to be a familial tendency. Immunologic factors may also play a role. Other risk factors may include vitamin deficiency, stress, smoking cessation, injury to the mouth, food allergies, menstruation, fatigue, some types of toothpaste, and some diseases.

Signs and Symptoms

Aphthous ulcers appear as small, painful ulcers on the inner lips, gums, or floor of the mouth; they have gray-yellow centers and reddened halos. More severe forms may appear as clusters of small ulcers or larger lesions (1 centimeter or more) that are intensely painful. The patient usually describes a burning or tingling sensation prior to ulcer formation that progresses to pain and tenderness once the ulcer forms. Occasionally the patient will also have enlarged, tender lymph nodes below the jaw and a mild fever.

Diagnosis

Diagnosis of aphthous ulcers is based upon the patient's description of symptoms and physical examination of the lesions.

Treatment

There is no cure for aphthous ulcers; however, a number of measures can be taken to reduce pain and discomfort, including using analgesic medication, rinsing the mouth with warm saltwater, and avoiding spicy or irritating foods and fluids. Vitamin B_{12} and zinc have also been found to provide some benefit. Individuals with severe ulcers may be treated with prescription corticosteroids. Patients may also be counseled to avoid toothpastes containing sodium dodecyl sulfate.

Prognosis

Prognosis for patients with aphthous ulcers is good, although recurrence is common.

Oral Herpes
ICD-9-CM: 054.9 (without complication)   [ICD-10: B00]

Flashpoint

Herpes simplex lesions are commonly called cold sores.

Herpes simplex lesions, also called *oral herpes, cold sores,* or *fever blisters,* are vesicular eruptions caused by the herpes simplex virus type 1 (HSV-1).

Incidence

Herpes simplex is extremely common because it is very contagious.

Etiology

HSV-1 is transmitted by contact with infected saliva or direct contact with fluid from a herpetic lesion. Contributors or triggers include fever, stress, mouth injury, hormones, and exposure to sun and wind.

Signs and Symptoms

The major symptoms of HSV-1 infection are lesions on the lips or in the mouth. They begin as tiny hard spots, usually on the lips, that tingle and develop into extremely painful vesicles (see Fig. 12-5). The condition can progress into gingivostomatitis, in which the gums and mouth become red and swollen and may bleed. Symptoms of gingivostomatitis may further include fever, pain, halitosis, and difficulty eating or drinking.

Diagnosis

Diagnosis is made by visual inspection and confirmed by culture of fluid from the lesions.

Treatment

Treatment includes antiviral medication, which does not cure the disorder but helps to shorten the course and lessen the severity of symptoms. Topical anesthetics and oral analgesics may help relieve pain. The patient is cautioned to avoid touching lesions, because the virus can spread via contact.

Prognosis

Once an individual is infected with HSV-1, that person remains infected for life. However, most people are able to manage outbreaks. Those with weakened immune systems may suffer more frequent outbreaks and more severe symptoms.

Flashpoint

Herpesviruses are easily spread by direct contact.

Dental Caries

ICD-9-CM: 521.00   [ICD-10: K20.9] (unspecified for both codes)

Dental caries, also called *tooth decay* or *cavities,* is a condition of erosion of parts of the teeth.

Incidence

The exact incidence of dental caries is unknown, since many people do not seek dental care. However, it is known to be extremely common in the United States and worldwide. It is especially prevalent in children and young adults, but it can affect individuals of any age.

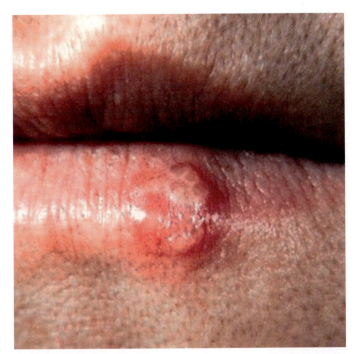

FIGURE 12-5 HSV-1 herpetic lesion (cold sore) (Courtesy of the Centers for Disease Control and Prevention and Dr. Hermann.)

Etiology

Dental caries develops when bacteria in the mouth convert foods into acids. The acids, bacteria, and bits of food act with saliva to form plaque. Plaque is a sticky substance that binds to teeth, especially along the gum line of molars, between teeth, around dental fillings, and in grooves of the teeth. If not removed, it develops into a mineral-like substance called tartar. Plaque and tartar both cause gum irritation and inflammation, resulting in gingivitis and erosion of tooth enamel. Once the protective enamel is eroded, the deeper structures of the teeth begin to erode as well. The rate of plaque buildup and tooth erosion is accelerated by frequent snacking on sticky foods high in carbohydrates (starchy, sugary foods).

Signs and Symptoms

People with cavities usually have no symptoms until the deeper structures of the teeth are involved. Once the nerve roots are affected or a tooth abscess (infection with pus collection) develops, the patient may complain of toothache and sensitivity to cold, heat, or sweets. Cavities may or may not be readily visible.

Flashpoint

People with cavities may have no symptoms until deeper structures are involved.

Diagnosis

Dental caries are diagnosed when the patient undergoes a dental examination. The dentist visually examines the teeth and probes the tooth surface with a sharp instrument, looking for pits and other types of damage. Some cavities are revealed only with x-rays.

Treatment

Dental caries are routinely treated by a dentist, who removes the eroded part of the tooth with a drill and replaces it with a filling or crown. These may be composed of gold, silver alloy, porcelain, or a composite resin. In cases where the tooth root has died, the patient may be referred to a specialist for a root canal. In this procedure the pulp, nerve, and any decaying matter are removed from the tooth center, and the tooth is filled and sealed. In cases where the tooth cannot be preserved, extraction (removal) may be necessary.

Prognosis

Prognosis for patients with dental caries is excellent if timely diagnosis and appropriate dental care occur. Regular dental hygiene will help to prevent or minimize further development of caries. However, if treatment does not occur, continued tooth erosion is likely. This can lead to abscesses and tooth loss.

Gingivitis

ICD-9-CM: 523.0 (acute), 523.1 (chronic)   [ICD-10: K05.0 (acute), K05.1 (chronic)]

Gingivitis is a condition of gum inflammation. It can progress into a form of periodontal disease that destroys the supportive structures of the teeth.

Incidence

The exact incidence of gingivitis is impossible to determine, since many people do not seek treatment. However, it is known to be extremely common, especially among teens and young adults.

Etiology

Gingivitis is caused by the buildup of plaque because of poor oral and dental hygiene. Plaque and tartar cause gum inflammation, and bacteria and bacterial toxins cause gum infection. Other contributors to gingivitis include poorly managed diabetes, hormonal fluctuations of pregnancy, misaligned teeth, poorly fitting appliances such as dentures or braces, and some medications. The part of the gums most affected is the gum line next to the teeth and between them. As the condition progresses, it may develop into periodontitis, in which deep pockets form between the gums and teeth; bone loss is possible. This can cause teeth to become loose and fall out.

Flashpoint

Gingivitis, which is easily prevented, can cause tooth loss if it worsens to periodontitis.

Signs and Symptoms

Gingivitis causes the gums to become shiny, swollen, tender, and redder than normal or even purple (see Fig. 12-6). Gums bleed easily with brushing and flossing and may also itch. Other symptoms include sores that emit purulent (pus-containing) drainage, and severe halitosis (foul breath).

Diagnosis

Diagnosis of gingivitis is based on physical examination of the mouth. The dentist may order x-rays to evaluate for dental caries and bone involvement.

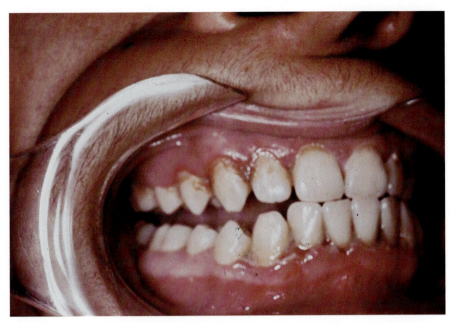

FIGURE 12-6 Gingivitis (From Goldsmith, LA, Lazarus, GS, and Tharp, MD. *Adult and Pediatric Dermatology: A Color Guide to Diagnosis and Treatment.* 1997. Philadelphia: F.A. Davis Company, with permission.)

Treatment

Treatment of gingivitis includes professional cleaning of the teeth by a dentist and initiation of regular dental hygiene. This should include brushing and flossing the teeth after meals. Saline or antibacterial rinses and analgesics may be advised when infection or tenderness is present. Other conditions, such as misaligned teeth or poorly fitting appliances, are corrected as needed.

Prognosis

Prognosis for patients with gingivitis is excellent if diagnosis and treatment occur before permanent damage develops. Recurrence is common, especially in patients with poor dental hygiene. Potential complications of gingivitis include periodontitis, gum and bone infection, and trench mouth (severe, ulcerative gingivitis).

Impacted Wisdom Teeth
ICD-9-CM: 520.6   [ICD-10: K01.1]

Impacted third molars, commonly known as *impacted wisdom teeth*, is a condition in which one or more of the third molars fail to erupt through the gums normally.

Incidence

The incidence of impacted third molars is very common. It is estimated that about 85% of the population eventually needs to have them removed due to impaction.

Etiology

Third molars were given the common name of wisdom teeth because they typically do not emerge until people are between 17 and 25 years old. It is believed that early humans had larger jaws and used all of their teeth to chew their tougher food, but that over the centuries, human jaws became smaller. Today most people's mouths cannot fully accommodate all of their teeth. Consequently, the third molars are often prevented from fully emerging by other teeth, bone, or overlying gum tissue. They may not erupt at all or may grow at odd angles within the jaw (see Fig. 12-7). This leads to crowding of all the teeth, trapping and subsequent decay of food, and inflammation. Crowding of the teeth can make good dental hygiene difficult, which further worsens the situation.

Signs and Symptoms

Many people with impacted third molars are symptom free. Others experience red, painful, swollen gums, jaw ache or headache, halitosis, an unpleasant taste in the mouth, and tender lymph nodes in the neck.

Flashpoint
Third molars are commonly known as wisdom teeth.

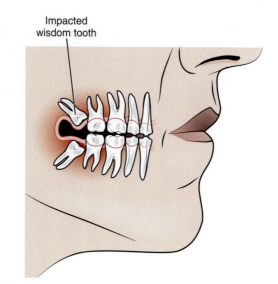

FIGURE 12-7 **Impacted third molars**

Diagnosis

Diagnosis is made by a dentist, who examines the patient's mouth, questions the patient about symptoms, and obtains dental x-rays.

Treatment

Conservative treatment for impacted third molars includes careful dental hygiene, analgesics for pain, mouthwashes or saline rinses as recommended by the dentist, and antibiotics if needed for infection. If symptoms do not improve, oral surgery is usually done to remove the third molars.

Because impaction is such a common problem, many experts recommend that patients have third molars removed as a preventive measure.

Prognosis

The prognosis for patients with impacted third molars is excellent if the condition is diagnosed and treated early. Delayed treatment can lead to a variety of complications, including further crowding of the teeth, periodontitis, tooth decay, pain, infection with abscess formation, cyst formation, and root damage. Furthermore, it has been noted that risk of complications increases as the patient ages.

Oral Thrush

ICD-9-CM: 112.0, 771.7 (newborn)   [ICD-10: B37.0]

Oral thrush, also called *oral candidiasis,* is an infection of the mouth with any species of *Candida,* but mainly *Candida albicans.*

Incidence

Oral thrush is rare in healthy people but more common in those with suppressed immune systems, including individuals with HIV and patients being treated with chemotherapy or immunosuppressive drugs.

Etiology

Oral thrush is caused by a disruption in the composition of the normal flora or a change in host defenses, which allows the *C. albicans* fungus to thrive. Infants are sometimes born with oral thrush because normal flora in the mouth have not yet been established. Risk factors for oral thrush include immune suppression, antibiotic treatment, tobacco smoking, and wearing dentures.

Signs and Symptoms

Symptoms of oral thrush include white-yellow patches in the mouth and red, tender oral mucous membranes (see Fig. 12-8). The tongue may have a white appearance. Individuals may also have "yeast" rashes on other parts of the body, including the groin and abdomen and under pendulous (drooping) breasts. The rash usually has a red, slightly raised appearance and may itch or burn.

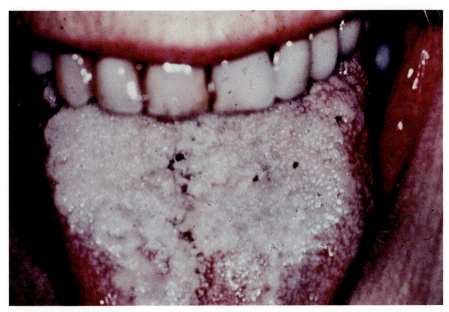

FIGURE 12-8 Oral thrush (From Goldsmith, LA, Lazarus, GS, and Tharp, MD. *Adult and Pediatric Dermatology: A Color Guide to Diagnosis and Treatment.* 1997. Philadelphia: F.A. Davis Company, with permission.)

Diagnosis

Diagnosis of oral thrush is established by visual inspection.

Treatment

Oral thrush is usually treated with antifungal medication. Forms include oral pills that have a systemic (whole-body) effect, an oral solution that can be applied to or swished around in the mouth and swallowed, and lozenges that can be held in the mouth.

Prognosis

The prognosis for individuals with oral thrush is usually good, since it is generally responsive to treatment. Complications include inadequate nutrition related to difficulty eating, and the spread of thrush to other areas.

Diseases and Disorders of the Upper Gastrointestinal Tract

The upper GI system contains structures from the esophagus through the first part of the small intestine. Diseases and disorders of these structures are common and can have a significant impact on quality of life. However, many can be successfully treated if they are detected early. Common upper GI diseases and disorders include esophagitis, gastroesophageal reflux disease, hiatal hernia, achalasia, esophageal varices, gastritis, chronic atrophic gastritis, peptic ulcer disease, and gastroenteritis.

Esophagitis

ICD-9-CM: 530.10   [ICD-10: K20]

Esophagitis is the inflammation of the lining of the lower esophagus. Those who suffer from esophagitis also usually have symptoms of gastroesophageal reflux disease.

Incidence

The incidence of esophagitis is unknown. It is frequently associated with gastroesophageal reflux disease, which is a common disorder.

Etiology

Esophagitis is caused by anything that irritates the lining of the esophagus. The most common cause is backflow of acidic fluids from the stomach, as is caused by gastroesophageal reflux and vomiting. Other contributors include bacterial, viral, and fungal infections; diseases that weaken the immune system; obesity; scleroderma; smoking; alcohol; radiation therapy; and medications such as aspirin and other NSAIDs.

Signs and Symptoms

The primary symptom of esophagitis is burning pain in the lower esophagus, commonly called heartburn. It is also sometimes felt as burning pain in the chest. Other symptoms may include nausea, vomiting, mouth sores, painful swallowing (dysphagia), and a feeling of something being stuck in the throat.

Diagnosis

After a medical history is obtained, the physician may order an upper GI series, which is a radiological study in which the patient usually drinks barium (see Box 12-2). This liquid causes the structures of the esophagus and stomach to show up well under x-ray. An **upper endoscopy** may also be done. In this procedure the physician examines the patient's esophagus, stomach, and other structures with a scope (see Box 12-3). This also allows obtainment of a tissue sample for biopsy.

Treatment

Mild cases of esophagitis may respond to conservative measures (see Box 12-4). Medication includes antacids and over-the-counter (OTC) or prescription-strength H_2 receptor antagonists or proton pump inhibitors. Surgical management is reserved for severe symptoms that do not respond to other measures and includes tightening of the lower esophageal sphincter (LES) by laparoscopic surgery.

Prognosis

Prognosis for patients with esophagitis is good if they receive adequate treatment. Chronic, severe esophagitis may result in stricture (narrowing) and precancerous cellular changes known as Barrett esophagus.

Gastroesophageal Reflux Disease
ICD-9-CM: 530.81   [ICD-10: K21.0]

Gastroesophageal reflux disease (GERD), commonly known as *heartburn*, is one of the most common disorders of the GI tract.

Incidence

As many as 44% of Americans suffer monthly symptoms of GERD, and 7% to 10% suffer daily symptoms. It is common in pregnant women because the enlarging uterus pushes upward, exerting pressure on the stomach and other structures.

Etiology

LES pressure that is lower than normal allows reflux of gastric contents into the esophagus (see Fig. 12-9). Unlike the stomach lining, the lining of the esophagus is not able to withstand the acidity of stomach fluid. When it enters the esophagus, the patient experiences a sensation of burning. Repeated exposure to stomach fluids can begin to erode the esophageal lining, leading

---

Box 12-2 Diagnostic Spotlight

UPPER GI SERIES

The upper GI series is a procedure in which x-rays are used to gather information about the GI tract. The patient drinks barium, a white, thickened liquid that coats the lining of the esophagus, stomach, and duodenum and makes them more visible on x-rays. The radiologist is able to study the x-rays and identify blockages, ulcers, hernias, and other problems. The procedure takes anywhere from 1 to 5 hours, depending upon how much of the small intestine is examined. It is not invasive or painful; however, the barium may cause constipation and light-colored stools. Therefore, patients may be advised to take laxatives for 1 or 2 days after the procedure.

Box 12-3 Diagnostic Spotlight

UPPER ENDOSCOPY

Upper endoscopy, also called *esophagogastroduodenoscopy* (EGD), is a procedure in which the physician visually examines the esophagus (esophagoscopy), stomach (gastroscopy), and duodenum (duodenoscopy) with a scope. Before the procedure, the patient's throat is sprayed with a topical anesthetic; medication may also be given to help the patient relax and to ease pain. The scope helps the physician carefully examine structures, take photos, remove tissue samples for biopsy, and perform certain treatments. The procedure usually takes 30 minutes or less; however, the patient will need to rest for 1 or 2 hours, until the medication wears off, and will not be able to drive home.

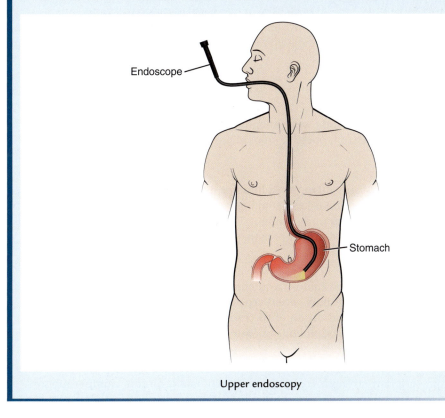

Endoscope

Stomach

Upper endoscopy

Box 12-4 Wellness Promotion

RELIEVING GERD

Disorders like esophagitis, GERD, and hiatal hernia share similar symptoms, caused by the effects of stomach acids in the esophagus. Therefore, some of the same simple measures can help to prevent or minimize symptoms for all of these conditions:

- stopping smoking
- losing weight
- eliminating or minimizing alcohol intake
- taking medications that worsen symptoms (like NSAIDs) with milk or food, if allowed
- eating small, frequent meals instead of large ones
- elevating the head of the bed 6 inches
- avoid high-fat foods, caffeinated beverages, and chocolate for 4 hours before bedtime

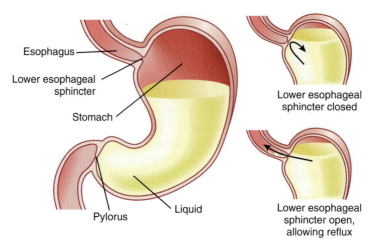

FIGURE 12-9 Lower esophageal sphincter (LES)

to esophagitis. Contributing factors include weak esophageal peristalsis, delayed gastric emptying, pyloric stenosis, hiatal hernia, obesity, smoking, alcohol, and medications such as aspirin and other NSAIDs.

Signs and Symptoms

Symptoms of GERD include heartburn, ***dysphagia*** (pain or difficulty with swallowing), chronic cough, upper abdominal pain, and asthma. Less common symptoms include laryngitis and tooth damage from enamel erosion. Symptoms worsen about 1 hour after meals, when the individual is lying down, and when intra-abdominal pressure increases, such as with coughing, belching, or physical strain.

> **Flashpoint**
>
> People who suffer from GERD also tend to suffer from esophagitis.

Diagnosis

Diagnosis of GERD is based upon history and clinical manifestations. Testing may include a barium swallow, which may reveal erosion or abnormalities of the esophagus. An upper endoscopy allows visualization of the esophagus, LES, and stomach, and allows testing of fluid pH and obtainment of tissue for biopsy.

Treatment

Mild cases of GERD may respond to conservative measures (see Box 12-4). Medication includes antacids and OTC or prescription-strength H_2 receptor antagonists or proton pump inhibitors. Surgical management is reserved for severe symptoms that do not respond to other measures, and includes tightening of the LES by laparoscopic surgery.

Prognosis

If conservative measures fail, symptoms can usually be managed effectively with drug therapy. Long-term complications may include esophagitis, dysphagia, and Barrett's esophagus.

Hiatal Hernia

ICD-9-CM: 553.3   [ICD-10: K44.9] (without obstruction or gangrene for both codes)

> **Flashpoint**
>
> A hernia is the protrusion of an organ or tissue through a wall or structure that contains it.

A hernia is defined as the protrusion of an organ or other tissue through a wall or structure that normally contains it. There are many different types and locations of hernias. In a hiatal hernia, the structures involved include the diaphragm, the esophagus, and the stomach.

Incidence

The incidence of hiatal hernia is greater in Western countries, increasing with age from 10% in those below the age of 40 to as high as 70% in those over 70 years of age.

Etiology

A hiatal hernia occurs when the part of the diaphragm around the base of the esophagus weakens and allows a portion of the stomach to slide upward into the thoracic cavity (see Fig. 12-10).

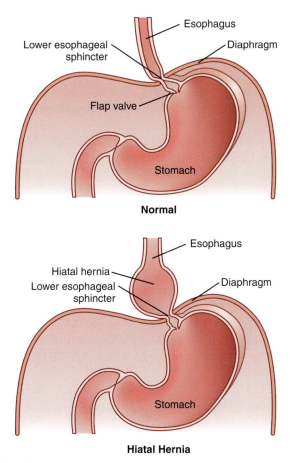

Normal

Hiatal Hernia

FIGURE 12-10 **Hiatal hernia**

The cause is not always clear, but contributing factors include obesity, trauma, advanced age, severe vomiting, coughing, pregnancy, lifting, or anything that increases intra-abdominal pressure.

Signs and Symptoms
Symptoms of hiatal hernia include heartburn, dysphagia, chronic cough, upper abdominal pain, and asthma. Symptoms worsen about 1 hour after meals, when the individual is lying down, and when intra-abdominal pressure increases, such as with coughing, belching, or physical strain. Other symptoms include chest pain and respiratory problems if aspiration occurs.

Diagnosis
Diagnostic studies include radiographic chest films and barium radiographic studies. Upper endoscopy may be done to confirm the diagnosis and check the pH of reflux fluid.

Treatment
Conservative management for patients with hiatal hernia includes weight loss; eating small, frequent meals instead of three large ones; and avoiding foods that exacerbate symptoms. Medications are similar to those used to treat esophagitis and GERD, including antacids and OTC or prescription-strength H_2 receptor antagonists or proton pump inhibitors. Cholinergic agents may be used to strengthen the LES. If conservative measures are not effective, surgical repair may be done.

Prognosis
Prognosis for patients with hiatal hernia is generally good. Complications such as a **strangulated hernia** (herniated tissue that has had the blood supply cut off, resulting in necrosis and possible septicemia) require prompt surgical intervention.

Achalasia

ICD-9-CM: 530.0   [ICD-10: K22.0]

Achalasia is the dilation and expansion of the lower esophagus due to pressure from food accumulation.

Incidence

Achalasia is an uncommon disorder, most prevalent in middle-aged and older adults.

Etiology

Achalasia develops when the LES fails to relax, and impedes passage of food into the stomach. As food accumulates in the lower esophagus, pressure builds; the result is distention of the lower esophagus.

Signs and Symptoms

Symptoms of achalasia include sharp lower-esophageal pain 10 to 15 seconds after swallowing, unpleasant taste, and aspiration (drawing in or out by suction) or regurgitation (backward flow) of undigested food.

Flashpoint

In achalasia, food collects in the lower esophagus rather than passing into the stomach.

Diagnosis

Diagnosis is based on presenting symptoms and the results of upper GI studies. Barium esophagography and esophageal manometry will reveal distention of the lower esophagus and failure of the LES to relax.

Treatment

Symptoms are minimized by eating small meals slowly with fluids and sleeping with the head elevated. Surgical correction includes dilation of the LES (see Fig. 12-11) and incision (myotomy) of the muscles of the lower esophagus.

Prognosis

Prognosis for patients with achalasia is good, with surgery. Dilation alone may provide only temporary improvement.

Esophageal Varices

**ICD-9-CM: 456.1 (without bleeding),   [ICD-10: I85.9 (without bleeding),
456.0 (with bleeding)   I85.0 (with bleeding)]**

Esophageal varices are varicose (abnormally enlarged) veins of the distal end of the esophagus.

Incidence

Esophageal varices are a common complication of liver disease. They develop in as many as 70% of those with cirrhosis (degenerative disease causing fibrosis and fatty tissue permeation) of the liver.

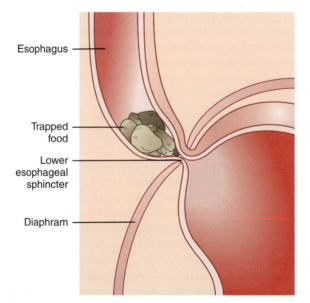

Esophagus

Trapped food

Lower esophageal sphincter

Diaphram

FIGURE 12-11 Achalasia

Etiology

Esophageal varices typically develop because of alcoholic or viral cirrhosis, or other conditions that affect blood flow through the liver. Cirrhosis causes scarring, which impedes circulation through the liver. **Portal hypertension** (increased pressure in the vein entering the liver) develops from blood backing up in the portal vein. Blood is then forced into smaller veins in the esophagus and stomach, causing them to become distended (stretched from overfilling). Another cause of esophageal varices is heart failure.

Signs and Symptoms

Patients may remain asymptomatic unless the varices rupture, causing hemorrhage, hematemesis (vomiting of blood), pain, and shock.

Diagnosis

Diagnosis is based upon a history of hepatic disease and radiographic studies, such as MRI or CT, which reveal obstruction of blood flow. Varices may also be noted incidentally during endoscopic examination.

Treatment

A priority of treatment is to prevent rupture and bleeding. Treatment usually includes upper endoscopy, which allows direct visualization of the bleeding site and immediate treatment in the form of sclerotherapy (injection of an irritating substance to fill, harden, or destroy the vessel) or banding (placement of a tiny rubber band over the varix). Antihypertensive medication may be prescribed to lower portal blood pressure. Application of direct pressure with epigastric balloon tamponade, a measure often used in the past, is now employed only as a temporary measure when endoscopy must be delayed for some reason. Other treatment includes administration of IV fluids and blood replacement. Ice-water **lavage** (irrigation or rinsing out of a body cavity) is seldom used, as it has been found to be of questionable value and may induce hypothermia.

> **Flashpoint**
> Treatment is aimed at preventing rupture and hemorrhage.

Prognosis

Prognosis for patients with esophageal varices is guarded. The risk of hemorrhage is 30% within the first year of diagnosis. The mortality rate is 40% with the initial episode of bleeding and 70% the second time.

> **Flashpoint**
> Esophageal varices are very dangerous, with a high mortality rate from rupture and hemorrhage.

Gastritis

ICD-9-CM: 535.00 (without hemorrhage), [ICD-10: K29.1 (without hemorrhage), 535.01 (with hemorrhage)   K29.0 (with hemorrhage)]

Gastritis is a condition of inflammation of the mucosal lining of the stomach.

Incidence

Chronic gastritis is most common in the elderly.

Etiology

Gastritis has many causes, including ingestion of alcohol, aspirin, or other NSAIDs and infection with *Helicobacter pylori* bacteria. Other contributors include caffeine, smoking, infectious disease, some immune disorders, and mechanical injury. In some cases the condition is idiopathic, meaning no direct cause is identifiable.

> **Flashpoint**
> Gastritis is most common in the elderly.

Signs and Symptoms

Common symptoms include indigestion, epigastric pain, anorexia, nausea, vomiting, cramping, belching, and bloating. Individuals may experience intolerance to fatty foods. If inflammation leads to bleeding, blood may be present in feces or vomit.

Diagnosis

A medical history is obtained to determine the pattern of symptoms and ingestion of potential irritants. Radiographic films may be done to identify any structural problems. Emesis (vomiting) or feces may be tested for the presence of blood. Gastroscopy may be done to visualize the stomach and obtain tissue samples for biopsy and fluid samples for pH testing and culturing for the presence of *H. pylori.*

Treatment

Antibiotics are prescribed if the presence of *H. pylori* is confirmed. Other treatment measures include elimination of irritating agents, and the use of medications such as H_2 receptor blocking agents, antacids, and proton pump inhibitors. Antiemetics may be prescribed if nausea and vomiting are significant complaints. Significant dietary changes are not usually needed; however, any food that seems to exacerbate symptoms should be avoided.

Prognosis

Prognosis for patients with gastritis is generally good but depends upon the cause and appropriate treatment.

Chronic Atrophic Gastritis
ICD-9-CM: 535.1   [ICD-10: K29.4]

Chronic atrophic gastritis is a group of disorders in which the mucosal lining of the stomach is chronically inflamed. Over time this leads to tissue changes in the stomach lining.

Incidence

Chronic atrophic gastritis usually occurs after 50 years of age. Some types are more common in individuals who live in developing countries while others are more common in northern European and Western populations. Most forms affect men and women equally, but autoimmune types affect females three times more often than males.

Etiology

Autoimmune metaplastic atrophic gastritis is inherited. It is caused by an autoimmune response aimed at the parietal cells of the stomach. Insufficient amounts of intrinsic factor then cause malabsorption of vitamin B_{12} and pernicious anemia. Environmental metaplastic atrophic gastritis is caused by dietary factors and *H. pylori* infection. Erosive and hemorrhagic gastritis are caused by alcoholism and medications like NSAIDS. Regardless of the cause, the result is a chronic inflammation of gastric mucosa and gradual replacement of normal tissue with a fibrous, intestinal type of tissue. These changes eventually result in atrophy (tissue wasting) of the mucosal lining of the stomach.

Flashpoint

Chronic inflammation causes fibrotic tissue changes in the stomach lining.

Signs and Symptoms

Patients with chronic atrophic gastritis may be asymptomatic. Symptoms depend on the type and cause of the condition but may include epigastric pain, feelings of fullness, anorexia, diarrhea, nausea, vomiting, weight loss, *flatulence* (gassiness), malaise, and fever.

Diagnosis

Environmental metaplastic atrophic gastritis can be diagnosed with a urea breath test, which identifies the presence of an *H. pylori* infection. Physical-examination findings are often normal; however, abdominal tenderness may be noted. The stool may be positive for occult (concealed or hidden) blood (see Box 12-5). Upper endoscopy may be done to visualize mucosal changes and to obtain tissue for biopsy and gastric secretions for culture.

Treatment

Treatment is aimed at eliminating the cause, relieving complications, and attempting to reverse the atrophy. Combination therapy has become popular. This combines two, three, or even four medications, including one or more antibiotics to treat the *H. pylori* infection as well as proton pump inhibitors to decrease stomach-acid production and promote healing. Individuals with erosive gastritis may undergo similar treatment and will be counseled to avoid using NSAIDS.

Prognosis

Flashpoint

Most cases of gastritis related to *H. pylori* can be completely cured.

The prognosis for patients with gastritis related to *H. pylori* is very good, with appropriate antibiotic treatment. Many cases can be completely cured. Others may be more chronic and result in permanent damage and complications such as pernicious anemia, gastric polyps, and gastric cancer. Erosive gastritis can result in significant blood loss and even death in some cases.

Peptic Ulcer Disease
ICD-9-CM: 531.90 (gastric), 532.90 (duodenal), 533.90 (peptic)   [ICD-10: K25.0 (gastric), K26.0 (duodenal), K27.0 (peptic)]

Peptic ulcer disease (PUD) is a condition in which sores develop in the lower esophagus (esophageal ulcers), stomach (gastric ulcers), or duodenum (duodenal ulcers) when an area of the protective mucous-membrane lining breaks down (see Fig. 12-12).

Box 12-5 Diagnostic Spotlight

FECAL OCCULT BLOOD TEST

The fecal occult blood test, sometimes called a *guaiac test,* identifies the presence of microscopic amounts of blood in the feces. It is a screening test that may indicate the need for further evaluation. Some potential problems it may signal include polyps, ulcers, cancer, and intestinal disorders that cause bleeding. Testing usually requires a collection of three separate samples, from three different days. After collecting the samples and applying them to the card, the patient returns the card to the health-care provider. In the medical clinic, a laboratory technician applies a developer solution to the specimen and notes the presence or absence of color changes that indicate the presence or absence of blood.

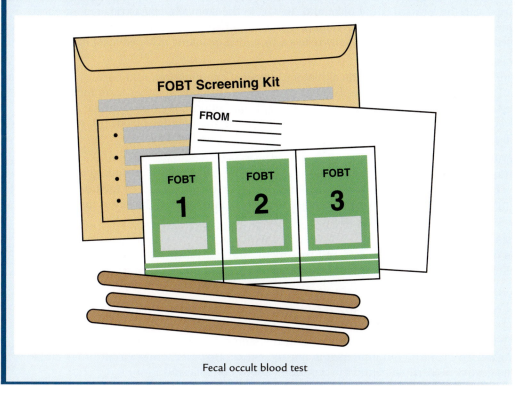

Fecal occult blood test

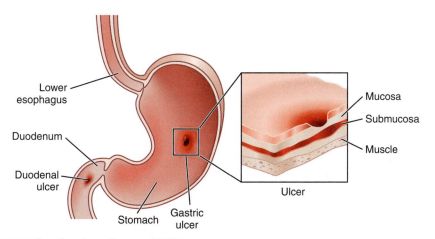

FIGURE 12-12 **Peptic ulcer disease (PUD)**

Incidence

Ten percent of Americans develop PUD at some point in their lives, and approximately 10% of emergency-department patients who complain of abdominal pain are diagnosed with PUD. An estimated 50% of the world's population is infected with *H. pylori*, the bacterium responsible for most cases of peptic ulcers, although the frequency of PUD in the developed world is decreasing.

Etiology

The majority of peptic ulcers are caused by *H. pylori* infection, which causes inflammation and breakdown of the mucosal lining. The next most common cause of ulcer formation is the use of NSAIDs. Other contributors include alcohol and tobacco use. While diet and stress may play a minor role for some individuals, they are not major risk factors as was commonly believed in the past.

Flashpoint

Most ulcers are caused by *H. pylori.*

Signs and Symptoms

Symptoms of gastric ulcers include indigestion, heartburn, and burning pain. The location varies with the location of the ulcer and may be in the stomach, epigastric area, or chest. Other symptoms include nausea and vomiting. Symptoms often peak about 2 hours after eating and may worsen at night. They are temporarily relieved by eating or taking acid-reducing medications.

Diagnosis

Information is obtained through medical history, physical examination, and barium radiographic studies. Blood may be tested for the presence of *H. pylori* antibodies. Other tests include a breath test, stool antigen test, and upper GI x-rays. Upper endoscopy may be done to visualize the involved structures and collect a specimen that can be analyzed for blood, pH, and the presence of *H. pylori*. Tissue biopsy may also be done to rule out malignancy.

Treatment

Combination therapy may be used; it employs two or more medications, including antibiotics to treat the *H. pylori* infection and promote healing. Other treatment measures include elimination of irritating agents. Significant dietary changes are not usually needed; however, any food that seems to exacerbate symptoms should be avoided.

Prognosis

Prognosis is good with early diagnosis and treatment, and mortality is low. Potential complications include mild or severe bleeding, infection, and formation of scar tissue.

Gastroenteritis
ICD-9-CM: 558.9   [ICD-10: A02.0 (due to salmonella), A03.9 (due to shigella), A08.0–A08.5 (due to specified viruses)]

Gastroenteritis is a condition of inflammation of the stomach and intestines. It is often referred to as the *stomach flu*, although influenza is not the cause. However, other viruses may cause contagious gastroenteritis, so contact precautions should be followed.

Incidence

The exact incidence of gastroenteritis is difficult to determine, since people often do not seek treatment unless their symptoms are severe. It most commonly affects infants and children under age 5.

Etiology

Numerous pathogens cause gastroenteritis. Common bacteria include salmonellae, *Escherichia coli*, campylobacters, and shigellae. Viral causes are many: adenoviruses, caliciviruses, rotaviruses, astroviruses, noroviruses, and Norwalk virus. Common parasitic infections include giardias and cryptosporidia. Other causes include irritating foods (alcohol, caffeine, dairy products), medications (NSAIDS, antibiotics, laxatives), exposure to heavy metals (mercury, lead, arsenic), and for some people, stress.

Flashpoint

The many causes of gastroenteritis include viruses, bacteria, food, and medications.

Signs and Symptoms

Symptoms of gastroenteritis depend upon the cause and may include watery diarrhea, abdominal cramps, anorexia, nausea, and vomiting. Other symptoms include headache, fever, chills, and weakness.

Diagnosis

Stool studies may reveal blood, white blood cells (WBCs), bacteria, and viruses. *Lower endoscopy* (visual examination of the lower digestive tract with a scope) may also be performed in select cases (see Box 12-6).

Box 12-6 Diagnostic Spotlight

LOWER ENDOSCOPY

Lower endoscopy is a procedure in which the physician visually examines the colon through a scope. It may include examination of the rectum (proctoscopy), sigmoid colon (sigmoidoscopy), and part or all of the colon (colonoscopy). Before the procedure, medication is given to help the patient relax. A nurse monitors the patient's vital signs and assists the physician. The scope helps the physician carefully examine structures, take photos, remove tissue samples for biopsy, and perform certain treatments. The procedure usually takes an hour or less; however, the patient will need to rest for 1 or 2 hours, until the medication wears off, and will not be able to drive home.

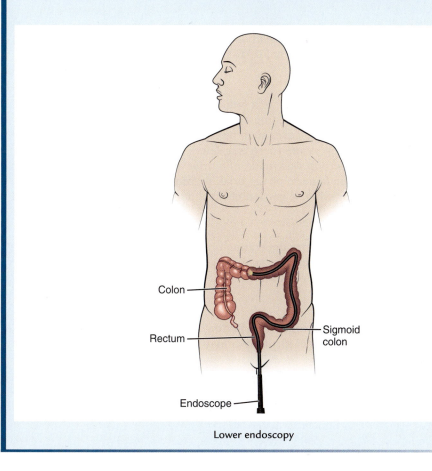

Lower endoscopy

Treatment

Treatment of gastroenteritis is aimed at removing causative factors and managing symptoms. It includes fluid and electrolyte replacement. Electrolytes are ionized substances in blood and tissue fluids, such as sodium, potassium, chlorine, magnesium, and calcium. Rehydration solutions such as Ricelyte and Pedialyte are good choices for children. Patients are instructed to eat a low-fiber diet such as the BRAT diet (bananas, rice, applesauce without sugar, toast) for several days. Prescription medications may include antiemetics, to help alleviate nausea and vomiting, and antibiotics, if appropriate, for an identified bacterial cause. Antidiarrheal agents are generally avoided unless toxins have been ruled out.

Prognosis

The typical course of gastroenteritis is 2 to 10 days, depending on the cause. Acute cases usually resolve without complications. Patients with chronic disease are at risk of infection, bowel perforation, dehydration, and electrolyte imbalances.

Flashpoint
People with diarrhea may find the BRAT diet helpful.

Diseases and Disorders of the Lower Gastrointestinal Tract

The lower GI system includes structures from the jejunum through the anus. Diseases and disorders of these structures are common and can have a significant impact on quality of life; however, many can be successfully treated if detection and treatment are early. Common lower GI diseases and disorders include abdominal hernia, small bowel obstruction, acute appendicitis, peritonitis, diverticulosis and diverticulitis, hemorrhoids, pseudomembranous enterocolitis, Crohn disease, ulcerative colitis, and irritable bowel syndrome.

Abdominal Hernia

ICD-9-CM: 553.9   [ICD-10: K45.8(without obstruction or gangrene)]

Abdominal hernias are hernias involving the abdominal wall and the structures enclosed within it (see Fig. 12-13).

Incidence

An estimated five million people in the United States have abdominal hernia, but only a percentage of these people seek treatment. Approximately 700,000 people undergo surgical repair of abdominal hernia each year.

Etiology

An abdominal hernia can develop anywhere there is a weakness in the containing structures of the abdominal cavity. When this occurs, the intestines protrude. Contributing factors include anything that increases intra-abdominal pressure, such as heavy lifting. Umbilical hernias are usually congenital. Some hernias develop where there is a defect in abdominal muscles. Incisional hernias develop where an incision was made in a prior abdominal surgery, leaving an area of weakness. Groin hernias can be femoral or inguinal. Inguinal hernias are the most common type of abdominal hernia, forming when a portion of the small intestine protrudes through the inguinal canal.

Signs and Symptoms

Signs and symptoms of abdominal hernia vary depending on the site and severity. Patients may notice a bulge that can be temporarily reduced by pushing on it. A person with an inguinal hernia may notice sharp pain when straining or standing. Severe pain, nausea, and vomiting may indicate a strangulated hernia.

Diagnosis

Diagnosis is usually based upon physical-examination findings and a description of the patient's symptoms. Radiographic studies of abdominal structures may be done as well.

Treatment

Treatment of an abdominal hernia depends on the type and location of the hernia, as well as patient factors such as age and general health status. Patients may wear a truss, which is a

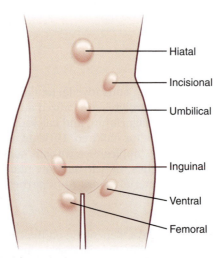

FIGURE 12-13 Abdominal hernia

device that holds the herniated tissue in place. If the patient is considered a good surgical candidate, surgical repair is done.

Prognosis

If untreated, a hernia may worsen over time. Therefore, evaluation by a health-care provider is recommended. Hernias may be surgically repaired, and prognosis is generally very good. A strangulated hernia is a medical emergency that requires prompt surgical intervention to prevent necrosis (tissue death), gangrene, and septicemia (presence of infectious organisms in the blood).

Small Bowel Obstruction
ICD-9-CM: 560.9   [ICD-10: K56.4]

Small bowel obstruction (SBO) is a condition in which intestinal contents are unable to move through the small intestine. The two types are mechanical obstruction and paralytic ileus.

Incidence

Small bowel obstruction occurs most commonly in middle-aged or elderly adults and accounts for 20% of acute surgical admissions.

Etiology

Paralytic ileus develops when the bowel stops functioning normally but no physical obstruction is present. Conditions leading to paralytic ileus include medications such as opiates, peritonitis, bowel ischemia, intra-abdominal surgery, some metabolic conditions, and some diseases. A mechanical SBO develops when the normal passage of intestinal contents is impeded. Adhesions, the most common cause, are scar tissue that develops after a previous abdominal surgery. As they develop, they may constrict an area of the bowel. Other causes include cancerous or benign masses, strictures (areas of narrowing), fecal *impaction* (tightly packed stool), *volvulus* (twisting of the bowel on itself), *intussusception* (telescoping of the bowel into itself), and strangulated hernias (see Fig. 12-14).

Signs and Symptoms

Severity of SBO symptoms depends on whether the obstruction is partial or complete. Patients with complete bowel obstruction present with nausea, vomiting, abdominal pain, and abdominal distention. Initially they may have hyperactive bowel sounds, but these diminish and eventually completely disappear. Other symptoms include inability to pass gas or stool, elevated WBC count, and electrolyte imbalances.

> **Flashpoint**
> A strangulated hernia is a medical emergency.

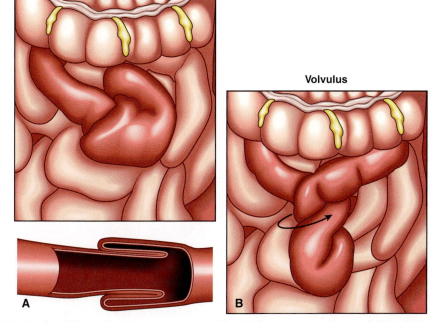

FIGURE 12-14 **Small bowel obstruction caused by (A) intussusception and (B) volvulus**

Diagnosis

Diagnosis of SBO is based upon symptoms and clinical presentation. Barium-swallow abdominal films or barium enema may be done, but should be avoided if bowel perforation or ischemia exists. Plain radiography may reveal dilated loops of small bowel with air-fluid levels and minimal or absent colonic gas. CT scan is useful to detect strangulated obstruction and more clearly identify the underlying cause, and it is considered the study of choice in many cases. Laboratory tests may include complete blood count (CBC), electrolytes, and others.

Treatment

Treatment of an SBO depends upon the cause. The patient is allowed nothing to eat or drink, and a nasogastric tube is inserted to decompress (empty) the stomach and relieve nausea and vomiting. If the cause of the SBO is nonmechanical, as with paralytic ileus, medications may be given to control nausea and promote abdominal peristalsis. Bowel motility and function often return spontaneously within 24 to 72 hours. If the cause of the SBO is mechanical, as with a tumor, adhesions, or a volvulus, surgery is indicated. IV fluid and electrolytes are administered and antibiotics are given to prevent or treat infection.

Flashpoint

A complete bowel obstruction is a surgical emergency.

Prognosis

Untreated strangulated obstructions, such as volvulus, result in tissue necrosis, which causes gangrenous bowel, perforation, and subsequent septicemia—with a 100% mortality rate. However, if surgical correction occurs within 36 hours, the mortality rate drops to 8%. Overall, prognosis for a patient with an SBO depends upon the underlying cause and the speed of accurate diagnosis and treatment. SBOs caused by malignant masses have a guarded prognosis, depending upon whether metastasis has occurred.

Acute Appendicitis

ICD-9-CM: 540.9   [ICD-10: K35.9] (without peritonitis for both codes)

When the appendix becomes inflamed, the result is the condition known as appendicitis.

Incidence

Nearly 7% of the population develops appendicitis at some time during their lives, and more than 300,000 Americans are hospitalized each year with this disorder. It is rare in those younger than 2 and is most common among those between ages 10 and 40. It is the second-most common cause of acute abdominal pain and surgery in the United States.

Etiology

Appendicitis occurs when the appendix becomes clogged with intestinal matter, small foreign bodies, or cancerous tumors. This results in inflammation and infection (see Fig. 12-15). In some cases the appendix may become swollen and filled with purulent matter, leading to rupture. When this happens, the matter spills into the abdomen and causes widespread infection.

Signs and Symptoms

Fewer than half of the patients with appendicitis develop the classic symptoms of nausea, vomiting, and severe periumbilical pain which eventually localizes to the right lower quadrant. Patients may exhibit rebound tenderness to palpation in this area. Other symptoms may include fever, diarrhea or constipation, and anorexia. In over half of cases, symptoms are less specific, with more generalized pain and tenderness.

Flashpoint

Fewer than 50% of people with appendicitis display the expected symptoms.

Diagnosis

Diagnosis is based primarily upon the patient's symptoms and physical-examination findings, which may include rebound tenderness in the right lower quadrant. An elevated WBC count is common. Radiological tests may include CT scan or ultrasound. Exploratory surgery may also be done.

Treatment

The most common treatment for appendicitis is an appendectomy, the surgical removal of the appendix. Antibiotics are also administered to prevent or resolve infection.

Prognosis

Prognosis for patients with appendicitis is good, and full recovery is expected in most cases. If the appendix ruptures before surgery, peritonitis develops, causing peritoneal abscess, infection of the reproductive organs, septicemia, and shock. In these cases the prognosis is more guarded.

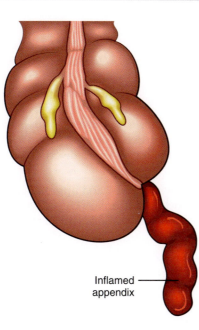

Inflamed appendix

FIGURE 12-15 Appendicitis

Peritonitis

ICD-9-CM: 567.9   [ICD-10: K65.9] (unspecified for both codes)

Peritonitis, sometimes called *acute abdomen*, is a condition of inflammation and infection of the membrane that lines the abdominal cavity and the organs and structures within it. It is classified as generalized or localized.

Incidence

The exact incidence of peritonitis is unclear. The risk of peritonitis is increased in individuals with liver or kidney disease, especially those undergoing peritoneal dialysis.

Etiology

Peritonitis is caused by infection and inflammation of the peritoneum, the serous membrane that covers the organs within the abdominal cavity. The most common causes are bacterial infection due to chronic liver disease, especially among patients with ascites, and complications of peritoneal dialysis. Infection also results when contamination from gastrointestinal contents occurs because of a ruptured appendix or other perforated structure (ulcer, gallbladder, or colon). In women it may be caused by a ruptured ovarian cyst or a fallopian-tube infection. Other causes include penetrating wounds and bloodborne infections.

Signs and Symptoms

Symptoms of peritonitis include severe abdominal distention, pain and tenderness, weakness, diaphoresis (severe sweating), anorexia, nausea, and vomiting. The patient's condition may worsen rapidly, with symptoms of tachycardia, hypotension, fever, and chills. Breathing is often shallow and rapid, and the abdomen may feel rigid and boardlike on examination. Paralytic ileus may develop, in which intestinal motion diminishes or ceases.

Diagnosis

Radiographic abdominal studies such as x-rays or CT scans may reveal gaseous distention and perforation of abdominal organs. Peritoneal fluid is aspirated and studied for bacteria. Serum WBC count will be elevated and electrolytes may be lowered.

Treatment

Treatment of peritonitis includes antibiotics, fluid and electrolyte therapy, analgesics, and possibly antiemetics to treat nausea. Laparoscopy (visual examination of the abdomen) may be performed. Surgical repair and peritoneal lavage with an antibiotic or saline solution may be necessary.

Prognosis

Peritonitis is a life-threatening condition that requires prompt intervention. Complications include septicemia, shock, and death.

> **Flashpoint**
> Peritonitis is a life-threatening condition.

Diverticulosis and Diverticulitis

ICD-9-CM: 562.10 (diverticulosis without hemorrhage), 562.12 (diverticulosis with hemorrhage), 562.11 (diverticulitis without hemorrhage), 562.13 (diverticulitis with hemorrhage)

[ICD-10: K57.3 (diverticulosis or diverticulitis without hemorrhage), K57.2 (diverticulosis or diverticulitis with hemorrhage)]

Diverticular disease includes both diverticulosis and diverticulitis. Diverticulosis is a disorder in which tiny pouchlike herniations called diverticula develop in the wall of the distal portion of the large intestine. Diverticulitis develops when one or more diverticula become inflamed.

Incidence

About 10% of those over age 40 have diverticulosis, and approximately half of those over age 60 have it. However, most people are not aware of it unless they develop symptoms associated with diverticulitis. It is estimated that 25% of those with diverticulosis will do so.

Etiology

Diverticula form in the intestinal wall when increased pressure causes small herniations around small vessels and other structures that transect the wall. Contributing factors include a low-fiber diet and chronic or recurrent constipation. When the diverticula become clogged with feces and become inflamed and infected, the diverticulosis becomes diverticulitis (see Fig. 12-16).

Flashpoint

A major risk factor for diverticular disease is chronic or recurrent constipation.

Signs and Symptoms

Patients with diverticulosis are usually asymptomatic. Symptoms of diverticulitis include fever, nausea, bloating, constipation, blood-streaked stools, and crampy pain in the left lower quadrant of the abdomen. Less commonly, individuals may also experience vomiting.

Diagnosis

Diagnosis is generally based upon a description of presenting symptoms when the patient has developed diverticulitis. Tests may include abdominal ultrasound, which reveals inflamed diverticula, and CT scan, which reveals complications such as abscesses and perforations. Lower endoscopy may also be done so that the physician can visually examine the colon. If diverticulitis is present, a CBC will show an elevated WBC count.

Treatment

Diverticulosis is treated with dietary measures, including adequate fluid and fiber, to prevent constipation, and avoidance of foods containing small seeds and nuts that might lodge in the diverticula. Supplemental fiber is often recommended. Diverticulitis is treated with antibiotics and analgesics. A liquid diet allows the bowel to rest. Surgery may be needed in cases of perforation. Additional measures include rest and stress reduction.

Prognosis

Prognosis for diverticulosis is good unless inflammation and infection (diverticulitis) develop. Mild cases of diverticulitis usually resolve without complications. However, more severe cases can lead to complications such as infection, bleeding, fistula formation, and bowel obstruction. Infection may lead to abscess and perforation, which in turn leads to peritonitis. Severe bleeding from diverticulitis is rare but possible. Fistulas form when an abnormal channel develops between two organs or structures. They can develop in any number of places, but most commonly form between the colon and the bladder. This results in a severe, chronic urinary tract infection unless surgically corrected. Intestinal obstruction can occur from adhesions left by infection and may require surgical repair.

Hemorrhoids

Flashpoint

Hemorrhoids are a type of varicose vein. While rarely serious, they can be quite uncomfortable.

ICD-9-CM: 455.6   [ICD-10: I84.2] (without complication for both codes)

Hemorrhoids are varicose veins of the anal area and lower rectum, and they may be either internal or external (see Fig. 12-17). While they are rarely serious, they are common and can be quite uncomfortable.

Incidence

Hemorrhoids are extremely common, and incidence increases with age. It is estimated that half of adults over the age of 50 suffer from hemorrhoids.

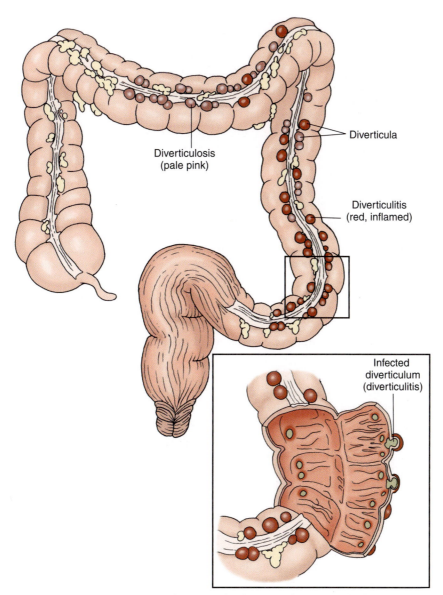

FIGURE 12-16 **Diverticulosis** (From Eagle, S. *Medical Terminology in a Flash! An Interactive, Flash-Card Approach.* 2006. Philadelphia: F.A. Davis Company, with permission.)

Etiology

Hemorrhoids result from a combination of constipation, which results in excessive straining during defecation, and other factors, such as pregnancy and obesity, that increase pressure on veins located in the anorectal area. Disorders that predispose people to the development of hemorrhoids are ulcerative colitis and Crohn disease.

Signs and Symptoms

Symptoms of hemorrhoids include small bulging areas in the anal region that may be painless. However, they can easily worsen with constipation and straining to defecate. Pain or tenderness may be present, as well as itching. Bleeding may occasionally occur after passing stool and is usually minor, although bright-red blood may be seen on the feces and on toilet tissue.

Diagnosis

Diagnosis is usually based upon the patient's description of symptoms and digital rectal examination. A ***proctoscopy*** (visual examination of the anus and rectum with a scope) may be done to examine the anal canal and rectum for internal hemorrhoids. Occasionally, a more extensive

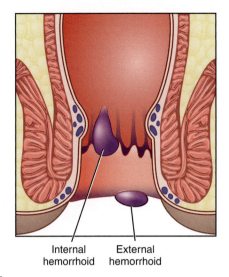

Internal   External
hemorrhoid   hemorrhoid

FIGURE 12-17 Hemorrhoids

examination, in the form of a sigmoidoscopy (visual examination of the sigmoid colon) or colonoscopy, may be done.

Treatment

Conservative measures are aimed at treating and preventing constipation by increasing dietary fluids and fiber and using stool softeners (see Box 12-7). Symptoms can be relieved by soaking in a warm bath and applying topical anesthetics or anti-inflammatory creams. When these treatments are ineffective, a variety of measures may be used to destroy or remove hemorrhoids. Hemorrhoidectomy is the surgical removal of the hemorrhoid. Ligation involves the placement of a tiny rubber band around the hemorrhoid, which cuts off circulation and causes the hemorrhoid to fall off within a few days. Sclerotherapy involves the injection of a chemical into the hemorrhoid that causes it to shrink. Coagulation therapy is treatment of the hemorrhoid with an infrared light or laser. Cryotherapy involves the application of a cold substance to the hemorrhoid to destroy it.

Flashpoint

Constipation can often be prevented or treated with conservative measures.

Prognosis

Prognosis for individuals with hemorrhoids is very good, with appropriate treatment. Complications are usually minor and include pain, bleeding, and infection.

Pseudomembranous Enterocolitis
ICD-9-CM: 008.45   [ICD-10: A04.7]

Pseudomembranous enterocolitis, also called *Clostridium difficile colitis* or *C. diff. colitis*, is an inflammatory condition of the small and large bowel resulting in severe watery diarrhea.

Box 12-7 Wellness Promotion

PREVENTING AND TREATING CONSTIPATION
Follow these measures to prevent or treat constipation:

- Drink plenty of alcohol-free and caffeine-free beverages.
- Eat a diet high in fiber, including fresh fruits, vegetables, and whole grains.
- Drink fruit juice, including prune juice.
- If you must use bowel medications, use bulk-forming nonchemical laxatives, such as Metamucil, or stool softeners instead of harsh chemical laxatives.

Incidence

Incidence of pseudomembranous enterocolitis is difficult to estimate. Antibiotic-associated diarrhea is common, occuring up to 40% of the time when patients undergo antibiotic treatment. Pseudomembranous enterocolitis makes up at least 10% of these cases. Incidence is greatest in hospitalized patients over age 60 who have undergone abdominal surgery and are currently on or have recently been on broad-spectrum antibiotics.

Etiology

Pseudomembranous enterocolitis is an acute inflammatory condition of the small and large bowel in which necrotic debris and mucus adhere to the mucosal lining in a plaque-like manner. Broad-spectrum antibiotic therapy used to destroy pathogenic (disease-causing) organisms may also destroy normal protective flora, which are microorganisms that normally reside within the intestines. This allows *C. difficile* to grow. This organism produces toxins that cause inflammation, ulceration, and necrosis of the bowel wall. The cellular debris and by-products of tissue inflammation combine to form what is known as the pseudomembrane.

> **Flashpoint**
> *C. diff.* colitis is usually associated with current or recent antibiotic use.

Signs and Symptoms

Symptoms of pseudomembranous enterocolitis typically begin several days after antibiotic treatment has ended and include mild to severe watery, foul-smelling diarrhea, abdominal cramping and tenderness, fever, leukocytosis (abnormal increase of white blood cells), weakness, anorexia, nausea, and vomiting. As the patient's condition worsens, tachycardia and hypotension may develop.

Diagnosis

Stool culture will be positive for *C. difficile* or its toxins. Serum WBCs may be elevated, serum electrolytes and protein may be low, and abdominal x-rays may reveal colonic distention. Lower endoscopy may be done to visualize the bowel lining and collect a tissue specimen for biopsy.

Treatment

Treatment includes replacement of fluid, electrolytes, and protein as needed. The antimicrobial of choice is usually metronidazole (Flagyl). Medications which reduce bowel motility are avoided because they may result in retention of toxins. In some cases, bile-acid resins may be given to bind the toxins.

Prognosis

Most people recover from pseudomembranous enterocolitis within 2 weeks, with appropriate treatment. Complications include severe dehydration, electrolyte imbalances, and perianal skin breakdown.

Crohn Disease

ICD-9-CM: 555.9   [ICD-10: K50.9] (unspecified site for both codes)

Crohn disease, also called *regional enteritis,* is a type of inflammatory bowel disease in which the lining of the GI tract becomes inflamed and edematous. It is chronic and can be debilitating.

Incidence

Crohn disease affects seven in 100,000 people in the United States. It is more prevalent in those of European and Jewish descent and is slightly more common in men than in women. It can affect individuals of any age, but most newly diagnosed patients are in their 20s.

Etiology

The cause of Crohn disease is not well understood. Current theories include an immune response to some bacteria; the condition has also been associated with the use of isotretinoin (Accutane), a medication used to treat severe acne. Other contributors may be genetics, infectious agents, and allergies. It is no longer thought to be caused by dietary factors or stress. Smoking increases a person's risk of developing Crohn disease and decreases a person's response to treatment.

> **Flashpoint**
> Smoking increases risk of developing Crohn disease and decreases response to treatment.

Signs and Symptoms

Symptoms of Crohn disease may be mild or severe. Symptoms include chronic diarrhea, fever, weight loss, fatigue, anorexia, abdominal pain, and cramping. Individuals may have periods of exacerbation, in which their symptoms worsen, and periods of remission, in which symptoms disappear.

Diagnosis

Diagnosis is based upon the patient's presenting signs and symptoms as well as the results of diagnostic tests. Visual examination by lower endoscopy is the preferred test, because it allows close inspection of the colon and biopsy of tissue. If this is not possible, barium enema may be done. In some cases a CT scan may also be done, because it can provide more detail than standard x-rays. Laboratory tests include CBC and stool studies.

Treatment

Treatment of Crohn disease is aimed at managing symptoms. Any number of medications may be used, depending upon the individual's specific symptoms. Anticholinergics may help reduce bowel motility; antimicrobials are used as needed for infection. A number of drugs may be used to reduce inflammation, which indirectly reduces pain, including immunosuppressant and anti-inflammatory medications. Opiate analgesics may help control pain not relieved by other medications. IV fluids and supplemental nutrition are used as needed to treat dehydration and malnutrition caused by severe episodes. If these measures are not sufficient, some patients may undergo surgery to remove involved portions of the colon. Patients may also find attending support groups to be helpful.

Prognosis

Crohn disease is chronic in nature, and there is currently no cure. However, it can usually be managed so that patients can have a normal or near-normal life expectancy. Potential complications include bowel obstruction, malnutrition, adhesions, abscess, fistula formation, and fluid and electrolyte imbalance. Patients with Crohn disease also have an increased risk of developing colon cancer.

Ulcerative Colitis

ICD-9-CM: 556.9   [ICD-10: K51.9] (unspecified for both codes)

Ulcerative colitis (UC) is a disorder of the innermost lining of the rectum and colon. Like Crohn disease, it is chronic and can sometimes be debilitating. It is sometimes categorized according to which part of the colon is most affected. Ulcerative proctitis affects only the rectum; left-sided colitis affects the descending colon and rectum; and pancolitis affects the entire colon. Fulminant colitis is a rare, life-threatening form of colitis that also affects the entire colon with much more severe symptoms.

Incidence

Ulcerative colitis affects more than 500,000 Americans, usually young adults in their 30s, men and women equally. Those of Caucasian, Jewish, and European descent have an incidence five times higher than that of other groups.

Etiology

The exact cause of UC is not fully understood. Like Crohn disease, it has been associated with use of isotretinoin (Accutane) to treat severe acne. It is no longer thought that stress causes this disorder, although stress might worsen symptoms. Theories of cause include heredity, viral or bacterial infection, and a possible autoimmune response.

Signs and Symptoms

People with UC usually exhibit a pattern of episodes of acute symptoms alternating with periods of remission. Symptoms include numerous episodes of bloody, mucoid diarrhea per day with pain, cramping, urgency to defecate, weight loss, fever, and malaise.

Flashpoint

The key feature of UC is episodes of bloody diarrhea.

Diagnosis

Diagnosis of UC is based upon the patient's presenting signs and symptoms and the results of diagnostic tests. Lower endoscopy allows the physician to visually examine the parts of the colon affected and obtain tissue for biopsy. Barium enema and small bowel x-ray may also be done. Results of a CBC may reveal anemia and infection.

Treatment

Treatment of UC includes following a nutritious, low-fiber diet and avoiding any foods that worsen symptoms. Other treatment is similar to that used for Crohn disease. Any number of medications may be used depending upon the individual's specific symptoms. Anticholinergics may help reduce bowel motility; antimicrobials are used as needed for infection. A number of drugs may be used to reduce inflammation, which indirectly reduces pain, including immunosuppressant and anti-inflammatory medications. Opiate analgesics may help control pain not relieved by other medications. IV fluids and supplemental nutrition are used as needed to treat dehydration and malnutrition caused by severe episodes. If these measures are not sufficient, some patients may undergo surgery to remove involved portions of the colon.

Prognosis
Ulcerative colitis is chronic in nature, and there is currently no cure. However, it can usually be managed so that patients can have a normal or near-normal life expectancy. Complications include infection and severe colitis, a form that causes severe pain, profuse diarrhea, hemorrhage, fluid and electrolyte imbalances, and shock. Other potential complications include toxic megacolon, a serious condition in which the colon becomes paralyzed. Patients with UC are also at increased risk of developing colon cancer.

Irritable Bowel Syndrome
ICD-9-CM: 564.1   [ICD-10: K58.0]
Irritable bowel syndrome (IBS) is a common condition in which the patient's bowel alternates between episodes of constipation and episodes of diarrhea, along with other GI symptoms.

Incidence
IBS is the most common gastrointestinal disorder in the United States, accounting for more than 10% of all doctor visits. It is estimated that 25 to 45 million Americans suffer from IBS, with young women most affected.

> **Flashpoint**
> People with IBS usually experience episodes of constipation alternating with episodes of diarrhea.

Etiology
The cause of IBS is not fully understood. Current theories include changes in motor or sensory nerves in the bowel causing hyper- or hypomotility, changes in the central nervous system, genetic factors, and hormonal influences. Symptoms may be aggravated by emotional stress and trigger foods such as chocolate, milk, and alcohol.

Signs and Symptoms
Patients with IBS complain of alternating episodes of diarrhea and constipation along with abdominal pain, bloating, gas, distention, cramping, and heartburn.

Diagnosis
Diagnosis is based upon excluding other disorders and identifying specific criteria associated with IBS. These include abdominal pain and discomfort that lasts for 12 weeks or longer plus two of the following:

- alteration in the consistency or frequency of stool
- urgency, straining, or the feeling of being unable to totally empty the bowels
- presence of mucus in the stool
- abdominal distention or bloating

   Diagnostic tests may include lower endoscopy and CT scan. Testing may be done to rule out lactose intolerance as an explanation for the patient's symptoms. Blood tests may also be done to rule out celiac disease.

Treatment
Treatment of IBS is aimed at symptom relief. Antispasmodics may help reduce hypermotility. Bulk fiber such as Metamucil helps minimize both diarrhea and constipation. The medication lubiprostone (Amitiza) has been approved to treat women over age 18 who suffer from IBS with constipation. Patients are also counseled to avoid identified trigger foods, in order to reduce the frequency of symptoms.

Prognosis
Prognosis is generally good but varies with the individual. IBS can worsen symptoms associated with hemorrhoids, may interfere with personal and professional activities, and increases risk of bowel cancer.

> **Flashpoint**
> Inflammatory bowel disease increases the patient's risk of developing bowel cancer.

Diseases and Disorders of Accessory Organs

A number of disorders affect the accessory organs of the GI system. Cholelithiasis and cholecystitis affect the gallbladder; acute and chronic pancreatitis affect the pancreas; and cirrhosis and various types of hepatitis affect the liver.

Cholelithiasis and Cholecystitis

ICD-9-CM: 574.20 (cholelithiasis, without obstruction), 575.12 (cholecystitis, unspecified)

[ICD-10: K80.5 (cholelithiasis, without obstruction), K81.9 (cholecystitis, unspecified)]

Cholelithiasis is a condition in which gallstones have developed and are present in the gallbladder, liver, or biliary ducts (see Fig. 12-18). When inflammation of the gallbladder exists, the condition is known as cholecystitis.

Incidence

Cholelithiasis affects 20 million people in the United States, with up to 3% becoming symptomatic with cholecystitis. It occurs in both genders but most commonly affects women of childbearing age. Incidence increases with age. Ethnic groups most commonly affected include those of fair-skinned northern European descent, Native Americans, and Hispanics.

Etiology

The cause of cholelithiasis is variable. One contributor is high cholesterol or bilirubin levels in the bile. Others are inadequate bile salts and improper emptying of the gallbladder. Risk factors include genetics, a high-calorie and high-fat diet, obesity, use of oral contraceptives, pancreatitis, and alcoholic cirrhosis. Gallstones most commonly develop from insoluble cholesterol but can also form from bile salts. The most common cause of cholecystitis is biliary-duct obstruction by gallstones or crystallized bile sludge. The resulting increased pressure creates inflammation within the gallbladder. Other contributors include infection, cirrhosis, gallbladder injury, and underlying diseases such as diabetes.

Signs and Symptoms

People with cholelithiasis are often asymptomatic and may not realize that they have gallstones. If bile ducts become obstructed by stones or sludge, biliary colic develops. This is intermittent pain in the epigastric area that radiates into the right upper quadrant, right shoulder, and back. It often occurs after, or is worsened by, a high-fat meal. Other symptoms include belching, bloating, intolerance of fatty food, nausea, vomiting, muscle guarding, fever, tachycardia, jaundice (yellowish skin and eyes), light-colored stools, dark urine, and pruritus (itching).

Flashpoint

Many people are unaware that they already have gallstones, because they are asymptomatic.

Diagnosis

Gallstones are often noted incidentally by CT or other tests when diagnostics are done for other reasons. Diagnosis of cholecystitis is based on presenting symptoms, ultrasound results that reveal thickening of the wall of the gallbladder, and testing of fluid from perforation or exudates. Numerous other tests are possible, including oral cholecystogram, plain abdominal x-ray, and IV cholangiogram. A complete blood count may indicate increased WBCs and increased serum bilirubin if obstruction is present.

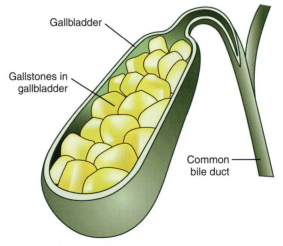

Gallbladder

Gallstones in gallbladder

Common bile duct

FIGURE 12-18 Cholelithiasis

Treatment

If patients are asymptomatic, no treatment is indicated. Diet should be modified to decrease fat intake. Treatment options are available to try to dissolve or disintegrate stones nonsurgically, but these are seldom used, because of their limited success. Elective surgery may be advised for people at high risk of complications, including those with cirrhosis and portal hypertension. The most definitive treatment is ***cholecystectomy*** (surgical removal of the gallbladder). Other measures include antibiotics to treat infection, antiemetics to relieve nausea, and analgesics to relieve pain.

Prognosis

Less than 50% of people with cholelithiasis become symptomatic with acute cholecystitis. For those who do, prognosis is good, with appropriate treatment. Complications of cholecystitis include biliary pancreatitis, perforation, and sepsis. Chronic cholecystitis may be a precursor to cancer of the gallbladder. The mortality rate for emergency cholecystectomy is 3% to 5%.

Acute Pancreatitis

ICD-9-CM: 577.0   [ICD-10: K85.9]

Pancreatitis is a condition in which the pancreas has become inflamed (see Fig. 12-19). It may be either acute or chronic.

Incidence

There are approximately 80,000 cases of acute pancreatitis in the United States each year. It is more common in men than women.

Etiology

The exact cause of acute pancreatitis is unclear. Enzymes commonly released by the pancreas may become active within the pancreas and begin to digest pancreatic tissue. This is called *autodigestion* and causes localized damage and inflammation. Acute pancreatitis is most commonly associated with alcoholism and with biliary-tract disease that includes the presence of gallstones or sludge lodged in the vessels leading from the gallbladder or liver through the pancreas to the duodenum. Other causes include infection, trauma, severe hypercalcemia (high blood calcium), hemorrhage, hyperlipidemia (high level of fat in the blood), endocrine disorders, and some drugs.

Signs and Symptoms

The primary symptom of acute pancreatitis is sudden onset of severe upper-abdominal pain and tenderness that often radiates into the back. Other symptoms may include nausea, vomiting, fever, tachycardia, hypotension, diaphoresis, and rapid, shallow respirations. Symptoms are usually worse after eating or drinking, especially after drinking alcohol. Illness usually lasts for just a few days.

Flashpoint

Acute pancreatitis is usually caused by alcoholism or gallstones.

Diagnosis

Diagnosis of acute pancreatitis is based on the patient's presenting signs and symptoms, physical examination, and diagnostic testing. Laboratory tests determine levels of digestive enzymes

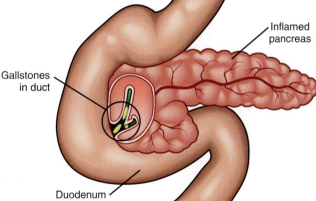

Gallstones in duct

Inflamed pancreas

Duodenum

FIGURE 12-19 Pancreatitis

such as serum amylase and lipase and urine amylase. Others may evaluate WBCs, hematocrit, electrolytes, serum calcium, and glucose. Radiological testing includes abdominal ultrasound, x-rays, CT scans, and MRI. In some cases, endoscopic retrograde cholangiopancreatography (ERCP) may be done to identify and remove stones from biliary vessels (see Box 12-8).

Treatment

Mild cases of acute pancreatitis may resolve without specific treatment. Severe cases require IV fluids and nutrition and gastric decompression, by placement of a nasogastric tube, so that the gastrointestinal tract can rest and heal. Other treatment includes analgesics, antibiotics, and anticholinergic medication. Laboratory tests are done to monitor levels of pancreatic enzymes. In some cases surgery may be done to ease pain and manage complications.

Prognosis

Prognosis for patients with acute pancreatitis is variable. Complications include damage to other organs, such as the heart, lungs, and kidneys, as well as paralytic ileus, bleeding, and infection.

Box 12-8 Diagnostic Spotlight

ERCP

Endoscopic retrograde cholangiopancreatography (ERCP) is a procedure in which the bile ducts and pancreatic ducts are x-rayed after dye is injected through an endoscope. Before the procedure, the patient's throat is sprayed with a topical anesthetic and the patient is given a mild sedative. During the procedure, the physician is able to remove gallstones that may be lodged in the main bile duct, widen a narrowed duct by making a small incision, place a small stent (tube), and gather tissue specimens for biopsy. The procedure usually takes 45 minutes or less. The patient may need to rest for 1 or 2 hours, until the medication wears off, and will not be able to drive home.

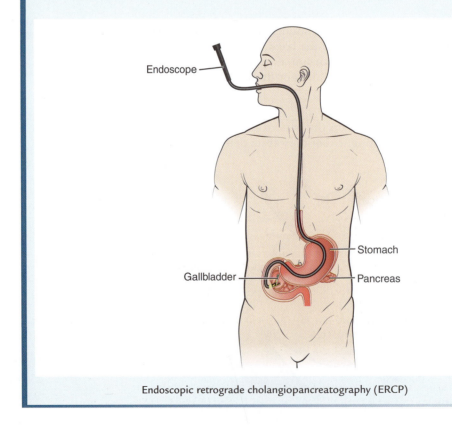

Endoscopic retrograde cholangiopancreatography (ERCP)

Chronic Pancreatitis
ICD-9-CM: 577.1 [ICD-10: K86.1]
Chronic pancreatitis is a long-term condition of inflammation within the pancreas that causes permanent damage to the pancreas.

Incidence
The alcoholic form of chronic pancreatitis is most common in men and develops around age 30 or 40. The hereditary form generally begins in childhood.

Etiology
The initial cause of chronic pancreatitis may be the same as for acute pancreatitis. In 70% of adults, alcoholism is the cause. Less commonly, heredity, cancer, or hyperparathyroidism may play a role. As in acute pancreatitis, autodigestion occurs, causing scarring and other destructive changes.

Signs and Symptoms
Symptoms of chronic pancreatitis may be similar to acute disease or may be more vague. In either case, they generally include abdominal and back pain which worsens with eating or drinking. Other symptoms include nausea, vomiting, and weight loss. As digestive enzymes decrease, food is less efficiently broken down and digested. This leads to signs of malnutrition. It may also cause **steatorrhea** which is unusual, light-colored, greasy, foul-smelling stools. Other disorders, such as diabetes, may be triggered.

Diagnosis
Diagnosis of chronic pancreatitis is based upon the patient's signs and symptoms, physical examination, and diagnostic testing. Laboratory tests determine levels of digestive enzymes such as serum amylase and lipase and urine amylase. Others may evaluate WBCs, hematocrit, electrolytes, serum calcium, and glucose. Radiological testing includes abdominal ultrasound, x-rays, and magnetic resonance cholangiopancreatography. The latter does a better job of revealing pancreatic ducts and bile than a standard CT scan does.

> *Flashpoint*
> Steatorrhea is the passage of light-colored, greasy, foul-smelling stool.

Treatment
Treatment may be the same as for acute pancreatitis. In addition, patients are monitored for signs of malabsorption and diabetes. If the cause is biliary, cholecystectomy may be indicated. Pain is managed with analgesics, and the patient is put on a diet high in carbohydrates and low in fat. Pancreatic enzymes may be taken with meals; insulin may be needed to manage elevated blood glucose. Surgery may be done to ease pain and manage complications. Alcohol must be avoided. If a pancreatic pseudocyst develops, it may need to be drained.

Prognosis
Complications of chronic pancreatitis include pain, nutritional deficiencies, and increased risk of developing pancreatic cancer. A collection of debris and fluid, known as a *pseudocyst*, may develop.

> *Flashpoint*
> A collection of debris sometimes develops in the pancreas—this is called a pseudocyst.

Liver Cirrhosis
ICD-9-CM: 571.2 (alcoholic), 571.5 (nonalcoholic) [ICD-10: K70.3 (alcoholic), K74.6 (nonalcoholic)]
Cirrhosis is an irreversible, chronic, degenerative disease that causes slow destruction of the liver as normal tissue is replaced with scarlike connective tissue (see Fig. 12-20). As a result, the normal functions of the liver are impeded.

Incidence
Approximately 5% of Americans develop cirrhosis and 25,000 die each year. It is more common in males than females.

Etiology
The two most common causes of cirrhosis are chronic alcoholism and hepatitis. Others include toxic chemicals, malnutrition, parasitic infections, heart failure, biliary obstruction, autoimmune reactions, and genetic disorders.

Signs and Symptoms
Patients may be asymptomatic or have only vague, mild symptoms in the early stages. As the condition worsens, symptoms may include anorexia, weight loss, ascites, abdominal

> *Flashpoint*
> The most common causes of cirrhosis are alcoholism and hepatitis.

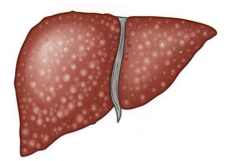

FIGURE 12-20 Cirrhosis

pain, fatigue, weakness, edema, nausea, and vomiting. Additional symptoms include easy bleeding and bruising, jaundice, pruritus, and increasing prominence of small, spiderlike veins in the face. In men, endocrine system changes can cause some feminization of features, such as gynecomastia (breast enlargement), testicular atrophy, and loss of chest hair.

Diagnosis

Diagnosis of cirrhosis is based upon physical-examination findings and results of diagnostic tests. The liver will be enlarged and firm to palpation. Diagnostic studies such as x-ray, liver scan, and MRI will confirm *hepatomegaly* (enlargement of the liver). A liver biopsy may confirm the presence of fibrotic tissue changes. A CBC will reveal anemia. Bilirubin and liver enzymes alanine aminotransferase (ALT) and aspartate aminotransferase (AST) will be elevated. Other testing may indicate vitamin deficiencies.

Treatment

Damage to the liver cannot be reversed, but treatment can arrest or slow the progression, depending upon the condition's underlying cause. Alcohol ingestion must be eliminated. Acetaminophen (Tylenol) and other damaging substances should be avoided. Antihypertensive medications may be given for portal hypertension, and antibiotics are given if infection is a factor. Other measures include a nutritious, low-sodium diet, rest, vitamin and mineral supplementation, and diuretics. In severe cases liver transplantation is considered.

Prognosis

In some cases, early disease can be reversed with appropriate treatment and lifestyle changes. In chronic or severe cases, the prognosis is poor. Complications include esophageal varices, bleeding, bruising, hepatic encephalopathy (decline in brain function), liver cancer, impotence, renal failure, osteoporosis, and portal hypertension resulting in severe ascites. The outlook is better for patients who undergo transplantation; they have a survival rate of around 90%, depending on the severity of the underlying disease.

Viral Hepatitis

ICD-9-CM: 070.00–070.90 (code by type and complications, and as acute or chronic)   **[ICD-10: B15.0–B19.9 (code by type and complications, and as acute or chronic)]**

Viral hepatitis is a condition of inflammation of the liver caused by infection with one of the hepatitis viruses. Types are A, B, C, D, and E.

Incidence

Incidence of viral hepatitis varies with the type (see Table 12-2).

Etiology

Viral hepatitis is caused by infection with one of the hepatitis viruses. In most cases it is spread through contaminated blood or body fluids; however, certain types, such as A and E, are spread through the fecal-oral route. This means that fecal matter, usually microscopic and not obvious to the naked eye, is transmitted by the hands to the mouth and ingested.

Signs and Symptoms

Hepatitis types A and E cause acute illness, but others may cause chronic, lifelong disease. In many cases infected individuals are symptom free. However, when evidence of illness develops,

TABLE 12-2

TYPES OF HEPATITIS

	Type A	Type B	Type C	Type D	Type E
Incidence	Estimates are that one-third of the U.S. population has evidence of past infection; over 30,000 new cases yearly	Estimates are that 1.5 million people are HBV carriers; estimated 300,000 to 750,000 with active infections	Estimates are that 3.2 million Americans are currently infected; 20,000 new cases yearly	Estimated 15 million people infected globally; co-infects about 5% of those with HBV	Rare in the United States; most common in 15- to 40-year-old age group
Duration	Acute (weeks to months)	Acute (several weeks) or chronic (lifelong)	Possibly acute (weeks), but usually chronic (lifelong)	Chronic (lifelong)	Acute
Etiology and Transmission	Hepatitis A virus (HAV) spread by fecal-oral route (fecal contamination of hands, food, and drinks)	Hepatitis B virus (HBV) spread by blood, bodily fluids (semen or breast milk), or needle-sharing	Hepatitis C virus (HCV) spread by blood, usually through needle-sharing, solid-organ transplant before July 1992, or transfusion of clotting factors before 1987	Hepatitis D virus (HDV) spread by similar means as HBV (can only coexist with HBV)	Hepatitis E virus (HEV) spread by similar means as HAV; often associated with a contaminated water supply
Treatment	Immune globulin (solution containing antibodies that provides short-term protection) given before exposure or within 2 weeks afterward	Antiviral drugs	Interferon and ribavirin; possible liver transplant	Supportive care; possible liver transplant	Supportive care
Prevention	Hepatitis A vaccination starting at 1 year and for those traveling abroad; hand washing after toileting and before eating	Hepatitis B vaccination for infants, children, and teens not already vaccinated and for adults at risk of infection	No vaccine available	No vaccine available; HBV vaccination recommended	No vaccine available

symptoms are similar for all forms. They often include joint pain, fatigue, abdominal pain, nausea, diarrhea, anorexia, fever, dark urine, clay-colored stools, and jaundice.

Diagnosis

Diagnostic tests to determine viral cause identify the presence of hepatitis antigens. For example, patients with hepatitis B will test positive for the hepatitis B antigen 1 to 2 months after exposure, those with hepatitis E will test positive for the hepatitis E antigen, those with hepatitis A will test positive for the hepatitis A antigen, and so on. Other tests are used to confirm a diagnosis of hepatitis C, including the enzyme immunoassay and the enhanced chemiluminescence test. Positive results are then confirmed with the recombinant immunoblot assay.

Treatment

Treatment depends upon the type of virus. Patients with hepatitis A may be given immune globulin; those with type B, antiviral medication; those with type C, interferon and ribavirin. Those with types D and E are given supportive care. Hepatitis C is the leading reason for liver transplants, although patients with type D may also occasionally receive transplants.

Prognosis

Flashpoint

Hepatitis C is the most common reason for liver transplantation.

Prognosis varies depending upon the type of virus and the patient's underlying health status. Most people recover from hepatitis B, but complications may include liver cancer and liver failure. The mortality rate for hepatitis C is fairly low, at 1% to 5%, but as many as 85% of patients will develop chronic infection or chronic liver disease. Patients with hepatitis D may develop cirrhosis, and up to 20% will develop liver failure.

Disorders of Nutrition

There are a number of disorders of nutrition, including malnutrition, short bowel syndrome, malabsorption syndrome, and celiac disease.

Malnutrition

ICD-9-CM: 262   [ICD-10: E42] (severe protein deficiency for both codes)

Malnutrition is a condition in which the body is not receiving enough protein, vitamins, minerals, or other vital nutrients.

Incidence

Malnutrition is a serious worldwide problem, especially among infants and children, because they have little or no ability to care for themselves. Others at risk include those who are pregnant, those who are elderly, those with chronic disease, those with alcohol- or substance-abuse issues, and those on extreme restrictive diets. Circumstances that contribute to malnutrition include poverty, political problems, natural disasters, and war.

Flashpoint

Those at greatest risk of malnutrition are those with a limited ability to care for themselves.

Etiology

Malnutrition is physically caused by insufficient intake, in quantity or quality, of food or nutrients. It may also be caused by inadequate absorption, metabolism, or utilization of food and nutrients—as occurs in some nutritional disorders—or by certain medications, such as corticosteroids. The sociopolitical causes of malnutrition are complex and difficult to resolve. Economic hardship leads to lowered productivity and decreased supply of food. Poverty leads to decreased access to food. Conditions are worsened by wars, natural disasters, and epidemics.

Signs and Symptoms

Symptoms of malnutrition are many and include weight loss, energy loss, hair loss, skin lesions, nails that are thin and brittle, generalized edema, diarrhea, muscle wasting, poor physical and mental growth, and delayed healing.

Diagnosis

Diagnosis is made through physical examination, including measurement of weight, body fat, and muscle mass. Laboratory tests include CBC, serum protein, electrolytes, and urine studies. Blood and urine tests may reveal anemia, decreased protein levels, and other abnormalities.

Treatment

Treatment of malnutrition is targeted at the underlying cause and includes nutritional supplements of protein, carbohydrates, fats, vitamins, and minerals. If patients are unable to ingest or absorb oral nutrition sufficiently, IV or enteral-tube feedings may be necessary.

Prognosis

Prognosis is variable depending upon the cause, the severity, and the timing of treatment. Patients with mild malnutrition should recover well, with appropriate treatment. Morbidity and mortality are high in severe cases.

Short Bowel Syndrome

ICD-9-CM: 579.3   [ICD-10: Q43.9 (congenital), K91.2 (postsurgical)]

Short bowel syndrome is the name given to the disorder of malabsorption and malnutrition created by the loss of a significant portion of functioning bowel.

Incidence

Patients with short bowel syndrome are usually children who were born with a congenital defect that required a surgical correction. Other patients are victims of trauma or ischemia that required removal of a significant portion of the bowel. As a result, there is inadequate bowel to absorb sufficient nutrients. Risk factors include intestinal diseases such as necrotizing enterocolitis and Crohn disease.

Etiology

Short bowel syndrome results from the loss of a significant portion of functioning small bowel secondary to resection that was necessitated by traumatic injury, congenital defect, or disease.

Signs and Symptoms

Patients suffer from malnutrition due to inadequate absorption of nutrients, fluids, vitamins, or minerals. Key symptoms include diarrhea, weight loss, weakness, fatigue, brittle hair and nails, and foul-smelling, pale, greasy stool.

Diagnosis

To diagnose short bowel syndrome, the physician reviews the patient's medical history for causes of lost bowel function due to disease or bowel resection. Numerous laboratory studies may be done for diagnostic purposes as well as for monitoring the patient's condition on an ongoing basis. Some of these include fecal fat test, serum electrolytes, CBC, triglycerides, cholesterol, and evaluation of nutritional status.

> **Flashpoint**
> People with short bowel syndrome suffer from malnutrition.

Treatment

Treatment depends on the underlying cause. Malnutrition is treated with a high-calorie, nutrient-dense diet and supplements as needed. Antidiarrheal medication may be used to manage diarrhea.

Prognosis

Prognosis is generally good, depending upon how well the bowel heals and absorbs nutrients. Complications include nervous system degeneration from vitamin B_{12} deficiency, gallstones, kidney stones, weight loss, osteoporosis, and general malnutrition. The most common cause of death in infants with short bowel syndrome is liver failure caused by extended IV nutrition.

Malabsorption Syndrome

ICD-9-CM: 579.9   [ICD-10: K90.9] (unspecified for both codes)

Malabsorption syndrome is a condition in which nutrients are not adequately absorbed in the intestines. Causes are numerous, and the condition may be congenital or acquired.

Incidence

The exact incidence of malabsorption syndrome is difficult to determine, since various disorders are involved. Those caused by celiac disease affect approximately 1% of the population. Those caused by enteropathy from allergies to milk protein are estimated to affect 3%. Individuals most commonly affected by malabsorption syndrome are children with cystic fibrosis, small children affected by toddler's diarrhea, and those with lactose intolerance. Only males are affected with autoimmune enteropathy (enterophathy caused by immune system malfunction).

Etiology

There are many causes of malabsorption syndrome, including viral infection, endocrine disorders such as diabetes, and hyperparathyroidism. Other possible causes include severe parasitic infestations, pancreatic disease, hepatic disease, autoimmune and allergic reactions, absence or deficiency of digestive enzymes, and impaired functioning of the cells of the small intestine's mucosa.

> **Flashpoint**
> Those affected by malabsorption syndrome are often children.

Signs and Symptoms

Symptoms vary depending upon the underlying cause. Most common is chronic or recurrent diarrhea of yellow-gray, greasy stools. Others include abdominal bloating, gas, pain, intermittent nausea and vomiting, weight loss, anemia, and other symptoms of nutritional deficiency.

Diagnosis

There is no specific test for malabsorption syndrome. Therefore, diagnosis is based on history, presenting symptoms, and serum tests. Anemia and deficits of protein and minerals are common findings. Stool samples may be tested for an abnormal increased presence of fat and the presence of parasites. Radiological studies may include barium follow-through or barium enema and magnetic resonance cholangiopancreatography. Biopsy of the small intestine may be done as well. Urine studies may reveal a high percentage of malabsorbed substances.

Treatment

Treatment includes dietary modification aimed at the specific cause. Most commonly, a diet high in calories, protein, vitamins, and minerals is needed. Consultation with a registered dietitian is recommended. Antimicrobials are prescribed for bacterial overgrowth. Oral supplements of pancreatic lipase are given to patients with enzyme deficiency.

Prognosis

Prognosis is generally good, with appropriate diagnosis and treatment. Complications include malnutrition and perianal skin breakdown.

Celiac Disease

ICD-9-CM: 579.0   [ICD-10: K90.0]

Celiac disease, also called *celiac sprue, gluten enteropathy,* and *nontropical sprue,* is a disorder in which the lining of the small intestine is damaged in response to gluten ingestion. Gluten is a type of protein found in barley, rye, and wheat. As a result of the damage, the person suffers from impaired nutrient absorption.

Incidence

An estimated 2.5 to 3 million Americans—one out of 133—have celiac disease, but only 150,000 have been diagnosed. Women are affected twice as often as men.

Etiology

Celiac disease describes an intolerance to the gluten found in wheat, wheat products, oats, and barley; it may be the result of an immunologic reaction. There is some evidence that genetic factors play a role as well. The mucosal lining of the small intestine becomes damaged, and nutrient absorption is hindered.

Flashpoint

Celiac disease involves intolerance to the gluten found in wheat and barley products.

Signs and Symptoms

Symptoms of celiac disease include abdominal distention, gas, anorexia, weight loss, cramping, and diarrhea of greasy, pale, foul-smelling stools. Other symptoms may include aphthous ulcers, fatigue, and bone or joint pain. Eventually, symptoms of malnutrition related to malabsorption appear.

Diagnosis

To be diagnosed with celiac disease, patients must be screened individually and a history of their symptoms obtained. Those with celiac disease have high levels of certain antibodies. Laboratory tests include WBC count, platelet count, glucose tolerance test, PT, and albumin level. Radiographic studies of the upper gastrointestinal system and small intestine may be done. Definitive diagnosis is determined through tissue biopsy and the improvement of symptoms upon adoption of a gluten-free diet.

Treatment

Patients are placed on a strict gluten-free diet. If symptoms do not sufficiently improve, corticosteroid medication may be used.

Prognosis

Patients generally recover by strictly adhering to dietary guidelines. Complications may include malnutrition, osteoporosis, lactose intolerance, infertility, nerve damage, seizures, depression, and abdominal cancer.

Food Poisoning

Food poisoning is a common lay term for a number of illnesses caused by eating food contaminated with bacterial or toxic organisms. Another term often used for similar illnesses is *dysentery,* which is defined as a group of disorders marked by intestinal inflammation and diarrhea. People of any age may be affected, but the very young and the elderly are more vulnerable to the adverse effects of dehydration caused by the associated vomiting and diarrhea. Food poisoning is caused by the ingestion of food that has spoiled or is contaminated by bacteria, toxins, insecticides, lead, mercury, and other substances. Common bacterial causes are *E. coli* O157:H7, campylobacters, and salmonellae.

E. coli O157:H7 Infection
ICD-9-CM: 008.04   [ICD-10: A04.3]

E. coli infection includes numerous strains of the bacterium, many of them quite harmless. Other strains are a frequent cause of intestinal and urinary tract infections. The name *E. coli* O157:H7 was given to a deadly strain because of chemical compounds found on the bacterium's surface. This strain produces toxins which can cause bloody diarrhea and severe damage to the intestinal lining.

Flashpoint

Food poisoning is the common term for illness caused by eating contaminated food.

Incidence

There are over 70,000 cases of *E. coli* infection each year in the United States. Those most vulnerable to it are the very young and the very old.

Etiology

The most common source of *E. coli* O157:H7 is cattle, but other mammals, domestic and wild, can harbor it. People are usually infected by ingesting undercooked or raw hamburger, as well as salami, alfalfa sprouts, lettuce, unpasteurized milk, apple juice, apple cider, and contaminated well water. Those who swim in contaminated water may become infected. Once infection occurs, the bacteria produce a toxin called Shiga toxin that damages the intestines.

Signs and Symptoms

Those with mild infection may be asymptomatic. Symptoms of severe infection typically begin 2 to 5 days after exposure and include bloody diarrhea, abdominal cramps, nausea, and fatigue. Other symptoms may include low-grade fever and vomiting.

Flashpoint

E. coli infection is usually contracted by eating undercooked hamburger or other foods contaminated by the bacterium.

Diagnosis

E. coli O157:H7 infection may be suspected based upon presenting symptoms. Diagnosis is confirmed with results of stool culture.

Treatment

Conservative treatment of rest and oral fluids is usually sufficient. In severe cases, hospitalization is needed for IV rehydration and treatment of complications.

Prognosis

Symptoms of infection with *E. coli* O157:H7 usually resolve within 8 days. Those whose primary symptom is diarrhea usually recover completely. Those with more serious infections may suffer kidney impairment or failure and the complications associated with it.

Campylobacteriosis
ICD-9-CM: 008.43   [ICD-10: A04.5]

Campylobacteriosis is infection with bacteria of the genus *Campylobacter.* It is the most common cause of foodborne bacterial illness of the intestines.

Incidence

According to the Centers for Disease Control and Prevention (CDC), more than 10,000 cases of campylobacteriosis are reported each year. However, most cases go unreported; it is estimated that two to four million people are affected by it annually. Most commonly affected are children under the age of 5 and young adults.

Flashpoint

Campylobacteriosis is the most common cause of food poisoning.

Etiology

There are several strains of *Campylobacter* bacteria, but *Campylobacter jejuni* is responsible for most cases of intestinal illness. It is spread by ingestion of contaminated food—most commonly undercooked poultry or drippings from raw poultry—contaminated water, and raw milk.

Signs and Symptoms

The most common symptom of campylobacteriosis is diarrhea, which may be bloody. Other frequent symptoms include abdominal cramps and pain, fatigue, and fever, usually within 2 to 5 days of exposure. Additional symptoms may include nausea, vomiting, headache, and muscle pain.

Diagnosis

Diagnosis is generally based upon the patient's presenting signs and symptoms and the results of a stool culture.

Treatment

Patients with campylobacteriosis usually respond well to conservative treatment, which includes rest and fluids. Antidiarrheal medication may also be helpful. Those with severe illness may be treated with macrolide or fluoroquinolone antibiotics.

Prognosis

Most people recover fully from campylobacteriosis after a week or so. Guillain-Barré syndrome (GBS) is a rare complication, but campylobacteriosis is nevertheless thought to account for up to 40% of GBS cases. See Chapter 6 for a discussion of GBS. Other potential complications include a type of arthritis, called Reiter syndrome, that usually affects the lower back or knees, as well as inflammatory conditions of the abdomen, heart, central nervous system, gallbladder, and urinary tract. Those with a weakened immune system may develop septicemia.

Salmonellosis

ICD-9-CM: 003.0   [ICD-10: A02.0]

Salmonellosis is an intestinal infection caused by *Salmonella* bacteria. Numerous types of salmonellae cause infections in animals and people, but *Salmonella typhimurium* and *S. enteritidis* are the most common ones found in the United States.

Incidence

Infections with salmonellae account for $1 billion in direct and indirect costs. Outbreaks usually occur in small, contained segments of the general population, but sometimes occur in the form of large outbreaks in hospitals, restaurants, or facilities for children or the elderly. Most cases are reported in North America and Europe. Approximately 40,000 cases are reported to the CDC annually. However, many milder cases go unreported. It is therefore estimated that actual incidence is around one and a half million cases each year, with approximately 500 related deaths. Those who are very young or very old and those who have impaired immune systems are most vulnerable.

Etiology

Salmonellae are spread via contaminated reptiles and mammals, undercooked poultry and beef, eggs, and the contaminated feces of those who are infected. Other sources may include unwashed fruits and vegetables grown in contaminated soil.

Flashpoint

Salmonellae are often spread by contaminated reptiles.

Signs and Symptoms

Those infected with salmonellae develop symptoms within 12 to 72 hours and report fever, headache, diarrhea, and abdominal cramps. Other symptoms may include nausea, vomiting, and anorexia.

Diagnosis

Diagnosis is based upon the patient's presenting signs and symptoms and the results of stool culture.

Treatment

Patients with salmonellosis are usually treated with fluid replacement and rest. Antimicrobials are usually not needed. However, individuals with severe cases may require hospitalization.

Prognosis

Illness usually lasts 4 to 7 days, and most people recover fully without treatment. However, in some cases severe diarrhea may result in dehydration and the need for hospitalization (see Box 12-9). Other potential complications include a type of arthritis, called Reiter's syndrome, that usually affects the lower back or knees, and septicemia.

Box 12-9 Wellness Promotion

PREVENT DEHYDRATION

Illnesses that cause vomiting and diarrhea can quickly lead to dehydration. To prevent or treat dehydration, be sure to drink plenty of fluids. Good choices include:

- water
- fruit juice (diluted with water if it causes stomach upset)
- rehydration solutions such as Pedialyte
- electrolyte sports drinks (diluted 50/50 with water for better absorption and less stomach irritation)
- Jell-O
- Popsicles
- broth

Avoid fluids which have a diuretic effect and worsen dehydration, such as caffeinated and alcoholic beverages.

STOP HERE.

Select the flash cards for this chapter and run through them at least three times before moving on to the next chapter.

Student Resources

American College of Gastroenterology: http://www.acg.gi.org
American Dental Association: http://www.ada.org
American Liver Foundation: http://www.liverfoundation.org
Celiac Disease Foundation: http://www.celiac.org
Centers for Disease Control and Prevention: http://www.cdc.gov
Crohn's and Colitis Foundation of America: http://www.ccfa.org
Merck Manual Medical Library: http://www.merckmanuals.com/professional

Chapter Activities

Learning Style Study Strategies

Try any or all of the following strategies as you study the content of this chapter:

Visual and auditory learners: Locate movies in which a lead character suffers from one of the disorders you are studying. Be careful to note that medical information is not always portrayed accurately in movies and films. However, this can still help you learn about the disorder and can provide powerful visual and auditory data to help you remember the disorder.

Kinesthetic learners: Play a Pictionary-like game with your study group in which you take turns drawing pictures that represent various diseases while your partners try to guess what they are.

Verbal learners: If you are self-conscious about speaking aloud while studying, find a private, secluded area like the back corner of the library, an empty classroom, or even the inside of your car.

Practice Exercises

Answers to Practice Exercises can be found in Appendix D.

Case Studies

CASE STUDY 1

You are a CMA working in the GI department at Valley Medical Clinic. Your next patient is Vivienne Richards, a 45-year-old woman who has been referred to the GI clinic with symptoms of pain and burning in her chest and throat. She describes the pain as sometimes worse after she drinks coffee or eats chocolate or spicy food. It occurs during the day but is often worse at night. She sometimes takes antacids, which seem to help but have been less effective recently. Possible differential diagnoses for Ms. Richards are GERD, esophagitis, achalasia, gastritis, PUD, and hiatal hernia.

1. What tests might the physician order to be able to correctly diagnose Ms. Richards?

2. Ms. Richards is eventually diagnosed with GERD and mild esophagitis. The physician prescribes Prilosec, a medication classified as a proton pump inhibitor that reduces the amount of acid her stomach produces. She voices confusion about how this medication will help, stating that the pain and burning are in her chest and throat, not her stomach. What explanation should you offer to help her better understand the cause of her symptoms and how the medication works?

3. Ms. Richards states that she doesn't want to take pills any longer than necessary and wonders whether there are any other measures she can use to relieve or minimize her symptoms. What do you tell her?

4. Ms. Richards comments, "The doctor said we should treat my symptoms in order to reduce my risk of getting throat cancer. I don't understand what one has to do with the other. Can you explain?" What do you tell her?

CASE STUDY 2

Danielle Davis, age 17, was brought to the urgent-care clinic by her mother. She reported a sudden onset of nausea and vomiting the night before, with onset of watery diarrhea this morning. She has not had any loose stools for the past 2 hours but describes feeling "totally wiped out" and complains, "My gut hurts really bad." She is unable to stand for more than a few minutes without help. Her heart rate is rapid, at 122, and her blood pressure is low, at 88/66.

1. What questions might be asked to further determine the severity of Danielle's dehydration?

2. What diagnostic tests is the physician most likely to order?

3. What types of disorders might cause symptoms such as Danielle's?

4. After several hours, during which she receives fluids and her pulse and blood pressure return to normal, Danielle is sent home with her mother, with instructions to return if she is not better in the next 12 hours. Her mother is concerned that Danielle may become dehydrated again and asks your advice to help prevent this. What do you tell her?

CASE STUDY 3

Maria Hernandez is a 65-year-old woman who was brought to the urgent-care clinic by her husband with complaints of acute abdominal pain and vomiting. Her symptoms began suddenly this morning and have worsened since. Her medical history includes an abdominal hysterectomy 10 years ago, appendectomy as a teenager, and partial colectomy secondary to complications from Crohn disease 2 years ago. As you help Mrs. Hernandez change into an examination gown, you notice that her abdomen is round and distended. She comments that she feels "bloated" and hasn't been able to pass stool or gas.

1. What diagnostic tests is the physician likely to order?

2. Based upon clinical presentation, physical-examination findings, and diagnostic-test results, Mrs. Hernandez is diagnosed with a small bowel obstruction (SBO) caused by adhesions. Mr. Hernandez pulls you aside and asks what adhesions are. What do you tell him?

3. Mr. Hernandez is concerned that his wife is becoming dehydrated and wants to give her some water to drink. What do you tell him?

4. Mrs. Hernandez is hospitalized for further treatment and monitoring. What treatment interventions is she likely to undergo in the hospital?

Multiple Choice

1. Which of the following disorders is matched with the correct information or definition?

    a. Gastroesophageal reflux disease (GERD): inflammation of the mucosal lining of the stomach

    b. Achalasia: may result in atrophy of the stomach lining

    c. Gastritis: dilation and expansion of the lower esophagus due to pressure from food accumulation

    d. Esophageal varices: varicose veins of the distal end of the esophagus

2. Which of the following disorders is matched with the correct information or definition?

    a. Peptic ulcer disease (PUD): commonly known as *heartburn*

    b. Gastroenteritis: most commonly caused by *H. pylori*

    c. Hiatal hernia: part of the diaphragm around the base of the esophagus weakens and allows a portion of the stomach to slide upward into the thoracic cavity

    d. Gastroesophageal reflux disease (GERD): common causes include salmonellae, *E. coli*, parasites such as giardias, and numerous viruses

3. Which of the following disorders is matched with the correct information or definition?

    a. Small bowel obstruction (SBO): occurs when the appendix becomes clogged with intestinal matter

    b. Peritonitis: potential complication of appendicitis

    c. Cirrhosis: remedy is surgical removal of affected part

    d. Appendicitis: commonly caused by adhesions

4. Which of the following disorders is matched with the correct information or definition?

    a. Crohn disease: the most common gastrointestinal disorder in the United States

    b. Diverticulosis: disorder of inflammation and edema deep into the layers of the lining of any part of the GI tract

    c. Ulcerative colitis: chronic inflammation of the innermost lining of the rectum and colon

    d. Irritable bowel syndrome (IBS): tiny pouchlike herniations develop in the wall of the distal portion of the large intestine

5. Which of the following disorders is matched with the correct information or definition?

    a.   Hepatitis B: cause is biliary-duct obstruction by gallstones or crystallized bile sludge

    b.   Cirrhosis: varicose veins of the anal area

    c.   Hepatitis C: the most common reason for liver transplantation

    d.   Cholelithiasis: irreversible, chronic, degenerative disease that causes slow destruction of the liver as normal tissue is replaced with scarlike connective tissue

Short Answer

1. **Poor oral and dental hygiene and inadequate dental care are risk factors for what disorders?**

2. **Fill in the table below to compare the cause and risk factors, descriptions, incidences, and treatments for a cold sore and an aphthous ulcer.**

	Cause and risk factors	Description	Incidence	Treatment
Apthous ulcer				
Cold sore				

3. **Explain the following statement: "Most ulcers can be cured with antibiotics."**

13 ENDOCRINE SYSTEM DISEASES AND DISORDERS

Learning Outcomes

Upon completion of this chapter, the student will be able to:

- Define and spell terms related to the endocrine system
- Identify key structures of the endocrine system
- Discuss the function of the endocrine system organs and key hormones

- Identify characteristics of common endocrine system diseases and disorders, including:
  - description
  - incidence
  - etiology
  - signs and symptoms
  - diagnosis
  - treatment
  - prognosis

KEY TERMS	
acromegaly	excessive growth of the bones and tissues of the face and extremities, caused by excessive levels of growth hormone
congenital hypothyroidism	congenital deficiency of thyroid hormones, characterized by arrested physical and mental development; formerly called *cretinism*
diabetic ketoacidosis	condition of severe hyperglycemia
diabetic neuropathy	damage to motor and sensory nerves from long-standing diabetes
diabetic retinopathy	diseased retina caused by poorly controlled diabetes
exophthalmos	protruding eyeballs
fasting	going without food or nutrition, usually for a specified period of time before laboratory tests or surgical procedures
gigantism	form of hyperpituitarism that results in an abnormal increase in height and size
glucometer	instrument used to measure glucose levels in the blood
goiter	enlarged thyroid gland
Graves disease	autoimmune form of hyperthyroidism
hirsutism	male pattern of body-hair development
hyperglycemia	high blood glucose
myxedema	collective symptoms of severe hypothyroidism, which include fatigue, hair that is dry and brittle, intolerance of cold, weight gain, constipation, mental apathy, physical sluggishness, muscle aches, and nonpitting edema
negative feedback system	system in which an increase or decrease in a substance stimulates an opposite response

KEY TERMS—cont'd

nephropathy	diseased changes of the kidneys, with eventual kidney failure
panhypopituitarism	condition of diminished secretion of all hormones secreted by the anterior pituitary gland
pituitary dwarfism	condition of reduced growth and development due to deficiency of growth hormone in childhood
polydipsia	excessive thirst
polyphagia	excessive appetite
polyuria	excessive urination
thyrotoxicosis	severe episode of worsening symptoms of hyperthyroidism
vasopressin	hormone that helps the body concentrate urine and conserve water

Abbreviations

Table 13-1 lists some of the most common abbreviations related to the endocrine system.

TABLE 13-1
ABBREVIATIONS

Abbreviation	Definition
ACTH	adrenocorticotropic hormone
ADH	antidiuretic hormone
BG	blood glucose; also called *blood sugar*
BS	blood sugar; also called *blood glucose*
Ca	calcium
DKA	diabetic ketoacidosis
DM	diabetes mellitus
FBG	fasting blood glucose; also called *fasting blood sugar*
FBS	fasting blood sugar; also called *fasting blood glucose*
FSH	follicle-stimulating hormone
GH	growth hormone
IDDM	insulin-dependent diabetes mellitus; also called *type 1 diabetes*
LH	luteinizing hormone
NIDDM	non–insulin-dependent diabetes mellitus; also called *type 2 diabetes*
PTH	parathormone; also called *parathyroid hormone*
T_3	triiodothyronine
T_4	thyroxine
TSH	thyroid-stimulating hormone

Structures and Functions of the Endocrine System

The endocrine system is made up of all of the hormone-producing and hormone-secreting structures of the body (see Fig. 13-1). It regulates many body functions through the action of these hormones.

Structures of the Endocrine System

The pituitary gland is a small, round, pea-sized structure attached to the lower surface of the hypothalamus in the brain. It has been nicknamed the *master gland* because it affects all of the

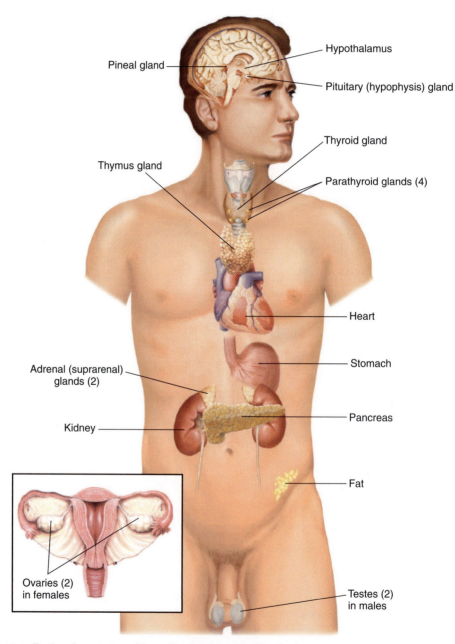

FIGURE 13-1 Endocrine system (From Eagle, S, et al. *The Professional Medical Assistant: An Integrative Teamwork-Based Approach.* 2009. Philadelphia: F.A. Davis Company, with permission.)

other glands in the body, but it is actually controlled by the hypothalamus. The pituitary gland is functionally divided into an anterior lobe and a posterior lobe, which each produce different hormones (see Fig. 13-2). The anterior lobe is responsible for secreting growth hormone, thyroid-stimulating hormone (TSH), follicle-stimulating hormone, luteinizing hormone, adrenocorticotropic hormone (ACTH), and prolactin. The posterior lobe is responsible for secreting oxytocin and antidiuretic hormone.

The thyroid gland, one of the largest endocrine glands, is highly vascular and is located in the base of the neck. It is shaped similar to the letter H, with two lobes (one on each side of the trachea) that are connected by a narrow band. Four tiny parathyroid glands lie on the posterior surface of the thyroid gland, within its connective tissue.

The thymus gland sits deep in the chest and encircles the lower portion of the trachea. It is comparatively smaller in infants and children and becomes smaller as individuals age.

The two triangular adrenal glands are located within the retroperitoneal cavity (in the back of the abdomen) on top of the kidneys. They are made up of an outer layer called the adrenal cortex and an inner part called the adrenal medulla. The two parts of the adrenal glands act separately.

The pancreas is located in the upper left quadrant of the abdomen. The endocrine portion of it is called the pancreatic islets or *islets of Langerhans*. The pancreas is also considered an accessory organ for the gastrointestinal system; for further discussion, see Chapter 12.

Flashpoint

The pituitary has been nicknamed the master gland because it affects all other glands in the body.

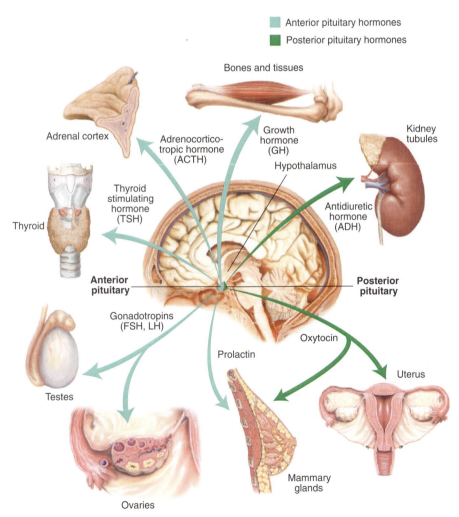

FIGURE 13-2 Pituitary hormones (From Eagle, S, et al. *The Professional Medical Assistant: An Integrative Teamwork-Based Approach.* 2009. Philadelphia: F.A. Davis Company, with permission.)

Flashpoint

The ovaries and testes are part of the reproductive and endocrine systems.

The pineal gland, sometimes referred to as the *pineal body*, is shaped like a pine cone and located in the brain, above and behind the thalamus.

The reproductive glands, sometimes called the *gonads*, are the ovaries and testes. The ovaries are located in the female reproductive tract, within the pelvis; the testes are located in the male reproductive tract, in the scrotum.

Functions of the Endocrine System

The pituitary gland controls many other glands in the body. The hormones secreted by the anterior lobe have the following functions:

- Growth hormone promotes the growth of body structures such as bones.
- Thyroid-stimulating hormone affects the growth and functioning of the thyroid gland.
- Follicle-stimulating hormone and luteinizing hormone act on the ovaries to produce an ovum and on the testes to produce sperm.
- Adrenocorticotropic hormone acts on the adrenal glands to secrete glucocorticoids, including cortisol.
- Prolactin acts on the mammary glands to produce milk.

The hormones secreted by the posterior lobe of the pituitary gland have the following functions:

- Oxytocin acts on the uterus to promote contractions during labor and delivery of a baby.
- Antidiuretic hormone acts on the kidneys to increase the absorption of water.

The thyroid gland produces two thyroid hormones, triiodothyronine and thyroxine, which are responsible for growth throughout childhood and regulation of body metabolism. It also produces calcitonin, which helps regulate blood calcium and phosphorus.

The parathyroid glands secrete parathormone (PTH), also called *parathyroid hormone*, which is responsible for regulating calcium and phosphorus levels in the blood.

The adrenal glands secrete several hormones:

- Epinephrine (also known as *adrenalin*) is released during the fight-or-flight response to increase the body's ability to cope with stress or trauma by helping convert glycogen into glucose for energy, opening the airways, and other changes.
- Aldosterone helps regulate fluid and electrolyte balance.
- Cortisol is the body's natural steroid, which helps decrease inflammation.
- Androgens are responsible for secondary sexual characteristics in females and males.

The pancreas secretes insulin and glucagon as needed to maintain optimal blood glucose levels and to aid in the metabolism of carbohydrates and other nutrients. Insulin acts to transport glucose from the blood to the cells of the body for energy. As a result, blood glucose levels are lowered. Glucagon is secreted as needed to increase glucose levels in the blood by stimulating the liver to release stored glucose, called *glycogen.* Glycogen is also stored in the muscles and can be converted into glucose during times of need, such as during exercise or prolonged periods without meals.

The pineal gland produces the hormone melatonin, which influences the body's natural circadian rhythm, or sleep-wake cycle.

Flashpoint

Insulin helps glucose move from the blood into the cells.

The main function of the thymus gland is to produce T lymphocytes for the immune system. It plays an active role in the immune system in children but shrinks and becomes less active as individuals age.

The two ovaries are responsible for producing an ovum during each menstrual cycle and secreting estrogen and progesterone. Estrogen is responsible for the development of sexual characteristics in the female, including breasts and pubic hair. It plays a vital role in the menstrual cycle and is important in the prevention of osteoporosis in postmenopausal women. Progesterone is necessary to prepare and maintain the uterus for a fertilized ovum.

The testes secrete testosterone, which is responsible for the development of male sex characteristics during puberty, such as deepening of the voice, facial and pubic hair, and body development. It is also necessary in the production of sperm.

Within the endocrine system, glands and hormones work together to maintain homeostasis in the body using a ***negative feedback system.*** The system is considered negative because it works in opposites to maintain an optimal level of certain substances in the body. Each gland produces a hormone that opposes another substance. The gland may increase or decrease production of the hormone to stimulate a corresponding decrease or increase in the other substance. Thus, this system works much like a thermostat, activating the production of heat in response to falling temperatures (a decrease in the normal level) or decreasing heat production in response to the optimal heat level or a level that is too high.

Flashpoint

A negative feedback system works in opposites to maintain a healthy level of certain substances.

Hormones of the Endocrine System

Table 13-2 contains a list of the hormones of the endocrine system, along with their descriptions.

TABLE 13-2
HORMONES OF THE ENDOCRINE SYSTEM

Term	Definition
adrenocorticotropic hormone (ACTH)	hormone secreted by the pituitary gland; acts on the adrenal gland to secrete cortisol
aldosterone	hormone secreted by the adrenal gland; responsible for increasing absorption of sodium in the kidneys
androgens	substances producing or stimulating the development of male characteristics, such as the hormone testosterone
antidiuretic hormone	hormone produced by the hypothalamus and stored in the pituitary gland; released to increase absorption of water by kidneys; also called *vasopressin*
calcitonin	hormone secreted by the thyroid gland; responsible for calcium-phosphorus balance in the blood
cortisol	hormone secreted by the adrenal glands; the body's natural steroid, closely resembling the medication cortisone
epinephrine	hormone produced by the adrenal gland; responsible for the fight-or-flight response; also called *adrenaline*
estrogens	natural or artificial substances that induce the development of female sex characteristics and female cyclic changes
follicle-stimulating hormone	hormone secreted by the pituitary gland; acts on the ovaries to produce an ovum and on the testes to produce sperm
glucagon	hormone secreted by the pancreas; increases blood glucose levels during times of fasting
glycogen	stored form of glucose, found in the liver and muscles
growth hormone	also known as *somatotropin*; produced and secreted by anterior pituitary gland, responsible for stimulating body growth
insulin	hormone secreted by the pancreas; aids in the utilization of glucose for the body's needs
luteinizing hormone	hormone secreted by the pituitary gland; stimulates the testes to release testosterone, stimulates ovulation
melatonin	hormone produced by the pineal gland; influences sleep-wake cycle

Continued

TABLE 13-2

HORMONES OF THE ENDOCRINE SYSTEM—cont'd

Term	Definition
oxytocin	hormone secreted by the pituitary gland; stimulates uterine contractions
parathormone (PTH)	hormone secreted by the parathyroid glands; works in concert with calcitonin and is responsible for calcium-phosphorus balance in the blood; also called *parathyroid hormone*
progesterone	steroid hormone produced by the ovaries and placenta; responsible for endometrial changes in the second half of the menstrual cycle
prolactin	hormone secreted by the pituitary gland; acts on the mammary glands to produce milk
testosterone	steroid sex hormone secreted by the testes; responsible for the growth and development of male characteristics
thyroid-stimulating hormone (TSH)	hormone secreted by the pituitary gland; stimulates the thyroid gland to function
thyroxine	one of two forms of the principal hormone secreted by the thyroid gland; responsible for food utilization and energy production
triiodothyronine	one of two forms of the principal hormone secreted by the thyroid gland; regulates growth and development, helps control metabolism and body temperature

Common Endocrine System Diseases and Disorders

There are many diseases and disorders of the endocrine system. They are often grouped according to the gland involved: diseases and disorders of the pancreas, the thyroid, the parathyroid glands, the adrenal glands, and the pituitary gland.

Diseases and Disorders of the Pancreas

As an endocrine gland, the pancreas secretes insulin and glucagon to regulate blood glucose. Consequently, disorders of this gland often result in alterations in blood glucose regulation and the complications caused by those alterations. Common disorders of the pancreas are type 1 and type 2 diabetes, gestational diabetes, and nondiabetic hypoglycemia.

Type 1 Diabetes

ICD-9-CM: 250.01 (controlled, without complications)　　　　**[ICD-10: E10.9 (without complications)]**

Diabetes mellitus is a chronic metabolic disorder characterized by **hyperglycemia** (high blood glucose). Type 1 diabetes is often referred to as *insulin-dependent diabetes mellitus* or sometimes *juvenile-onset diabetes.* However, people can develop type 1 diabetes into early adulthood.

Flashpoint

People with type 1 diabetes require insulin injections.

Incidence

An estimated 9 to 12 million Americans have type 1 diabetes. Onset usually occurs during childhood but can be later. High-risk groups include Native Americans, African Americans, Pacific Islanders, and Mexican Americans; incidence may be as high as 20% in these groups.

Etiology

Type 1 diabetes is caused by autoimmune destruction of the beta cells in the pancreas, which are responsible for producing insulin. As a result, the individual is left with an absence of insulin. This causes blood glucose levels to rise out of control while the cells of the body starve for lack of glucose.

Signs and Symptoms

Onset of type 1 diabetes is often acute. Individuals usually experience ***polydipsia*** (excessive thirst), ***polyphagia*** (excessive appetite), ***polyuria*** (excessive urination), and weight loss. Often, an initial diagnosis is made after the individual has been hospitalized with ***diabetic ketoacidosis,*** a condition of severe hyperglycemia (see Table 13-3). Diabetic ketoacidosis often has a gradual onset preceded by infection or illness. Symptoms include abdominal pain; cramps; nausea; vomiting; headache; irritability; tachycardia; hypotension; flushed, dry skin; and fruity breath odor. Many of these symptoms are related to the severe dehydration that occurs. The condition will deteriorate into a diabetic coma if not treated, and it can be fatal.

Diagnosis

Diagnosis of diabetes mellitus is based upon a medical history, signs, symptoms, and results of diagnostic testing. A variety of tests may be done, including a random blood glucose level, fasting blood glucose level, and glycosylated hemoglobin level (see Box 13-1). The glucose tolerance test is no longer recommended to confirm diagnosis; instead, diagnosis is based upon the presence of the classic symptoms along with two separate fasting blood glucose levels over 126 mg/dL or a random blood glucose level over 200 mg/dL. Individuals with blood glucose values from 100 to 125 mg/dL are identified as having prediabetes.

Treatment

Treatment for type 1 diabetes includes dietary modification, regular exercise, careful foot and eye care (see Box 13-2), and supplemental insulin. The insulin must be administered by injection because it is broken down by gastric juices (stomach acid) and therefore cannot be taken orally. Therapy must be individualized. Some people do well with one or two injections per day of long-acting insulin, but others may require several injections per day of shorter-acting insulin. Another option is continuous infusion of short-acting insulin with an insulin pump. This

Flashpoint

Classic symptoms of diabetes are the *polys*: polydipsia, polyphagia, and polyuria.

TABLE 13-3

HYPOGLYCEMIA VERSUS HYPERGLYCEMIA

This table lists the most common signs and symptoms of hyperglycemia and hypoglycemia, with the onset, cause, and most common treatment of each condition. Note: Severity of symptoms depends upon how abnormally high or low the blood glucose levels become.

	Hypoglycemia (glucose < 70 mg/dL)	Hyperglycemia (glucose > 100 mg/dL)
Onset	Acute	Gradual
Signs and symptoms	Fatigue, restlessness, hunger, dizziness, irritability, tremulousness, clammy skin, combativeness, heart palpitations, confusion, eventual loss of consciousness	Fruity breath odor, deep rapid respirations, polydipsia, polyphagia, polyuria, glycosuria, weight loss, dry and flushed skin, lethargy, confusion, eventual coma
Cause	Too much insulin, not enough food, overexercise, vomiting, diarrhea	Not enough insulin or missed insulin doses, too much food, lack of activity, stress, illness, infection
Treatment	If patient is conscious and has a gag reflex, give some form of simple sugar (glucose tablets, orange juice, nondiet soda, hard candy, etc.); if patient is not conscious, call 911 and inject glucagon (if available). After blood glucose rises, provide a follow-up snack or meal of complex carbohydrates and protein.	Administer insulin after checking blood glucose level or administer oral hypoglycemic agents per physician recommendation.

Box 13-1 Diagnostic Spotlight

GLYCOSYLATED HEMOGLOBIN

Blood glucose binds with hemoglobin on red blood cells in a process known as glycosylation. The higher the level of blood glucose, the more that is available to bind with hemoglobin. The glycosylated hemoglobin test is a blood test that measures this as a percentage. Since this test isn't affected by short-term fluctuations in blood glucose, and since red blood cells live for about 4 months, the test reveals the patient's average blood glucose levels for that amount of time. Some patients even call it the "tattletale" test, because it tells the truth about just how well they have (or have not) managed their blood glucose level for the past several months. A value of 6% or lower is considered normal for the average nondiabetic person. A value of 8% reflects fair blood glucose control. A value of 10% reflects poor blood glucose control. A value of 12% or higher reflects very poor control and indicates that the patient is at very high risk of complications of diabetes. Most patients are advised to have their glycosylated hemoglobin checked every 3 to 6 months.

Box 13-2 Wellness Promotion

DIABETIC FOOT CARE

Following these measures will significantly reduce the risk of limb amputation from wounds and ulcers that do not heal.

- Inspect your skin daily, paying special attention to your feet; use a mirror to inspect your soles.
- Wash your feet daily with a mild soap and lukewarm water; dry gently and thoroughly.
- Apply lotion to keep skin soft and supple.
- Trim toenails carefully, clipping straight across to avoid ingrown nails; if this is too difficult, have your physician trim your toenails.
- Have a podiatrist treat corns and calluses.
- Always wear good-fitting shoes, even in the house.
- Break in new shoes very carefully to avoid blisters.
- Change stockings daily.
- Avoid wearing stockings with tight tops.
- Never go barefoot.
- Inspect shoes before putting them on to make sure there is nothing inside.
- Wear house slippers and keep a night-light on when getting up during the night, to prevent foot injury.
- Report any redness, sores, or breaks in the skin to your physician as soon as possible.

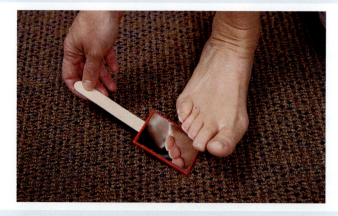

Diabetic foot care (From Eagle, S, et al. *The Professional Medical Assistant: An Integrative Teamwork-Based Approach.* 2009. Philadelphia: F.A. Davis Company, with permission.)

device, attached to a catheter that is inserted into the abdomen, releases a steady amount of insulin into subcutaneous tissue. This closely mimics the body's natural way of infusing insulin from the pancreas. The management goal is to maintain a balanced blood glucose level without great fluctuations.

Prognosis

In years past, the prognosis for those with type 1 diabetes was grim; few lived beyond childhood. As treatment options have improved, life expectancy has increased significantly. Many individuals still continue to suffer from devastating long-term consequences, though. An example is blindness caused by *diabetic retinopathy,* a diseased retina caused by poorly controlled diabetes (see Fig. 13-3). Another is limb loss caused by peripheral *diabetic neuropathy,* in which motor and sensory nerves have been damaged from long-standing diabetes. Yet another long-term complication of diabetes is *nephropathy,* diseased changes of the kidneys, with eventual kidney failure. Fortunately, diabetes is much better understood today and treatment options much more effective. The risks of these disabling long-term complications, while still real, have lessened considerably. In fact, research indicates that those who develop good self-care habits and maintain tight control over blood glucose levels on a daily basis can now lead long, productive, reasonably healthy lives (see Box 13-3).

> **Flashpoint**
> Insulin must be administered by injection because stomach acid destroys it.

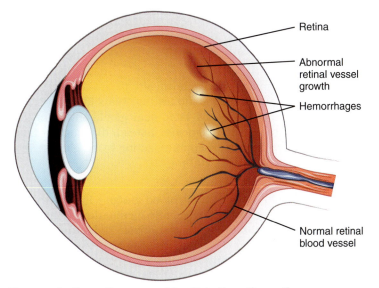

Retina

Abnormal retinal vessel growth

Hemorrhages

Normal retinal blood vessel

FIGURE 13-3 **Changes to the retina caused by diabetic retinopathy**

Box 13-3 Wellness Promotion

DIABETIC SELF-CARE

Following these measures, as recommended by a physician, will help manage blood glucose levels and maintain an optimal level of health.

- Consult with a dietitian to determine dietary guidelines that best meet your needs.
- Eat frequent, small, well-balanced meals throughout the day rather than three large meals.
- Monitor your intake of carbohydrates and calories.
- Engage in moderate, regular physical exercise.
- Check your blood glucose levels faithfully.
- Find and use a glucometer that best fits your lifestyle and personal needs.
- Consider using a system that maps injection sites, to prevent overuse of any one site.
- Develop a habit of regularly inspecting and caring for your skin and feet.
- Keep a list of resources handy for when you have questions or concerns.

Type 2 Diabetes

ICD-9-CM: 250.00 (controlled, without complications)   **[ICD-10: E11.9 (without complications)]**

Type 2 diabetes, also referred to as *non–insulin-dependent diabetes mellitus* and *adult-onset diabetes*, usually appears after the age of 40 but can occur at any age.

Incidence

It is estimated that nearly 20 million Americans have type 2 diabetes and that many of them remain undiagnosed. This is because they are usually asymptomatic in the early years. Those at greatest risk are obese middle-aged people with sedentary lifestyles. Sadly, the incidence of type 2 diabetes is rapidly growing in this country, due to childhood and adult obesity.

Flashpoint

Because type 2 diabetes often begins in adulthood, it has been called adult-onset diabetes.

Etiology

Type 2 diabetes is caused by decreased insulin production and decreased sensitivity of the body to the insulin that is produced. As a result, individuals develop hyperglycemia. The development of type 2 diabetes is linked to family history, obesity, and sedentary lifestyle.

Signs and Symptoms

In the early stages, most individuals with type 2 diabetes are asymptomatic and may therefore be unaware that they have diabetes. As hyperglycemia worsens, the individual will begin to exhibit many of the same symptoms as with type 1 diabetes. These may include polydipsia, polyphagia, polyuria, and blurred vision. In addition, the person may notice weight gain and delayed healing of wounds. Onset of symptoms is more gradual in type 2 diabetes than in type 1, and the development of diabetic ketoacidosis is less likely.

Diagnosis

Diagnosis of type 2 diabetes is made similarly to diagnosis of type 1 diabetes, based on medical history, signs and symptoms, and results of diagnostic testing. Tests include a random blood glucose level, fasting blood glucose level, and glycosylated hemoglobin level. The glucose tolerance test is no longer recommended to confirm diagnosis; instead, diagnosis is based upon the presence of the classic symptoms along with two separate fasting blood glucose levels over 126 mg/dL or a random blood glucose level over 200 mg/dL.

Treatment

Some patients with type 2 diabetes can control their blood glucose level with diet and regular exercise, while others may need to take oral hypoglycemic medications that stimulate the pancreas to produce insulin or make the body more responsive to insulin. Glucose is thus made available to the cells of the body, and the blood glucose level normalizes. In some individuals the pancreas eventually stops producing insulin. When this happens, they must begin injecting insulin to manage their blood glucose levels. (Regardless of whether insulin production ceases altogether, the diabetes type remains type 2; it does not change to type 1.)

Flashpoint

Many people with type 2 diabetes can control their disease with diet and exercise.

Prognosis

Diabetes is a chronic disease for which there is no identified cure. However, with proper diagnosis and management, most diabetics can lead long, healthy lives. The key is daily management to prevent the destructive changes that gradually occur over time.

Complications include retinopathy leading to blindness, nephropathy leading to kidney failure, and neuropathy and peripheral vascular disease leading to delayed wound healing, tissue necrosis, and limb loss. Diabetics are also at increased risk of heart disease, which in turn puts them at risk of heart attack.

Gestational Diabetes

ICD-9-CM: 648.80   **[ICD-10: O24.9] (unspecified for both codes)**

Gestational diabetes is diabetes that begins during pregnancy because of insulin resistance and altered metabolism of glucose.

Incidence

Gestational diabetes affects 135,000 to 270,000 American women each year. Those at greatest risk include those over age 25, those with a history of gestational diabetes during a previous pregnancy, those with a family history of diabetes, and those who are overweight at the start of pregnancy. Additional risk factors include African American, Native American, Pacific Islander, or Hispanic ethnicity and a previous stillbirth or a baby weighing more than 9 pounds.

Etiology

The cause of gestational diabetes is not fully understood. It is known that placental hormones, which help the baby grow, cause insulin resistance in the mother's body. Subsequently, the mother develops hyperglycemia as glucose levels rise in her blood. Gestational diabetes usually subsides after delivery. However, women who develop gestational diabetes have a 50% chance of developing type 2 diabetes later in life.

Signs and Symptoms

Gestational diabetes usually doesn't begin until before the 24th week of pregnancy (fifth or sixth month), and most women are asymptomatic. Those who do experience symptoms most likely exhibit polydipsia, polyphagia, and polyuria, as well as fatigue, sudden weight gain or loss, and dehydration.

> **Flashpoint**
> Women with gestational diabetes have a 50% chance of developing diabetes later in life.

Diagnosis

Screening for gestational diabetes is just one of the many reasons women should seek health care before and during pregnancy. Measuring blood glucose levels and screening for diabetes are part of routine prenatal care. Diagnosis of gestational diabetes is made similarly to that of other types of diabetes. Many physicians recommend a glucose challenge test between 24 and 28 weeks of pregnancy.

Treatment

Treatment of gestational diabetes includes a calorie-restricted diet, regular moderate exercise, blood glucose monitoring, and possibly insulin injections (depending on severity) to maintain normal blood glucose levels. Oral hypoglycemic medications are contraindicated during pregnancy and should not be administered.

Prognosis

With careful management, the woman with gestational diabetes can experience a normal, healthy pregnancy and delivery. However, there are complications that can arise, especially when maternal hyperglycemia is poorly controlled. The most life-threatening of these is pregnancy-induced hypertension, which can cause eclampsia—the woman may experience severe hypertension, convulsions, and coma. Another complication is the need for a cesarean-section delivery due to macrosomia, which is an abnormally large baby. This is caused by the transfer of maternal glucose across the placenta, giving the baby hyperglycemia. In response, the baby's pancreas makes more insulin, which then causes the excess glucose to be stored in the baby's body in the form of fat. As a result, the baby may suffer shoulder injury at birth and may have severe hypoglycemia. The baby may also have a higher risk of respiratory problems, jaundice, and stillbirth. In addition, such babies are at risk of obesity and development of type 2 diabetes in the future.

> **Flashpoint**
> Women with gestational diabetes often need to deliver by cesarean section because of a very large baby.

Nondiabetic Hypoglycemia

ICD-9-CM: 251.2   [ICD-10: E16.2] (hypoglycemia, unspecified)

Nondiabetic hypoglycemia is a condition in which a nondiabetic person experiences low blood glucose levels and is mildly symptomatic.

Incidence

The incidence of nondiabetic hypoglycemia is unknown. It primarily occurs in older adults, women more often than men. It rarely occurs in infants and children.

Etiology

Simply stated, the cause of hypoglycemia is low blood glucose. But exactly what causes the blood glucose level to be low in a nondiabetic person is not always clear. Hypoglycemia may be categorized as either *reactive hypoglycemia,* which occurs postprandially (after meals) and is not caused by any disease processes, or as *fasting hypoglycemia,* which is caused by some type of disease process. Examples include Addison disease, pancreatic tumors, hypopituitarism, certain medications, heavy alcohol use, sepsis, liver disorders, and renal failure. Newborn infants of diabetic mothers may experience transient neonatal hypoglycemia. Though rare in children, hypoglycemia can occur; deficiencies in enzymes or hormones are usually to blame.

Signs and Symptoms

Signs and symptoms of hypoglycemia are similar in those who are nondiabetic and those who are diabetic. Individuals may complain of hunger, stomachache, nausea, headache, dizziness, or fatigue. In addition, they often become tachycardic, irritable, and confused, have slurred speech and poor coordination, and break out in a cold sweat.

Diagnosis

Fasting hypoglycemia is defined as a blood glucose level of 50 mg/dL or lower after exercising or after *fasting* (going without food or nutrition) for a specified period of time. Reactive hypoglycemia is a blood glucose level of 70 mg/dL or lower that develops within 4 hours of a meal; its symptoms are relieved by eating. Testing must be done when the patient is experiencing symptoms. Other tests may be done to check liver function. Abdominal computed tomography (CT) may be done to screen for tumors.

Treatment

Treatment of fasting hypoglycemia is aimed at treating the underlying cause, such as surgery to remove a tumor. Reactive hypoglycemia can usually be corrected by supplying the patient with an oral form of a simple carbohydrate, such as fruit juice, 1 to 2 cups of milk, or a piece of fruit. Individuals who are not able to safely swallow should be given a dose of intramuscular or subcutaneous glucagon. For most individuals, episodes of hypoglycemia can be prevented or minimized by the adjustment of eating patterns (see Box 13-4).

Flashpoint

Most people can avoid reactive hypoglycemia by adjusting their eating pattern.

Prognosis

Prognosis for patients with fasting hypoglycemia depends upon the underlying cause and the success of treatment. Prognosis for patients with reactive hypoglycemia is excellent, particularly if they adopt lifestyle and dietary changes aimed at preventing symptoms.

Diseases and Disorders of the Thyroid Gland

The thyroid gland produces the hormones triiodothyronine and thyroxine, which are responsible for growth throughout childhood and for regulation of metabolism. Disorders of the thyroid gland include hypothyroidism and Hashimoto thyroiditis, conditions in which too little of these hormones is produced, and hyperthyroidism, in which too much is produced.

Box 13-4 Wellness Promotion

PREVENTING REACTIVE HYPOGLYCEMIA

Nondiabetic people who experience reactive hypoglycemia can prevent or minimize symptoms by following some simple guidelines.

Dietary Modification
- Eat several (five or six) small meals each day instead of three large ones.
- Eat high-fiber foods.
- Eat a variety of foods.
- Eat meat and other high-protein foods regularly.
- Avoid simple carbohydrates (sugary foods), especially when snacking.
- Avoid fasting.
- Keep a source of carbohydrates handy (such as fruit) for hypoglycemic episodes.
- Eat complex-carbohydrate foods such as whole grains, rice, potatoes, and pasta.

Other Measures
- Get moderate, regular exercise.
- Avoid unnecessary stress.
- Develop effective strategies to cope with stress; see a counselor if necessary.

Hypothyroidism

ICD-9-CM: 243 (congenital hypothyroidism), 244.9 (myxedema)   **[ICD-10: E03.0 (congenital hypothyroidism), E30.9 (myxedema)]**

Hypothyroidism is a condition of inadequate levels of thyroid hormones in the body. There are several types of hypothyroidism. ***Congenital hypothyroidism,*** formerly called *cretinism,* is a congenital deficiency of thyroid hormones, characterized by arrested physical and mental development (see Fig. 13-4). The term *cretin* originated in the 18th century and was used widely in the 19th and 20th centuries. It has taken on a negative, judgmental meaning, however, and is sometimes used in a derogatory manner, so it is not commonly used in medicine today. ***Myxedema*** is a severe form of hypothyroidism that develops in the older child or adult.

Incidence

Congenital hypothyroidism is rare in industrialized countries due to early diagnosis and treatment of newborns. However, in many countries where diets are often deficient in iodine, the problem is much more prevalent.

Etiology

Congenital hypothyroidism results from abnormal functioning of the fetal thyroid gland. In many cases, an underlying cause of hypothyroidism is a dietary deficiency of iodine, an essential trace element that is required for synthesizing thyroid hormones. Other causes of hypothyroidism include surgical removal of the thyroid gland, and some medications.

Signs and Symptoms

General hypothyroidism causes diminished basal metabolism. Myxedema describes the collective symptoms of severe hypothyroidism, which include fatigue, hair that is dry and brittle, intolerance

Flashpoint

Myxedema is a severe form of hypothyroidism that develops in the older child or adult.

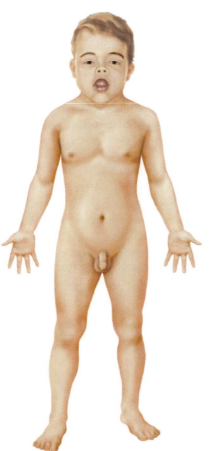

FIGURE 13-4 Congenital hypothyroidism (From Eagle, S, et al. *The Professional Medical Assistant: An Integrative Teamwork-Based Approach.* 2009. Philadelphia: F.A. Davis Company, with permission.)

of cold, weight gain, constipation, mental apathy, physical sluggishness, and muscle aches. The character of the skin changes due to infiltration by mucopolysaccharides, giving it a waxy or coarsened appearance with nonpitting edema. If it is left untreated, hypothermia, coma, and death may result. Another common symptom of hypothyroidism is enlargement of the thyroid gland, sometimes called *goiter.* Congenital hypothyroidism causes poor growth and results in a very short adult. In addition, bone growth and maturation are impeded, sexual development is severely delayed, and infertility is common.

Flashpoint

An enlarged thyroid gland is sometimes called a goiter.

Diagnosis

Hypothyroidism is detectable long before symptoms become apparent, through the use of thyroid function tests. A high level of plasma TSH and a low index of free thyroxine confirm the diagnosis.

Treatment

Treatment of most forms of hypothyroidism consists of lifelong administration of synthetic thyroid hormones. The addition of iodine to packaged table salt in many countries has alleviated the incidence of diet-related hypothyroidism, thereby reducing the incidence of goiter.

Prognosis

Prognosis for those with hypothyroidism is generally good, depending upon how early diagnosis is made and treatment begun. In most cases symptoms will improve or resolve.

Hyperthyroidism
ICD-9-CM: 242.9   [ICD-10: E05.9] (unspecified for both codes)

Hyperthyroidism is a condition of excessive thyroid hormones in the body. The most common form of hyperthyroidism is *Graves disease,* which is an autoimmune form. When production of thyroid hormones increases, the body's metabolism is increased, resulting in physical and mental symptoms.

Incidence

Hyperthyroidism is 10 times more common in women than in men, and it is more common after the age of 15. Incidence is about one per 1,000 women. Eighty percent of patients may develop goiter.

Etiology

There are several causes of hyperthyroidism, including nodular goiter (an enlargement of the thyroid with one or more nodules, which are small, tumorlike growths), hyperemesis gravidarum (extreme nausea and vomiting during pregnancy), excessive thyroid replacement, excessive iodine intake, and pituitary adenoma. Graves disease is caused by an autoimmune response in which the body's immune system begins attacking the thyroid gland.

Flashpoint

The most common type of hyperthyroidism, Graves disease, is caused by an autoimmune response.

Signs and Symptoms

The symptoms of hyperthyroidism are related to the stimulation of the sympathetic nervous system and to an increase in circulating thyroxine; both stimulate the metabolism. Symptoms include tachycardia, palpitations, hypertension, tremor, anxiety, nervousness, insomnia, hyperreflexia, depression, weight loss in spite of increased food intake, intolerance of heat, hair thinning, and *exophthalmos* (protruding eyeballs—see Fig. 13-5). Hypertrophy (excessive growth) of the thyroid gland may also cause goiter. *Thyrotoxicosis* is an episode of sudden worsening of symptoms and may be life-threatening.

Diagnosis

Thyroid disorders are easily detected by medical examination and blood tests; early detection is vital for successful treatment. Blood tests may show a decreased TSH level and increased levels of thyroid hormones.

Treatment

Treatment of hyperthyroidism consists of medications to suppress thyroid function and surgical removal of part or all of the thyroid gland. Prevention, early detection, and treatment are the keys to minimizing the impact of the disorder. Therefore, annual physical examinations for adults and scheduled well-baby visits for infants and children are encouraged.

Prognosis

Prognosis for those with hyperthyroidism is generally good but varies somewhat depending upon the underlying cause. In most cases, a balanced level of thyroid hormones can be restored.

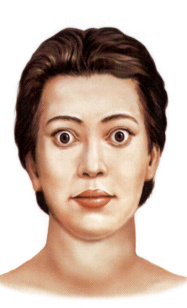

FIGURE 13-5 **Exophthalmos caused by Graves disease** (From Eagle, S, et al. *The Professional Medical Assistant: An Integrative Teamwork-Based Approach.* 2009. Philadelphia: F.A. Davis Company, with permission.)

Hashimoto Thyroiditis
ICD-9-CM: 245.2 [ICD-10: E06.3]

Hashimoto thyroiditis, also called *chronic lymphocytic thyroiditis,* is the most common type of thyroiditis. It is a chronic, inflammatory condition that leads to underactive thyroid.

Incidence

It is estimated that between 100,000 and 450,000 Americans are diagnosed with Hashimoto thyroiditis each year. It affects both genders and all age groups, but it most commonly affects middle-aged women.

Etiology

Hashimoto thyroiditis is thought to be caused by a combination of genetics and an autoimmune response that leads to inflammation and slow destruction of the thyroid gland (see Fig. 13-6). As more thyroid tissue is destroyed over time, the thyroid gland becomes unable to produce enough

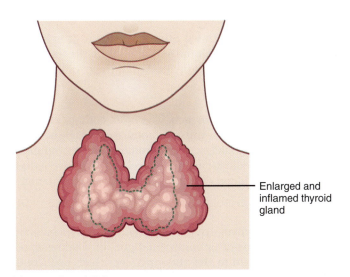

Enlarged and inflamed thyroid gland

FIGURE 13-6 **Hashimoto thyroiditis**

thyroid hormones. In response to lower levels of thyroid hormones, the pituitary gland produces more TSH in an attempt to stimulate the thyroid gland to increase production. This causes the thyroid gland to enlarge.

Signs and Symptoms

Individuals with Hashimoto thyroiditis are usually symptom free in the early stages. Consequently, enough destruction of thyroid tissue may occur that the individual begins to experience symptoms of hypothyroidism. In addition to enlargement of the thyroid gland, patients may note fatigue, weight gain, stiffness and pain of the joints, constipation, sensitivity to cold, depression, weakness, and increased menstrual flow. Changes in the texture of the skin and hair may be noted as hair becomes drier and more brittle and skin becomes paler and rougher. Occasionally, patients also note a feeling of pressure in the throat, some difficulty swallowing, and a hoarse voice.

Diagnosis

Diagnosis of Hashimoto thyroiditis may be suspected based upon the patient's signs and symptoms; it is confirmed based upon the results of thyroid function tests. Blood tests identify the presence of antibodies. Thyroid hormones may be low while TSH is elevated. Needle biopsy may also be done to evaluate thyroid tissue. Cholesterol and triglyceride levels will also be elevated.

Treatment

There is no cure for Hashimoto thyroiditis. However, treatment consisting of lifelong supplementation with synthetic thyroid hormones is very effective. With treatment, the thyroid gland is likely to decrease in size.

Prognosis

Prognosis for patients with Hashimoto thyroiditis is excellent if diagnosis and treatment occur in a timely fashion. Untreated conditions lead to an enlarged thyroid (goiter), increased risk of heart disease from elevated cholesterol, depression, myxedema, and increased risk of birth defects in children of pregnant women.

Diseases and Disorders of the Parathyroid Glands

The parathyroid glands secrete parathormone (PTH) and calcitonin, which help regulate calcium and phosphorus levels in the blood. Disorders of the parathyroid glands are caused by too little or too much of these hormones.

Hypoparathyroidism
ICD-9-CM: 252.1   [ICD-10: E20.9 (unspecified)]

Hypoparathyroidism is a condition in which the parathyroid glands are hypoactive; as a result, the level of PTH is too low.

Incidence

The incidence of hypoparathyroidism in the United States is unclear. It is listed as a "rare disease" by the Office of Rare Diseases Research of the National Institutes of Health, which means that it affects fewer than 200,000 Americans. In Japan the prevalence is estimated to be about 10 per million.

Etiology

There are a number of causes of hypoparathyroidism. The most common is thought to be an autoimmune response; others include surgical trauma, abnormally high or low blood magnesium levels, thyroid cancer, iron accumulation, DiGeorge syndrome (a congenital disorder caused by chromosome defects), heredity, some medications, and, rarely, radioactive iodine therapy. Low levels of PTH lead to hypocalcemia (low blood calcium) and hyperphosphatemia (high blood phosphorus).

Signs and Symptoms

Signs and symptoms of hypoparathyroidism are actually related to hypocalcemia. They are many and include muscle tetany (spasms or cramping), fatigue, or weakness; overactive reflexes; tingling in the fingers, toes, and lips; pain in the abdomen, legs, feet, or face; dry hair and skin; brittle nails; absent teeth or delayed tooth formation; cataracts; and, in severe cases, diminished consciousness and seizures. Women may complain of more painful menses. Other symptoms can include headaches, bradycardia, respiratory difficulties, anxiety, depression, and memory problems.

Diagnosis

Hypoparathyroidism is diagnosed by testing levels of blood PTH and calcium, both of which will be low. Blood phosphorus level will be elevated and blood magnesium level may be low. Electrocardiogram (ECG) may identify bradycardia or other rhythm disturbances. A dual energy x-ray absorptiometry (DEXA) scan may be done to test bone strength (see Box 13-5). Tooth development in children may be evaluated. The patient's eyes may be examined to detect cataract formation. Patients with hypocalcemia will demonstrate Trousseau sign 94% of the time. In this test, a blood-pressure cuff is placed on the patient's arm and inflated to a pressure higher than the patient's systolic blood pressure; it is kept inflated for 3 minutes. If the patient is experiencing hypocalcemia, this test will cause spasms of the hand and forearm muscles (see Fig. 13-7).

Flashpoint

Signs and symptoms of hypoparathyroidism are related to hypocalcemia.

Treatment

Treatment of hypoparathyroidism usually involves lifelong supplementation with calcium, vitamin D, and phosphorus, and regular blood testing. In severe cases, IV calcium is given and

Box 13-5 Diagnostic Spotlight

DUAL ENERGY X-RAY ABSORPTIOMETRY SCAN

The dual energy x-ray absorptiometry (DEXA) scan is a test that has proven reliable as an indicator of whether patients have osteoporosis. It produces two x-ray beams, one at high energy and one at low energy. Bone density is determined by the difference between the amounts of the two x-rays that pass through the bone. Measurement is usually done at the spine or the hip and takes only 10 to 20 minutes. The patient must lie still, but the test is noninvasive and painless. Smaller DEXA scanners can also be used to measure bone density at the heel, shin, or knee. The patient may be advised to avoid taking calcium supplements for 24 hours before the test, but no other special preparation is needed.

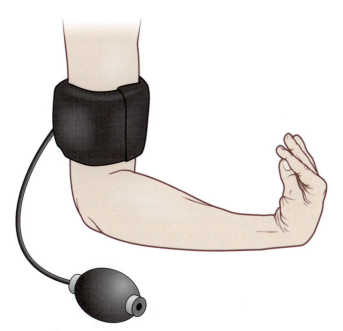

FIGURE 13-7 Trousseau sign

precautions are taken to monitor and respond to seizures or laryngospasm. A calcium-rich diet may be recommended. If these measures are not sufficient, some patients may be started on a thiazide diuretic. Unlike other diuretics, it actually increases blood calcium.

Prognosis

Prognosis for individuals with hypoparathyroidism depends upon the underlying cause but is usually very good, if timely diagnosis and treatment occur. Patients with this disorder have an increased risk of developing Parkinson disease and Addison disease. Complications of untreated hypoparathyroidism include poor growth, slowed mental functioning, and cardiomyopathy.

Hyperparathyroidism
ICD-9-CM: 252.0   [ICD-10: E21.0]

Hyperparathyroidism is a condition in which the parathyroid glands produce excessive PTH. Because PTH regulates the level of calcium and phosphorus in the body, an excess of it leads to an imbalance in these substances. This can result in problems that affect many parts of the body, including the bones, teeth, muscles, kidneys, and nervous system.

Flashpoint

Because hyperparathyroidism affects calcium levels, it can lead to problems with bones and teeth.

Incidence

Hyperparathyroidism is common in the elderly and is twice as common in women as in men. It is estimated that two in 1,000 elderly women will develop this disorder.

Etiology

Primary hyperparathyroidism is the most common type of hyperparathyroidism. It is caused by hyperplasia (excessive growth) of one or more parathyroid glands or by a tumor on one of the parathyroid glands. These tumors are usually benign, but may occasionally be malignant. Secondary hyperparathyroidism is less common; it is caused by conditions, such as kidney failure and malabsorption problems, that produce hypocalcemia (low blood calcium). It may also be caused by rickets (softening of children's bones that is caused by a deficiency of vitamin D and possibly calcium). Hypocalcemia stimulates the parathyroid glands to increase production of PTH in an effort to correct the calcium levels. Vitamin D deficiency is a risk factor, and genetics also play a role.

Signs and Symptoms

Many people with hyperparathyroidism are asymptomatic until the disease becomes severe. Loss of calcium from the bones eventually leads to signs and symptoms related to osteoporosis, including bone pain, fractures, back pain, and decrease in height. Hypercalcemia can cause hypertension, kidney stones, increased thirst, and urinary frequency. Other signs and symptoms of hyperparathyroidism include fatigue, heartburn, abdominal pain, anorexia, nausea and vomiting, depression, confusion, memory deficits, muscle and joint aches, and itchy skin. Severe conditions can lead to decreased consciousness and coma.

Diagnosis

A diagnosis of hyperparathyroidism may be suspected based upon high blood calcium, often noted when testing is done for other reasons. Diagnosis is confirmed when blood tests reveal an increased PTH level. A sestamibi scan will detect abnormal growths on the parathyroid glands. In this test, the patient is given a small dose of a radioactive substance that is absorbed by abnormally active parathyroid tissue. A 24-hour urine test will reveal the amount of calcium being excreted from the body. Bones may be x-rayed to identify fractures. A DEXA scan, which evaluates bone density, may identify osteoporosis.

Treatment

Individuals with mild primary hyperparathyroidism may not need treatment, but they are advised to see their health-care provider on a regular basis for ongoing evaluation, to make sure the condition is not worsening. For those with moderate or severe symptoms caused by a parathyroid tumor, surgical removal usually resolves the condition. A procedure known as a minimally invasive parathyroidectomy is less invasive than traditional surgery. It may be done as a 1-day surgical procedure using localized anesthesia rather than general anesthesia. In this procedure, the surgeon locates the abnormal tissue with a sestamibi scan and removes it through a small incision. Patients with general hyperplasia of parathyroid tissue may have three of the four glands removed. Other treatment may include medication to treat or minimize osteoporosis, such as estrogen replacement in women. Treatment of secondary disease is aimed at the underlying cause.

Prognosis

Prognosis for most patients with hyperparathyroidism is quite good, but it depends upon the underlying cause and the effectiveness of treatment. Complications of hyperparathyroidism include osteoporosis and bone fractures, urinary tract infections, kidney stones, peptic ulcer disease, pancreatitis, hypertension, and pseudogout (a form of arthritis marked by pain and swelling of one or more joints). Potential risks of parathyroid surgery include damage to the vocal cords and chronic hypocalcemia.

> *Flashpoint*
>
> Complications of hyperparathyroidism include osteoporosis, fractures, and kidney stones.

Diseases and Disorders of the Adrenal Glands

The adrenal glands secrete epinephrine to increase the body's ability to cope with stress and aldosterone to help regulate fluid and electrolytes. Disorders of the adrenal glands are caused by too little or too much production of these hormones.

Addison Disease
ICD-9-CM: 255.4   [ICD-10: E27.1]

Addison disease, also called *hypoadrenalism,* is an illness characterized by gradual failure of the adrenal glands resulting in insufficient production of steroid hormones.

Incidence

It is estimated that approximately 9,000 Americans suffer from Addison disease.

Etiology

Addison disease is characterized by failure of the adrenal glands. The most common cause is an autoimmune response in which the body's immune system attacks the cells of the adrenal glands, slowly destroying them over a period of months or years. Other causes of adrenal failure include some types of chronic infections and cancers that spread to the adrenal glands.

Signs and Symptoms

Patients with Addison disease are often asymptomatic until most of the adrenal tissue is destroyed. However, early symptoms might include vague complaints of weakness or fatigue. Later manifestations include anorexia, weight loss, nausea, vomiting, abdominal pain, dizziness, postural hypotension, and increased skin pigmentation, causing a bronze coloration of the skin. Addison disease can also cause hyponatremia (low blood sodium), and hyperkalemia (high blood potassium), which can become life-threatening if severe enough.

Diagnosis

Diagnosis is based upon presenting signs and symptoms and is confirmed with the results of tests that measure the levels of cortisol and aldosterone in the blood and urine. There will be a lack of normal increase in these hormones when ACTH is administered by injection. A check of electrolytes may reveal hyperkalemia and hyponatremia.

> *Flashpoint*
>
> Patients with Addison disease develop a bronze coloration of the skin from increased pigmentation.

Treatment

Addison disease is treated with the administration of corticosteroids, such as prednisone, on a regular basis to serve as a replacement for missing steroid hormones. Temporary dosage increases may be needed during times of physical or emotional stress, such as during episodic illness or surgery. Patients should be under the care of an endocrinologist, who specializes in the diagnosis and treatment of this type of illness.

Prognosis

Individuals who receive timely diagnosis and treatment have an excellent prognosis. Those who go untreated may experience progressively worsening symptoms and may experience life-threatening shock during major illnesses.

Cushing Syndrome
ICD-9-CM: 255.0   [ICD-10: E24.9]

Cushing syndrome, sometimes called *hypercortisolism* or *hyperadrenalism,* is a disorder caused by prolonged excessive levels of the hormone cortisol.

Incidence

Cushing syndrome is most common among adults between the ages of 20 and 50. It affects between 3,000 and 4,500 Americans each year. Some forms affect women more than men.

Etiology

Cushing syndrome results from chronic exposure to high levels of cortisol. One common cause is taking glucocorticoids to treat disorders such as asthma, lupus, or rheumatoid arthritis or to suppress the immune system after organ transplantation. Another cause is overproduction of cortisol in response to overproduction of corticotropin-releasing hormone and ACTH; both hormones normally stimulate the production of cortisol. Other causes include pituitary tumors (benign and cancerous) and adrenal tumors, both of which cause increased secretion of ACTH. There is also a very rare type of Cushing syndrome that is inherited.

Signs and Symptoms

A common symptom of Cushing syndrome is increased fat distribution on the upper body, including the face, neck and torso; the extremities tend to be thin. The skin becomes thin and fragile, bruising and injuring easily and healing poorly. Pink-purple striae (stretch marks) may appear on the thighs, buttocks, arms, breasts, and abdomen (see Fig. 13-8). Osteoporosis develops, causing bones to become weak and fracture easily. Most individuals experience fatigue, weakness, anxiety, irritability, and depression. High blood sugar and hypertension are also common. Women develop **_hirsutism_** (male pattern of body-hair development) and their menses becomes irregular or may cease altogether. Men experience decreased libido and fertility. Children with Cushing syndrome are usually obese and demonstrate slow growth rates.

Flashpoint

Cushing syndrome can cause thin, fragile skin; stretch marks; and hirsutism, which is a male pattern of body hair in women.

Diagnosis

Diagnosis of Cushing syndrome is based upon a review of the patient's signs, symptoms, and medical history, as well as results of examination and laboratory tests. X-rays may indicate

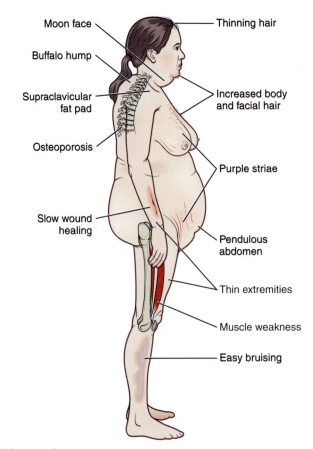

Moon face

Buffalo hump

Supraclavicular fat pad

Osteoporosis

Slow wound healing

Thinning hair

Increased body and facial hair

Purple striae

Pendulous abdomen

Thin extremities

Muscle weakness

Easy bruising

FIGURE 13-8 Cushing syndrome

the presence of tumors. A variety of tests may indicate increased levels of the hormones involved. These include a 24-hour urinary free cortisol level, a dexamethasone suppression test, and a corticotropin-releasing hormone stimulation test. Radiological tests including CT scan and magnetic resonance imaging (MRI) may be done to visualize the adrenal glands.

Treatment

Treatment of Cushing syndrome is based on the underlying cause and may include surgery, chemotherapy, radiation, or medications that suppress the release of cortisol. When the cause is a pituitary tumor, a transsphenoidal adenomectomy is usually done to remove it surgically. If the cause is an adrenal tumor, an adrenalectomy is performed. If the cause is long-term corticosteroid use to treat other disorders, the dosage amount or schedule may be modified in an effort to minimize the cushingoid side effects.

Prognosis

Prognosis for patients with Cushing syndrome is variable depending upon the underlying cause and the timeliness of diagnosis and treatment. In many cases it is very good; however, when the underlying cause is cancer, the prognosis is poor.

> **Flashpoint**
> Surgery may be done if the condition is caused by a tumor.

Hyperaldosteronism

ICD-9-CM: 255.1   [ICD-10: E26.0]

Hyperaldosteronism, also called *Conn syndrome,* is a condition in which the adrenal glands release excessive amounts of aldosterone. Aldosterone is a hormone responsible for increasing the absorption of sodium in the kidneys.

Incidence

Hyperaldosteronism is twice as common in women as in men. The primary form is most common in those ages 30 to 50 years old.

Etiology

Hyperaldosteronism may be classified as primary disease, which is caused by a problem within the adrenal gland, or as secondary disease, which is caused by a problem external to the adrenal gland. Primary hyperaldosteronism is usually caused by a benign adrenal tumor. Very rarely, it may be caused by adrenal cancer. Secondary disease is usually related to liver cirrhosis, nephrotic syndrome, or heart failure.

Signs and Symptoms

Signs and symptoms of hyperaldosteronism are caused by excess aldosterone, which stimulates the kidneys to conserve sodium and excrete potassium. The resulting elevated sodium level further promotes water retention. Hypokalemia (low blood potassium) and hypernatremia (high blood sodium) are responsible for many of the other symptoms experienced by patients with primary hyperaldosteronism. These include muscle weakness, fatigue, headache, numbness, and changes of heart rhythm. Patients with adrenal cancer may also develop hypertension or experience symptoms of Cushing syndrome.

Diagnosis

Patients with hyperaldosteronism often exhibit electrolyte abnormalities, including low levels of potassium and magnesium and high levels of sodium. They may also experience acid-base imbalances, which are revealed by analysis of arterial blood gases. Serum and urine aldosterone levels will be increased. Suppressed renin levels are another important diagnostic finding. ECG may indicate heart-rhythm disturbances related to hypokalemia. Abdominal CT will likely reveal an adrenal mass. Most patients will have a single adrenal tumor, but some may have multiple tumors.

> **Flashpoint**
> Hypokalemia and hypernatremia cause many of the symptoms associated with hyperaldosteronism.

Treatment

As many as 90% of patients with a single adrenal tumor will experience relief of their symptoms by having the tumor surgically removed. Others may continue to require treatment for hypertension. Surgery is not effective for secondary hyperaldosteronism, but symptoms can usually be managed with dietary modifications and medications.

Prognosis

Prognosis for patients with hyperaldosteronism depends upon the underlying cause. Those with primary disease will usually experience resolution of symptoms with surgical removal of the tumor. Those with secondary disease can generally manage symptoms with diet and medications.

Pheochromocytoma
ICD-9-CM: 255.6   [ICD-10: C74.1]

Pheochromocytoma is a tumor of the adrenal medulla, the central part of the adrenal gland. The tumor is usually benign but can cause fluctuations of stress hormones, such as epinephrine.

Incidence

The incidence of pheochromocytoma is unknown. It is listed as a "rare disease" by the Office of Rare Diseases Research of the National Institutes of Health, which means that it affects fewer than 200,000 Americans. It most commonly develops in middle-aged people.

Etiology

The adrenal glands produce epinephrine (adrenaline) and norepinephrine (noradrenaline), which help the body maintain blood pressure and respond to challenging situations. It is not clear why tumors develop in the adrenal glands, although genetics are thought to play a role. Pheochromocytoma occasionally occurs as a part of another disorder, called multiple endocrine neoplasia. Pheochromocytoma may affect one or both adrenal glands and occasionally develops in areas other than the adrenal glands, such as the bladder, neck, heart, abdomen, or spine.

Signs and Symptoms

Signs and symptoms of pheochromocytoma are related to excess production of stress hormones, such as epinephrine. They are episodic, usually lasting up to an hour, and include hypertension, tachycardia, palpitations, headache, sweating, anxiety, and chest pain. Over time the patient may also experience weight loss. Symptoms may be triggered by emotional distress or by physical triggers such as exercise, change in body position, lifting, or defecation. They can also be triggered by certain medications and by tyramine-rich foods like processed cheese and meats, beer, and wine.

Flashpoint

Signs and symptoms of pheochromocytoma are caused by excess production of stress hormones.

Diagnosis

Pheochromocytoma is frequently discovered accidentally when imaging studies are done for other reasons. If this condition is suspected, the physician will order an abdominal CT scan, an MRI, or another type of scan called a metaiodobenzylguanidine scan. Blood and urine tests may also be done to reveal increased levels of epinephrine, norepinephrine, and their metabolic products called metanephrines.

Treatment

The most common and most curative form of treatment for pheochromocytoma is surgery to have the affected adrenal gland removed. This may be done laparoscopically, with tiny incisions made and a laparoscope inserted with a tiny camera. Tiny instruments are inserted through the scope to perform the surgery. Patients generally recover more quickly from this type of surgery than from one that involves larger incisions. In some cases, such as with a cancerous tumor that has metastasized, surgery isn't an option; in those cases, radiation or chemotherapy may be used. Other treatment may include antihypertensive medication to manage blood pressure.

Prognosis

Pheochromocytoma frequently causes hypertension, which can damage the arteries and organs if it remains uncontrolled for an extended period of time. This can lead to stroke, heart attack, dementia, and damage to the kidneys or eyes. A sudden release of epinephrine can cause a hypertensive crisis, in which blood pressure rises as high as 250/150. This also puts the patient at risk of a stroke. Most pheochromocytomas are benign; however, malignant ones can spread to other parts of the body.

Diseases and Disorders of the Pituitary Gland

The pituitary gland exerts hormonal control over many other glands of the body. Disorders of the pituitary gland involve the secretion of too much or too little of these hormones and include diabetes insipidus, hyperpituitarism, hypopituitarism, and precocious puberty.

Flashpoint

The name diabetes insipidus can be confusing, because the disorder has nothing to do with diabetes.

Diabetes Insipidus
ICD-9-CM: 253.5   [ICD-10: E23.2]

Diabetes insipidus is an endocrine disorder characterized by the output of abnormally large amounts of dilute urine. In spite of the name, diabetes insipidus is completely unrelated to other forms of diabetes.

Incidence

It is estimated that 41,000 Americans have diabetes insipidus.

Etiology

There are several different causes of diabetes insipidus. The most common is a lack of antidiuretic hormone, also known as **vasopressin,** a hormone that helps the body concentrate urine and conserve water. This deficiency is sometimes attributed to damage to the posterior pituitary gland, which is responsible for vasopressin production. Trauma to the brain from accidental injury or surgery may be the cause. Other causes include hypothyroidism, some drugs, and destruction of vasopressin during pregnancy because of gestational diabetes and kidney disease.

Signs and Symptoms

Symptoms of diabetes insipidus include urinary frequency, nocturia (frequent need to urinate during the night), and enuresis (involuntary urination during sleep). Large volumes of very dilute, pale-colored urine are excreted, sometimes as much as 10 liters (approximately 10 quarts) per day. By comparison, normal urine excretion is around 1.5 liters per day. This makes it difficult for the individual to drink enough water to replace fluids, and can result in severe dehydration.

Diagnosis

Diagnosis of diabetes insipidus is based upon signs and symptoms, analysis of urine, and measurement of fluid intake compared with urine output. The urine will be very dilute, with a specific gravity below 1.005 (the specific gravity of urine is normally 1.005 to 1.035).

Treatment

Treatment of diabetes insipidus usually involves replacement of vasopressin—often in the form of lypressin (Diapid) or desmopressin acetate (DDAVP)—monitoring of daily fluid intake and urine output, checking of daily weight, and watching for signs of dehydration. The individual should also wear a medical-alert bracelet.

Prognosis

Prognosis for diabetes insipidus is very good with appropriate diagnosis and treatment. Complications are most commonly related to severe dehydration. Those at greatest risk of complications are those who are not able to provide their own self-care, such as the very young, the very elderly, and those with disabilities.

Hyperpituitarism
ICD-9-CM: 253.0   [ICD-10: E22.0]

Hyperpituitarism takes two forms. **Gigantism** occurs when the pituitary gland secretes excessive amounts of human growth hormone (GH), also called *somatotropin,* during childhood. This results in an abnormal increase in height and size (see Fig. 13-9). The largest person documented to have gigantism was a young man who was nearly 9 feet tall when he died in his mid-20s. **Acromegaly** occurs when the pituitary gland becomes overactive after the individual has reached adulthood, and it causes abnormal continued growth of the bones and tissues of the face and extremities.

Incidence

Gigantism and acromegaly are rare. There have been approximately 100 cases of gigantism ever reported in the United States. Acromegaly is somewhat more common, with an incidence between 12,000 and 21,000.

Etiology

The underlying cause of gigantism and acromegaly is the same: Usually a tumor of the pituitary gland has caused increased secretion of growth hormone. The difference is that in gigantism, the tumor develops early in childhood, while the individual's body is still growing. In acromegaly, the tumor develops after the individual reaches adulthood.

Signs and Symptoms

With gigantism, the individual experiences excessive growth that is proportional, meaning that most parts of the body are enlarged but normally propotioned with respect to one another. However, sexual and mental development may be slowed. In contrast, the individual with acromegaly experiences excessive growth of the bones and tissues of the face and extremities that is disproportionate to the size of the trunk. In addition, the bony features of the face become coarser and more prominent over time. Such features become even more prominent after years of growth, as the individual reaches the age of 40 or so. Individuals may become

Flashpoint
Without proper treatment, people with diabetes insipidus can quickly die from dehydration.

Flashpoint
Gigantism develops in childhood; acromegaly develops in adulthood.

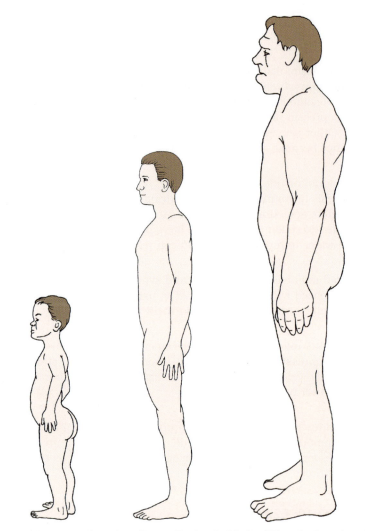

FIGURE 13-9 **Dwarfism and gigantism** (From Eagle, S. *Medical Terminology in a Flash! An Interactive, Flash-Card Approach.* 2006. Philadelphia: F.A. Davis Company, with permission.)

aware of these changes as they notice that they need increasingly larger shoes and gloves. Other complaints may include headache, muscle pain, and weakness.

Diagnosis

Noticing abnormal growth patterns may lead the individual or health-care provider to pursue diagnostic testing for growth disorders. Levels of GH will be elevated, and radiographic studies such as CT scan may reveal a pituitary tumor. Bone studies will reveal abnormal thickening of the cranium and long bones.

Treatment

Treatment is aimed at reducing the amount of GH secreted. Options include removal of all or a portion of the pituitary gland, radiation, and medication therapy. Children with gigantism may also need supplementation of gonadal hormones to help with sexual maturation.

Prognosis

Reduction in the amount of GH secreted in children helps to normalize growth and prevent further effects of gigantism. Reduction in the amount of GH in adults with acromegaly results in improvement of their symptoms.

Hypopituitarism
ICD-9-CM: 253.2; 253.3 (dwarfism) [ICD-10: E23.0; Q77.4 (achondroplasia)]

Hypopituitarism, also called *underactive pituitary gland,* is a condition of diminished secretion of pituitary hormones. **Panhypopituitarism** results from diminished secretion of all hormones secreted by the anterior pituitary gland. **Pituitary dwarfism** is a condition of reduced growth and development due to deficiency of growth hormone in childhood (see Fig. 13-9).

Incidence

Hypopituitarism is listed as a "rare disease" by the Office of Rare Diseases Research of the National Institutes of Health. Therefore, it has been identified as affecting fewer than 200,000 Americans.

Etiology

Causes of hypopituitarism fall into two categories: those that directly affect the pituitary gland and those that affect it indirectly through the hypothalamus. The most common direct causes include pituitary tumors, infection or disease, impaired circulation, radiation therapy, surgical excision, and autoimmune disease. Causes that indirectly affect the pituitary gland through the hypothalamus include hypothalamic tumors, head injuries, and inflammatory disease.

Signs and Symptoms

Symptoms of hypopituitarism vary widely depending on which hormones are deficient, and they may develop gradually or suddenly. When gonadotropins (gonad-affecting hormones) are deficient in women, common symptoms include vaginal dryness and absence of menses; when they are deficient in men, common symptoms include decreased sperm production, impotence, and atrophy of the testes. In both genders there may be infertility and loss of some of the secondary sex characteristics. When growth hormone is deficient in adults, there are usually no symptoms; however, when it is deficient in children, the result is stunted growth and hypopituitary dwarfism. When there is a deficiency of TSH, the result is symptoms of hypothyroidism. A deficiency of prolactin may result in the inability of some women to produce breast milk after giving birth.

Diagnosis

Diagnosis of hypopituitarism is based upon a thorough medical history, physical examination, and diagnostic testing. A CT scan and MRI may detect tumors or other lesions that do not show up on typical x-rays. Blood tests will reveal abnormal hormone levels, thus identifying specifically which hormones are involved.

Treatment

Treatment of hypopituitarism depends on the underlying cause and the extent of the disease. It usually involves hormone-replacement therapy, surgical excision of tumors, and possible radiation therapy.

Prognosis

Prognosis is variable depending upon the type of hypopituitarism, the extent of the disease, and the age of the individual at the time of diagnosis. In many cases a normal balance of hormones can be achieved, with some degree of symptom resolution.

Precocious Puberty
ICD-9-CM: 259.1 [ICD-10: E30.1]

Precocious puberty is the premature onset of puberty in young children, with the appearance of secondary sex characteristics. There are several variations, which sometimes go by different names: *familial testotoxicosis, pubertas praecox,* and *gonadotropin-independent familial sexual precocity.* This disorder is generally defined as premature puberty in boys 9 years or younger and in girls 8 years or younger.

Incidence

Precocious puberty occurs more frequently in girls than in boys, although hereditary precocious puberty is more common in males.

Flashpoint
Deficiency of growth hormone during childhood can cause pituitary dwarfism.

Flashpoint
Precocious puberty is the onset of puberty in girls 8 years or younger and in boys 9 years or younger.

Etiology

In most cases of precocious puberty, the cause is unknown. Some cases are linked to brain tumors or injuries, brain infections, hypothyroidism, and hormonal disorders. Regardless of the triggering cause, hormones that produce sexual maturation are produced and released prematurely. The process may begin in the brain, where the hypothalamus produces gonadotropin-releasing hormone, which signals the pituitary gland to release luteinizing hormone and follicle-stimulating hormone. These hormones then stimulate the ovaries to produce estrogen and the testicles to produce testosterone. Estrogen and testosterone are the sex hormones responsible for causing development of the sex characteristics. Changes in the adrenal glands, such as with adrenal hyperplasia, or abnormalities in the ovaries or testicles may also cause production of the sex hormones. Genetics may play a role in some cases of precocious puberty, since familial cases have been identified. Other risk factors include African American heritage, childhood obesity, and exposure to estrogen or testosterone creams or medications.

Signs and Symptoms

Signs and symptoms of precocious puberty primarily include the premature development of secondary sex characteristics. In girls, this means breast development, underarm and pubic hair, and early onset of menstruation. In boys, it is facial, underarm, and pubic hair; growth of the penis and testicles; sperm production; deepening of the voice; and more aggressive behavior. In both genders, symptoms have been documented as early as 3 years old. Both genders may also experience acne and adult body odor. They may be taller than their peers during childhood but are often shorter than their peers in adulthood, since closure of bone-growth plates occurs prematurely.

Flashpoint

Children diagnosed with precocious puberty may be taller than their peers during childhood but shorter than their peers in adulthood.

Diagnosis

Diagnosis of precocious puberty is made through a combination of the child's or parent's description of symptoms, physical-examination findings that reveal premature sexual development, and blood tests that reveal elevated levels of sex hormones. Bone x-rays are done in some cases to identify bone age; this reveals whether the child is growing too quickly. Other tests may be done to identify the type and cause of the disorder. These may include brain MRI, thyroid function tests, and pelvic ultrasound in girls.

Treatment

Treatment of precocious puberty depends upon the underlying cause. Conditions caused by tumor growth may sometimes be corrected with surgical removal of the tumor. Conditions caused by hypothyroidism usually respond to thyroid-hormone supplementation. In many cases children may be given a modified type of gonadotropin-releasing hormone that temporarily stops puberty and slows the rate of bone maturation.

Prognosis

Prognosis for children with precocious puberty depends on the underlying cause and the timeliness of diagnosis and treatment. Girls who experience early onset of menstruation are at increased risk of developing polycystic ovary syndrome. Children who are treated with gonadotropin-releasing hormone may experience a temporary increase in sexual maturation before symptoms begin to lessen.

STOP HERE.
Select the flash cards for this chapter and run through them at least three times before moving on to the next chapter.

Student Resources

American Diabetes Association: http://www.diabetes.org
Cushing's Support and Research Foundation: http://www.csrf.net
The Endocrine Society: http://www.endo-society.org

EndocrineWeb: http://www.endocrineweb.com
The Magic Foundation (Major Aspects of Growth in Children): http://www.magicfoundation.org
Parathyroid.com: http://www.parathyroid.com
Pituitary Network Association: http://www.pituitary.org
Society for Endocrinology: http://www.endocrinology.org

Chapter Activities

Learning Style Study Strategies

Try any or all of the following strategies as you study the content of this chapter:

Visual and kinesthetic learners: Take turns in your study group creating scenarios that depict patients with one or more of the disorders you are studying. It is
OK to be silly. The funnier your skits are, the more likely you will be to remember them.
Auditory and verbal learners: Create silly rhymes to help you memorize key data about the diseases you are studying. Repeating the rhymes aloud appeals to your auditory and verbal senses, and it will be extremely effective in helping you remember the data.

Practice Exercises

Answers to Practice Exercises can be found in Appendix D.

Case Studies

CASE STUDY 1

Alex Andersen is a 12-year-old boy who was recently diagnosed with type 1 diabetes. He is in the clinic today with his mother for a follow-up visit. He is still feeling confused and overwhelmed by this new diagnosis, and he has several questions. These questions need to be answered in a way that both he and his mother can understand. How should the medical assistant do this?

1. How did I get this disease?

2. When I got sick and went to the hospital, I remember feeling hungry and thirsty all the time and just feeling really lousy. My mom says there are certain symptoms that I should look out for when my blood sugar is too high and others that I should look out for when my blood sugar is too low. I'm supposed to ask you what they are.

3. So what should I do if I notice those symptoms?

4. What would cause my blood sugar to go too high or too low?

5. Can't I just take some type of pills instead of giving myself injections?

6. My mom also told me to ask you about special care that I'm supposed to take of my feet. What does that mean?

CASE STUDY 2

Martha and Ana are both regular patients in the endocrinology clinic. Martha has hypothyroidism and Ana has hyperthyroidism. Given their two diagnoses, they might be expected to exhibit some interesting differences. Complete the comparison table here using key words found in the entries for these two disorders.

	Hypothyroidism (Martha)	Hyperthyroidism (Ana)
Cause (thyroid level)		
Metabolism		
Energy level and mental state		
Hair changes		
Body weight		
Temperature sensitivity		
Thyroid-gland size		
Diagnostic-test results		
Treatment focus		

CASE STUDY 3

Scott is a certified medical assistant who has just been hired to work in an endocrinology office. His prior work experience was in a sports-medicine clinic, and he knows that the patient population in his new job will be very different. Therefore, he is studying and reviewing information about endocrine disorders so that he will be prepared to do his best. Today he is studying disorders of the adrenal glands, and he is currently comparing and contrasting Addison disease and Cushing syndrome.

1. How might Scott briefly describe these two conditions?

2. How might Scott briefly describe the most common causes of these two conditions?

3. How might Scott describe the symptoms commonly seen with these two disorders?

4. How might Scott describe the key differences in how these two disorders are treated?

Multiple Choice

1. Which of the following terms is matched to the correction definition?

    a. Acromegaly: severe form of hypothyroidism that develops in the older child or adult

    b. Goiter: hormone that helps the body concentrate urine and conserve water

    c. Myxedema: excessive growth of the bones and tissues of the face and extremities

    d. Hirsutism: male pattern of body-hair development

2. All of the following terms are matched with the correct definition **except:**

    a. Exophthalmos: protruding eyeballs

    b. Diabetic ketoacidosis: condition of severe hyperglycemia

    c. Graves disease: diseased retina caused by poorly controlled diabetes

    d. Goiter: enlarged thyroid gland

3. Polydipsia is a condition of:

    a. Increased thirst

    b. Increased hunger

    c. Increased urination

    d. Increased sweating

4. All of the following are potential complications of diabetes mellitus **except:**

    a. Nephropathy

    b. Retinopathy

    c. Neuropathy

    d. Pancreatopathy

5. Which of the following statements is true?

    a. Acromegaly and gigantism are both related to diabetes insipidus.

    b. Vasopressin is a hormone that helps the body concentrate urine and conserve water.

    c. Cushing syndrome is a condition in which the parathyroid glands produce an excessive amount of parathyroid hormone.

    d. People with type 2 diabetes usually need to take supplemental insulin.

Short Answer

1. List and define the three potential long-term complications of poorly controlled diabetes.

2. Define pituitary dwarfism.

3. Explain the difference between gigantism and acromegaly.

MUSCULOSKELETAL SYSTEM DISEASES AND DISORDERS 14

Learning Outcomes

Upon completion of this chapter, the student will be able to:

- Define and spell terms related to the musculoskeletal system
- Identify key structures of the musculoskeletal system
- Discuss the roles the musculoskeletal system plays in facilitating movement

- Identify characteristics of common musculoskeletal diseases and disorders, including:
  - description
  - incidence
  - etiology
  - signs and symptoms
  - diagnosis
  - treatment
  - prognosis

KEY TERMS	
abduction	motion away from the midline of the body
adduction	motion toward the midline of the body
adhesive capsulitis	loss of range of motion in the shoulder; also called *frozen shoulder*
arthrodesis	surgical procedure to fuse a joint
atrophy	decrease in mass of a muscle or organ; also called *wasting*
cholinergic crisis	episode of respiratory failure, paralysis, salivation, and sweating that can occur if a patient takes too much anticholinesterase medication
circumduction	motion of a body part in a circle
ergonomics	study of human ability relative to work demands
eversion	motion that turns a body part outward
exacerbation	aggravation of symptoms or increase in severity
extension	motion that straightens a body part
flexion	motion that bends a body part
gait	manner of walking
goniometry	process of measuring joint movements and angles
hematopoiesis	production and development of blood cells
hyperextension	extension of a body part beyond its normal limits
inversion	motion that turns a body part inward
myasthenic crisis	potentially life-threatening episode of worsening of myasthenic symptoms
pathological fracture	breaking of diseased, weakened bone from the stress of normal, everyday activities
pronation	act of lying facedown or turning the hand so the palm faces downward
range of motion	normal range through which a joint moves

Continued

KEY TERMS—cont'd	
reduction	manual manipulation of a bone to return it to its normal position
remission	period of improvement or absence of disease activity
rotation	motion that turns a body part about its axis
sciatica	condition in which compression of the sciatic nerve causes pain that radiates down the leg to the ankle
supination	act of lying faceup or turning the hand so the palm faces upward

Abbreviations

In orthopedics, as in other areas of health care, abbreviations are commonly used. Abbreviations such as the ones listed in Table 14-1 save time and effort in documentation and written communications.

Structures and Functions of the Musculoskeletal System

The musculoskeletal system consists of muscles, bones, ligaments, and tendons. Together, these structures facilitate body movement and protect the internal organs.

TABLE 14-1
ABBREVIATIONS

Abbreviation	Meaning	Abbreviation	Meaning
ADL	activities of daily living	ortho	orthopedic; straight
AK	above the knee	OT	occupational therapy
AKA	above-the-knee amputation	PT	physical therapy
BK	below the knee	RLE	right lower extremity
BKA	below-the-knee amputation	ROM	range of motion
C1–C7	first cervical vertebra, second cervical vertebra, etc.	RUE	right upper extremity
DTR	deep tendon reflex	S1–S5	first sacral vertebra, second sacral vertebra, etc.
Fx	fracture	T1–T12	first thoracic vertebra, second thoracic vertebra, etc.
IM	intramuscular	THA	total hip arthroplasty; also called *total hip replacement*
L1–L5	first lumbar vertebra, second lumbar vertebra, etc.	THR	total hip replacement; also called *total hip arthroplasty*
LLE	left lower extremity	TKA	total knee arthroplasty; also called *total knee replacement*
LUE	left upper extremity	TKR	total knee replacement; also called *total knee arthroplasty*
ORIF	open reduction and internal fixation		

Structures of the Musculoskeletal System

The structures of the musculoskeletal system are the bones, muscles, tendons, and ligaments.

Bones

Bones comprise the framework of the body (see Fig. 14-1). They consist of a type of dense connective, osseous tissue with a high mineral content that makes them strong. In spite of their hard appearance they are actually living, dynamic tissues with their own nerves and blood vessels.

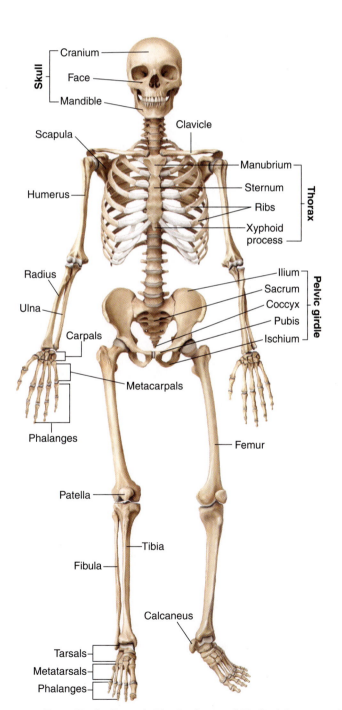

Skull — Cranium, Face, Mandible

Scapula
Clavicle
Manubrium
Sternum
Humerus
Ribs
Xyphoid process
Thorax
Radius
Ulna
Ilium
Sacrum
Coccyx
Pubis
Ischium
Pelvic girdle
Carpals
Metacarpals
Phalanges
Femur
Patella
Tibia
Fibula
Calcaneus
Tarsals
Metatarsals
Phalanges

FIGURE 14-1 Skeletal system (From Eagle, S, et al. *The Professional Medical Assistant: An Integrative Teamwork-Based Approach.* 2009. Philadelphia: F.A. Davis Company, with permission.)

Muscles

Muscles are connective tissues made up of contractile fibers. They are covered by a fibrous membrane called a fascia. The fascia is connective tissue, arranged in sheets or bands, that covers, separates, and supports muscle. Because the muscle and fascia are connected, these structures are commonly referred to as one structure: *myofascial*, muscle and fascia. There are three types of muscle tissue: skeletal, smooth, and cardiac (see Fig. 14-2).

Skeletal Muscle

Striated muscles are found in the tongue, the pharynx, the upper portion of the esophagus, and all skeletal muscles. The striations, or stripes, in this type of muscle are created by the structure of the muscle, which is bundled fibers surrounded by a sheath of connective tissue.

Smooth Muscle

Smooth muscle is found principally in the internal organs of the digestive tract and in the respiratory passages, the urinary bladder, and the walls of the blood vessels. No striations appear on these muscles; this type of muscle is arranged in sheets or layers.

Cardiac Muscle

The muscles of the heart branch and connect, forming a continuous network. Cardiac muscle cells are quadrangular in shape and have a single central nucleus. The muscle fibers contain striations as in skeletal muscle, but they are arranged in a branching network, not a linear bundle.

Tendons and Ligaments

A tendon is fibrous connective tissue structured like a cord or strap that usually attaches to a small area of bone. A tendon that attaches to a larger area of a bone is called an aponeurosis; it is flat or ribbonlike and larger than a typical tendon. Ligaments are bands or sheets of strong, fibrous connective tissue. This type of tissue attaches from bone to bone across joints.

Functions of the Musculoskeletal System

The musculoskeletal system, including bones, muscles, tendons, and ligaments, provides movement, protection, and a framework for the body.

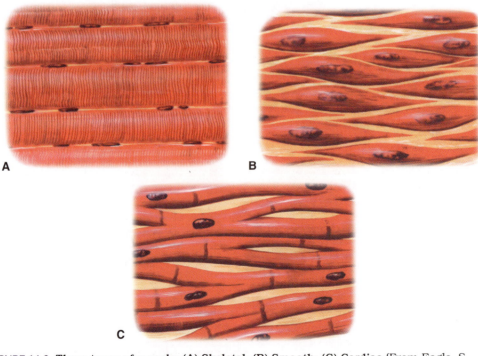

FIGURE 14-2 **Three types of muscle: (A) Skeletal; (B) Smooth; (C) Cardiac** (From Eagle, S, et al. *The Professional Medical Assistant: An Integrative Teamwork-Based Approach.* 2009. Philadelphia: F.A. Davis Company, with permission.)

Bones

There are 206 bones in the skeletal system. They provide a framework for the body and protect internal organs. For example, the skull protects the brain and the rib cage protects the heart and lungs.

Bones enable movement at joints through their attachments to muscles and tendons. There are three types of joint:

- A synarthrosis is an immovable joint, such as the sutures of the skull.
- An amphiarthrosis is a slightly movable joint, such as those between vertebrae.
- A diarthrosis is a freely movable joint, such as the knee joint.

Bone marrow within the bone produces red and white blood cells in a process called **hematopoiesis.** Bones also serve to store essential minerals, such as calcium and phosphorus. When dietary intake of calcium and phosphorus is inadequate or the need for these minerals increases, as in puberty or pregnancy, the bones release their stores into the bloodstream for use. This leaves the bones vulnerable to deterioration and increases the risk of osteoporosis.

Flashpoint
Blood cells are produced inside of the bone marrow.

Muscles

The primary function of muscles is to provide movement, using contractile cells or fibers. Movement depends on the force of the contraction and the type of muscle. Muscle fasciae support and separate muscles and subcutaneous tissues, such as fat and the internal organs. The movement of muscles depends on the type of muscle.

Skeletal Muscle

Movement of skeletal muscles is under conscious control (voluntary). Skeletal muscles work with tendons, ligaments, and bones to help the body move (see Fig. 14-3). Examples of skeletal muscles are the tongue and those that move the arms, legs, and eyeballs. The brain and spinal cord tell muscles to move, or *contract.* Nerves at motor points within the muscle tissue receive these signals from the brain and spinal cord and initiate muscle movement (see Fig. 14-4). Skeletal muscles facilitate a variety of complex movements that allow people to perform many activities. Many of these types of movement can be measured and evaluated by a physician or physical therapist in a process called **goniometry** (see Box 14-1). Common types of body movement include:

abduction: motion away from the midline of the body, such as moving a straightened leg outward at the hip joint

adduction: motion toward the midline of the body, such as moving a straightened leg inward at the hip joint

eversion: motion that turns a body part outward, such as moving the ankle so that the sole of the foot turns outward

inversion: motion that turns a body part inward, such as moving the ankle so that the sole of the foot turns inward

flexion: motion that bends a body part, such as moving the hand up to the shoulder by flexing at the elbow

extension: motion that straightens a body part, such as moving the hand away from the shoulder by elongating or extending the elbow joint

pronation: twisting to face downward, such as turning the wrist so the palm faces down

supination: twisting to face upward, such as turning the wrist so the palm faces up

rotation: motion that turns a body part about its axis, such as turning the head by looking left and right

circumduction: motion of a body part in a circle, such as at the shoulder or hip joint

Skeletal muscle responds to exercise by increasing in strength, size, and definition. If a person does not use the skeletal muscles (for example, a comatose patient), they will **atrophy,** or decrease in size.

Smooth Muscle

Smooth muscle, which is not under conscious control (involuntary), is found in the internal organs, such as the digestive tract, urinary bladder, gallbladder, and the walls of the blood vessels. In the digestive tract, smooth-muscle contractions create peristalsis, which

Flashpoint
Exercise causes skeletal muscles to increase in strength and size.

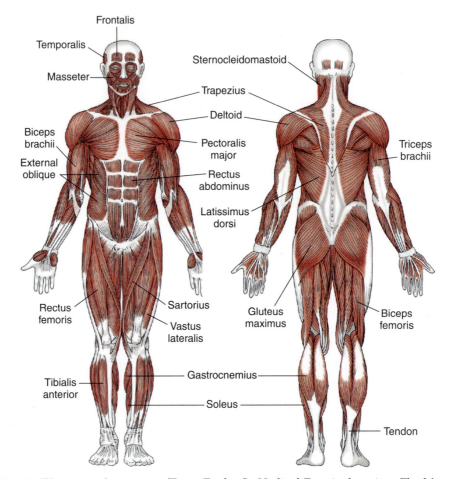

FIGURE 14-3 **The muscular system** (From Eagle, S. *Medical Terminology in a Flash! An Interactive, Flash-Card Approach.* 2006. Philadelphia: F.A. Davis Company, with permission.)

propels food through the alimentary canal to aid in the process of digestion and absorption. Smooth muscle provides strength to blood vessels and allows them to relax or contract as needed to keep vascular tone at an optimal level. The structure of smooth muscle, arranged in sheets or layers, is determined by its function. Because movement is not directed along a single axis, the structure of this type of muscle must allow for movement in many directions. Unlike with skeletal muscle, the size and strength of smooth muscle are not affected by exercise.

Cardiac Muscle

Cardiac muscle is located only in the heart. It works to pump blood through the heart and out to the body. The strong contractions of cardiac muscle push blood through the circulatory system, supplying blood, nutrients, and oxygen to all the tissues of the body. As blood is returned to the right side of the heart, it is pumped to the lungs, where it is reoxygenated, and then returns to theleft side of the heart. Like with skeletal muscle, the efficiency of cardiac muscle improves with use. Exercise that increases the heart rate increases the efficiency of the cardiac muscle.

Tendons and Ligaments

A tendon attaches muscle to bone. A tendon does not contract or elongate with the movement of the muscle, but facilitates the bone's movement. In some places where an aponeurosis attaches muscle to bone, it covers such a large area of bone that it also serves as a protective fascia.

Ligaments attach bone to bone across joints, to limit the motion of the joint and provide strength and stability. Ligaments prevent **hyperextension,** which is the extension of a body part beyond its normal limits. They essentially hold the joint together, providing joint stability while allowing the attached muscles to move the bones by contracting (see Fig. 14-5).

Flashpoint

Tendons attach muscle to bone, and ligaments attach bone to bone.

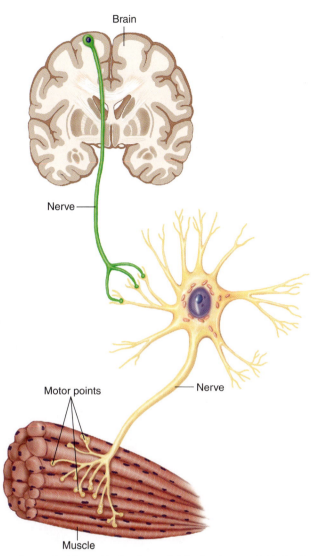

FIGURE 14-4 **Motor point of muscle** (From Eagle, S, et al. *The Professional Medical Assistant: An Integrative Teamwork-Based Approach.* 2009. Philadelphia: F.A. Davis Company, with permission.)

Common Musculoskeletal System Diseases and Disorders

There are numerous diseases and disorders of the musculoskeletal system. Some, like the spinal-curvature disorders, may be congenital. Others are related to trauma or overuse during physical activities such as work or athletics. Many primarily affect the joints, yet others affect various structures of the body and are related to many possible causes, including autoimmune disorders, mineralization defects, and poorly fitting footwear.

Spinal-Curvature Disorders

Spinal-curvature disorders can be congenital or may develop secondary to a variety of other disorders. They include scoliosis, kyphosis, and lordosis.

Scoliosis
ICD-9-CM: 737.43   [ICD-10: M41.9]
Scoliosis is an abnormal lateral, S-shaped curvature of the spine (see Fig. 14-6).

Box 14-1 Diagnostic Spotlight

GONIOMETRY

Goniometry is the process of measuring joint movements and angles. A goniometer is a device used to perform these measurements.

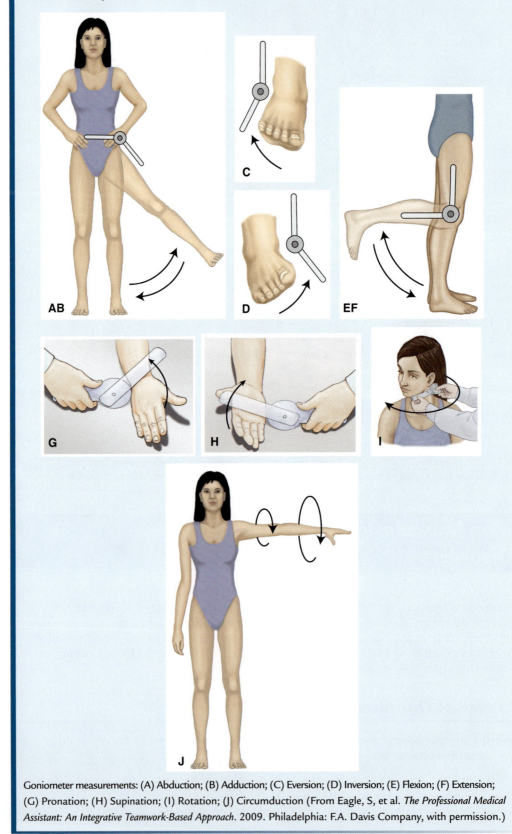

Goniometer measurements: (A) Abduction; (B) Adduction; (C) Eversion; (D) Inversion; (E) Flexion; (F) Extension; (G) Pronation; (H) Supination; (I) Rotation; (J) Circumduction (From Eagle, S, et al. *The Professional Medical Assistant: An Integrative Teamwork-Based Approach*. 2009. Philadelphia: F.A. Davis Company, with permission.)

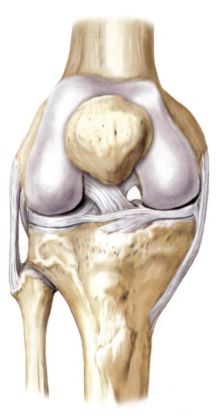

FIGURE 14-5 **Knee joint, including the bones, tendons, and ligaments that provide joint stability** (From Eagle, S, et al. *The Professional Medical Assistant: An Integrative Teamwork-Based Approach.* 2009. Philadelphia: F.A. Davis Company, with permission.)

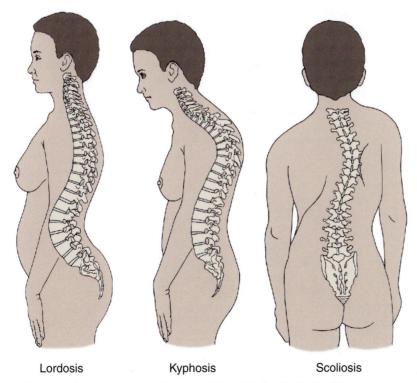

Lordosis   Kyphosis   Scoliosis

FIGURE 14-6 **Abnormal curvatures of the spine** (From Eagle, S. *Medical Terminology in a Flash! An Interactive, Flash-Card Approach.* 2006. Philadelphia: F.A. Davis Company, with permission.)

Incidence

Approximately six million Americans have some degree of scoliosis. It is more common in adolescents because the adolescent spine is still developing, and it is more common in girls than in boys.

Etiology

Some cases of scoliosis are congenital; the condition can run in families. However, it can also be caused by abnormalities of the spinal cord or brain stem, muscle paralysis or degeneration, and unequal-length legs. Idiopathic scoliosis (having an unknown cause) is the most common form. It develops in individuals with previously straight spines.

Signs and Symptoms

Signs and symptoms of scoliosis include lateral spinal deformity and back pain. Mild scoliosis generally causes no problems and is usually not noticeable. Severe scoliosis can cause significant back pain, fatigue, uneven shoulders or hips, and possibly heart or lung problems, because of the decreased space in the thoracic cavity on one side.

Diagnosis

Diagnosis of scoliosis is often suspected based on a physical examination. Routine screening tests during well-child examinations and school physicals identify a large percentage of the children with scoliosis in the United States (see Box 14-2). Spinal x-rays confirm the diagnosis.

Flashpoint

Scoliosis is often noted during routine school physicals.

Treatment

Most children with scoliosis don't require extensive treatment, though they should be examined regularly to make sure the problem isn't worsening. Treatment considerations include the child's age, gender, family history, curve size, and likely future growth. Children who are still growing and have a curve of 25 to 40 degrees may benefit from wearing a brace to prevent further progression of the curvature. The brace must be worn consistently during the day and night. Braces are of little help if the child has stopped growing or the curve is greater than 40 degrees. Surgery may be needed for more severe curvatures. This usually involves the fusing

---

Box 14-2 Diagnostic Spotlight

SCOLIOSIS SCREENING TEST

The scoliosis screening test (forward bend test) is surprisingly simple. The child is instructed to remove his shirt, stand in front of the examiner, and bend over as if to touch his toes. As he does this, the examiner positions herself so that her eyes are at the level of the child's back and notes whether one side of his back is higher than the other or whether there is any asymmetry.

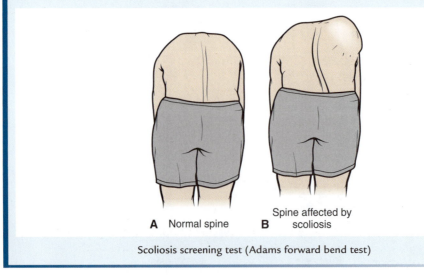

A Normal spine   **B** Spine affected by scoliosis

Scoliosis screening test (Adams forward bend test)

of vertebrae together and the use of metal hardware to hold them together while they heal. Bracing and asymmetrical exercise may be used to correct muscle imbalances, where one side is stronger than the other.

Prognosis

Prognosis for patients with scoliosis depends upon the type and severity of the curvature and the timeliness of diagnosis and treatment. Severe untreated scoliosis can result in heart and lung damage, increased risk of lung infections, chronic back pain, and spinal arthritis. Those who undergo bracing or surgery generally do very well and can experience significant improvement in their scoliosis. Complications of surgery can include pain, bleeding, infection, and nerve damage. Children with scoliosis often feel isolated and may struggle with body image and self-esteem issues.

Kyphosis

ICD-9-CM: 737.0 (adolescent), 737.1 (acquired)   [ICD-10: M40.0 (adolescent), M40.1 (acquired)]

Kyphosis is an exaggerated outward curvature (more than 40 degrees) of the thoracic region of the spine (see Fig. 14-6). It is sometimes referred to as *hunchback.*

Incidence

Approximately 300,000 individuals in the United States suffer from kyphosis. It is most common in older women.

> **Flashpoint**
> Kyphosis is commonly known as hunchback.

Etiology

Kyphosis may be due to a congenital abnormality, arthritis, syphilis, malignancy, compression fractures related to osteoporosis, or disease such as tuberculosis. Risk factors include being an adolescent female with poor posture and having a connective-tissue disorder such as Marfan syndrome.

Signs and Symptoms

The primary symptom of kyphosis is a stooped posture. Others include fatigue, pain, tenderness or stiffness in the back, and in severe cases, breathing difficulties.

Diagnosis

Examination of the patient suspected of having kyphosis may include the forward bend test, in which the patient is asked to bend forward from the waist. When the physician views the patient from the side, the kyphotic curvature will be more obvious in this position. Diagnosis is confirmed with spinal x-rays.

Treatment

Congenital kyphosis may require surgery while the individual is young. Osteoporosis can be prevented or improved with supplemental calcium, vitamin D, and medications to slow the progression of bone loss. Postural kyphosis may improve on its own or in response to postural training and exercises to strengthen back muscles. Severe cases may require bracing or even surgery. Pain and tenderness may be treated with analgesics, physical therapy, massage, and acupuncture.

Prognosis

Prognosis for patients with kyphosis depends upon the underlying cause, the severity, and the timeliness of diagnosis and treatment. Preventing and treating osteoporosis helps prevent many cases of kyphosis in the elderly. Patients with kyphosis may suffer pain and fatigue as well as body-image and self-esteem problems.

Lordosis

ICD-9-CM: 737.20 (acquired), 754.2 (congenital)   [ICD-10: M40.5 (acquired), Q76.4 (congenital)]

Lordosis, sometimes called *swayback* or *saddleback,* is an excessive curvature in the lumbar portion of the spine (see Fig. 14-6).

> **Flashpoint**
> Lordosis is sometimes called swayback or saddleback.

Incidence

The incidence of lordosis is unknown. This is likely due in part to the fact that people with mild cases do not seek medical treatment. However, abnormal curvatures of the spine are thought to be common.

Etiology

The cause of lordosis is not always clear. Some cases are related to achondroplasia (a genetic cause of dwarfism) and spondylolisthesis (anterior displacement of a vertebra over the one below it). Other cases are thought to be congenital or associated with poor posture, back surgery, hip dysplasia, diskitis (inflammation of the disk space), obesity, osteoporosis, or pregnancy.

Signs and Symptoms

Lordosis is usually an asymptomatic condition. However, it can cause low back pain due to strain on supporting muscles and ligaments. The individual with lordosis will display an exaggerated low back curve, with a more prominent abdomen and buttocks.

Diagnosis

Lordosis is commonly diagnosed in childhood; school nurses may notice it when conducting scoliosis screening. Diagnosis is confirmed with spinal x-rays and physical examination, including observation of the patient's standing posture.

Treatment

The goal of treatment is to stop the progression of the abnormal curve and prevent deformity. Exercises conducted at home or with a physical therapist can correct postural abnormalities. If underlying hip abnormalities are the cause of lordosis, correction of the hip pathology will help decrease abnormal curvature.

Prognosis

Prognosis for most individuals with lordosis is very good, depending upon the underlying cause and the severity.

Injuries Related to Overuse and Trauma

Many musculoskeletal disorders are caused by trauma and by wear and tear from overuse. A large number of these disorders affect the joints; however, most involve multiple structures and tissues, including bones, joints, tendons, ligaments, and muscles. Common disorders include sprains and strains; dislocation; fractures; torn or inflamed ligaments, tendons, bursas, and fasciae; and herniated disks.

Sprains and Strains
ICD-9-CM: 840–848   [ICD-10: S13.0–S93.6] (sprain; code by site for both codes)

A sprain is traumatic injury to a joint that causes a brief, partial dislocation, resulting in tearing of the ligaments that stabilize the joint. A strain is traumatic injury to a muscle or sometimes a tendon from violent contraction or excessive forcible stretching.

Flashpoint

A sprained joint is one that was briefly, partially dislocated.

Incidence

It is impossible to estimate the exact incidence of sprains and strains, since there are many kinds and people often do not seek medical treatment for mild conditions. However, it is known that many forms of sprain are very common; for example, it is estimated that 850,000 Americans suffer ankle sprain every year and that 80% of the population suffers back strain at some time in their lives.

Etiology

Sprains and strains are almost always caused by some form of trauma or repetitive motion.

Signs and Symptoms

People with sprains may also have suffered injury to surrounding tissue, including blood vessels, nerves, muscles, and tendons. Thus, the patient commonly complains of pain, heat, localized swelling, and decreased functioning. Symptoms of sprain include pain, weakness, decreased function, and possible numbness. Strain may be moderate to severe, with similar symptoms to sprain; the most common are pain and decreased functioning.

Diagnosis

With most types of joint injury, the patient's condition is typically unclear at first. Thus, most medical-office protocols include sending the patient for an immediate x-ray before consultation with the physician, to help determine whether the injured body part is fractured or sprained. An x-ray also helps to rule out an avulsion fracture of the ligament's attachment.

Treatment

The treatment of strain injuries depends upon the anatomy involved. Most cases involve resting the body part and gently stretching the involved muscle groups. Analgesics, NSAIDs, and muscle relaxants may be used to help alleviate pain and muscle spasms. Sprains involving the extremities, such as ankle sprain, include resting of the injured part, application of cold, compression, and elevation. This is often called the RICE approach (see Box 14-3). These measures help to minimize inflammation and swelling, which in turn helps minimize pain and dysfunction. Other treatment for severe sprains may include physical-therapy measures such as ultrasound and electrical muscle stimulation.

> **Flashpoint**
> Sprains and strains will often respond to RICE treatment.

Prognosis

Prognosis for patients with sprain and strain injuries is usually excellent if appropriate treatment occurs. Most injuries heal completely, with a full return of function.

Dislocation

ICD-9-CM: 830–839   [ICD-10: S03.0–S93.5] (code by specific site for both codes)

Dislocation is the displacement or separation of a bone from its normal position where it articulates with another bone (see Fig. 14-7). The most frequently dislocated joints are of the fingers, wrists, elbows, shoulders, and knees.

Box 14-3 Wellness Promotion

RICE

The *RICE* approach to treating sprains is easy to remember and involves measures that are simple enough for patients to begin at home as soon as injury occurs:

- **R**est (to the greatest extent possible, avoid using the injured part)
- **I**ce (apply cold to the injured area—but do not apply ice directly to the skin, as this might cause frostbite; place at least one layer of cloth between the ice and the skin)
- **C**ompression (apply a stretchable material, such as an elastic bandage, to create gentle compression without impeding circulation)
- **E**levation (if possible, position the injured part higher than the heart, or at least higher than the rest of the extremity, to promote good blood return and lymphatic drainage and to minimize swelling)

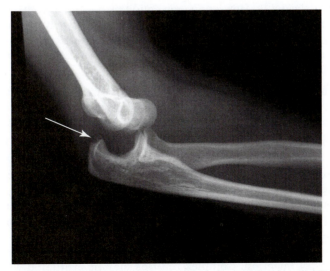

FIGURE 14-7 X-ray of a dislocated elbow (From McKinnis, L. *Fundamentals of Musculoskeletal Imaging*, 3rd Edition. 2010. Philadelphia: F.A. Davis Company, with permission.)

Incidence

The incidence of joint dislocation is difficult to estimate, given the many different types that occur. However, it is known to be very common.

Etiology

Dislocations are caused by traumatic force to the joint, such as might occur with a fall, a blow, or other physical force.

Signs and Symptoms

Dislocated joints are often deformed, bruised, and swollen. Patients usually describe them as very painful and are usually unable to use them.

Diagnosis

Joint dislocation is often evident upon visual inspection but in some cases may be difficult to identify without radiological testing. An x-ray confirms the diagnosis.

Treatment

Reduction (manual manipulation of a bone to return it to its normal position) of dislocated joints should never be attempted by laypeople, since it can increase injury to the joint and surrounding tissues. The dislocated joint must be manually repositioned by a physician in the medical office or, if anesthesia is required, in the operating room.

Flashpoint

Reduction of a dislocated joint should only be attempted by a physician.

Prognosis

Prognosis for patients with joint dislocation is generally very good but depends upon the joint involved and the timeliness of diagnosis and treatment. Complications include temporary or permanent damage to surrounding blood vessels, nerves, ligaments, and other tissues. Joints that have been dislocated have a greater risk of repeated dislocation in the future.

Fractures

> **ICD-9-CM: 800–829**   **[ICD-10: M80.0–M94.9] (code by site, type, and other factors for both codes)**

A fracture is a condition in which a bone is broken or cracked. There are many different types of fractures, each with its own name (see Fig. 14-8).

Incidence

It is difficult to estimate accurate numbers of fractures, given the many different types; however, they are known to be very common. For example, hip fractures are all too common among the elderly, with risk being highest among the frail elderly (over 85 years old). It is estimated that nearly one million women and over 400,000 men in this age group suffer a hip fracture annually.

Etiology

Fractures are almost always caused by some form of physical trauma, such as falls, sports injuries, and motor vehicle accidents. However, some conditions—such as osteoporosis or bone tumors—may weaken the bone, making it much more vulnerable to fracture injuries. In some cases the bone may become so fragile that *pathological fractures* occur. This is the breaking of diseased, weakened bone from the stress of normal, everyday activities.

Flashpoint

Diseased bone can suffer pathological fractures.

Signs and Symptoms

Signs and symptoms of bone fractures are caused by trauma to the bone as well as the surrounding tissue, including blood vessels, nerves, muscles, and tendons. Thus, the patient commonly complains of pain and decreased functioning, and may exhibit deformity, swelling, and bruising. However, not all of these signs and symptoms are always present.

Diagnosis

It is often unclear, when patients first appear, whether they suffer from a sprain or a fracture. Therefore, most medical-office protocols include sending the patient for an immediate x-ray before consultation with the physician, to help determine whether the injured body part is fractured or sprained. However, if the patient has an obvious compound (open) fracture, in which the bone is protruding from the skin, the physician must evaluate the patient immediately. Such a fracture can cause severe pain, hemorrhage, numbness, and circulation impairment, and has a high risk of infection. Complex injuries may be evaluated with magnetic resonance imaging (MRI) or bone scan.

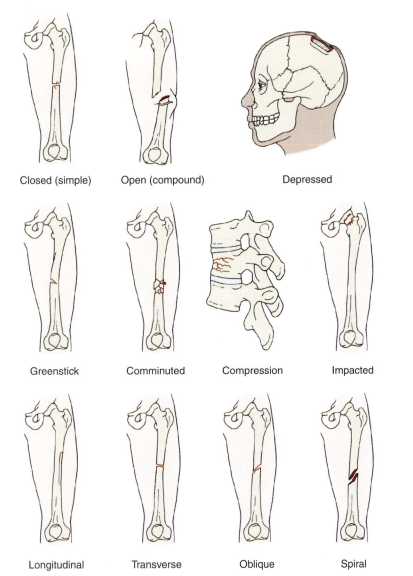

FIGURE 14-8 **The many different types of bone fractures** (From Eagle, S. *Medical Terminology in a Flash! An Interactive, Flash-Card Approach.* 2006. Philadelphia: F.A. Davis Company, with permission.)

Treatment

Treatment of bone fractures depends upon the bone involved. Fractures involving the arms, legs, hands, and feet are usually immobilized with splints to provide stability and prevent further injury while healing occurs. Before and after applying a splint, the health-care provider must evaluate the body part by checking circulation, motion, and sensation (see Box 14-4). Application of cold and elevation help minimize swelling. Analgesics, NSAIDs, and muscle relaxants may be used to manage pain and reduce muscle spasms. Once edema has subsided, a cast may be applied to the body part. Patients with casts must be educated about proper cast care to avoid further complications (see Box 14-5). Fractures that are very unstable or badly displaced, or have compromised circulation, may require surgery. This allows the surgeon to realign the bones, apply hardware to stabilize them, and repair injury to soft tissue as necessary.

Prognosis

Prognosis for patients suffering from bone fractures is generally good but depends upon what anatomy is involved and whether injury to vessels and nerves occurred. In some cases there may

Box 14-4 Wellness Promotion

CHECKING CMS

Checking *CMS* before and after applying a splint helps to prevent damage from tissue ischemia (impaired circulation).

- **C**irculation is evaluated by checking pulses and capillary refill (compressing nailbeds just enough to cause blanching, then noting whether color returns within 3 seconds).
- **M**otion is evaluated by asking the patient if she can wiggle her fingers or toes.
- **S**ensation is evaluated by asking the patient to close her eyes and verify when you touch her fingers or toes.

Box 14-5 Wellness Promotion

PROPER CAST CARE

The health-care provider must be sure to explain proper cast care to the patient. Key points include:

- Cover the cast with waterproof material while bathing. Some casts can change shape if they get wet.
- Elevate the injured body part to reduce swelling and pain.
- Observe fingers or toes for changes in color or temperature or decreased sensation. This could indicate that the cast is too tight. Contact the health-care provider immediately if changes are noted.
- Contact the health-care provider if a foul odor, loss of sensation, numbness, tingling, or bleeding is noted.
- Do not stick anything down the cast to scratch the skin—this could cause infection. If itching is a problem, applying cold may help; if it doesn't, contact the health-care provider.
- Clean the cast with a damp cloth; decorate if desired with felt-tipped pens or paints, but do not cut or puncture the cast for any reason.

---

be permanent loss of some function or sensation. Damage to epiphyseal plates (growth plates) in children may result in stunted growth.

Flashpoint

If a fracture damages the growth plate in a child, the bone may not grow normally.

Torn Anterior Cruciate Ligament
ICD-9-CM: 717.83   [ICD-10: M23.1]

A tear of the anterior cruciate ligament (ACL) is an injury to the stabilizing ligament of the knee that originates on the anterior portion of the femur, in the intercondylar notch (see Fig. 14-9).

Incidence

This injury is most common in athletes, especially those involved in basketball and skiing. It is also more common in females.

Etiology

The ACL usually tears from a twisting force applied to the knee when the person's foot is placed firmly on the ground. It can also be caused by a blow to the outer aspect of the knee, as often happens in sports such as rugby or football.

Flashpoint

ACL tears are usually caused by a twisting force to the knee.

Signs and Symptoms

Symptoms of ACL tear include severe pain, tenderness to palpation, swelling, instability, and an inability to bear weight. The patient may also report having heard a crack or popping sound at the time of the injury.

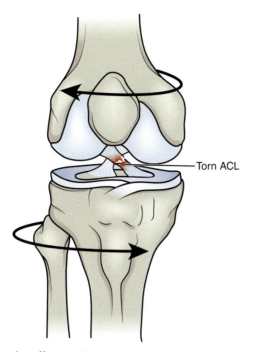

Torn ACL

FIGURE 14-9 Anterior cruciate ligament tear

Diagnosis

Diagnosis of ACL tear is based on the patient's report of injury, presenting signs and symptoms, examination findings, and test results. Physical examination reveals functional instability of the knee, which is confirmed by MRI or computed tomography (CT) scan. The patient may also report tenderness on the inside of the joint from cartilage injury.

Treatment

Treatment involves surgical reattachment of the ligament followed by rest and physical therapy to strengthen and stabilize the knee joint. A knee brace is commonly used for return to contact sports.

Prognosis

Prognosis for patients with ACL tear is generally good, with appropriate treatment. Athletes are usually able to return to full competition within 6 to 9 months.

Torn Meniscus

ICD-9-CM: 731.0   [ICD-10: M23.3]

The menisci are two C-shaped cartilage structures within each knee joint that serve to cushion and stabilize it. This cartilage can become torn during activities in which the knees twist forcefully (see Fig. 14-10).

Incidence

Those at greatest risk are athletes who play sports that require sudden twists, turns, and stops. The risk increases with age, as the structures within the knee joint slowly degenerate.

Etiology

The menisci can tear as a result of any forceful rotation of the knee, particularly when the person's full weight is placed on it. Activities that commonly result in a meniscal tear include football, basketball, and tennis. Other activities that may cause this injury include heavy lifting, kneeling, and squatting.

Signs and Symptoms

Patients with meniscal tears will most likely describe a popping sensation and complain of pain, particularly with turning or rotating the knee and with weight-bearing activities. They may have difficulty fully extending the knee and may have some knee swelling.

Diagnosis

Meniscal tear is suspected from the patient's description of injury and symptoms. Upon physical examination, the physician will manipulate the leg to see if symptoms are

> **Flashpoint**
> Meniscal tears are frequently caused by a twisting force to the knee.

> **Flashpoint**
> The patient often describes a popping sensation in the knee.

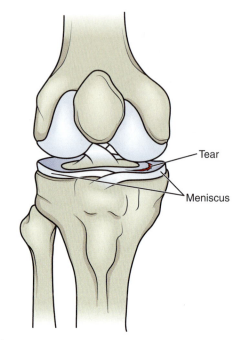

FIGURE 14-10 Torn meniscus

reproduced and to note whether a popping sound occurs and the knee locks in place. Diagnosis may be confirmed and other injuries ruled out by means of x-ray or MRI. The inner structures of the knee may be visually examined by means of arthroscopy. Repair can also be done at this time, with tiny surgical instruments inserted through the arthroscope or other small incisions.

Treatment

Some patients with a torn meniscus respond adequately to conservative treatment. This includes rest, application of cold several times each day, and analgesics. The patient may be advised to use crutches for a time to avoid full weight-bearing. Physical therapy may be useful to help the patient increase the strength and stability of the joint. In some cases, orthotics are useful in helping to distribute the patient's weight more equally around the knee. Patients who do not respond adequately to conservative care may undergo surgical repair or removal of the meniscus.

Prognosis

A patient with a meniscal tear who does not undergo treatment or who does not respond well to conservative care may experience worsening joint instability and chronic pain. Those who undergo surgery usually recover fully within several weeks or months.

Torn Rotator Cuff
ICD-9-CM: 727.61   [ICD-10: M75.1] (complete tear for both codes)

The rotator cuff is made up of four muscles and their tendons that wrap around the front, back, and top of the shoulder joint. Together, the rotator cuff muscles help guide the shoulder through many motions and provide stability to the joint. At the ends of the rotator cuff muscles, tendons attach to the humerus. Traumatic injury to the shoulder can result in tearing of one or more structures of the rotator cuff (see Fig. 14-11).

Incidence

Rotator cuff tears are seen in patients of all ages; however, they are more common in older patients. It is estimated that more than 30% of individuals over age 70 have some degree of tearing, but not all are symptomatic. Less than 40% of those affected individuals seek treatment.

Flashpoint

As muscles and tendons lose elasticity, the risk of rotator cuff tear increases.

Etiology

As a person ages, the muscles and tendons of the rotator cuff lose some elasticity, causing an increased susceptibility to tears. In younger patients, the cause of a tear in the rotator cuff is usually a traumatic injury or excessive use of the shoulder (as seen in athletes).

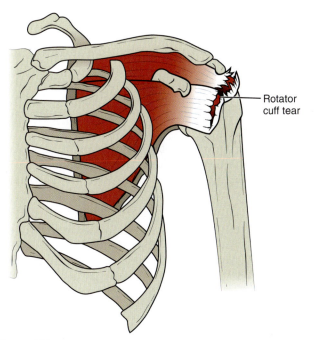

Rotator cuff tear

FIGURE 14-11 Rotator cuff tear

Signs and Symptoms

The most common symptom of a rotator cuff tear is generalized pain exacerbated by shoulder movement. Depending on the severity of the tear, loss of motion and decreased strength may also occur.

Diagnosis

Diagnosis of a rotator cuff tear is based on patient history and physical examination, which will reveal loss of strength and **range of motion** (normal degree of movement). Diagnosis is confirmed by an arthrogram after injection of a contrast dye into the joint capsule (see Box 14-6). If a tear is present, the dye will leak out of the joint capsule, confirming the diagnosis.

Treatment

Conservative treatment for rotator cuff tear includes physical therapy to strengthen the muscles and maintain normal function. Medications include NSAIDs and cortisone injection, to decrease inflammation and pain. If conservative measures are ineffective, surgical repair is necessary.

Prognosis

Prognosis is generally good for patients with rotator cuff tear, if adequate treatment is administered. However, prognosis depends upon the severity of the injury, the presence of any other underlying pathologies, and the patient's age. If the patient suffers a large tear and has arthritis, the condition is more likely to become chronic. It may not heal or improve without surgical repair or total joint replacement.

Box 14-6 Diagnostic Spotlight

ARTHROGRAM

An arthrogram is a radiological procedure in which a series of images of a joint are created with x-rays, CT, or MRI scan. First a local anesthetic is applied, and then a type of dye or contrast is injected into the joint to enhance the picture. The images created allow the radiologist to examine details of the joint and identify any number of problems, such as muscle or tendon tears. Treatment, such as corticosteroid injection, may also be done at the same time. A variation of this procedure is magnetic resonance arthrography.

Epicondylitis

ICD-9-CM: 726.32 (lateral), 726.31 (medial)   [ICD-10: M77.1 (lateral), M77.0 (medial)]

Lateral epicondylitis, commonly called *tennis elbow*, is tiny tears and inflammation along the lateral side of the joint, particularly the epicondyle, caused by trauma or overuse of the elbow (see Fig. 14-12). A similar condition, medial epicondylitis, is the same injury except that it affects the medial side of the joint. Medial epicondylitis is also called *golfer's elbow*, because the repeated motion of driving the golf club is the most common cause.

Incidence

Lateral epicondylitis develops in up to 50% of tennis players. It also occurs in individuals who develop overuse injury from other activities, such as weight lifting. Most commonly affected are people ages 35 to 55 who are recreational athletes or who participate in demanding daily activity.

Etiology

Epicondylitis is caused by activities that involve extension or supination of the wrist and overuse of the muscles that originate at the epicondyle. Risk increases with age, frequency of the activity, and improper technique. Theories of exact cause vary, but most include the idea that overuse causes inflammation. Another idea is that microscopic tearing and repair leads to damage and structural failure of the involved tissues.

Signs and Symptoms

Signs and symptoms of both types of epicondylitis include tenderness, stiffness, inflammation, pain around the elbow, and sometimes pain that radiates down the arm. Symptoms are worse when the patient extends or supinates the arm against resistance.

Diagnosis

Diagnosis is determined mainly through the patient's report of symptoms and physical-examination findings that reveal tenderness to palpation. The patient may also be asked to perform the *chair-raise test*. In this test the patient is asked to stand behind a chair and lift it by putting her hands on the top of the chair back. The results are positive if this causes a painful response.

Treatment

Treatment includes immobilization with a splint, strapping (using a strap positioned around the arm 2 to 3 inches below the elbow joint to take pressure off the extensor tendons of the wrist), ultrasound, acupuncture, NSAIDs, RICE therapy, and muscle relaxants. Cortisone injections may be administered if the injury does not respond to other treatments. The majority of patients respond to conservative treatment; those who do not may need surgery.

Prognosis

The prognosis for patients with epicondylitis is very good. Most respond well to conservative treatment.

Tendonitis

**ICD-9-CM: 726 (use fourth and   [ICD-10: M70.0–M76.9 (code by site)]
fifth digit to code by site)**

Tendonitis is a condition of inflammation of a tendon due to overuse. There are many types of tendonitis, and the names vary depending upon the location involved. Most commonly affected

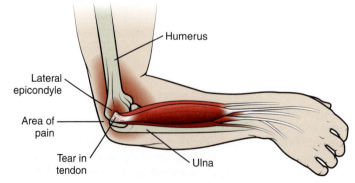

FIGURE 14-12 Lateral epicondylitis (tennis elbow)

are tendons of the upper extremities, including the elbow, wrist, shoulder, and biceps. This is followed by inflammation of the tendons of the lower extremities, including the hip, leg, knee, ankle, and Achilles tendon.

Incidence

It is difficult to estimate the incidence of tendonitis, since there are many different types and many patients do not seek treatment for mild cases.

Etiology

The most common cause of tendonitis is overuse. It can also be caused by age-related changes due to less efficient circulation, and other changes, as tendons lose elasticity and fail to slide smoothly.

Signs and Symptoms

Signs and symptoms of tendonitis can be moderate to severe and include sensations of stiffness, tenderness, aching, or burning over the tendon. Symptoms usually worsen with use and improve with rest.

> **Flashpoint**
> The most common cause of most forms of tendonitis is overuse.

Diagnosis

Diagnosis is often based upon physical-examination findings and the patient's report of symptoms. X-rays may be done to rule out the possibility of a fracture or other disorders.

Treatment

Treatment of tendonitis includes resting the affected part by avoiding the causative activity or wearing a splint. Other measures include application of cold and use of NSAIDs and analgesics. Corticosteroid medications may be taken orally or administered directly to the affected site through local injections. Physical therapy may include ultrasound, electrical muscle stimulation, and strengthening range-of-motion exercises.

Prognosis

Prognosis for patients with tendonitis is very good if they are able to abstain from the causative activity and get appropriate treatment. It generally takes 3 to 6 weeks for healing to occur.

Carpal Tunnel Syndrome
ICD-9-CM: 354.0   [ICD-10: G56.0]

Carpal tunnel syndrome, also called *median neuropathy at the wrist*, is a condition in which the median nerve is compressed at the wrist due to inflammation and edema of the structures within the carpal tunnel (see Fig. 14-13).

Incidence

Incidence of carpal tunnel syndrome is difficult to identify, since many individuals do not seek treatment. However, it is estimated that 90,000 Americans suffer from it at any given time. It is most common among adults and affects women more often than men. Those at greatest risk are those who perform repetitive assembly-line work in industries such as meatpacking, cleaning, sewing, and manufacturing.

> **Flashpoint**
> At greatest risk of carpal tunnel syndrome are people who perform repetitive work such as meatpacking, cleaning, sewing, or manufacturing.

Etiology

The carpal tunnel is a narrow passageway of bones and ligaments within the wrist. When irritation and edema occur, the pressure within this passageway increases, causing compression on these structures—including the median nerve. It is thought that some people have a congenital predisposition for this disorder simply because they have a smaller carpal tunnel than do other people. Factors that cause inflammation include injuries, such as fractures or sprains, and work stress from repetitive motion or the use of vibrating power tools. Other contributors include tumors or cysts, diabetes, thyroid disorders, rheumatoid arthritis, and conditions that cause hormone fluctuations, such as pregnancy and menopause.

Signs and Symptoms

The median nerve has both sensory and motor functions. It provides sensation to the thumb, the index finger, the middle finger, and the medial side of the ring finger. Therefore, symptoms associated with carpal tunnel syndrome frequently affect these areas. Symptoms include sensations of itching, numbness, burning, tingling, or pain; onset is usually gradual. Symptoms are felt within the wrist but may also radiate into the hand and fingers or up the arm into the shoulder. In the beginning, symptoms are usually worse at night, but eventually they become constant. Motor

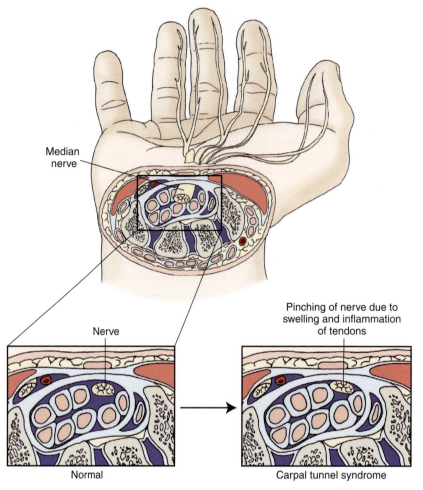

Median nerve

Nerve

Pinching of nerve due to swelling and inflammation of tendons

Normal

Carpal tunnel syndrome

FIGURE 14-13 Carpal tunnel syndrome (From Eagle, S. *Medical Terminology in a Flash! An Interactive, Flash-Card Approach.* 2006. Philadelphia: F.A. Davis Company, with permission.)

symptoms include decreased range of motion, feelings of weakness, and difficulty grasping objects firmly.

Diagnosis

Diagnosis is suspected based upon the patient's presenting report of symptoms. Physical-examination findings help to differentiate this disorder from others. X-ray may be done to rule out fractures and arthritis. Specific tests may be done to elicit carpal tunnel symptoms. The Tinel test produces a shocklike sensation or tingling when the physician taps on the median nerve. During the Phalen (wrist-flexion) test the patient is instructed to hold the forearms upright, with fingers pointed downward, and press the backs of the hands together. A positive reaction occurs when symptoms of numbness or tingling are felt within 1 minute. Electromyography and nerve conduction velocity studies may also be done to evaluate the speed with which nerves are able to transmit messages (see Box 14-7). Ultrasound imaging can also be used to reveal impaired movement of the median nerve.

Treatment

Conservative treatment of carpal tunnel syndrome includes resting the wrist and hand by wearing a splint for 2 or 3 weeks. If splinting is not possible during the daytime, it is still beneficial at night. This allows the wrist to rest in a neutral position, rather than curling inward as often happens during sleep. Other treatment measures include application of cold and medications such as NSAIDs, analgesics, and corticosteroids. Physical therapy may include stretching and strengthening exercises. An occupational therapist may provide an

Box 14-7 Diagnostic Spotlight

ELECTROMYOGRAPHY

Electromyography (EMG), also called *myography*, is a procedure that measures and records the electrical activity generated by muscles. There are two types: needle and surface. In needle EMG, a very thin needle electrode is inserted into the muscles. Electrical activity generated by the muscle is recorded as the needle is inserted, when the muscle is at rest, and during muscle contraction. In surface EMG, a surface electrode is used to record general muscle activity. EMG is usually performed along with a nerve conduction velocity study.

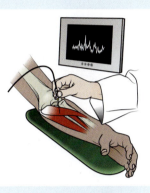

Electromyography

NERVE CONDUCTION VELOCITY

A nerve conduction velocity study is a test that measures the speed with which signals are transmitted through a nerve. Surface electrodes are applied to the skin at several locations along the route of a nerve. Each electrode stimulates the nerve with a very minor electrical impulse, which is recorded by the other electrodes. The speed of impulse conduction is determined by the distance between electrodes and the time required for the impulses to travel between them. This test is usually performed along with electromyography.

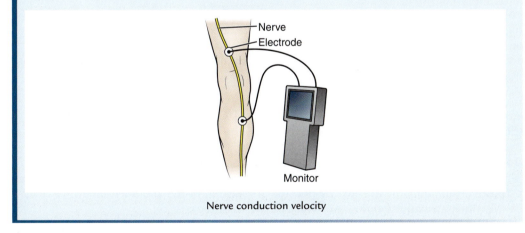

Nerve conduction velocity

evaluation of the ***ergonomics*** (study of human ability relative to work demands) of the situation in which the repetitive activity occurs and help the patient modify the work environment or physical movements to lessen injury (see Box 14-8). Complementary therapies include acupuncture, chiropractic care, and yoga. Patients who do not respond to conservative treatment may be candidates for surgery. The carpal tunnel release procedure involves cutting the carpal ligament to enlarge the tunnel. It may be done as an open procedure or as an endoscopic surgery (through a small

Box 14-8 Wellness Promotion

CTS PREVENTION THROUGH GOOD ERGONOMICS
Follow these guidelines to prevent or minimize CTS:

- Change body position frequently. This allows muscle groups to rest.
- Take regular breaks (10 minutes for each hour) to let the arm rest.
- Stretch the arms, wrists, hands, and fingers regularly to improve circulation and relieve tension.
- Minimize stress to internal structures by working with your forearm and wrist in the natural position.
- Type with the keyboard at or just below elbow level.

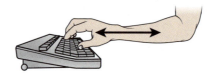

Type with your keyboard at or below elbow level

- Avoid working with your joints extremely flexed.
- Keep your wrists, arms, hands, and fingers strong and flexible so they are less vulnerable to injury.
- Use tools (golf clubs, shovels, hammers, etc.) with a comfortable-size grip.
- Work with your hands a comfortable distance from your body, so that your trunk and shoulders can share the workload.

Flashpoint

Wearing a wrist splint at night allows the wrist to rest in a neutral position.

telescope instrument). Both are done under local anesthesia. Physical therapy is recommended after surgery to help the patient regain wrist strength.

Prognosis

Prognosis for patients with carpal tunnel syndrome depends upon how severe the condition is and whether treatment occurs. Those who undergo surgery usually recover fully over a period of several months. Recurrence is rare. Potential complications include nerve damage, infection, and loss of strength.

Bursitis

ICD-9-CM: 727.30, 727.20 (specific, of   [ICD-10 M70.0–M76.6 (code occupational origin; use fifth digit to specify site)   by site)]

Bursitis is a condition of inflammation of a bursa (see Fig. 14-14). A bursa is a tiny sac filled with fluid that acts as a cushion and provides lubrication to decrease friction and irritation between structures such as bone, tendons, muscle, and skin. There are more than 150 bursas in the body. Those most commonly affected by bursitis are located in the shoulder, elbow, base of the thumb, hip, knees, Achilles tendon, and base of the great toes.

Incidence

Bursitis affects nearly nine million Americans. It is most common among adults over the age of 40.

Etiology

Bursitis is a repetitive-motion disorder but can also be caused by acute injury. Risk increases with age, since tendons withstand stress less well as they age, lose elasticity, and injure more easily. Common overuse activities include working in a poor posture, throwing, carpentering, gardening, shoveling, painting, scrubbing, prolonged walking, wearing poorly fitting shoes, and playing sports such as golf or tennis. Contributing conditions include rheumatoid arthritis, gout, infection, thyroid disorders, and rotator cuff injury.

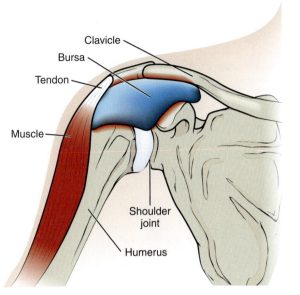

FIGURE 14-14 Bursitis

Signs and Symptoms

The most common symptom of bursitis is pain. It may develop gradually or suddenly. Other signs and symptoms include stiffness, burning, swelling, warmth, and occasionally redness. ***Adhesive capsulitis,*** also called *frozen shoulder*, may result if the joint is not fully used. This is indicated by loss of range of motion in the shoulder.

Diagnosis

Diagnosis is suspected based on the patient's description of symptoms. Physical examination reveals a painful joint and tenderness in the area of the bursa. X-ray may be done, and fluid aspirated from the bursa for testing, to rule out other injuries and disorders.

Flashpoint

Moving and using the shoulder joint helps to reduce the risk of adhesive capsulitis.

Treatment

Conservative treatment of bursitis includes resting the affected body part, providing support and protection with a brace, applying cold, and taking NSAIDs. If these measures do not provide adequate relief, corticosteroid injections may be given and physical therapy offered. In rare cases, surgery is needed to drain the fluid or remove the bursa.

Prognosis

Prognosis for patients with bursitis is generally very good, with proper care. Pain should decrease over several weeks, but healing may take at least 6 to 8 weeks. Symptoms of 6 months' duration or more indicate a more chronic condition that may respond less well to treatment.

Medial Tibial Syndrome
ICD-9-CM: 844.9   [ICD-10: M76.8]

Medial tibial syndrome, more commonly called *shin splints*, is a painful condition involving the anterior tibias (shins) and the muscles and tendons that attach to them (see Fig. 14-15).

Incidence

The exact incidence of shin splints is unknown, since many people do not seek treatment. However, it is known to be fairly common among runners and is estimated to be responsible for 6% to 16% of all running injuries.

Etiology

Shin splints is caused by irritation of muscles, tendons, and tissues along the anterior tibia and periosteum (tissue layer covering the bone) related to overuse and physical trauma. This is caused by physical activities such as running, jumping, jogging, or even walking; running

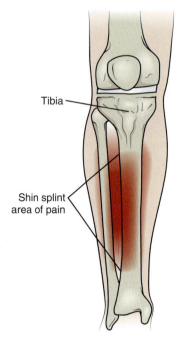

FIGURE 14-15 Medial tibial syndrome, or shin splints

downhill, playing sports with frequent stops and starts (such as tennis), and wearing poorly fitting shoes can also cause or worsen the condition. Shin splints often occurs in new athletes or those who increase the intensity and duration of their activities. It is worsened or aggravated by overpronation of the feet, which increases stress on the muscle along the front of the leg. This is commonly caused by flat arches.

Signs and Symptoms
Shin splints causes patients to experience aching pain along the inner aspect of the anterior tibia. The area may be tender to the touch and may or may not be swollen.

Diagnosis
A presumptive diagnosis may be based upon the patient's history of physical activities and description of symptoms, along with physical-examination findings. Diagnostic imaging may include standard x-ray or bone scan; the latter is better able to identify stress fractures or other subtle problems and differentiate them from shin splints.

Treatment
Most patients with shin splints respond to conservative treatment of rest, elevation, compression, NSAIDs, and application of cold through ice massage several times each day. Properly fitting shoes are important; orthotic shoe inserts can help individuals with flat arches. A change to low-impact exercise, such as swimming or bicycling, is often recommended. Some people also find it useful to tape the lower legs and ankles, to provide stability.

Prognosis
Most people with shin splints respond well to conservative treatment. However, if the condition progresses it can lead to stress fracture of the tibia.

Plantar Fasciitis
ICD-9-CM: 728.71   [ICD-10: M72.2]
Plantar fasciitis is a painful condition of the structures that support the arch of the foot. It primarily involves the plantar fascia, which is a band of tissue that connects the heel with the toes (see Fig. 14-16).

Incidence
Plantar fasciitis is one of the most common causes of foot pain. It develops most often in recreational runners between ages 40 and 60. It affects women slightly more often than men. It is

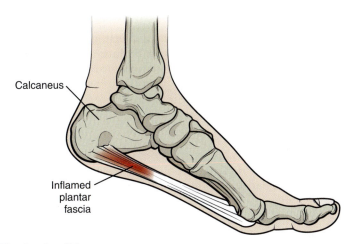

Calcaneus

Inflamed
plantar
fascia

FIGURE 14-16 Plantar fasciitis

also common in ballet dancers and those who spend long hours working and walking on hard surfaces.

Etiology

Plantar fasciitis is sometimes confused with a calcaneal (heel) spur. Although the two often occur together, they are different conditions. Plantar fasciitis develops when the plantar fascia, a band of thick connective tissue that extends from the heel across the arch, becomes inflamed from overuse (tendonitis). The plantar fascia bears a large amount of weight and stress when a person walks or runs, and it suffers minor tearing and stretching. A calcaneal spur is a protrusion of bone that forms on the calcaneus (heel bone). As many as 70% of those with plantar fasciitis also have a calcaneal spur. Risk factors for plantar fasciitis include obesity, pregnancy, rapid weight gain, flat feet or very high arches, poorly fitting shoes (such as high heels) and loose, thin-soled shoes that lack arch support (such as flip-flops).

Flashpoint
Plantar fasciitis is one of the most common reasons for foot pain.

Signs and Symptoms

The primary symptom of plantar fasciitis is tenderness or sharp pain in the heel and bottom of the foot that is often most intense when the individual first stands in the morning. The pain usually resolves quickly but may recur after prolonged weight-bearing activities. Symptoms of plantar fasciitis usually develop slowly and may affect one or both feet.

Diagnosis

Diagnosis of plantar fasciitis is generally based upon the patient's description of the pattern of symptoms and physical activity. Physical examination reveals tenderness along the bottom of the foot, particularly the heel. Radiological testing such as x-ray or MRI may be done to rule out other pathology, such as stress fractures or bone spurs. Although spur formation is a common finding, it is rarely the cause of the pain and rarely requires surgical removal, contrary to what was commonly thought in the past.

Treatment

Most individuals with plantar fasciitis respond well to conservative treatment. This involves resting, applying cold, wearing foot splints at night, using orthotic shoe inserts, and taking NSAIDs. Physical therapy may include stretching the plantar fascia and Achilles tendon and strengthening the muscles of the lower legs. Stretching the plantar fascia before getting out of bed in the morning can help reduce morning pain. Corticosteroid medication may be administered locally through injection or iontophoresis. The latter uses a painless electrical current to aid the absorption of medication into the tissues. Weight loss is encouraged if obesity is a contributing cause. The patient should avoid wearing flip-flops, sandals, or open-back shoes. In severe cases, surgery may be done to disconnect the fascia from the calcaneal bone.

Flashpoint
Wearing good shoes and using orthotics can help to prevent plantar fasciitis.

Prognosis

Approximately 90% of patients with plantar fasciitis respond well to conservative treatment and experience resolution of symptoms within 3 to 12 months. Failure to treat symptoms may result in a more chronic condition. Potential complications of corticosteroid injection include atrophy of the fat pad within the heel and rupture of the plantar fascia. Approximately 90% of those who undergo surgery experience improvement in their symptoms.

Herniated Disk

ICD-9-CM: 722.00–722.93   [ICD-10: M50.0–M53.9] (code by specific site and conditions for both codes)

A herniated disk, also called a *slipped* or *ruptured disk,* is a prolapse of the nucleus pulposus of an intervertebral disk into the spinal canal (see Fig. 14-17).

Incidence

It is estimated that three to six million Americans suffer from symptomatic disk herniation each year. Men are affected more often than are women, and those ages 20 to 50 are affected most often.

Etiology

Disk herniation most commonly involves disks near the fifth lumbar (L5) and first sacral (S1) vertebrae. It is caused by some form of traumatic injury.

Signs and Symptoms

Patients with a herniated disk complain of back pain and pain or weakness of the extremities. The most common symptom of a herniated disk is **sciatica,** a condition in which compression of the sciatic nerve causes leg irritation and can produce pain radiating down the back of the leg as far as the ankle. The pain may be described as sharp, stabbing, shooting, or electric; the patient may alternatively complain of numbness and weakness in the leg. Over time the patient may exhibit decreased or absent deep reflexes of the tendons and weakness or atrophy of muscles.

Flashpoint

A herniated disk often causes painful sciatica.

Diagnosis

Procedures used to diagnose a herniated disk include CT and MRI.

Treatment

Conservative treatment for a herniated disk may include rest, application of cold, NSAIDs or corticosteroids, analgesics, muscle relaxants, chiropractic adjustment, physical therapy, traction,

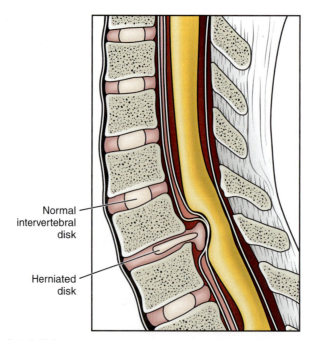

Normal intervertebral disk

Herniated disk

FIGURE 14-17 Herniated disk

and acupuncture. Such treatments are palliative, not curative, and may offer the patient some pain relief. Surgical treatment may be necessary for patients whose symptoms are not responsive to conservative measures. Diskectomy involves the removal of most of the disk. Laminectomy involves the removal of a part of the vertebra over the nerve root to allow the disk and nerve root more space (see Fig. 14-18).

Prognosis

Prognosis for patients with disk herniation is generally good, regardless of the treatment options employed.

Gout

ICD-9-CM: 274.0 (acute)   [M10.0–M10.9 (code by cause)]

Gout is a disease caused by a congenital or acquired disorder of uric-acid metabolism.

Incidence

The estimated incidence of gout in the United States is approximately 600,000. Rates are much higher in those over 75 years old. Gout is most prevalent among African American males, in whom the incidence is twice that in white males.

Etiology

A family history of gout is present in 20% of patients. Risk factors for acquiring the disease include obesity; alcohol abuse; lead exposure; and a high-purine, high-protein diet, including such foods as cream, meats, and fish. Underlying medical conditions such as renal insufficiency, high blood pressure, and hypothyroidism may also increase risk. Medications that can contribute to gout in some people include diuretics, niacin, cyclosporines, and salicylate-containing drugs such as aspirin.

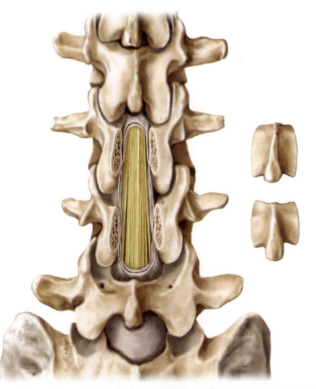

FIGURE 14-18 **Laminectomy** (From Eagle, S, et al. *The Professional Medical Assistant: An Integrative Teamwork-Based Approach.* 2009. Philadelphia: F.A. Davis Company, with permission.)

Signs and Symptoms

People with gout are unable to clear uric acid from the bloodstream. Subsequently, crystals of uric acid deposit in the articular cartilage of joints, most commonly the knee and great toe (see Fig. 14-19). The deposits provoke an inflammatory response in the affected joints, causing pain and restriction of the range of motion of the joint. The deposits commonly increase in size and burst through the skin, causing a chalky white material to appear. Affected joints will appear red, swollen, and painful to the touch. The patient may have a fever during an acute episode. Gout is commonly chronic, with episodes of acute attacks.

Diagnosis

Diagnosis of gout is based upon physical-examination findings, patient history, and levels of blood uric acid greater than 7.0 mg/dL in men and 6.0 mg/dL in women (hyperuricemia).

Treatment

Treatment is directed at pain relief, with NSAIDs and intra-articular injections (into the joint) of corticosteroids to reduce inflammation. Aspirin should never be used for pain relief, because it can worsen the condition. Patients with a history of gout can elect to take allopurinol, a medication that directly reduces the production of uric acid. Allopurinol is a lifelong medication and cannot be initiated during an attack, because it will make the acute gout worse. Patients should be advised about dietary changes that can help prevent further attacks (see Box 14-9).

Prognosis

There is no cure for gout. The prognosis varies with the person, but with adequate treatment most people lead a good quality of life. Some individuals have only one episode and then never have any more problems; others have multiple episodes over time and suffer permanent damage and pain. Left untreated, gout may advance and cause tophi, which are nodules of urate crystals that form beneath the skin. During gout episodes, the tophi become tender and swollen. Urate crystals may also form in the urinary tract and cause kidney stones.

Osteoarthritis

ICD-9-CM: 715.9 (use fifth digit to code by site)   [ICD-10: M15.0–M19.9 (code by site)]

Osteoarthritis, also called *degenerative joint disease*, is the most common form of arthritis, a condition of joint inflammation characterized by pain, stiffness, redness, warmth, swelling, deformity, and decreased range of motion. Most commonly affected are the weight-bearing joints in the body.

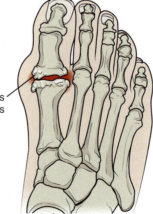

Urate crystals in a tophus

FIGURE 14-19 Gout affecting the great toe

Box 14-9 Wellness Promotion

ANTIGOUT DIET
The patient with gout should be educated about foods that can help or hurt the condition.

Good for Gout
These foods will help reduce production of uric acid and should be included in the diet:

- mushrooms
- spinach
- asparagus
- cauliflower
- cherries
- strawberries

Bad for Gout
These foods contain elements, such as purine, that should be limited or avoided in the diet:

- alcohol
- cream
- meat
- fish
- pinto, kidney, and red beans

Incidence
Arthritis affects approximately 43 million Americans and is more common in women than men. Incidence of arthritis increases with age. Risk factors include obesity, overuse or abuse of joints in sports or strenuous occupations, and trauma.

Etiology
Osteoarthritis is caused by erosion of the joint's cartilage and eventual erosion of the bone surface. The joints most commonly affected are the shoulder, elbow, hip, wrist, finger, knee, ankle, and toe. Bone spurs may develop, causing increased pain with movement (see Fig. 14-20).

Signs and Symptoms
Patients with osteoarthritis complain of gradually increasing pain and gradually decreasing range of motion in the affected joint.

Diagnosis
Diagnosis of osteoarthritis is based on physical-examination findings, description of symptoms, and results of radiological studies. X-rays and possibly MRI studies reveal eroded cartilage, narrowing of the joint space, and formation of bone spurs.

Treatment
There is no cure for osteoarthritis. Treatment with medication such as corticosteroids and analgesics, rest, heat, acupuncture, and weight reduction can minimize symptoms and slow the progression of the disease. Other treatment measures include joint protection, exercise, and application of cold. If joint deterioration is severe, joint-replacement surgery may be necessary. Physical and occupational therapy are common with or without surgery. Regardless of the treatment strategy, the goal is to promote function, comfort, and safety.

Prognosis
Osteoarthritis is not life-threatening but commonly impairs quality of life by causing chronic pain and decreasing mobility. For some patients it is a mild annoyance; for others, it may force them to leave work and may severely limit everyday activities such as walking.

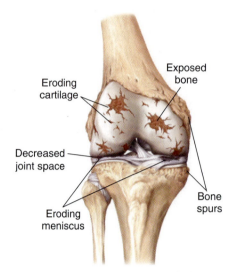

FIGURE 14-20 The degenerative changes of osteoarthritis (Adapted from Eagle, S, et al. *The Professional Medical Assistant: An Integrative Teamwork-Based Approach.* 2009. Philadelphia: F.A. Davis Company, with permission.)

Rheumatoid and Juvenile Rheumatoid Arthritis

ICD-9-CM: 714.0 (rheumatoid arthritis), 714.30 (juvenile rheumatoid arthritis)	[ICD-10: M05.0–M06.9 (rheumatoid arthritis; code by sites of involvement and additional organ system involvement), M08.0 (juvenile rheumatoid arthritis)]

Rheumatoid arthritis (RA) is a condition of chronic systemic inflammation of the joints and synovial membranes that also involves elevated levels of serum rheumatoid factor. It shares some similarities with osteoarthritis in that it causes pain, stiffness, and loss of function in the joints. However, it differs in that its effects are usually more severe and it can affect other tissues in the body. There are several variations of juvenile rheumatoid arthritis (JRA), but overall it is similar to adult-onset RA with earlier onset and more severe symptoms.

> **Flashpoint**
> RA affects joints but can also affect many other tissues in the body.

Incidence
RA is up to three times more common in women than in men, and it often begins in young or middle adulthood. However, it can affect young children and older adults as well.

Etiology
RA is an autoimmune disease that may be triggered by any number of things, including viral infections, genetic susceptibility, smoking, and other environmental factors. The immune response causes inflammation and the release of certain proteins that affect the synoviums of joints, causing them to thicken. Inflammatory changes also damage bones, cartilage, tendons, and ligaments. Over time, the affected joints lose function and may move out of alignment, becoming dislocated.

Signs and Symptoms
Symptoms of rheumatoid arthritis usually affect several joints of the body in a bilateral pattern (on both sides). Signs and symptoms include severe joint pain, swelling, stiffness, tenderness, redness, joint deformity, and loss of range of motion and function. RA can affect many joints (wrists, hands, ankles, feet, shoulders, elbows, knees, hips, jaw) but most commonly involves the wrists and fingers (see Fig. 14-21). Rheumatoid nodules (firm bumps) may appear beneath the skin on the patient's arms. Patients with RA also frequently experience generalized symptoms of fatigue, fever, and weight loss. Patients often experience ***exacerbations*** (periods of worsening or flare-up) and relative ***remission*** (period of improvement or absence of disease activity).

> **Flashpoint**
> RA usually has a bilateral, symmetrical pattern, affecting matching joints on both sides of the body.

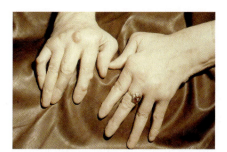

FIGURE 14-21 **Rheumatoid arthritis** (From Dillon, PM. *Nursing Health Assessment.* 2003. Philadelphia: F.A. Davis Company, with permission.)

Diagnosis

Diagnosis of RA is based upon the patient's presenting signs and symptoms, examination findings, and results of certain tests. Blood tests include antinuclear antibody and erythrocyte sedimentation rate. Other tests check for the presence of rheumatoid factor and anti-cyclic citrullinated peptide antibodies. However, these two tests are not conclusive, since these substances are not always present in people with RA. Fluid may be drawn from the affected joint and tested. X-rays are done to track the progression of the disease.

Treatment

There is no cure for rheumatoid arthritis; however, there are many treatment options. Patients must work with their physician to create an individualized management plan. A number of medications can be used to relieve symptoms and slow the progression of the disease. These include NSAIDs, corticosteroids, disease-modifying antirheumatic drugs, immunosuppressants, and TNF-alpha inhibitors. Medication choice depends upon many factors, including the severity and duration of the illness and the patient's other medical conditions. Surgery may also be considered, to repair severely damaged joints, reduce pain, and improve appearance and function. Examples of surgical repair include total joint replacement and synovectomy (removal of the inflamed synovial lining).

Prognosis

There is no cure for RA. Patients often experience periods of improvement and periods of worsening of symptoms. The disease is usually chronic, progressive, and lifelong. It can cause debilitating and disfiguring joint damage that makes daily activities difficult and affects body image and self-esteem. Early, aggressive treatment may slow joint damage and limit disability.

> **Flashpoint**
> There is no cure for RA, but there are many different treatments available.

Osteitis Deformans

ICD-9-CM: 731.0   [ICD-10: M88.9]

Osteitis deformans, also called *Paget disease*, is a chronic condition in which the usual process of bone destruction and regrowth occurs abnormally. As a result, bones become weak, fragile, enlarged, and misshapen.

Incidence

Estimates of the incidence of osteitis deformans vary widely by country; in the United States, estimates are between four and 24 million affected people. Osteitis deformans most commonly affects people over age 40, men more than women.

Etiology

The exact cause of osteitis deformans is unknown, although a combination of genetics and certain viral infections may be a factor. Even though individuals stop growing after reaching young adulthood, bones continue a process of renewal called remodeling. In this process, old bone is broken down and replaced by new bone tissue. In patients with osteitis deformans, old bone tissue is broken down faster than it can be replaced by new tissue. The body tries to keep up by producing new bone even faster; however, the new bone that is produced is weaker and softer than normal. This leads to fractures, deformities, and bone pain. Risk factors include advancing age and heredity.

Signs and Symptoms

Osteitis deformans can affect bones throughout the body or it may only affect a few. The bones most commonly involved are those of the spine, pelvis, arms, legs, and clavicles. Some patients have no symptoms. When they do occur, typical signs and symptoms include aching bone pain, headache, neck pain, tooth pain, joint pain, and warmth over the affected area. Deformities may occur, including bowing of the legs, curvature of the spine, skull deformities, bone fractures, and reduced height. Deterioration of joint cartilage can lead to osteoarthritis. Neurological symptoms such as hearing loss and, rarely, vision loss may also occur.

Diagnosis

In addition to gathering data through physical examination and patient interview, the physician may order bone x-rays and a bone scan. A bone scan will usually detect bone changes before they are detectable on x-ray. Blood tests can reveal an elevated level of alkaline phosphatase isoenzyme.

Treatment

Patients with very mild disease and no symptoms may not need treatment. Those more likely to need treatment are those who have deformities, those who are symptomatic, and those who are not yet symptomatic but are at risk for future complications. The latter includes those with involvement of weight-bearing bone, the skull, or the spine. Medications such as bisphosphonates and calcitonin may be used to prevent continued breakdown of bone. Bisphosphonates are also given to people with osteoporosis to increase bone density. Calcitonin is a hormone normally produced in the body that is important in the regulation of calcium and bone metabolism. NSAIDs or analgesics may help manage pain. Surgery may be needed to correct problems related to fractures, severe arthritis, and deformities. Other treatment guidelines usually include up to 1,500 milligrams of daily calcium, vitamin D, regular exercise, optimal weight maintenance, and adequate exposure to sunshine.

Prognosis

There is no cure for osteitis deformans. However, the prognosis for patients with this disorder is generally good, especially if they receive treatment before major complications develop. Potential complications include spinal stenosis, fractures, arthritis, deafness, paraplegia, deformities, heart failure, kidney stones, and, rarely vision loss or a form of bone cancer called osteogenic sarcoma or *osteosarcoma.*

Osteomalacia

ICD-9-CM: 268.2   [ICD-10: M83.9]

Osteomalacia is a condition of softening and weakening of the bones. When it occurs in children it is called *rickets.*

Incidence

Osteomalacia is rare in the United States and other developed countries because of the availability of milk fortified with vitamin D; the current incidence is 0.1%. However, in some countries it affects up to 15% of the population. Rickets is most likely to develop in children ages 6 to 24 months when they are going through growth spurts.

Etiology

The body uses minerals such as calcium and phosphorus to build strong bones. Osteomalacia develops when the supply of these minerals is inadequate or other factors interfere with the bone's ability to use them. In many cases the cause of osteomalacia is a poor supply of vitamin D, which is an important vitamin for calcium utilization. A patient's poor supply of vitamin D can occur because of low amounts in the diet, impaired absorption in the intestines, or inadequate exposure to sunlight. Risk factors for osteomalacia include liver disease, kidney failure, cancer, celiac disease, certain antiseizure medications, and gastrectomy (surgical removal of the stomach) or removal of part of the small intestine.

Signs and Symptoms

Patients with mild osteomalacia may be symptom free. Developing symptoms may include bone pain (especially in the hips, spine, and legs), fractures, and muscle weakness. Patients may also begin to walk with a waddling type of *gait* (manner of walking) due to an abnormal curvature in the leg bones (see Fig. 14-22). Other symptoms related to low calcium levels may be present in some people. These include muscle spasms in the hands and feet, numbness of the extremities or around the mouth, and irregular heart rhythm.

Diagnosis

A variety of tests may be done to diagnose osteomalacia. Blood tests may reveal low levels of calcium, vitamin D, and phosphorus. X-rays and bone scans may reveal bone loss and fractures. Bone biopsy allows direct examination of bone tissue and reveals softening due to a mineral deficit.

Treatment

Prevention and treatment of osteomalacia includes sunlight exposure and adequate dietary intake of vitamin D, calcium, and phosphates. Individuals with intestinal malabsorption may need larger amounts than the average person. If the condition is caused by other disorders, such as renal failure, the treatment plan is modified according to those needs. Occasionally, patients may be advised to wear braces to minimize or prevent irregularity of the bone structure, or they may undergo surgery to repair deformity.

Prognosis

The prognosis for patients with osteomalacia is excellent if the disorder is diagnosed and treated before significant bone loss, fractures, or deformity occurs. Improvement is seen within several weeks, and complete healing occurs within 6 months.

Flashpoint

The prognosis for patients with osteomalacia is excellent if treatment begins early.

Osteoporosis

ICD-9-CM: 733.00   [ICD-10: M81] (unspecified for both codes)

Osteoporosis is a condition characterized by loss of bone mass throughout the skeleton.

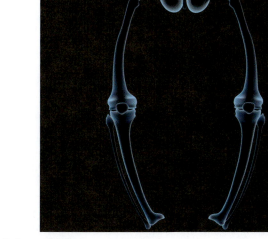

FIGURE 14-22 **Osteomalacia**

Incidence

Osteoporosis affects an estimated eight million American women and two million American men. Those of northern European or Asian descent and those with a family history of osteoporosis are at increased risk.

Etiology

Osteoporosis develops when bones lose mass and density as bone resorption (removal) exceeds new bone development. This is caused by insufficient intake of minerals. Contributing factors include postmenopausal decrease in hormones, nutritional deficiencies (lack of calcium, magnesium, and vitamin D), immobility and sedentary lifestyle, excess of thyroid hormones, parathyroid abnormalities, corticosteroid use, some anticonvulsant medications, and use of alcohol and tobacco. Also at increased risk are those of advanced age and those with a family history of osteoporosis.

Signs and Symptoms

Individuals with osteoporosis are often asymptomatic until bone fractures occur. Most common are vertebral and hip fractures. Subsequent immobility exacerbates the condition. Thoracic vertebral changes can cause kyphosis, vertebral compression fractures, or even vertebral collapse, with subsequent pain and disability. Loss of bone density in the vertebrae causes changes in posture and decreased height (see Fig. 14-23).

Diagnosis

Diagnosis of osteoporosis usually does not occur until the individual suffers a related injury, such as a hip fracture. Diagnosis is based upon results of radiological tests such as x-rays, CT scan, and dual energy x-ray absorptiometry scan, all of which reveal decreased bone density. Blood tests may be done to check levels of serum calcium and estrogen.

Flashpoint

Many people do not know they have osteoporosis until they suffer a bone fracture.

Treatment

Treatment of osteoporosis is aimed at preventing or minimizing further bone loss and disability. Dietary modification includes mineral and vitamin supplements. Also considered are estrogen replacement, weight-bearing exercise, and bisphosphate medications to foster bone density. Treatment for injury and disability from osteoporosis includes surgery, physical therapy, and analgesics and muscle relaxants for pain.

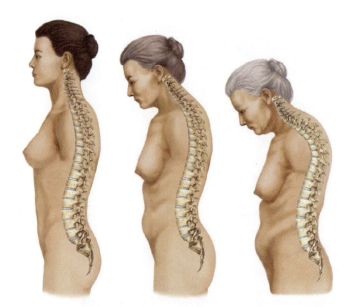

FIGURE 14-23 **Osteoporosis causes loss of bone density in the vertebrae, which results in changes in posture and decreased height.** (From Eagle, S, et al. *The Professional Medical Assistant: An Integrative Teamwork-Based Approach.* 2009. Philadelphia: F.A. Davis Company, with permission.)

Prognosis

Prognosis for patients with osteoporosis depends upon the severity of the disease and the timeliness of diagnosis and treatment. Osteoporosis puts a person at greater risk of vertebral and hip fractures. As with many other disorders, prevention is the wisest course of action. Good self-care should begin in childhood (see Box 14-10).

Fibromyalgia

ICD-9-CM: 729.1   [ICD-10: M79.7]

Fibromyalgia is a chronic condition marked by pain in the muscles, tendons, ligaments, and soft tissues of the body.

Incidence

Fibromyalgia affects about six million Americans of all ages. It is more common in women than in men.

Etiology

The exact cause of fibromyalgia is not well understood. Genetics may play a role. It is also thought that individuals with this disorder may develop changes in their brains that result in an abnormal increase in certain neurotransmitter chemicals that signal pain; as a result, their brains' pain receptors become more sensitive. Fibromyalgia often follows physical trauma such as an automobile accident, bacterial or viral infection, or an underlying medical condition such as rheumatoid arthritis, lupus, or hypothyroidism. It can even follow emotional trauma. However, in many cases no triggering event is identified. It is associated with numerous other conditions, including sleep disorders, irritable bowel syndrome, chronic fatigue syndrome, chronic headaches, depression, endometriosis, temporomandibular-joint problems, osteoarthritis, increased chemical sensitivity, and other musculoskeletal complaints. Fibromyalgia is aggravated by monthly hormonal variations and changes in weather or temperature, stress, anxiety, and depression.

Box 14-10 Wellness Promotion

OSTEOPOROSIS RISK AND PREVENTION

Good self-care, including preventive measures, is the best way to prevent or minimize osteoporosis. Such preventive measures should begin in childhood. This table contains a list of the most common risk factors for osteoporosis, along with related preventive measures.

Risk factor	Preventive measure
Immobility or sedentary lifestyle	Regular weight-bearing exercise, such as walking (30–60 minutes three or four times per week) and modest weight lifting
Diet poor in calcium, magnesium, and vitamin D	Consistent intake of adequate amounts of calcium, magnesium, and vitamin D
Excessive thyroid hormones	Timely, appropriate treatment of hyperthyroidism
Decrease in sex hormones	Hormone replacement therapy
Excessive alcohol use	Elimination or minimization of alcohol consumption
Tobacco use	Elimination of tobacco use
Medications such as corticosteroids and phenytoin (Dilantin)	Administration of the smallest therapeutic dose of such medications (determined in consultation with a physician, with the risks and benefits carefully weighed)

Signs and Symptoms

Signs and symptoms of fibromyalgia differ depending upon variables such as physical activity, stress, and the weather. They include diffuse, dull muscle aches and pains all over the body, with specific points of tenderness, and general fatigue (see Fig. 14-24).

Diagnosis

Diagnosis of fibromyalgia is made by eliminating any other cause of the symptoms, identifying pain that lasts 3 months or longer, and finding 11 of 18 specific points to be extremely tender to touch. Diagnostic testing may be done to exclude other diagnoses but there is no specific diagnostic test for fibromyalgia.

Treatment

There is no known cure for fibromyalgia. Treatment includes NSAIDs, nutritional and herbal support, exercise, and massage. Trigger-point injections may also be beneficial. This is a procedure in which anesthetic or corticosteroid medication is injected through a small needle into trigger points, which are knots of muscle under the skin that may be irritating nerves and causing referred pain (pain felt elsewhere).

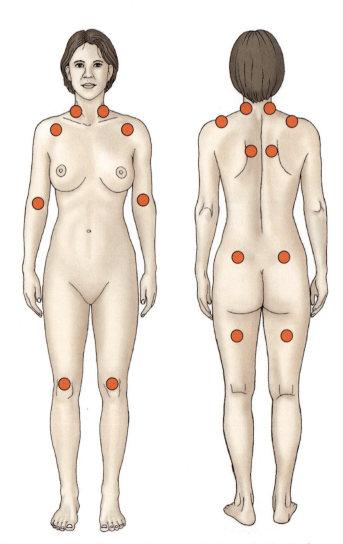

FIGURE 14-24 **Fibromyalgia tender points** (From Eagle, S, et al. *The Professional Medical Assistant: An Integrative Teamwork-Based Approach.* 2009. Philadelphia: F.A. Davis Company, with permission.)

Prognosis

The prognosis for patients with fibromyalgia is generally good, since the condition is not progressive, but it varies with each individual. The symptoms can interfere with the person's ability to function professionally and socially and may interfere with personal relationships.

Myasthenia Gravis

ICD-9-CM: 358.0   [ICD-10: G70.0]

Myasthenia gravis (MG) is a neuromuscular disorder characterized by muscle weakness and muscle fatigue.

Incidence

Myasthenia gravis is three times more common in women than in men, with a peak onset between ages 20 and 30.

Etiology

Myasthenia gravis is thought to be the result of an abnormal immune reaction in which antibodies inappropriately attack and gradually destroy certain receptors in muscles that receive nerve impulses. It is also associated with tumors of the thymus gland. Patients with other immune disorders, such as rheumatoid arthritis and systemic lupus erythematosus, are at increased risk. There also may be a relationship with hyperthyroidism.

Signs and Symptoms

Although myasthenia gravis usually becomes apparent during adulthood, symptom onset may be gradual and can occur at any age. The condition may be generalized, involving multiple muscle groups, or restricted to certain muscle groups, particularly those of the eyes; in this case it is called *ocular myasthenia gravis.* Most individuals with myasthenia gravis develop blepharoptosis (drooping of the eyelids—see Fig. 14-25), weakness of eye muscles, inability to maintain a steady gaze, diplopia (double vision), and weakness of facial muscles. Dysphasia (difficulty speaking), dysphagia, shallow respirations, difficulty holding up the head, and weakness of the upper arms and legs are also common. Patients will have difficulty climbing stairs and lifting heavy objects, due to muscle weakness. A general defining feature is fatigue and weakness of the skeletal muscles that worsens with use but is partially relieved by short rest periods.

Diagnosis

Diagnosis of myasthenia gravis is made by physical examination, including muscle-strength assessment, and diagnostic tests. Laboratory testing reveals that up to 90% of patients have antibodies to acetylcholine receptors. An electromyogram may help to differentiate between disorders of muscle weakness and those involving a deficit of nerve-impulse transmission. A test using anticholinesterase drugs such as edrophonium (Tensilon) can be used to make a definitive diagnosis of MG. This medication blocks the action of enzymes that break down the neurotransmitter acetylcholine, thereby briefly increasing its availability. This results in brief improvement of symptoms.

Flashpoint

A key feature of MG is muscle fatigue and weakness that worsens with use but is partially relieved by rest periods.

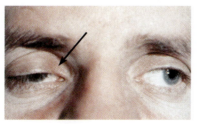

FIGURE 14-25 **Myasthenia gravis can cause blepharoptosis (drooping of the eyelids)** (From Morton, PG. *Health Assessment in Nursing,* 2nd Edition. 1993. Philadelphia: F.A. Davis Company, with permission.)

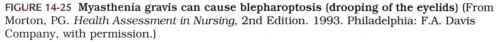

Treatment

There is no known cure for MG. Treatment is directed at reducing symptoms of muscle weakness and fatigue. The health-care provider should advise patients of general measures to manage the disease and avoid complications (see Box 14-11). Patients should avoid stress and exposure to heat, because those can exacerbate symptoms. The patient may want to wear an eye patch if diplopia is problematic. Anticholinesterase medications can improve communication between nerves and muscles and can decrease weakness. Thymectomy (surgical removal of the thymus) may cause permanent remission or decrease the need for medication; it is most effective if done within the first two years of diagnosis. A procedure called plasmapheresis may be done to remove antibodies from the blood, but this provides only temporary improvement.

Prognosis

Periods of improvement and worsening are common with myasthenia gravis. In about 10% of cases, affected individuals may develop **myasthenic crisis,** a potentially life-threatening episode of worsening of myasthenic symptoms. It may be caused by undermedication or triggered by an infection, and it must be immediately treated with anticholinesterase medications. A **cholinergic crisis** can occur if the patient takes too much anticholinesterase medication. This causes respiratory failure, paralysis, salivation, and sweating. Treatment of cholinergic crisis involves withholding the regular medication and administering atropine.

Flashpoint

Myasthenic crisis is a potentially life-threatening episode in which the MG symptoms get worse.

Osteomyelitis

ICD-9-CM: 730.00 [ICD-10: M86.9] (unspecified for both codes)

Osteomyelitis is an acute or chronic infection within the bone (see Fig. 14-26). It most commonly affects long bones, such as those in the legs and arms, in addition to those in the pelvis and spine.

Incidence

Osteomyelitis affects approximately 60,000 Americans each year, children more frequently than adults, and males four times more often than females. Children more frequently suffer infection within the long bones, while adults more often suffer infection within bones of the spine, pelvis, and feet.

Etiology

Bones are normally not vulnerable to infection. However, bacteria or fungi can spread to the bone from other areas of the body. They can also enter the bone through openings created by

---

Box 14-11 Wellness Promotion

ENERGY CONSERVATION WITH MYASTHENIA GRAVIS

Patients with myasthenia gravis should follow these measures to enjoy the best quality of life and minimize potential complications:

- Take medication approximately 1 hour before meals.
- Plan important physical activities for early in the day, when energy and strength are greatest.
- Sit upright when eating.
- Pace activities (take your time).
- Plan frequent rest periods.
- Rearrange your home environment for convenience and energy conservation; the main living area, bedroom, and laundry should all be on the same floor.
- Arrange to live where yard maintenance is not needed, or find someone to manage these chores.

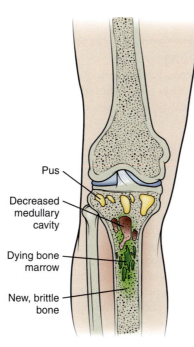

FIGURE 14-26 Osteomyelitis

fracture, punctures, surgery, or other trauma. This is especially true when the injured site is open at the skin, which allows environmental pathogens to enter the wound. Conditions that make people more vulnerable to osteomyelitis include immune suppression, diabetes, some types of anemia, poor circulation, use of illegal injectable drugs, undergoing dialysis, and the presence of central IV catheters and urinary catheters. When infection occurs, the bone deteriorates and an abscess may form. This can impede circulation, which further complicates the situation and may prevent healing. Some infections are resistant to treatment and become chronic.

Flashpoint
Osteomyelitis may be either acute or chronic.

Signs and Symptoms
Signs and symptoms of acute osteomyelitis include redness, heat, edema, fever, and chills. Signs and symptoms of chronic infection include skin ulceration and formation of a sinus tract (abnormal, narrow passage) with drainage. Both forms of infection cause fatigue, malaise, and pain that is sometimes severe.

Diagnosis
Diagnosis of osteomyelitis is based upon the patient's presenting signs and symptoms, examination findings, and test results. A complete blood count (CBC) will reveal increased white blood cells in patients with acute osteomyelitis, while an elevated erythrocyte sedimentation rate is indicative of chronic osteomyelitis. Needle aspiration or biopsy may be done to collect a specimen for microscopic examination as well as culture and sensitivity testing. X-rays, MRI, and CT may also be done to evaluate bone damage.

Treatment
Patients with osteomyelitis are treated with prolonged antibiotic therapy, first intravenously and then orally. Surgery is also often done to remove the damaged and infected tissue, especially with chronic osteomyelitis. Chronic infection that doesn't resolve with these measures may require amputation of the affected body part.

Prognosis
Osteomyelitis was once considered incurable. However, now the prognosis is usually good for those with acute infection if they receive aggressive treatment. Prognosis is more guarded for those with chronic infection, and complications are more likely. Those include septicemia and the need for amputation.

Hallux Valgus

ICD-9-CM: 727.1   [ICD-10: M20.1]

Hallux valgus, also called *bunion*, is a condition in which the big toe is improperly aligned and points laterally toward the second toe. This creates a large bump on the inner edge of the foot at the base of the big toe (see Fig. 14-27).

Incidence

According to the American Orthopaedic Foot and Ankle Society, 88% of American women wear shoes that are too small and 55% of American women have hallux valgus. This strongly suggests a connection between the two and explains why this condition is much more frequent in women than in men.

Etiology

Hallux valgus is caused by a combination of factors. Certain types of foot structure may run in families, making some individuals more prone to the development of hallux valgus. In such people, a malfunction or malformation of tendons, ligaments, and bones within the feet predispose them to this condition. Wearing certain types of shoes, especially high heels with narrow toes, is a significant contributor. Experts disagree, however, whether the shoes actually cause the condition or simply worsen it. Other contributors include arthritis and polio.

Flashpoint

Wearing narrow, pointed high-heeled shoes makes bunions worse.

Signs and Symptoms

Patients with hallux valgus have a reddened, visible deformation (a large bump) on the inner aspect of the base of the great toe. They often report pain with walking, tenderness, burning, or numbness. Calluses may form on the big toe, sores may develop between the toes, and ingrown toenails are more likely.

Diagnosis

Hallux valgus is easily diagnosed based upon appearance. However, a thorough evaluation will include x-rays. Referrals to a podiatrist (specialist in disorders of the feet) and a surgeon may be necessary.

Treatment

Treatment required for hallux valgus depends upon the severity of the deformation and the patient's symptoms. If the condition is mild, conservative measures may be sufficient. These include wearing appropriate shoes that do not aggravate the condition, using padding over the bunion to reduce pain, resting, and modifying physical activities that worsen pain. Discomfort can be further managed with application of cold, use of NSAIDs, or injection of corticosteroids to reduce inflammation. Some patients may benefit from the use of custom-fitted orthotics inserted in the shoes to help realign the foot and toes. Patients with severe

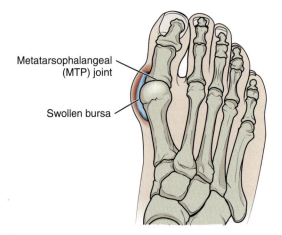

Metatarsophalangeal (MTP) joint

Swollen bursa

FIGURE 14-27 Hallux valgus

conditions may require corrective surgery to realign, shorten, lengthen, or otherwise reposition the first metatarsal bone; reduce bony enlargements; or reposition bones beneath the metatarsal bone.

Prognosis

Prognosis for patients with hallux valgus depends upon the severity of the condition and the timeliness of proper treatment. Potential complications include foot deformity, foot stiffness, and chronic pain. Most people do well after surgery, and healing usually occurs within 6 to 8 weeks. Potential complications include infection, nerve damage, and recurrence.

Hallux Rigidus

ICD-9-CM: 735.2   [ICD-10: M20.2]

Hallux rigidus is a condition in which degenerative arthritis affects the metatarsophalangeal (MTP) joint at the base of the big toe. It leads to pain, stiffness, and difficulty moving the toe.

Flashpoint
Hallux rigidus causes the big toe to become stiff and painful.

Incidence

Hallux rigidus is nearly as common as hallux valgus. It usually, though not always, affects both great toes, and commonly affects both men and women.

Etiology

The exact cause of hallux rigidus is not clear, although there seem to be several potential contributors. Injury to the toe can trigger a degenerative process in the joint. Genetics seems to play a role, since this disorder runs in families. It is thought that individuals in such families have features of the foot anatomy that make the MTP joint less able to withstand the repetitive stress of walking and other activities. Repetitive activities that place stress on the great toe, such as stooping or squatting, can trigger the condition. Other risk factors include rheumatoid arthritis and gout.

Signs and Symptoms

The most common complaints from patients with hallux rigidus are pain and loss of flexibility of the MTP joint. This leads to pain and difficulty walking, running, jumping, or performing any activities that require flexion of this joint. Symptoms are worsened with cold, damp weather. Because the condition is progressive, the patient's history reflects increasing pain and loss of function over time. Eventually the patient also experiences pain at rest and may struggle to find comfortable shoes. The joint may become swollen, and calluses may form because of its changed shape. Eventually the MTP joint may become completely "frozen," or rigid. The patient may also complain of pain in the knees, hips, and lower back as walking patterns change.

Flashpoint
As toe pain causes the patient to walk differently, pain may also develop in the knees, hips, or back.

Diagnosis

Diagnosis of hallux rigidus is suspected based upon the patient's description of symptoms and physical-examination findings. X-rays will reveal degeneration of the MTP joint and may identify bone spurs.

Treatment

Treatment of hallux rigidus usually begins with conservative measures. These include NSAIDs to manage pain and reduce inflammation. Specific types of shoes with stiff or "rocker-bottom" soles may be recommended to reduce the need for toe flexion. In some cases, custom-designed orthotics (shoe inserts) can help. Corticosteroids may be administered to the MTP joint by injection to reduce inflammation. Physical therapy may provide ultrasound or other treatments to reduce pain and improve function.

   Patients with severe conditions may benefit from surgery. Cheilectomy is the removal of bone spurs at the top of the joint. This reduces pain and provides for better flexion. **Arthrodesis** is a surgical procedure to fuse a joint. This eliminates any flexion of the MTP joint, which relieves pain but requires wearing special shoes. Joint-replacement surgery may also be considered. This relieves pain while preserving motion and function; however, the procedure may need to be repeated after several years.

Prognosis

Prognosis for patients with hallux rigidus depends upon the severity of the disorder and the timeliness of treatment. Most people will experience some improvement with conservative measures. However, the condition is often progressive, and those with severe symptoms may eventually need surgery.

Hammertoe, Mallet Toe, and Claw Toe

ICD-9-CM: 735.4 (hammertoe),   [ICD-10: M20.4 (hammertoe), M20.6
735.8 (mallet toe), 735.5 (claw toe)   (mallet toe), M20.5 (claw toe)]

Hammertoe, mallet toe, and claw toe are deformities of a toe (see Fig. 14-28). Hammertoe is a condition in which the toe is bent downward at the proximal interphalangeal joint. Mallet toe is a condition in which the toe is bent downward at the distal interphalangeal joint. Claw toe is similar to hammertoe except that the MTP joint is dorsiflexed (bent upward) while the other joint or joints in the toe are plantar flexed (bent downward). In other respects these conditions are similar.

> **Flashpoint**
>
> Hammertoe and mallet toe are very similar except for the joint involved.

Incidence

As many as 20% of Americans are believed to suffer from toe deformities such as hammertoe, claw toe, and mallet toe. Incidence of these disorders increases with age; they are most common among people in their 70s and 80s.

Etiology

Hammertoe may be congenital and inherited or may develop from wearing poorly fitting shoes that are too tight, too short, too narrow, or too high in the heels. If the toes are pushed against the front of the shoe, an abnormal bend can form. Over time, the tendons may shorten and the condition become permanent. Other possible causes include toe injuries, diabetic neuropathy, and other disorders that cause nerve and muscle damage.

Signs and Symptoms

Signs and symptoms of hammertoe, mallet toe, and claw toe include toe deformities, calluses on the soles, corns on the tops of the toes, and toe and foot pain.

Diagnosis

Hammertoe, mallet toe, and claw toe are diagnosed by physical-examination findings.

Treatment

Conservative treatment for all three types of toe deformity includes wearing appropriately fitting shoes with spacious toe boxes and using orthotics and pads to reposition the toes and relieve pressure. If the toe is still flexible, it can be splinted. Corns and calluses must be treated and the area protected from further aggravation. Surgery may be required for severe conditions. This can involve releasing (cutting) tendons or fusing affected joints.

Prognosis

Prognosis for patients with hammertoe, mallet toe, or claw toe is very good if the condition is treated early. Possible complications include foot deformity and changes to gait and posture because of difficulty walking.

Ganglion Cyst

> **Flashpoint**
>
> Ganglion cyst has sometimes been called a *Bible cyst* because of the old home remedy that involves smashing the cyst with a heavy book.

ICD-9-CM: 731.0   [ICD-10: M67.4]

A ganglion cyst, sometimes called a *Bible cyst*, is one or more small benign tumors that develop over a joint or tendon. They are most frequently located on the wrist or back of the hand (see Fig. 14-29) but may also arise on the shoulders or fingertips, at the base of the fingers, on the lateral aspect of the ankles and knees, and on top of the feet. Within the cyst is a thick, colorless, gelatinous substance which sometimes gives the cyst a spongy texture. This substance is similar to the fluid found within joint capsules.

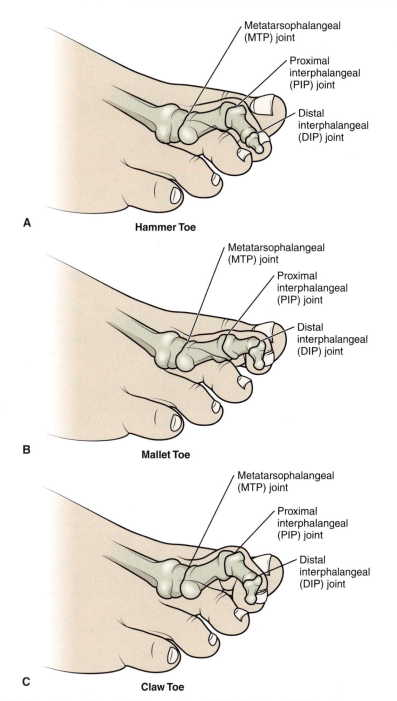

Metatarsophalangeal (MTP) joint

Proximal interphalangeal (PIP) joint

Distal interphalangeal (DIP) joint

A **Hammer Toe**

Metatarsophalangeal (MTP) joint

Proximal interphalangeal (PIP) joint

Distal interphalangeal (DIP) joint

B **Mallet Toe**

Metatarsophalangeal (MTP) joint

Proximal interphalangeal (PIP) joint

Distal interphalangeal (DIP) joint

C **Claw Toe**

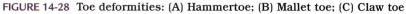

FIGURE 14-28 Toe deformities: (A) Hammertoe; (B) Mallet toe; (C) Claw toe

Incidence

Ganglion cysts are common, usually developing in people ages 15 to 40. They are more common in women than in men.

Etiology

The cause of ganglion cysts is unknown. They may be related to defects in structures such as tendon sheaths or joint capsules that cause joint tissue to bulge out. They may also be related to injury that results in breakdown of joint tissues. Contributing factors are thought to include injury or inflammation, overuse activities, and degeneration related to arthritis.

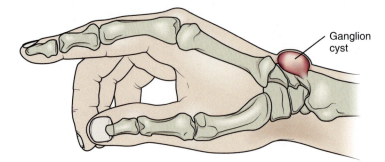

FIGURE 14-29 **Ganglion cyst**

Signs and Symptoms

Ganglion cysts may develop slowly or suddenly; they appear as nonmovable, spongy bumps that may be firm or soft. Sizes vary but usually range between 1 and 3 centimeters. Cysts may be painless or may be tender and cause an aching pain. Because cysts can sometimes exert pressure on nerves, patients occasionally complain of tingling, numbness, or weakness in the affected body part. In some people the cysts may impede joint motion or cause cosmetic concern.

Diagnosis

Diagnosis of a ganglion cyst is usually based upon physical examination. Needle aspiration may be done to remove a fluid specimen for examination. Ultrasound may also be used to determine whether the cyst is filled with fluid or solid material and to identify any vascular involvement. Occasionally, x-ray may be done to rule out other disorders, such as arthritis or tumors.

Treatment

Up to 60% of ganglion cysts will resolve spontaneously and require no treatment. If a cyst is a cause for discomfort or is cosmetically unacceptable, it may be surgically removed. Other treatment may include immobilization by splinting, massage, or aspiration of contents and injection of a steroid medication.

Prognosis

Prognosis for patients with ganglion cyst is excellent. Many cysts disappear without treatment. Recurrence rate is as high as 80%, whether treatment is done or not, but repeated treatment eventually reduces risk of recurrence.

Thoracic Outlet Syndrome

ICD-9-CM: 353.0   [ICD-10: G54.0]

Thoracic outlet syndrome (TOS) is a group of painful disorders involving compression of the nerves or vessels in the neck and arms (see Fig. 14-30).

Incidence

TOS most commonly affects individuals between ages 20 and 50, women more often than men.

Etiology

TOS occurs when the nerves of the brachial plexus or the subclavian artery or vein are compressed between the clavicle and the first rib. The cause of TOS is not always readily apparent. It may be congenital, with the presence of an extra cervical rib above the first rib or a tight band between the spine and rib. It can be caused by poor posture or traumatic injury, as might occur in motor vehicle accidents. It can also develop in people who perform repetitive motions with the upper extremities. Examples include using a computer; lifting weights; swimming; playing volleyball, tennis, or baseball; and playing musical instruments. Frequent carrying of heavy backpacks or bags may also contribute to the disorder.

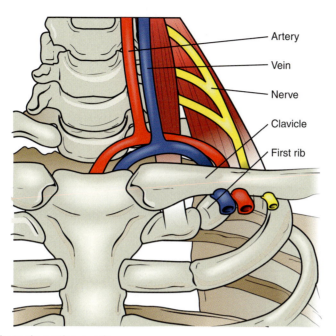

FIGURE 14-30 Thoracic outlet syndrome

Signs and Symptoms

Individuals with TOS often complain of pain or aching in the neck, shoulders, and axillae (armpits); numbness; tingling; or a feeling of heaviness in the fingers, hand, or forearm. Other symptoms may include a weak grip, poor pulses, coolness, and a pale or blue appearance of the involved extremity. Some individuals may experience the formation of a thrombosis (blood clot) in the subclavian vein, a throbbing lump near the clavicle, or tiny dark spots on the fingers.

Diagnosis

Diagnosis of TOS can be challenging, since patients have varying symptoms and the disorder can be confused with a number of others. However, it is generally diagnosed from a combination of the patient's description of signs and symptoms, physical-examination findings, and results of various diagnostic tests. During examination the physician may use one or more provocation tests that indicate the presence of TOS. During these tests, the patient is instructed to move the upper extremities in specific ways. If TOS symptoms are reproduced, a diagnosis of TOS is suspected. Diagnostic tests may include nerve conduction studies, electromyography, x-ray, and MRI.

> **Flashpoint**
> Patients with TOS often complain of neck, shoulder, or arm pain, or feelings of numbness, heaviness, or tingling.

Treatment

Most patients with TOS respond to conservative treatment, which includes physical therapy, relaxation exercises, stretching, massage therapy, application of heat or cold, improvement of posture, and chiropractic or osteopathic treatments. Some patients benefit from NSAIDs or muscle relaxants. Treatment may also be given with corticosteroid injection or the injection of botulinum toxin type A into selected muscles. Up to 15% of patients require surgical decompression of the thoracic outlet. This procedure relieves pressure by removing specific structures, such as certain muscles, the first rib, or fibrous tissue.

Prognosis

The prognosis for patients with TOS is generally good but depends upon the specific type and the severity of symptoms. If treatment does not occur, the individual may eventually suffer permanent nerve damage.

 STOP HERE.
Select the flash cards for this chapter and run through them at least three times before moving on to the next chapter.

Student Resources

About Orthopedics: http://orthopedics.about.com
Arthritis Foundation: http://www.arthritis.org
Back.com: http://www.back.com
National Osteoporosis Foundation: http://www.nof.org
SpineUniverse: http://www.spineuniverse.com

Chapter Activities

Learning Style Study Strategies

Try any or all of the following strategies as you study the content of this chapter:

Visual and kinesthetic learners: With the help of your study group, create fictional characters that each have one of the diseases you must learn about. Create these characters' life stories with careful attention to how their illnesses were diagnosed, the effect their symptoms have on their daily lives, and the type of treatments and coping strategies they use to manage the diseases and improve the quality of their lives. Feel free to make the stories as funny or dramatic as you wish; this will help you to recall the details later.

Auditory and verbal learners: Instruct each member of your study group to write at least 10 "test" questions. Require at least half of them to be multiple-choice questions. Members must bring their lists to your next study session so you can all take turns completing the tests provided by one another. Be sure to provide correct answers with rationales (after the tests are completed).

Practice Exercises

Answers to practice exercises can be found in Appendix D.

Case Studies

CASE STUDY 1

Elvira Jamison is a 47-year-old regular patient at the Family Medical Clinic. She is concerned about the possibility of developing osteoporosis. She is 5 feet 3 inches tall, weighs 108 pounds, and is currently perimenopausal. Her elderly mother has severe osteoporosis with kyphosis and has recently been hospitalized with a pathological hip fracture. Ms. Jamison wants to know what she can do to avoid the same fate. How should the medical assistant answer her questions so that she can understand the answers?

1. What exactly causes osteoporosis?

2. What signs of osteoporosis should I watch out for?

3. Is there some type of test we can do to let me know if I am getting osteoporosis before it gets so bad?

4. What kinds of things should I be doing now to keep from getting osteoporosis later?

CASE STUDY 2

Brian Williams is a 17-year-old high-school student who has been running on his school's cross-country team. He is at the Family Medical Clinic today complaining of severe pain in his shins. The physician has diagnosed Brain with medial tibial syndrome. Brian has some questions about this disorder; how should the health-care provider answer them?

1. I've never heard of medial tibial syndrome before. What is it?

2. What exactly causes this?

3. My mom says I have flat feet. How would that make any difference?

4. What can I do to make this better so I can keep running?

CASE STUDY 3

Wayne Reynolds is a medical assistant at Family Medicine Clinic. It is Saturday, and he is enjoying a day off from work in his backyard when he is approached by his neighbor over the back fence. She is a 44-year-old woman who states that her doctor recently diagnosed her with something called "hallux valgus." She has a few questions for Wayne about this. After tactfully telling his neighbor that he cannot make a diagnosis nor dispense medical advice, Wayne says that he can share some general information about hallux valgus in answer to her questions.

1. There is another name for this foot problem, but I can't remember what it is. Do you know?

2. What makes the big bump on the inside of the foot?

3. My husband said that wearing high heels causes bunions. Is that true?

4. Aren't there some other things that a person can do to help prevent or improve bunions?

Multiple Choice

1. All of the following terms are matched to the correct definition **except:**

   a. Adduction: motion toward the midline of the body

   b. Circumduction: motion of a body part in a circle

   c. Eversion: motion that turns a body part outward

   d. Pronation: movement of the arm so the palm is up

2. Which of the following terms is matched to the correct definition?

   a. Myasthenic crisis: episode of respiratory failure, paralysis, salivation, and sweating that can occur if a patient takes too much anticholinesterase medication

   b. Range of motion: manual manipulation of a bone to return it to its normal position

   c. Rotation: motion that turns a body part about its axis

   d. Extension: motion that bends a body part

3. In which of the following disorders will the patient experience pain?

   a. Remission

   b. Sciatica

   c. Hematopoiesis

   d. Atrophy

4. All of the following are caused by some type of trauma **except:**

   a. Rheumatoid arthritis

   b. Bursitis

   c. Herniated disk

   d. Torn meniscus

5. All of the following disorders involve the feet **except:**

   a. Hallux valgus

   b. Gout

   c. Plantar fasciitis

   d. Kyphosis

Short Answer

1. **Describe the three types of abnormal spinal curvatures.**

2. **Describe at least five key ways in which RA differs from osteoarthritis.**

3. **Complete this table by filling in the similarities and differences between acute and chronic osteomyelitis.**

	Similarities	Differences
Symptoms		
Diagnosis		
Treatment		
Prognosis		

15 SENSORY SYSTEM DISEASES AND DISORDERS

Learning Outcomes

Upon completion of this chapter, the student will be able to:

- Define and spell terms related to the sensory system
- Identify key structures of the eyes, ears, mouth, nose, and throat
- Discuss the functions of the eyes, ears, mouth, nose, and throat

- Identify characteristics of common sensory system diseases and disorders, including:
  - description
  - incidence
  - etiology
  - signs and symptoms
  - diagnosis
  - treatment
  - prognosis

KEY TERMS	
accommodation	ability of the eye to see objects in the distance and then adjust to a close object
acute glaucoma	form of glaucoma in which a sudden blockage of outflow of the aqueous humor causes a rapid increase in intraocular pressure; also called *closed-angle glaucoma*
astigmatism	abnormality of the eye in which the refraction of a ray of light is spread over a diffuse area rather than sharply focused on the retina
central scotoma	blind spot in the center of the visual field surrounded by an area of normal vision
chronic glaucoma	form of glaucoma in which the aqueous humor drains too slowly, leading to gradually increased intraocular pressure; also called *primary open-angle glaucoma*
conductive hearing loss	partial or complete hearing loss caused by factors that interfere with sound transmission from the outer to the inner ear
dynamic equilibrium	sense of balance when in motion
equilibrium	sense of balance
esotropia	form of strabismus in which one or both eyes are turned inward
exotropia	form of strabismus in which one or both eyes are turned outward
gustation	sense of taste
hypertropia	form of strabismus in which one or both eyes are turned upward
hypotropia	form of strabismus in which one or both eyes are turned downward

KEY TERMS—cont'd

legal blindness	vision that is worse than 20/200 in the better eye with correction
mastication	chewing
myringotomy	procedure in which a tiny tube is placed in the tympanic membrane
olfaction	sense of smell
ophthalmoscope	handheld device used to examine the interior of the eye
otoscope	handheld device used to view the outer ear canal and tympanic membrane
sensorineural hearing loss	partial or complete hearing loss caused by degeneration of or damage to the sound pathway from the hair cells of the inner ear to the auditory nerve and brain
static equilibrium	ability to maintain a steady position of the head and body in relation to gravity
tinnitus	ringing or other abnormal sounds in the ears
vertigo	sensation of moving around in space and extreme dizziness

Abbreviations

Table 15-1 lists some of the most common abbreviations related to the sensory system.

TABLE 15-1
ABBREVIATIONS

Abbreviation	Meaning	Abbreviation	Meaning
ARMD	age-related macular degeneration	OM	otitis media
EENT	eyes, ears, nose, and throat	PERRLA	pupils are equal, round, reactive to light and accommodation
ENT	ears, nose, and throat	PND	postnasal drip; postnasal drainage
EOM	extraocular movement	PO, po	by mouth
HEENT	head, eyes, ears, nose, and throat	T&A	tonsillectomy and adenoidectomy
IOP	intraocular pressure	TM	tympanic membrane
LASIK	laser-assisted in situ keratomileusis	TMJ	temporomandibular joint
NPO, npo	nothing by mouth		

Structures and Functions of the Eyes, Ears, Mouth, Nose, and Throat

The organs of the sensory system are the eyes, ears, mouth, nose, and throat. They enable the special senses: vision, hearing, balance, taste, and smell.

Structures of the Eyes, Ears, Mouth, Nose, and Throat

The key structures of the eyes are the sclera, cornea, choroid, and retina. The key structures of the ears are the auricle, tympanic membrane, and cochlea. The mouth and throat are made up of the teeth, gums, tongue, nasopharynx, and oropharynx. The nose comprises the nares and olfactory neurons.

Eyes

> **Flashpoint**
> The layers of the eye are the sclera, choroid, and retina.

The eye is a globe-shaped organ that consists of three layers: the sclera, the outer portion; the choroid, the middle portion; and the retina, the inner portion (see Fig. 15-1).

Sclera and Cornea

The outermost layer of the eye includes the sclera and cornea. The sclera is opaque and has a distinctive white color. At the front of the eye, it bulges forward to become the cornea, which is transparent. A thin mucous membrane called the conjunctiva covers the outer surface of the eye and lines the eyelids.

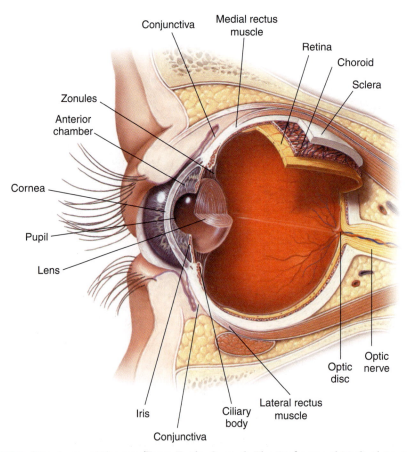

FIGURE 15-1 Structures of the eye (From Eagle, S, et al. *The Professional Medical Assistant: An Integrative Teamwork-Based Approach.* 2009. Philadelphia: F.A. Davis Company, with permission.)

Choroid

The middle layer of the eyeball is the choroid, a dark-blue vascular layer between the sclera and the retina. The optic nerve, also called the *second cranial nerve,* is attached to the retina at one end and the diencephalon of the brain at the other. An opening in the choroid allows the optic nerve to enter the inside of the eyeball. Other structures in the anterior (front) choroid include the iris, ciliary body, lens, and suspensory ligaments. The iris is a colored structure that surrounds the pupil, which is a hole in the iris. The ciliary body is a circular muscle that lies posterior to (behind) the iris. It is attached to a capsular structure that contains the lens (a clear, hard, transparent disk) and suspensory ligaments.

Retina

The innermost layer of the eye is the retina (see Fig. 15-2). The retina is further divided into two layers. The thin outer layer is red due to blood flow from its main central artery. This outer layer lies next to the choroid. The thicker inner layer is the visual portion and contains two types of visual receptors, called rods and cones. Rods and cones are elongated nerve cells that are lined up along the posterior portion of the retina (see Fig. 15-3). They contain photopigments that undergo chemical changes when light strikes them.

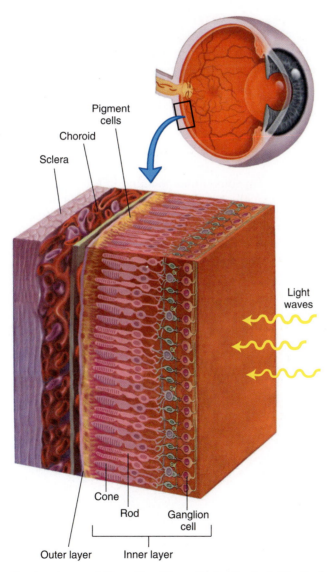

FIGURE 15-2 Microscopic structures of the retina (From Eagle, S, et al. *The Professional Medical Assistant: An Integrative Teamwork-Based Approach.* 2009. Philadelphia: F.A. Davis Company, with permission.)

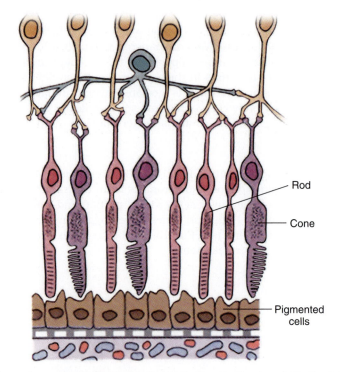

FIGURE 15-3 **Rods and cones** (From Eagle, S, et al. *The Professional Medical Assistant: An Integrative Teamwork-Based Approach.* 2009. Philadelphia: F.A. Davis Company, with permission.)

Other Structures

The eye contains two fluids. The aqueous humor is found in the posterior and anterior chambers. It drains through a small opening called the canal of Schlemm. The posterior chamber contains aqueous humor and a jellylike substance called vitreous humor.

Lacrimal glands are located on the lateral, posterior side of the eye, above the eyelids. The nasolacrimal canal, which drains tears into the nasal cavity, is located at the medial or inner corner of the eye, next to the nose (see Fig. 15-4).

Flashpoint

The terms aqueous and vitreous humor are remnants of an ancient name given to all fluids in the body.

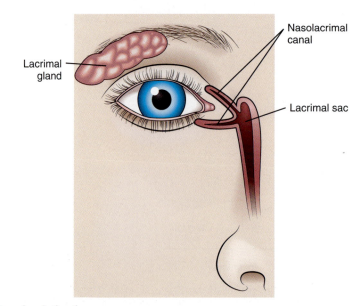

FIGURE 15-4 **Lacrimal glands**

Ears

The ear consists of three major sections: the outer or external ear; the middle ear, which comprises the tympanic membrane and tympanic cavity; and the inner ear or labyrinth (see Fig. 15-5).

External Ear

The external ear consists of the auricle, or *pinna,* which sits visibly outside of the head. It is made up of cartilage covered with skin and is connected to the external auditory canal, a slender tube that leads to the middle ear. The auditory canal is lined with modified sweat glands called *ceruminous glands.*

Middle Ear

At the inner end of the external auditory canal is the tympanic membrane (TM), an irregularly shaped, membranous structure that forms a thin wall between the external and internal ears. It is connected to the first of three tiny ossicles (bones) of the middle ear. These bones are, in order, the malleus (hammer), incus (anvil), and stapes (stirrups). These tiny articulating bones are located in the tympanic cavity.

Inner Ear

The first structure of the inner ear is the cochlea, a snail-shaped structure filled with a fluid called perilymph. The inner surface of the cochlea is lined with a highly sensitive hearing structure called the organ of Corti. The organ of Corti contains nerve endings called hair cells, which are long, hairlike projections. The hair cells transmit impulses to the auditory nerve, located behind the ossicles.

> **Flashpoint**
> The TM acts like a closed window between the external and internal ear.

   The last of the three ossicles, the stapes, fits into an opening on the cochlea called the oval window. In the lower part of the temporal bone is an opening called the round window, covered with a thin membrane. The semicircular canals, located behind the ossicles and two windows, contain perilymph and endolymph, a pale, transparent fluid. Together with the cochlea, these structures make up the vestibular system. Connecting the tympanic cavity and the oropharynx is a structure called the eustachian tube.

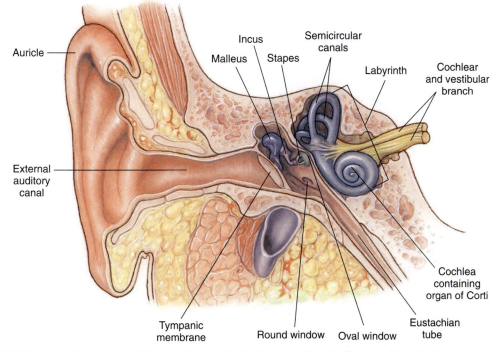

FIGURE 15-5 Structures of the ear (From Eagle, S, et al. *The Professional Medical Assistant: An Integrative Teamwork-Based Approach.* 2009. Philadelphia: F.A. Davis Company, with permission.)

Mouth

The mouth, or *oral cavity,* contains the teeth, gums, and tongue (see Fig. 15-6). The tongue is a muscular organ that lies partly in the floor of the mouth and partly in the pharynx. The surface of the tongue contains papillae (taste buds).

Nose and Throat

The nose is a triangular structure made up of bone and cartilage (see Fig. 15-7). It is covered with skin and lined with a mucous membrane. It contains two openings called nares (nostrils). The nares are separated by a cartilage portion called the nasal septum. Behind and above the nasal cavity are the sinuses, which are hollow, mucus-lined cavities. The sinuses are grouped by their location into the frontal sinuses (above the eyebrows in the frontal bone of the skull), maxillary sinuses (the largest sinuses, located on either side of the nose), sphenoid sinuses (located in the sphenoid bone), and ethmoid sinuses (located between the nose and eyes in the ethmoid bone). Olfactory neurons are located among the epithelial cells of the nasal cavity.

Flashpoint

There are four different sets of sinuses.

The nasal cavity is connected to a muscular tube called the pharynx, or throat. The pharynx is divided into three sections: the nasopharynx, oropharynx, and laryngopharynx. The nasopharynx, the first portion of the pharynx, is a rigid muscular tube that is open to the eustachian tube on either side. The top and sides of the nasopharynx contain the adenoids, also called *pharyngeal tonsils,* which are lymphatic tissues. The nasopharynx continues inferiorly and becomes the oropharynx, which is softer. It begins at the level of the soft palate and ends at the epiglottis. Located on both side of the oropharynx are the palatine tonsils, collections of lymphatic tissue. Inferior to the oropharynx is the laryngopharynx, the lowest portion of the pharynx. It begins at the base of the tongue and is also made up of soft tissue. The inferior end of the laryngopharynx divides into the larynx, which leads to the lungs, and the esophagus, which leads to the stomach.

Functions of the Eyes, Ears, Mouth, Nose, and Throat

The eyes, ears, mouth, nose, and throat serve several important functions in the body. These include providing the special senses of vision, hearing, balance, taste, and smell and protecting against injury.

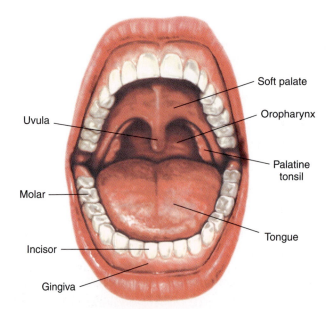

FIGURE 15-6 Structures of the mouth (From Eagle, S, et al. *The Professional Medical Assistant: An Integrative Teamwork-Based Approach.* 2009. Philadelphia: F.A. Davis Company, with permission.)

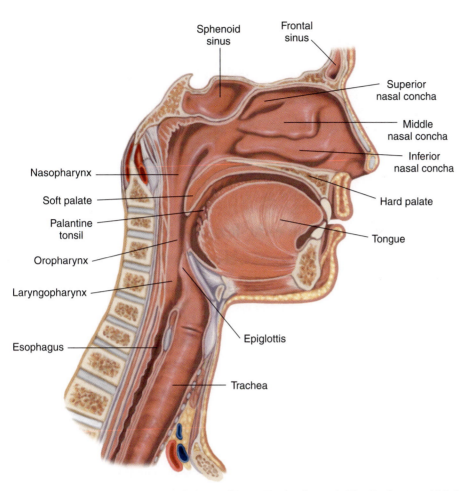

FIGURE 15-7 Structures of the nose and throat (From Eagle, S, et al. *The Professional Medical Assistant: An Integrative Teamwork-Based Approach.* 2009. Philadelphia: F.A. Davis Company, with permission.)

Eyes

The eyes are the sensory organs responsible for sight. Each of the layers of the eye functions to protect the eye, provide vision, or communicate that vision to the brain.

Sclera and Cornea

The sclera, or white of the eye, provides the strength, structure, and shape of the eye. The transparency of the cornea allows light into the eye. The conjunctiva protects the cornea from dust and debris. Blinking, which normally occurs 12 to 20 times per minute, helps to protect the cornea from microscopic injury by keeping foreign debris out and spreading tears across the surface of the eye.

Choroid

In the middle layer of the eyeball, the vascular choroid supplies blood to the entire eye. The colored iris surrounding the pupil expands and contracts to modify the quantity of light entering the pupil. When light is low, the pupil dilates, appearing bigger to allow more light into the eye. In a brightly lit environment the iris expands, causing the pupil to constrict and limiting the amount of light entering the eye. The ciliary body produces aqueous humor and changes the shape of the lens to accommodate near and far vision. For near vision, the ciliary muscles contract, causing increased rounding of the lens; for far vision, the ciliary muscles expand, causing flattening of the lens. This process of adjusting the thickness of the lens to see near and far objects is called *accommodation.* The suspensory ligaments attach the ciliary body to the lens and keep the lens in place.

Flashpoint
The cornea is like a closed, transparent window that lets light into the eye.

Retina

The innermost layer of the eye, the retina, is responsible for the reception of visual impulses through the lens and the transmission of these impulses to the brain. The retina has two layers with individual functions. The thin outer layer contains pigment that protects the choroid and sclera from light at the back of the eye. The thick inner layer of the retina contains rods and cones. Rods detect the presence of light; they function in dim light and produce images that are only in black and white. Cones function in bright light and detect color. A deficiency of cones results in color deficiency, a genetic or acquired inability to distinguish colors. As light waves from the anterior portion of the eye hit the retina, they stimulate the rods and cones. The visual information from the rods and cones is directed to the optic nerve fibers located on the inner surface of the thick inner layer of the retina. The optic nerve fibers transmit visual information via ganglion neurons, which converge at the optic disc. The optic disc contains no rods or cones and is commonly called the *blind spot.* The optic nerve gathers visual stimuli from the ganglion neurons and then transmits the visual information to the brain for interpretation.

Other Structures

Aqueous humor in the anterior chamber provides nourishment for the lens and cornea. Vitreous humor in the posterior chamber gives shape to the eye. The aqueous humor, vitreous humor, and lens are all refractory structures; they bend light rays to focus them sharply onto the retina. Lacrimal glands keep the eye moist by producing tears that bathe and lubricate the eye. If needed, the lacrimal glands produce a larger amount of tears to flush foreign debris from the eyes. The anterior mucous membrane, the conjunctiva, produces clear, watery mucus that allows the eyelid to slide smoothly over the eye when a person blinks.

Flashpoint

Tears are produced to bathe and lubricate the eyes and flush away foreign debris.

Ears

The structures in the three major sections of the ear function together to protect internal structures and provide hearing.

External Ear

The auricle of the external ear collects sound waves traveling through the air and channels them into the external auditory canal. Ceruminous glands that line the canal secrete cerumen, a waxy substance that traps tiny foreign particles and prevents them from entering the deeper structures.

Middle Ear

In the middle ear, the tympanic membrane vibrates when sound waves hit it. Vibration of the tympanic membrane causes movement of the ossicles. Sound, in the form of vibration, is transmitted from the tympanic membrane to the malleus, then the incus, then the stapes, and from there to the cochlea of the inner ear.

Inner Ear

The cochlea receives vibration from the stapes through the oval window. Vibration from the stapes causes a disturbance of the perilymph, which disturbs the hair cells on the organ of Corti. The hair cells transmit impulses to the auditory nerve, where they are interpreted as sound.

Flashpoint

Your ears pop when air moves in or out of your eustachian tubes, equalizing pressure between your middle ear and the external atmosphere.

Because the eustachian tube connects the middle ear to the pharynx, it allows air pressure in the middle ear to equalize with air pressure in the mouth and, therefore, the external atmosphere. This occurs, for example, when individuals drive their car over a mountain and notice their ears "popping" (see Box 15-1).

The inner ear also functions to provide **equilibrium,** which is the sense of balance. **Static equilibrium** is the ability to maintain a steady position of the head and body in relation to gravity; **dynamic equilibrium** refers to the sense of balance when in motion.

The vestibular system controls both forms of equilibrium. Endolymph, the pale, transparent fluid within the labyrinth, responds to changes in body position based on gravity. The vestibulocochlear nerve transmits this information to the brain, and the brain interprets the body's position in space.

Mouth

The mouth contains the teeth, gums, and tongue. The teeth are used for **mastication,** or chewing. The anterior teeth, the incisors, tear food; the posterior teeth, the molars, grind it. The gums anchor the teeth in place. **Gustation,** the sense of taste, is a function of the tongue. The tongue

Box 15-1 Wellness Promotion

RESPONDING TO PRESSURE

When pressure changes suddenly, such as in an airplane, it can be equalized by deliberate swallowing. Many people chew gum because it causes frequent swallowing. Patients who are planning to travel by airplane can be advised to bring chewing gum, especially for children, because the anatomy of the head and eustachian tubes can cause pain when external pressure changes. Babies can be bottle-fed or breastfed on an airplane to equalize pressure and prevent pain in their ears.

contains papillae, or taste buds, which detect the flavors of sweet, salty, sour, and bitter. The muscular nature of the tongue also aids in swallowing food after chewing.

Nose and Throat

Hairs just inside of the nostrils block the entrance of dust and small insects into the nasal cavity. The nasal cavity filters, moistens, and warms inhaled air to prepare it for entrance to the lungs. Olfactory neurons function as receptors for *olfaction* (sense of smell). The sinuses, located behind and around the nose, are normally filled with air; they further warm and humidify inhaled air and provide resonance to the voice. Sinuses are lined with mucous membranes that drain secretions via the nasal passages.

After air is inhaled, filtered, moistened, and warmed, it enters the pharynx. The pharynx serves as a passageway for air, food, and liquids. The adenoids in the nasopharynx and the palatine tonsils produce white blood cells to fight infection in the throat. They sometimes respond to infection by temporarily increasing in size. The lower sections of the pharynx, the oropharynx and the laryngopharynx, are muscular and act to push food down into the esophagus during swallowing.

> **Flashpoint**
> Small hairs in the inside of the nose help to filter inhaled air.

Diseases and Disorders of the Eyes

Many eye diseases and disorders involve the structures at the anterior and posterior portions of the eye globe. Refractive disorders, which affect vision, involve the actual shape of the eye globe. Other eye conditions involve the eyelid.

Keratitis

ICD-9-CM: 370.20   [ICD-10: H16.9] (superficial, unspecified for both codes)
Keratitis is a condition in which the cornea of the eye is inflamed.

Incidence

Keratitis occurs in people of all ages; however, it is most prevalent in those ages 21 to 30, men more than women.

Etiology

Keratitis is commonly caused by fungal or viral infections. Herpes simplex virus type 1 is a common cause. Other causes include disorders that cause decreased tear production, foreign objects in the eye, overuse of contact lenses, vitamin A deficiency, allergic reactions, and injury from sunlight. Those at greatest risk of keratitis include smokers and welders (see Box 15-2).

> **Flashpoint**
> There are many potential causes of keratitis.

Signs and Symptoms

Individuals with keratitis complain of eye pain, blurred vision, and the sensation of something in the eye. They also have redness of the eye and eyelid, increased tearing, and mucopurulent eye drainage.

Box 15-2 Wellness Promotion

BE KIND TO YOUR EYES

Many eye injuries and disorders are preventable. Following these guidelines will help protect your eyes:

- Never look directly at the sun.
- Wear sunglasses with good UVA and UVB protection.
- Use protective eyewear (goggles) when performing any activities that can cause objects or debris to fly into the eyes.
- Flush the eyes immediately with sterile saline or clean water if exposure to foreign objects occurs.
- Avoid touching the eyes with unclean hands and fingers.
- Don't smoke.
- Maintain an optimal weight.
- Eat a healthy diet, including fruit, vegetables, and fish.
- Visit an eye doctor annually for an eye examination and vision screening.
- Don't sleep with daily-wear contact lenses, and don't use extended-wear lenses longer than recommended.
- Don't share eye makeup.
- Buy new eye makeup at least every 6 months.

Diagnosis

Diagnosis of keratitis is based on physical examination and possible vision testing. The pupil is likely to be constricted due to ciliary spasm and iritis. Purulent drainage may be noted.

Treatment

Treatment of keratitis includes antiviral or antibiotic eyedrops or ointment. Contact lenses should not be worn until the condition clears; a temporary eye patch may be recommended.

Prognosis

The prognosis for patients with keratitis is usually good with early intervention but depends upon the underlying cause and the speed with which treatment is initiated. Potential complications include ulceration, scarring, vision loss, and development of glaucoma.

Hypertensive Retinopathy

ICD-9-CM: 362.11   [ICD-10: H35.0]

Hypertensive retinopathy is a condition in which the retina of the eye develops destructive changes from hypertension. The degree of retinal damage is graded on a scale of I to IV, with grade I being the least severe and grade IV the most severe.

Incidence

Typical patients with hypertensive retinopathy are middle-aged or older, and African American more often than Caucasian. The number of individuals with this disorder is unknown. Over 23% of the American population is estimated to have hypertension.

Etiology

Hypertension is generally caused by atherosclerosis and arteriosclerosis, both of which narrow and harden the tiny blood vessels in the eyes. Microscopic infarcts (areas of tissue that die after losing blood supply), superficial hemorrhages, and edema develop. Increased blood pressure also pushes more blood into the vessels of the retina. Increased blood volume and pressure causes leakage of fluid and cellular debris from blood vessels into the retina that then dries, forming deposits on the retina.

Signs and Symptoms

Individuals with hypertensive retinopathy suffer from hypertension, which may run as high as 250/150. However, such individuals may have no eye or vision symptoms.

Diagnosis

Because individuals with hypertensive retinopathy are often symptom free, diagnosis may not occur until they undergo routine vision examination. The condition is also discovered when high blood pressure is noted, which prompts the physician to examine the patient's eyes. The physician may note cotton-wool spots (white or gray opacity in the retina), flame-shaped hemorrhages, hard exudates caused by fatty deposits, AV nicking (caused when an arteriole crosses and compresses a venule), and occasionally retinal or macular edema. In severe cases, a macular star (ring of exudates) and disk edema will also be noted.

Flashpoint

Physicians often examine a patient's eye to look for damaging effects of hypertension.

Treatment

Treatment for hypertensive retinopathy involves treatment of high blood pressure. Regular eye screening is recommended to monitor changes (see Fig. 15-8).

Prognosis

Retinal changes caused by hypertension resolve over a matter of weeks or months if hypertension is brought under control. However, some vision changes may be permanent.

Flashpoint

The best way to treat hypertensive retinopathy is to treat the patient's high blood pressure.

Amblyopia

ICD-9-CM: 368.00   [ICD-10: H53.0] (unspecified for both codes)

Amblyopia, sometimes called *lazy eye*, is a disorder in which the eyes are used unequally by the brain. As a result, the brain disregards images from the weaker eye and relies on those from the stronger eye. Amblyopia may affect both eyes but usually affects just one. The most common types of amblyopia are anisometropic and strabismic.

Incidence

Amblyopia affects up to 5% of the population and is most common in infants and children through age 7. It is the most common vision disorder in young people that affects one eye. Amblyopia is more common in those who were born prematurely or with low birth weight and those with a family history of amblyopia or strabismus.

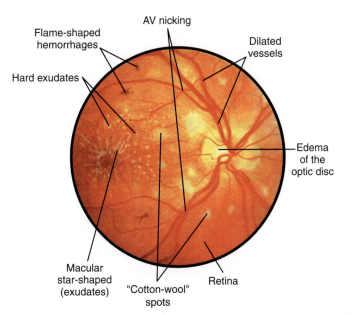

FIGURE 15-8 Retinal changes due to hypertension (From Eagle, S, et al. *The Professional Medical Assistant: An Integrative Teamwork-Based Approach.* 2009. Philadelphia: F.A. Davis Company, with permission.)

Etiology

Amblyopia is really a problem of inadequate development of a part of the brain which corresponds to the visual system, rather than a problem of the eyes, although some eye problems can induce amblyopia. With *strabismic amblyopia* there is a lack of alignment of the eyes; as a result, one eye is used by the brain more than the other. Because the nondominant eye is inadequately stimulated, related parts of the brain do not develop normally. With *anisometropic amblyopia*, the refractive power of the eyes differs. One may be farsighted and the other nearsighted. This discrepancy makes it challenging for the brain to balance the information, so the brain ends up favoring the dominant eye. If both eyes are very farsighted or very nearsighted, amblyopia can develop in both eyes. Less common forms of amblyopia are caused by conditions that prevent light from entering the eye, such as cataracts and cornea defects.

Signs and Symptoms

Many people with amblyopia have no symptoms, although some will complain of headaches related to eyestrain. Some children appear to have one eye that doesn't move with the other one. Others are observed to squint or have an upper eyelid that droops. Those with severe amblyopia may have other visual disturbances, such as poor depth perception or reduced motion sensitivity. In those with strabismic amblyopia, an obvious sign is a crossed eye.

Diagnosis

Diagnosis of amblyopia is made based upon an eye examination. Specific age-appropriate vision tests are used to identify strabismus and unequal vision. Ophthalmic examination is done to evaluate eye structures. An examination technique called photoscreening is sometimes used on small children, in which a video or camera is used to create images of the eyes and their reflexes.

Treatment

Amblyopia is treated by forcing the weaker eye to get stronger. This is done by covering the strong eye with a patch or instilling eyedrops that blur its vision. This forces the brain to rely on the weaker eye. As a result, the eye and the associated part of the brain are strengthened.

Treatment is most effective when initiated before the child's eyes are fully developed, preferably before age 5. However, it is still beneficial for older individuals as well.

Flashpoint

The weak eye may be strengthened by placing a patch over the strong eye.

Prognosis

The prognosis for patients with amblyopia is excellent if the condition is identified and treated early. Individuals treated later in life may experience less improvement but may still benefit from treatment.

Strabismus

ICD-9-CM: 378.00   [ICD-10: H49.9] (unspecified for both codes)

Strabismus, commonly called *crossed eyes,* is a condition in which the eyes are misaligned, adversely affecting depth perception (see Fig. 15-9). Variations include **esotropia** (one or both eyes are turned inward), **exotropia** (one or both eyes are turned outward), **hypertropia** (one or both eyes are turned upward) or **hypotropia** (one or both eyes are turned downward).

Flashpoint

Strabismus is often referred to as *crossed eyes.*

Incidence

Approximately 2% of American children have strabismus; of those, half are born with it.

Etiology

Strabismus is caused by paralysis or unequal functioning of the eye muscles. The resulting lack of coordination prevents the eyes from focusing on the same point.

Signs and Symptoms

Newborn infants have poorly developed vision, which may give the appearance of strabismus. This generally disappears as they grow. However, if it does not disappear, they should be evaluated. If the condition doesn't resolve, they can experience blurred vision.

Diagnosis

The cover test is typically used to check for strabismus. A strabismic eye will fixate on the object being viewed only after the stronger eye is covered. During the Hirschberg test, the

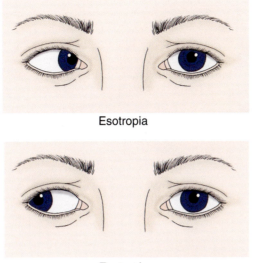

Esotropia

Exotropia

FIGURE 15-9 **Strabismus** (From Eagle, S. *Medical Terminology in a Flash! An Interactive, Flash-Card Approach.* 2006. Philadelphia: F.A. Davis Company, with permission.)

physician shines a light into the patient's eye. When the patient looks at the light, a reflection will be seen on the front of the pupil; if the patient has strabismus, the reflection will be in a different spot on each eye.

Treatment
Strabismus is treated similarly to amblyopia, including the use of eye patches, visual exercises, corrective lenses, eyedrops to aid focus, and surgery to correct the misalignment. In some cases botulinum toxin (Botox) may be used.

Prognosis
Strabismus can lead to the development of amblyopia. The earlier treatment is initiated, the lower the risk that will happen.

Cataracts

ICD-9-CM: 366.10   [ICD-10: H25.9] (senile cataract, unspecified for both codes)
Cataracts are opacities of the lens of the eye that develop as a gradual clouding.

Incidence
Cataracts are the leading cause of blindness in adults worldwide. After age 65, 90% of adults have some cataract formation.

Etiology
Cataracts are caused by gradual clouding of the lens from age-related deterioration (see Fig. 15-10). Other contributors include traumatic injury, drug toxicity, diabetes, and prolonged high-dose corticosteroid therapy.

Signs and Symptoms
As cataracts develop, the pupil takes on a milky, white appearance. Symptoms of cataracts include gradual loss of visual acuity, blurring, loss of acuity at night, sensitivity to light, and a blue or yellow tint to the visual field.

Diagnosis
Diagnosis of cataracts is determined by visual examination and a vision test.

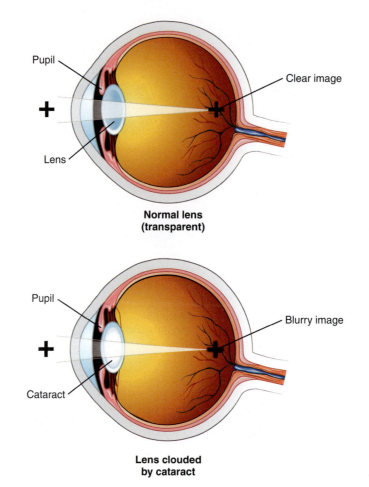

FIGURE 15-10 Cataracts

Treatment

Wearing sunglasses, contact lenses, or glasses can improve vision for patients with cataracts; however, these are not curative measures. The most effective form of treatment is surgical removal of the lens and replacement with an artificial lens.

Prognosis

Cataracts usually worsen with time, resulting in worsening of vision. Surgical lens replacement has a 95% success rate, with recovery in approximately 4 weeks.

Glaucoma

ICD-9-CM: 365.00–365.89   [ICD-10: H40.0–H40.9 (code by type)]
(code by type)

Glaucoma is a group of disorders in which increased intraocular pressure (IOP) results in atrophy of the optic nerve, leading to loss of peripheral vision and eventual blindness (see Fig. 15-11).

Incidence

Flashpoint

Glaucoma is a common cause of blindness worldwide.

Glaucoma is the second-most common cause of blindness in the world, with an estimated incidence of 65 million cases. It affects more than three million Americans; over 100,000 of them are already blind. It affects people in all age groups, although the elderly are at increased risk. African Americans have a much higher incidence of glaucoma than Caucasians.

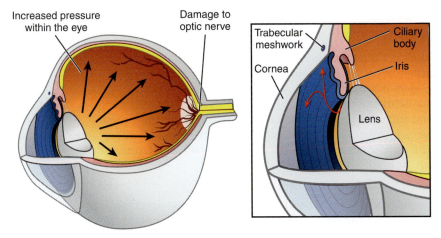

FIGURE 15-11 Glaucoma

Etiology

The actual cause of glaucoma varies with the type. In all types, damage to the optic nerve occurs, usually secondary to abnormally increased IOP. However, there is also a form of glaucoma in which IOP is normal. The cause of this type of glaucoma is not known.

Normally, the aqueous humor is produced and circulates through the anterior chamber of the eye and then drains out through a tiny channel called the canal of Schlemm. In healthy eyes, the continuous production and flow of aqueous humor maintains normal pressure. However, when fluid drainage is impeded, IOP increases and damage occurs to the optic nerve. As a result, blind spots develop in the visual field. In **chronic glaucoma,** also called *primary open-angle glaucoma*, the aqueous humor drains too slowly, leading to gradually increased intraocular pressure. The exact reason this occurs is unclear.

Acute glaucoma, also known as *closed-angle glaucoma*, often has a rapid onset. Its cause is a sudden blockage of outflow of the aqueous humor, which causes a rapid increase in intraocular pressure. This form is usually associated with a canal of Schlemm that has a very narrow drainage angle, which means it is more easily blocked. Risk factors for this type of glaucoma are aging and farsightedness. Triggers for angle closure include anything that causes the pupils to become dilated, such as darkness, stress, certain medications, and excitement.

Signs and Symptoms

Patients with chronic glaucoma are often asymptomatic until significant peripheral vision is lost. Both eyes are affected, although vision loss may initially progress more rapidly in one eye. Acute glaucoma usually develops rapidly; loss of vision may occur within 1 day. Signs and symptoms include severe eye pain, blurred vision, eye redness, light halos, nausea, and vomiting.

Diagnosis

For all types of glaucoma, the eye is carefully examined with an **ophthalmoscope** (handheld device used to examine the interior of the eye) to identify damage to the optic nerve. The optic disk of the eye is where the nerve fibers join at the back of the eyeball. An optic disk damaged by glaucoma takes on an indented appearance; this is called *cupping*. Other signs of damage include changes in disk color and contour. The eye is also evaluated to determine whether the angle of the eye where drainage occurs is open, narrow, or closed. This helps determine diagnosis and appropriate treatment. Diagnostic findings for primary open-angle glaucoma include an open angle, obvious damage to the optic nerve, and loss of peripheral vision evidenced on a visual-field test. During evaluation, a variety of tests may be done. A tonometer is an instrument that measures IOP; a reading of 22 mm Hg or higher indicates a high risk of glaucoma. A perimetry test is done to evaluate the visual field. Pachymetry is a test in which ultrasound waves are used to measure the thickness of the cornea; this is done because thick corneas may lead to high pressure readings and give a false impression of glaucoma. Gonioscopy and tonography may be done to determine how rapidly fluid drains from the eyes.

Treatment

Treatment of glaucoma includes reduction of IOP by reducing the production of aqueous humor or making the outflow of aqueous humor more efficient with miotic eyedrops. Other forms of treatment include systemic medications, laser treatment, and surgery.

Acute glaucoma is an emergency in which blindness can develop rapidly. Therefore, treatment is urgent and includes use of medication to reduce IOP and probable iridotomy. This is a type of laser surgery in which a small hole is created in the iris to allow aqueous humor to flow into the anterior chamber of the eye, where it can then flow out through the canal of Schlemm.

Flashpoint

Acute glaucoma is an emergency because blindness can occur very quickly.

Prognosis

There is no cure for glaucoma, and any vision loss that develops is permanent. Left untreated, glaucoma causes blindness. Even with treatment, approximately 10% of affected individuals still lose their vision. However, the prognosis for those who get early diagnosis and treatment is very good, and further damage can usually be prevented or minimized. Glaucoma is a chronic condition which can change over time; therefore, ongoing management and regular medical checks are important.

Macular Degeneration

ICD-9-CM: 362.50   [ICD-10: H35.3 (unspecified)]

Macular degeneration is also sometimes called *age-related macular degeneration* (ARMD). It is a disorder in which the macula of the retina, located at the back of the eye, deteriorates, resulting in progressive vision loss in the center of the visual field (see Fig. 15-12). It is categorized as either atrophic (dry) or exudative (wet).

Incidence

Macular degeneration is a common cause of blindness among those over age 55. It is much more common among Caucasians than other ethnic groups and is more frequent in women than in men.

Etiology

In atrophic macular degeneration, the macula develops irregular pigmentation, but there is no scarring, hemorrhage, or exudate. In exudative macular degeneration, hemorrhaging or fluid accumulation occurs, causing elevation of part of the macula and eventual scarring. Contributors include inflammation, injury, and infection. Risk factors include advancing age, genetics, obesity, cigarette smoking, cardiovascular disease, high cholesterol, hypertension, nutritional deficiencies, light eye color, and exposure to ultraviolet light.

Signs and Symptoms

Atrophic macular degeneration usually manifests slowly and painlessly. The exudative form progresses more quickly. It causes rapid vision loss, although color and peripheral vision

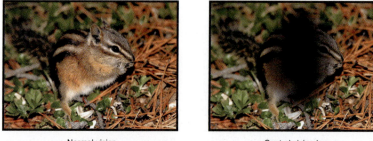

Normal vision   Central vision loss

FIGURE 15-12 Macular degeneration (From Gylys, BA, and Wedding, ME. *Medical Terminology Systems: A Body Systems Approach,* 6th Edition. 2009. Philadelphia: F.A. Davis Company, with permission.)

may remain intact. In either case, vision loss occurs and may develop faster in one eye than the other. Tasks requiring sharp vision become difficult and then impossible. *Legal blindness* may occur, which is defined as vision that is worse than 20/200 in the better eye with correction.

Diagnosis

Diagnosis is established by inspecting the maculae of the retina with an *ophthalmoscope* and noting tiny yellow deposits under the macula, called drusen. Vision testing identifies vision loss. Angiography may be done to evaluate the blood vessels in the eye. The optical coherence tomography test helps identify retinal thinning or thickening, or the abnormal presence of fluid. Through funduscopy, the eye doctor may identify pigment changes and tiny hemorrhages. Other noted changes may include scarring, atrophy, retinal detachment, and lipid (fatty) exudates. An Amsler grid may be used to identify the visual distortion that rapidly occurs in exudative macular degeneration (see Box 15-3). A **central scotoma** (blind spot in the center of the visual field surrounded by an area of normal vision) may be noted in atrophic macular degeneration.

Treatment

There is no cure for macular degeneration. However, vitamin therapy may be beneficial; daily supplements of beta carotene, vitamin E, vitamin C, zinc oxide, and copper are recommended. Individuals should consult with their ophthalmologist regarding specific dosages. Treatment of exudative disease may prevent or delay blindness. In addition to vitamin therapy, laser therapy or phototherapy may be used. Those who have lost central vision may find adaptive devices helpful, including reading glasses, magnifiers, telescopic lenses, and computer monitors for some types of work.

Prognosis

The prognosis for patients with macular degeneration depends upon the type of disease involved. In most cases, mild to moderate vision loss is experienced over time. In some cases blindness occurs, due to complications of retinal detachment or scarring. Ninety percent of these cases involve exudative disease. Atrophic disease causes mild to moderate vision loss but rarely causes blindness.

Box 15-3 Diagnostic Spotlight

AMSLER GRID
The Amsler grid test is a screening test used to evaluate the macula. It is designed with vertical and horizontal lines that create a grid of 5-millimeter boxes. The patient is instructed to hold the grid 30 centimeters away and note whether any of the lines appear distorted or any areas on the grid are missing. A variety of grids may be used; the most common one is shown here.

Amsler grid

Nystagmus

ICD-9-CM: 379.50   [ICD-10: H55] (unspecified for both codes)

Nystagmus is a condition in which the eyes move continually and involuntarily in a rapid, rhythmic, oscillating fashion. Most commonly it causes the eyes to swing from side to side, but some forms cause an up-and-down movement. Various types of nystagmus include congenital (present at birth), manifest (present at all times), latent (present when one eye is covered), manifest-latent (constantly present, but worse when one eye is covered), and acquired (caused by trauma, neurological deficit, or disease).

Flashpoint

Nystagmus is a condition of continual, involuntary, rhythmic eye movement.

Incidence

Congenital nystagmus comprises 80% of all cases and affects one in every several thousand infants born. Therefore, it is estimated to affect approximately 100,000 Americans. It is two times more common in males than in females.

Etiology

Nystagmus is usually present at birth. It is caused by instability of the muscles that control the eyes. It may be inherited or may be associated with another sensory deficit. Acquired nystagmus develops secondary to trauma or disease affecting the nervous system.

Signs and Symptoms

The signs and symptoms of nystagmus worsen with stress and fatigue. They include visual deficits such as blurring, difficulty with depth perception, and difficulty with balance and coordination. In some cases vision is so impaired that individuals are considered legally blind. Their eyes display characteristic rapid back-and-forth, up-and-down, or circular movements. Individuals with nystagmus often display an odd stance, in which their head is tilted or turned at an angle. This is because they find that they are better able to focus by turning their head and locking their eyes into the null point, which is an angle at which the eyes are most stable and vision becomes most clear.

Diagnosis

Congenital nystagmus is often detected at birth or during infancy when the characteristic eye movements are noted. Development during childhood should be carefully evaluated, since progressive vision loss or a pale optic disk indicates acquired, rather than congenital, nystagmus. Furthermore, any patients who develop new-onset nystagmus without a clearly identifiable cause should undergo magnetic resonance imaging (MRI) along with a thorough history and physical examination. A test known as electronystagmography may also be done, which records contractions of the eye muscles to aid in determining the velocity and direction of nystagmus. This information is useful in determining the best treatment.

Treatment

There is no cure for nystagmus, although some types improve during childhood. There are various forms of treatment. Specialty corrective contact lenses generally work better than eyeglasses, since they move with the eye. Surgical procedures help minimize the need for null positioning of the head. Other forms of treatment that are sometimes helpful include biofeedback and injection of botulinum toxin into specific eye muscles, though repeated injections are needed as the effect wears off.

Prognosis

Vision loss associated with congenital nystagmus is usually stable and does not worsen. Other types of nystagmus can be improved through the use of corrective lenses or surgery, so that individuals can lead a productive life.

Flashpoint

Retinal detachment is an emergency because blindness may quickly occur.

Retinal Detachment

ICD-9-CM: 361.00   [ICD-10: H33.0]

Retinal detachment is a disorder in which part or all of the retina separates from the underlying layer of tissue (see Fig. 15-13). It may be localized or may rapidly progress to total detachment, leading to partial or total blindness. It is considered a medical emergency.

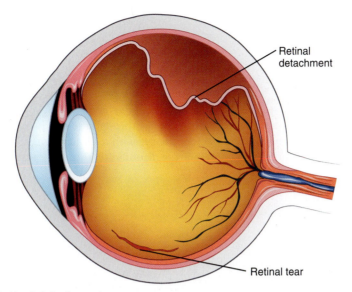

Retinal detachment

Retinal tear

FIGURE 15-13 **Retinal detachment**

Incidence

Approximately 15,000 to 20,000 individuals in the United States experience a detached retina each year. Incidence is greatest among adults ages 20 to 50. Retinal detachment is more common in Caucasians than in other ethnic groups and in men more than women.

Etiology

The retina is a layer of light-sensitive tissue that lines the inside back wall of the eye and sends visual messages to the brain. Occasionally, a tear in the retina develops secondary to eye or head trauma and allows vitreous humor to leak through and collect beneath it. This causes the retina to begin to separate and peel away from the underlying tissue. If a blood vessel is included in the tear, bleeding may occur. As more fluid accumulates, the degree of detachment increases. Risk factors for retinal detachment include the use of pilocarpine (an eyedrop medication for glaucoma), uveitis, myopia, recent cataract surgery, retinopathy, and a family history of retinal detachment.

Signs and Symptoms

Patients with retinal detachment often describe seeing flashing lights and a sudden increase in the number of *floaters* (specks or cobwebs that appear to float in the visual field). Some individuals see a ring of floaters and experience a slight feeling of heaviness in the eye. A shadow in the peripheral vision that progresses across the visual field or toward the center, like a veil or curtain being drawn over the visual field, indicates progression of retinal detachment and must be evaluated immediately.

Diagnosis

Diagnosis is based upon the results of eye examination performed with the eyes dilated. A slit-lamp microscope may be used to aid the doctor in viewing parts of the eye under magnification (see Box 15-4). An Amsler grid test may reveal the appearance of curved lines that should appear straight. A standard test of visual acuity may also be done.

Treatment

Individuals experiencing possible symptoms of retinal detachment should be evaluated by an ophthalmologist immediately, so that diagnosis and treatment can be initiated before the macular area of the retina becomes detached. Several options for treatment exist. Cryotherapy (freezing) and laser photocoagulation create scar tissue around the retinal tear that prevents fluid from flowing through the hole and collecting behind the retina. Scleral buckling is a surgical procedure in which tiny bands of silicone, plastic, or sponge are sewn to the outer surface of the eyeball. They act like a belt and pull the eye wall inward against the hole, thereby compressing it and helping the retina to reattach. Some of the fluid that has collected behind the retina is also drained though a small slit in the sclera. Vitrectomy is a

Flashpoint

Symptoms of retinal detachment include flashing lights, floaters, a feeling of heaviness in the eye, and a curtainlike shadow moving over the visual field.

Box 15-4 Diagnostic Spotlight

SLIT-LAMP MICROSCOPE

The slit-lamp microscope is used to examine the eye. The patient's chin is placed on a chin rest, and the forehead against a support. This stabilizes the patient's head so that it doesn't move. The examiner then uses the slit-lamp microscope to shine a thin sheet of light into the patient's eye and views the structures of the eye through the microscope lens. By examining structures in the front and back of the eye with a slit-lamp microscope, the examiner is able to identify many different eye disorders.

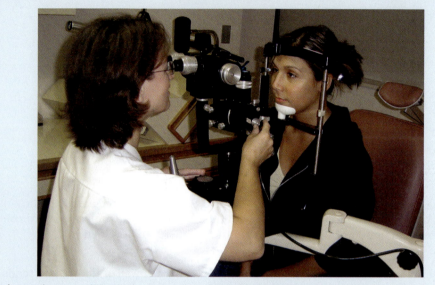

Slit-lamp microscope (From Gylys, BA, and Wedding, ME. *Medical Terminology Systems: A Body Systems Approach,* 6th Edition. 2009. Philadelphia: F.A. Davis Company, with permission.)

procedure in which vitreous humor is removed. It is usually combined with a procedure called pneumatic retinopexy, in which a gas bubble is injected into the eye. Afterward, the patient maintains a specified position (often facing downward) over the next several days or weeks so that the bubble pushes against the retinal tear. The bubble expands initially and then is absorbed over the next several weeks. As this occurs, the eye produces vitreous fluid and refills the posterior chamber.

Prognosis

The prognosis for patients with retinal detachment is very good if treatment is initiated in a timely fashion. Over 90% of reattachments are successful, although a second treatment is needed in some cases. Some permanent changes in vision may occur. Individuals who have experienced retinal detachment have a 9% risk of recurrence.

> **Flashpoint**
>
> The prognosis for patients with retinal detachment is very good if they receive treatment right away.

Uveitis

ICD-9-CM: 364.3   [ICD-10: H20.9] (unspecified for both codes)

Uveitis is inflammation of the inner eye, including the choroid, the ciliary body, where the lens is located, and the iris. It usually affects only one eye. The most common form, called *iritis*, makes up 90% of cases.

Incidence

Estimates regarding the incidence of uveitis are quite variable, with some sources indicating that over two million people in the United States may suffer from it annually. Although it strikes individuals of all ages, the average patient is between 40 and 50 years old.

Etiology

The exact cause of uveitis is not known. It has been associated with bacterial, viral, and parasitic infections. It has also been associated with autoimmune responses, psoriasis, ankylosing spondylitis, inflammatory bowel disease, certain types of arthritis, sarcoidosis, and other disorders.

Signs and Symptoms

Signs and symptoms of uveitis include eye pain, sensitivity to light, redness, blurred vision, floaters, and itching.

Diagnosis

Diagnosis is based upon the patient's description of signs and symptoms in addition to a slit-lamp ophthalmic examination. Laboratory tests associated with related disorders may be done as well; examples include tests for syphilis, tuberculosis, Lyme disease, juvenile arthritis, and sarcoidosis.

Treatment

Treatment for uveitis is tailored specifically to the underlying cause. In most cases, topical or systemic corticosteroids and other agents are used to relieve pain and photophobia.

Prognosis

The prognosis for uveitis is variable depending upon the underlying cause and the timeliness of diagnosis and treatment.

Disorders of Refraction

ICD-9-CM: 367.1 (myopia), 367.0 (hyperopia), 367.4 (presbyopia), 367.20 (astigmatism)	[ICD-10: H52.1 (myopia), H52.0 (hyperopia), H52.4 (presbyopia), H52.2 (astigmatism)]

Refractive disorders are very common. They involve abnormalities in the shape of the eye globe, cornea, or lens surface. Common types of refractive disorders are myopia, hyperopia, presbyopia, and astigmatism (see Fig. 15-14).

Myopia, commonly called *nearsightedness*, is an error of refraction caused by a misshapen eyeball. Hyperopia is the condition commonly called *farsightedness*. Presbyopia is the loss of visual acuity with advancing age. **Astigmatism** is an abnormality of the eye in which the diffraction of a ray of light is spread over a diffuse area rather than sharply focused on the retina. This causes the light coming into the eye to be focused on more than one point on the retina. The patient may see more than one image or a blurred image.

> **Flashpoint**
>
> Hyper- means *excessive or far*. Therefore, hyperopia means farsightedness.

Incidence

Myopia is estimated to affect 70 to 80 million Americans, men and women equally. Hyperopia affects approximately 25% of the U.S. population. Incidence increases with age; about half of all people over age 65 have it. It affects men and women equally. Presbyopia is estimated to affect nearly 25 million Americans. Astigmatism affects an estimated 45 million Americans.

Etiology

Errors of refraction other than presbyopia are thought to be largely genetic, since most people are born with them. There are other contributors for each of the errors, though.

In myopia, the eyeball is more elongated than normal or the cornea has an excessive curvature, which causes light rays to focus in front of the retina. Risk factors may include visual stress from excessive close work and other health conditions, such as diabetes. In hyperopia: the eyeball is shorter than normal or the lens is not rounded enough, causing parallel light rays to come into focus behind the retina.

Presbyopia is changes in the accommodation ability of the crystalline lens from aging, retinal damage, cornea changes, or reduced pupil size.

In astigmatism, the cornea of lens has one or more defective curvatures. The exact cause of astigmatism is unknown, but it often occurs along with farsightedness or nearsightedness.

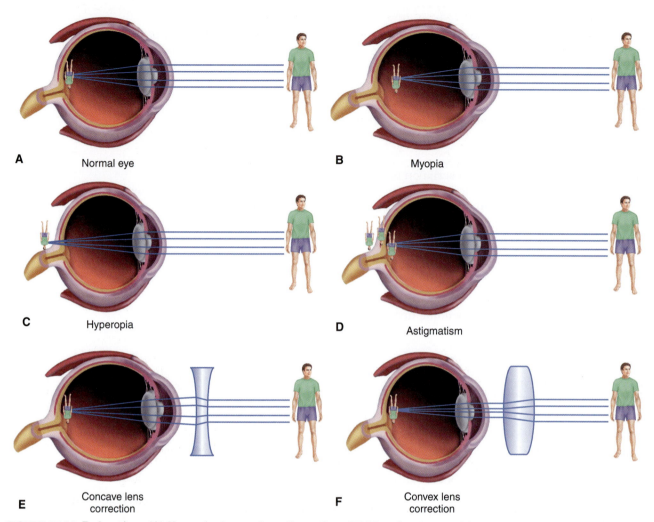

A Normal eye **B** Myopia

C Hyperopia **D** Astigmatism

E Concave lens correction **F** Convex lens correction

FIGURE 15-14 Refraction: (A) Normal—focused on the retina; (B) Myopia—focused in front of the retina; (C) Hyperopia—focused behind the retina; (D) Astigmatism—multiple images on the retina; (E) Correction by a concave lens for myopia; (F) Correction by a convex lens for hyperopia (From Eagle, S, et al. *The Professional Medical Assistant: An Integrative Teamwork-Based Approach.* 2009. Philadelphia: F.A. Davis Company, with permission.)

Signs and Symptoms

Many signs and symptoms are the same for all types of refractive disorders. These include poor vision, headaches, eyestrain, fatigue, and burning. There are also some signs and symptoms specific to each type of refractive disorder:

- Myopia: blurred vision and squinting when looking at distant objects
- Hyperopia: difficulty focusing on nearby objects
- Presbyopia: increasing difficulty focusing on nearby objects or reading material with advancing age; dry, irritated eyes; sensitivity to light; decreased visual acuity in the dark; reduced ability to discriminate between greens, blues, and pastel colors
- Astigmatism: difficulty focusing on fine detail near or far

Diagnosis

Myopia, hyperopia, and presbyopia are diagnosed with a standard eye examination. This generally includes an ophthalmic examination, testing of visual acuity, and refractive testing. Snellen and Jaeger charts are commonly used (see Box 15-5). Other tests may include slit-lamp testing and evaluation of color vision.

Astigmatism is diagnosed by an ophthalmic examination including retinoscopy (visual examination of the retina), corneal topography (imaging technique for mapping the surface curvature

Flashpoint

All types of refractive disorders cause headaches, poor vision, eyestrain, fatigue, and burning.

of the cornea), and keratometry (measurement of the curvature of the anterior surface of the cornea), or by the use of an astigmatometer (device that measures the degree of astigmatism).

Treatment

Myopia may be corrected with the use of a negative, or concave, lens of the proper strength to counter the effects of the defect and sharpen focus at far distances. Hyperopia may be corrected with the use of a positive, or convex, lens. Astigmatism may be corrected with glasses or hard contact lenses. Presbyopia is corrected with contact lenses, reading glasses, or bifocal lenses.

A variety of procedures may also be useful in correcting refractive disorders. Orthokeratology is a nonsurgical procedure in which the patient wears a series of rigid contact lenses that slowly change the shape of the cornea. Astigmatic keratotomy and laser-assisted in situ keratomileusis

Box 15-5 Diagnostic Spotlight

EYE-EXAMINATION CHARTS

The Snellen chart comes in three variations: one using letters, one using objects, and one using the letter E rotated in various positions.

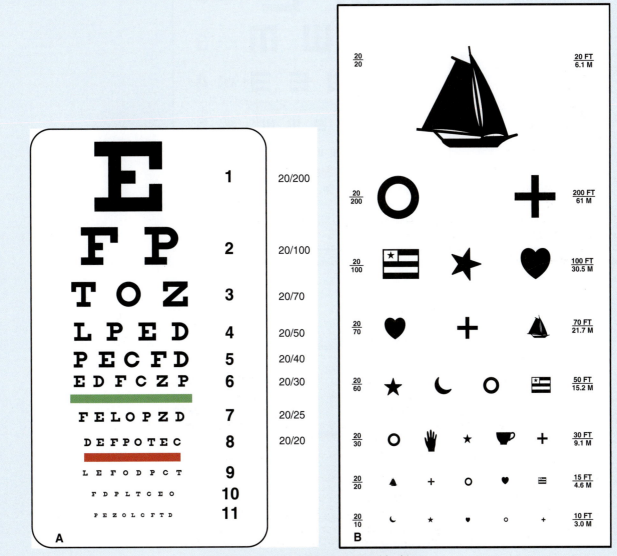

Snellen charts: (A) With letters; (B) With objects;

Continued

Box 15-5 Diagnostic Spotlight—cont'd

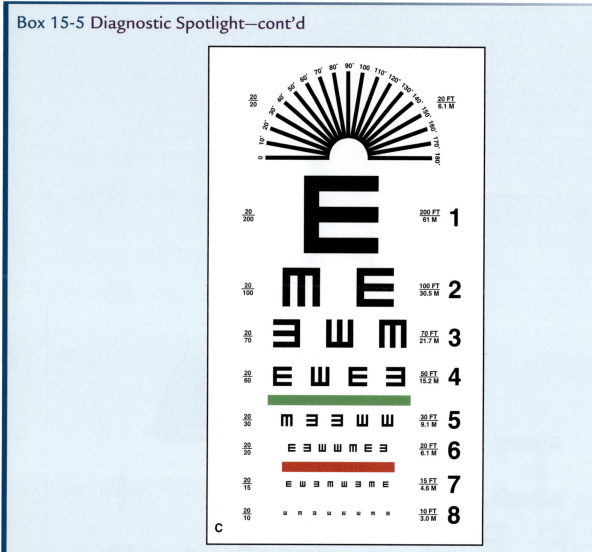

(C) With rotating E (From Eagle, S, et al. *The Professional Medical Assistant: An Integrative Teamwork-Based Approach.* 2009. Philadelphia: F.A. Davis Company, with permission.)

The Jaeger chart is for evaluating close vision.

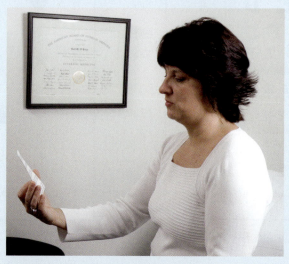

Ask the patient to hold the Jaeger card 30 centimeters away from the eyes (From Eagle, S, et al. *The Professional Medical Assistant: An Integrative Teamwork-Based Approach.* 2009. Philadelphia: F.A. Davis Company, with permission.)

Box 15-5 Diagnostic Spotlight—cont'd

The Ishihara test is used to evaluate color vision.

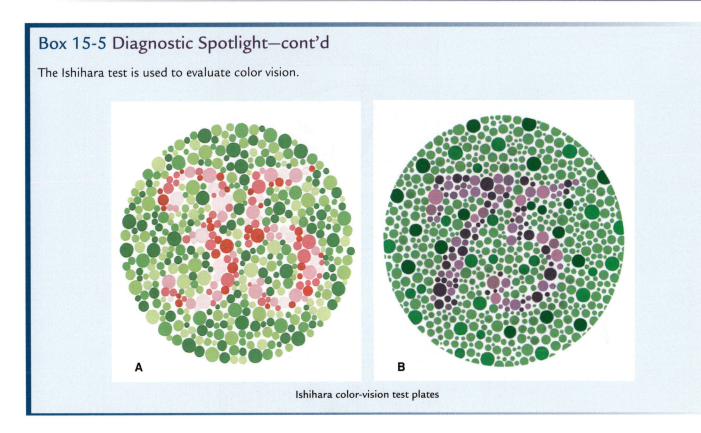

A   B

Ishihara color-vision test plates

are surgical procedures that correct the shape of the lens. A phakic intraocular lens implant involves the implantation of a small lens next to, or in place of, the patient's native lens.

Prognosis

The prognosis for patients with refractive disorders is very good if they receive appropriate treatment. Rare complications of myopia are retinal detachment and retinal degeneration.

Disorders of the Eyelid

There are numerous diseases and disorders that affect the eyelids, including chalazion, hordeolum, blepharitis, entropion, ectropion, and conjunctivitis.

Chalazion and Hordeolum

ICD-9-CM: 373.2 (chalazion), 373.00 (hordeolum, unspecified), 373.11 (hordeolum externum), 373.12 (hordeolum internum), 373.13 (abscess of the eyelid)

[ICD-10: H00.1 (chalazion), H00.0 (hordeolum)]

Because of their similarities, chalazion and hordeolum are discussed together. A hordeolum, commonly called a stye, is an infection of a sebaceous gland at the base of an eyelash. A chalazion, also called a *meibomian-gland lipogranuloma*, is a small cyst in the eyelid (see Fig. 15-15). It differs from a hordeolum in that it is usually larger and less painful. Over time it develops into a small, nontender nodule in the center of the eyelid. In contrast, a hordeolum localizes to the edge of the eyelid and remains painful (see Fig. 15-16).

Incidence

Chalazion and hordeolum are both extremely common lesions. They affect individuals of all ages in all ethnic groups.

Flashpoint

Chalazion and hordeolum are similar. One is an infected sebaceous gland near an eyelash, and the other is a small nodule in the middle of the eyelid.

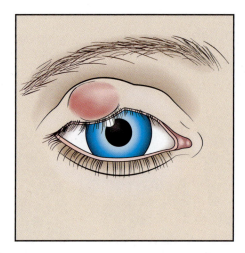

FIGURE 15-15 Chalazion

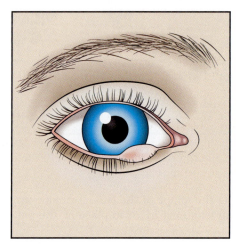

FIGURE 15-16 Hordeolum

Etiology

Hordeola are caused by bacterial infection, usually *Staphylococcus aureus*, and may also be caused by blepharitis. Risk factors include stress and poor nutrition. A chalazion is usually located on the upper eyelid and is caused by a blocked meibomian gland that then becomes inflamed.

Signs and Symptoms

Signs and symptoms of chalazion and hordeolum are quite similar, and initially the two conditions may be impossible to distinguish from one another. Both include redness, edema, and tenderness of the eyelid along with sensitivity to light and increased tear production.

Diagnosis

Diagnosis of chalazion and hordeolum is based upon a physical examination and the patient's description of signs and symptoms.

Treatment

Treatment of chalazion and hordeolum is similar and includes application of warm compresses and antimicrobial eyedrops or ointment. A chalazion may also be injected with corticosteroids. In some cases a surgical procedure may be done to remove a chalazion or drain a hordeolum.

Prognosis

Prognosis for both types of lesions is very good; both are likely to disappear on their own, with conservative treatment. A recurring chalazion in the same area may need to be biopsied to rule out sebaceous cell carcinoma.

Blepharitis
ICD-9-CM: 373.00   [ICD-10: H01.9] (unspecified for both codes)

Blepharitis is a noncontagious inflammation of the eyelash follicles and tiny oil glands along the margins of the eyelids. Anterior blepharitis develops at the outer, front edge of the eyelid, where the eyelashes are located. Posterior blepharitis develops along the inner surface of the eyelid, where it touches the eyeball.

Incidence

The exact incidence of blepharitis is unclear. However, it is known to be very common and affect individuals of all ages.

Etiology

The most common cause of blepharitis is bacterial infection secondary to excessive oil production in the glands along the eyelid, which creates an environment conducive to bacterial growth. Other causes include allergies and pediculosis (lice infestation).

Signs and Symptoms

Symptoms of blepharitis include itching, burning, gritty sensation, red-rimmed eyelids, greasy scales, photophobia, loss of eyelashes, and sticky, crusted eyelids (see Fig. 15-17). Eyelids may also be swollen or ulcerated on the margins, and in the case of pediculosis, lice eggs may be present on the eyelashes.

> **Flashpoint**
> Blepharitis causes itching, burning, a gritty sensation, sensitivity to light, and sticky, crusted eyelids.

Diagnosis

Diagnosis of blepharitis is usually made based upon visual inspection under a magnifying lens. A sample of skin cells and exudate (fluid containing protein, cells, or debris) may be examined for the presence of bacteria.

Treatment

Treatment includes daily cleansing of the eyelids to remove skin oils and bacteria and application of warm saline compresses. Medications include antibiotic eyedrops or ointment and possibly steroids. Artificial tears may be used to treat dryness. Petroleum jelly may be applied along the base of the eyelashes to remove lice, if necessary.

Prognosis

Prognosis is good with appropriate treatment, although blepharitis is often a chronic or recurring condition. Possible complications include the development of hordeolum, chalazion, corneal ulceration, conjunctivitis, scarring of the eyelids, and loss of the eyelashes.

Entropion and Ectropion
ICD-9-CM: 374.00 (entropion),   [ICD-10: H02.0 (entropion), H02.1
374.10 (ectropion)   (ectropion)]

Entropion is a condition in which the edges of the eyelid are turned inward and rub the surface of the eye. It usually affects the lower eyelid (see Fig. 15-18). Ectropion is a condition in which the lower eyelid is turned outward and droops more with aging.

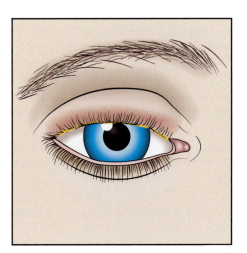

FIGURE 15-17 Blepharitis

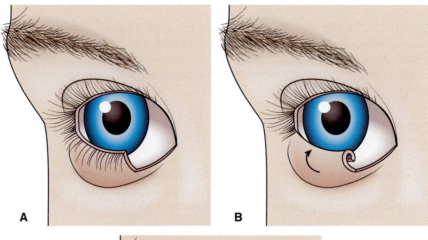

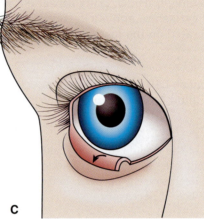

FIGURE 15-18 Eyelids: (A) Normal; (B) Entropion; (C) Ectropion

Incidence

Entropion and ectropion affect patients of all ages but are most commonly seen in older adults. Entropion is more common in women.

Etiology

Both disorders may be congenital and may also be caused by aging and scarring. Other contributors include allergies, palsy of the facial nerves, and skin disorders.

Signs and Symptoms

Symptoms of entropion and ectropion are similar and include redness, pain, sensitivity to wind and light, excessive tearing, and sagging of the eyelids. Ectropion is more likely to cause dryness than entropion is.

Diagnosis

Diagnosis of entropion and ectropion is based upon physical examination and the patient's description of symptoms. A slit lamp may also be used for eye examination.

Treatment

Treatment for entropion and ectropion involves surgical removal of excess skin to relieve symptoms and improve the field of vision. Artificial tears may be used to ease dryness and irritation.

Prognosis

The prognosis for both disorders is good if treatment is initiated before permanent damage occurs.

Conjunctivitis

ICD-9-CM: 372.00 (acute), 372.10 (chronic)   **[ICD-10: H10.3 (acute, unspecified), H10.4 (chronic, unspecified)]**

Conjunctivitis, commonly called *pinkeye,* is an inflammation or infection of the conjunctiva, which is the transparent membrane that lines the eyelid and part of the eyeball. As a result of the inflammation, the normally white surface of the eye takes on a reddened, bloodshot appearance (see Fig. 15-19).

Incidence

Conjunctivitis is very common, with increased incidence in early spring and late fall. It is estimated to be responsible for 30% of all eye complaints. Conjunctivitis is common in all age groups but is most prevalent in children. Approximately 4% of schoolchildren and 6% of high schoolers see a physician for conjunctivitis each year.

Etiology

Conjunctivitis is usually caused by allergic reactions or infection with a variety of bacteria or viruses. Other causes include the presence of a foreign object in the eye and the splashing of an irritating substance into the eye. Newborn babies are susceptible to bacteria normally present in the mother's birth canal. They also sometimes have tear ducts that are not fully open. These two factors make them vulnerable to eye infection. The name *pinkeye* comes from the pink or red appearance of the conjunctiva as inflammation causes small blood vessels to become more prominent.

Signs and Symptoms

Usual signs and symptoms of conjunctivitis include eyes that are reddened, swollen, teary, sensitive to light, and itchy, with a gritty feeling. Individuals with allergic conjunctivitis may also sneeze and produce a watery nasal discharge. Bacterial or viral conjunctivitis may affect only one eye; however, since it is spread easily, both eyes often become involved. The discharge may change from clear to a thicker yellow or green color. This is especially true of bacterial conjunctivitis, which produces a purulent (pus-containing) discharge that causes the eyelids to become matted and stuck together after sleeping. Conjunctivitis caused by a foreign object or chemical splash may be quite painful and may produce a mucuslike discharge.

Diagnosis

Diagnosis of conjunctivitis is usually made by visual inspection; testing is usually not necessary. However, the Schirmer test may be done in some cases to helps diagnose dry eye. In this test, the moisture from each eye is collected on a filter paper for 5 minutes. Visual deficits not caused by the presence of mucus should be investigated. A purulent discharge suggests a bacterial

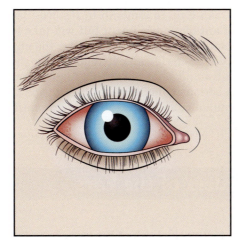

FIGURE 15-19 **Conjunctivitis**

Box 15-6 Wellness Promotion

STOP THE SPREAD

When being treated for bacterial conjunctivitis, patients must be told how to keep from spreading the infection to their other eye or to other people. Following these guidelines will help:

- When using eye ointment or drops, be careful not to touch the tip of the container to the infected eye.
- Wash hands frequently, especially before and after touching the eyes.
- Cleanse the eyes with a clean washcloth moistened with warm (not hot) water; use a separate cloth for each eye.
- Avoid touching the infected eye.
- Avoid sharing items that come into contact with the face, such as towels, face cloths, pillowcases, eye makeup, eye medications, and sunglasses.
- Keep a child with conjunctivitis out of school or day care until treatment has been ongoing for 24 hours.

cause; swabbing may be done for culturing to identify the causative organism, but low-grade infections often test negative.

Treatment

Treatment of conjunctivitis varies with the cause. Symptoms of allergic and viral conjunctivitis respond to application of cool, moist compresses and artificial tears. Severe cases may be treated with anti-inflammatory medications, antihistamines, decongestants, mast-cell stabilizers, and topical-steroid eyedrops. Conjunctivitis that is thought to have a bacterial cause is treated with broad-spectrum antibiotic eyedrops or ointments. Some forms are highly contagious through direct contact with infected eye secretions. Therefore, patients are instructed in ways to avoid spreading the infection (see Box 15-6).

Flashpoint

Some forms of conjunctivitis are very contagious.

If a chemical splash is the cause, the eyes must be immediately and thoroughly irrigated with sterile saline, or water if saline is not available. Depending upon the type of chemical and the severity of the burn, treatment may include the use of topical steroids and referral to an ophthalmologist for further care.

Prognosis

Most individuals with conjunctivitis recover fully, although some forms of the disorder may last for months, especially if not treated. Viral conjunctivitis may worsen in the first 5 days and then gradually clear, taking up to a month to resolve. Bacterial cases should begin to improve within 2 days of antibiotic treatment but will take longer to fully resolve. It is important that individuals continue using medication for the entire time indicated, to prevent recurrence. In rare cases, bacteria can cause infants to develop a serious form of conjunctivitis known as *ophthalmia neonatorum*, which requires immediate treatment to preserve sight. To prevent this serious complication, most hospital policies require the administration of a preventive antibiotic, such as erythromycin ointment, to the eyes of every newborn.

Diseases and Disorders of the Ears

Many diseases and disorders involve the structures of the ears. Disorders involving the outer ear include otitis externa and foreign bodies. Disorders of the middle ear include otitis media, hearing loss, otosclerosis, and cholesteatoma. Disorders of the inner ear include labyrinthitis and Ménière disease.

Otitis Externa

ICD-9-CM: 380.10   [ICD-10: H60.3]

Otitis externa, also called *swimmer's ear,* is inflammation or infection of the external auditory canal (see Fig. 15-20). It may be an acute infection of short duration or a chronic infection, defined as one lasting for more than 4 weeks or recurrence of more than four episodes in a year.

Incidence

An estimated 300,000 individuals in the United States are affected by otitis externa each year. Those most commonly affected are children between ages 7 and 12.

Etiology

Otitis externa develops when excessive moisture is retained in the ears, often after swimming. This creates a hospitable environment for the growth of microorganisms, such as *pseudomonads, staphylococci, streptococci,* and some types of fungi. Other contributors include dermatitis, allergies, and trauma.

Signs and Symptoms

Patients with otitis externa usually complain of ear pain, decreased hearing, itching, and a feeling of pressure. There may also be purulent discharge coming from the ear canal.

Diagnosis

Diagnosis is usually based upon a combination of data. These include the patient's description of symptoms, recent history of being in the water, and physical-examination findings. The physician examines the patient's ears with an **otoscope,** a handheld device used to view the outer ear canal and tympanic membrane (see Box 15-7). Examination of the ear canal reveals a reddened, inflamed, tender outer ear as well as narrowing of the ear canal due to swelling. Moist debris and fungal growth may be seen within the canal. Ear-canal discharge may be stained and cultured to confirm a fungal cause. Rarely, computed tomography (CT) may be used when bone involvement is suspected.

Treatment

The health-care provider may gently cleanse the ear canal with a small suction catheter or plastic curette. If the tympanic membrane is intact, the ear canal may be irrigated with a mix of water and peroxide. Antibiotic eardrops are usually administered, often with wick placement to facilitate delivery. Acetic acid solution or a topical antifungal may be used to treat fungal infections. Analgesics may be needed to relieve pain, and topical steroid drops may be applied to decrease inflammation. Antipruritics and antihistamines may be used to relieve itching.

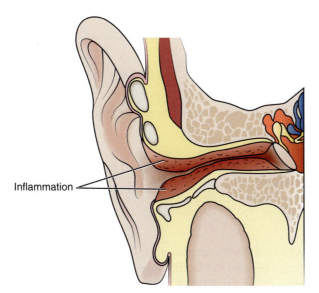

Inflammation

FIGURE 15-20 Otitis externa

Box 15-7 Diagnostic Spotlight

OTOSCOPY

Otoscopy is a procedure in which an examiner uses a handheld device called an otoscope to look into a patient's ears and view the outer ear canal and the tympanic membrane (TM). The otoscope includes a magnifying lens and a light to help illuminate structures of the ear. It also allows for the attachment of a small tube with an air bulb. This lets the examiner send a small puff of air toward the TM to test it for movement. The portion of the otoscope inserted into the ear canal is the speculum. Specula come in a variety of sizes for different-size patients. By examining the patient's ears, the examiner can identify infections of the outer and middle ear and numerous other disorders.

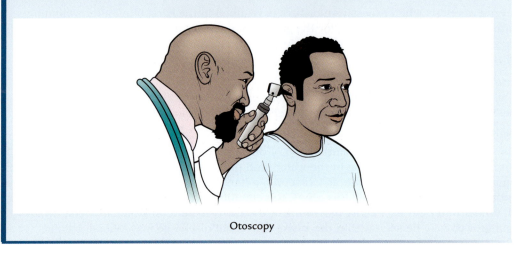

Otoscopy

Prognosis

Prognosis for individuals with otitis externa is generally very good. More than 90% of cases resolve with proper treatment. Individuals who have diabetes or weak immune systems are at risk of complicated infections involving deeper structures of the ear and surrounding bones. Such complications include cellulitis and osteomyelitis, both of which are serious disorders with mortality rates as high as 50%.

Foreign Bodies

ICD-9-CM: 931   **[ICD-10: T16]**

Foreign bodies in the ears and nose are typically placed there by bored or curious children.

Incidence

> Flashpoint
>
> Patients with foreign bodies in the ears and nose are usually children.

Incidences of foreign bodies in the ears and nose are common, especially among children under 5 years of age.

Etiology

Foreign bodies in the ears and nose are often placed there by curious or bored children in an attempt to entertain themselves or explore their bodies. The children may also be attempting to imitate others. Objects vary and include food, beans, seeds, buttons, crayons, small toys, and beads.

Signs and Symptoms

Individuals with foreign objects in the ears or nose may be asymptomatic. However, inflammation and infection may develop. This can cause irritation, redness, purulent or bloody drainage, and foul odor. Impaired hearing may also occur if the ear canal becomes blocked or an infection develops.

Diagnosis

Diagnosis of a foreign body is based upon a description of events from the patient or care provider, along with physical-examination findings.

Treatment

Treatment involves the prompt removal of the foreign object by a qualified health-care provider. Antibiotic drops may be prescribed for the ears if infection is present.

Prognosis

Prognosis for children with foreign bodies in their ears or nose is very good if appropriate treatment is initiated.

Otitis Media

ICD-9-CM: 381.0 (acute nonsuppurative), 382.0 (acute suppurative)	[ICD-10: H65.1 (acute nonsuppurative), H65.0 (acute suppurative)]

Otitis media is inflammation or infection of the middle ear (see Fig. 15-21). It is the most common cause of earache, is commonly associated with respiratory infections, and is responsible for a large number of health-care visits. In isolated cases it is called *acute otitis media (AOM)*. Repeated cases of three or more infections within a 6-month period are called *recurrent otitis media*. Infections that persist for weeks are called *chronic otitis media*.

Incidence

Ear infections are responsible for 30 million doctor visits annually and cost approximately $3 billion a year to treat. Most commonly affected are small children between the ages of 6 months and 3 years. Members of the American Indian and Inuit ethnic groups are affected more than others. Males are affected more than females. Children with cleft palate have an especially high risk. Overall incidence is highest during the autumn and winter.

Etiology

Otitis media is usually preceded by some type of upper respiratory infection (URI). The inflammation and increase in secretions within the middle ear create an environment conducive to bacterial growth. Organisms most commonly involved are *Haemophilus influenzae, Streptococcus pneumoniae, Moraxella* species, and *mycoplasmas*. Small children are most commonly affected because the tiny eustachian tubes that connect the middle ear and the throat are positioned horizontally during early growth and development. Usually, excess fluid can escape through the eustachian tube; however, during a URI the eustachian tube may become swollen, impairing its effectiveness. Risk factors for otitis media include immune suppression, chronic respiratory disease such as asthma and allergies, bottle feeding, pacifier use, prematurity, genetics, gastroesophageal reflux disease, and the presence of adenoids. Environmental risk factors include day-care attendance and secondhand smoke.

Signs and Symptoms

Some individuals with otitis media are symptom free. Individuals most likely to suffer from otitis media are those least able to communicate their symptoms, since most have not yet mastered

Flashpoint
Otitis media, infection of the middle ear, is the most common cause of earache in children.

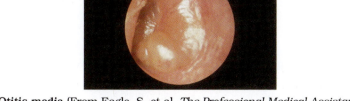

FIGURE 15-21 Otitis media (From Eagle, S, et al. *The Professional Medical Assistant: An Integrative Teamwork-Based Approach.* 2009. Philadelphia: F.A. Davis Company, with permission.)

language skills. Therefore, in infants and toddlers the primary signs may be increased fussiness, difficulty sleeping, poor appetite, and fever. Occasionally the children may be observed tugging at their ears. Older children may complain of mild to severe ear pain. Hearing may be diminished in all age groups.

Diagnosis

Diagnosis is established based upon otoscopic examination of the tympanic membrane (TM) and patient history. The TM may appear red and inflamed. It may appear to be bulging outward or retracted (pulled inward). Because the TM is translucent (semitransparent), fluid or bubbles are sometimes seen behind it. In severe cases it may have ruptured, as evidenced by a hole and traces of blood or other drainage. Tympanometry tests the TM for movement in response to air pressure. Tympanocentesis is done rarely to remove fluid for culture and sensitivity testing. Laboratory tests are rarely done, but an elevated count of white blood cells may indicate infection.

Treatment

In mild cases or when diagnosis is uncertain, the patient may be observed for 48 to 72 hours, since 80% of ear infections resolve on their own. Patients are given symptomatic treatment, including analgesics for pain and decongestants to reduce congestion and inflammation. If symptoms do not improve, or if they worsen, a repeat evaluation is done. When diagnosis is certain, or when children appear very ill or are under age 2, antibiotics are usually prescribed. Children who suffer severe chronic or frequently recurring ear infections may be candidates for *myringotomy,* a procedure in which a tiny tube is placed in the tympanic membrane (see Fig. 15-22). The tube acts as an open window, allowing excess air or fluid to escape, and significantly reduces the risk of infection and damage from increased pressure. Tubes remain in place for up to a year and then fall out on their own. Children with tubes in place must be prevented from getting water into their ears. In some cases adenoidectomy (surgical removal of the adenoids) is also done.

Flashpoint

Very mild cases of otitis media may not require antibiotic treatment.

Prognosis

Prognosis is very good for individuals who suffer from otitis media if timely diagnosis and treatment occur. Potential complications include mastoiditis (inflammation and infection of the surrounding bone), hearing loss, perforated TM, meningitis, paralysis of the facial nerve, and Ménière disease.

Hearing Loss

Flashpoint

Presbycusis is a type of hearing loss that occurs due to aging.

ICD-9-CM: 389.1 (sensorineural hearing loss), 388.01 (presbycusis)   [ICD-10: H90.5 (sensorineural hearing loss), H91.1 (presbycusis)]

Hearing loss affects individuals of all ages and may affect one or both ears. It may be categorized as sensorineural loss or conductive loss. *Presbycusis* is progressive, age-related hearing loss that typically begins after age 55. It usually affects both ears equally and begins with the loss of high-pitched sounds.

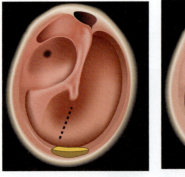
A small incision is made in the tympanic membrane

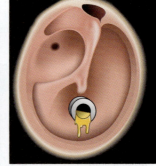
A tiny tube is inserted to drain fluid

FIGURE 15-22 **Myringotomy**

Incidence

An estimated four million Americans currently are deaf or have profound hearing loss. As many as 12,000 children each year experience hearing loss. Incidence of hearing loss further increases with age; as many as 50% of individuals over age 75 have hearing loss. Internationally, incidence varies widely. It is higher in westernized countries than others, possibly due to industrial noise.

Etiology

Sensorineural hearing loss is partial or complete hearing loss caused by degeneration of or damage to the sound pathway from the hair cells of the inner ear to the auditory nerve and brain. Causes include age-related degeneration, traumatic injury to hair cells, Ménière disease, and bacterial or viral infections, such as meningitis or mumps, that damage hair cells or the auditory nerve.

Conductive hearing loss is partial or complete hearing loss caused by factors that interfere with sound transmission from the outer to the inner ear. Causes include severe or chronic otitis media, fluid collection in the middle ear, impacted cerumen (earwax), otosclerosis, acoustic neuroma (a benign tumor), and nervous system disorders such as stroke or multiple sclerosis. Trauma to the TM or the tiny bones within the middle ear is another cause. Some medications, such as antibiotics, can cause permanent hearing loss; toxic doses of aspirin cause temporary tinnitus. Other factors contributing to presbycusis are stress and genetics. Some individuals suffer from a combination of conductive and sensorineural hearing loss. General contributors include daily noise from traffic, construction, music, and various types of equipment, as well as side effects of medication (see Box 15-8). Underlying physical disorders that affect circulation to structures of the ear may also be a factor. These include diabetes, hypertension, and atherosclerosis.

Signs and Symptoms

Early hearing loss is often not detected until family or friends notice the need to repeat things or observe their loved one turning up the TV or radio. Individuals with presbycusis may complain that others mumble too much or speak too quietly. They have greater difficulty hearing when background noise is present. The ability to hear high-pitched sounds and "*s*," "*sh*," and "*ch*" sounds is the first to go. Individuals with presbycusis may find a man's lower-pitched voice easier to hear and understand than a woman's higher-pitched voice. They may also complain of **tinnitus** (ringing or other abnormal sounds in the ears), which compounds their hearing difficulties.

Diagnosis

Diagnosis is based upon otoscopic examination of the ear, a variety of hearing tests, and other tests such as CT scan and MRI. The Weber and Rinne tuning-fork tests help to differentiate between conductive and sensorineural hearing loss (see Box 15-9). Presbycusis is diagnosed when other possible causes of hearing loss are excluded.

Flashpoint

The ability to hear high-pitched sounds is lost first.

Box 15-8 Wellness Promotion

BE KIND TO YOUR EARS

These guidelines can help people protect themselves from some types of hearing loss as well as some types of injury and disease that harm the ears:

- Avoid exposure to loud noises whenever possible.
- Wear ear protection such as earplugs when you must be around loud noise.
- Take medications only as directed by a qualified health-care provider.
- Consult with a physician if tinnitus or hearing loss is noticed.
- Obtain vaccinations for children as recommended by your health-care provider.
- Wear protective headwear, such as helmets, when playing contact sports or bicycling.
- Use seat belts when riding in motor vehicles.
- Follow recommended precautions when scuba diving.
- Do not insert anything into the ear canals to clean or scratch them.
- Dry the ears after bathing or swimming.

Box 15-9 Diagnostic Spotlight

TUNING-FORK TESTS

In the Weber test, the examiner holds a tuning fork at it base and strikes it against the palm of the hand, causing the fork to vibrate. The fork is then held on the center of the patient's head. If the patient hears the sound equally in both ears, the test result is normal. If the patient has conductive hearing loss, the sound will be stronger in the problem ear. Sensorineural hearing loss will cause the sound to be heard faintly or not at all in the affected ear.

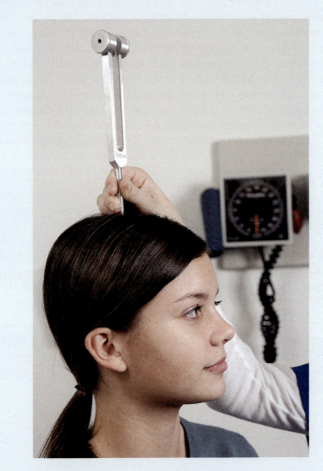

Weber test (From Eagle, S, et al. *The Professional Medical Assistant: An Integrative Teamwork-Based Approach.* 2009. Philadelphia: F.A. Davis Company, with permission.)

In the Rinne test, the examiner places the base of a vibrating tuning fork on the patient's mastoid bone and asks the patient to report when the sound is no longer audible. The examiner then moves the tuning fork near the patient's ear without touching it and asks whether the patient can still hear it. If the patient hears the tuning fork, the test result is normal, because air-conduction hearing should be better than bone-conduction hearing. Conductive hearing loss will cause the patient to hear the sound longer through bone conduction, so when the turning fork is then placed next to the ear, no sound is heard. If the patient has a sensorineural hearing loss, the sound will still be audible longer through air conduction than through bone conduction, but not twice as long.

Box 15-9 Diagnostic Spotlight—cont'd

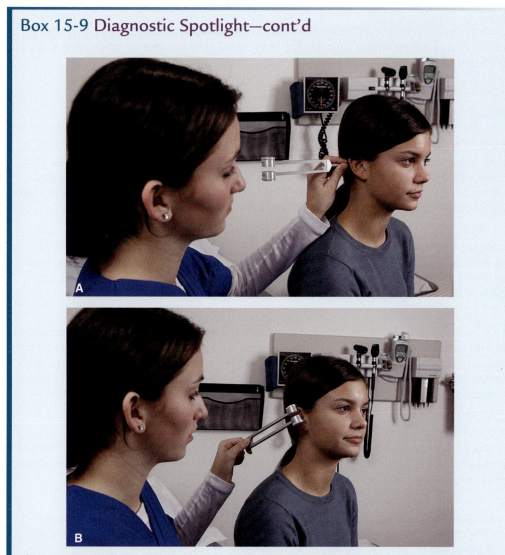

Rinne test: (A) On the mastoid bone; (B) Beside the patient's ear (From Eagle, S, et al. *The Professional Medical Assistant: An Integrative Teamwork-Based Approach.* 2009. Philadelphia: F.A. Davis Company, with permission.)

Treatment

Conductive hearing loss can often be treated through surgical procedures such as stapedectomy or tympanoplasty. Sensorineural hearing loss is permanent; hearing aids or other devices may be needed. A variety of strategies and technological devices are currently available to improve hearing and understanding. Many individuals benefit from hearing aids. Amplification devices can be used for telephones. Some technology makes sounds clearer with or without the use of hearing aids. Many individuals benefit from learning lipreading. Some also benefit from cochlear implants, which are surgically implanted electronic devices that stimulate auditory nerves within the cochlea with electrical impulses. This provides a sense of sound for individuals with severe hearing loss.

Prognosis

There is currently no cure for presbycusis. However, with appropriate diagnosis and treatment, most individuals can continue to live high-quality lives using hearing aids or other devices that improve their ability to hear and understand the sounds around them.

Otosclerosis

ICD-9-CM: 387.9   [ICD-10: H80.9] (unspecified for both codes)

Otosclerosis is a condition in which hearing is lost due to microscopic bone growth on the tiny ossicles (bones) called the malleus, incus, and stapes. Hearing is lost as these bones become fixed in place rather than being allowed to vibrate to facilitate sound transmission. This is a progressive form of conductive hearing loss that affects both ears in 85% to 90% of cases.

Incidence

It is estimated that as many as 30 million Americans have otosclerosis; however, most of them do not become symptomatic. Women are affected more often than men. Onset is typically during young adulthood. Individuals of Caucasian or Asian descent are affected more than members of other ethnic groups.

Etiology

Otosclerosis is considered an autosomal dominant inherited disorder. This means that a child of someone with otosclerosis has a 50% chance of inheriting the gene. However, not all individuals with the gene develop symptoms. There is also evidence that viruses, such as the measles virus, may be a contributing factor. Otosclerosis may cause either conductive or sensorineural hearing loss, depending upon whether the ossicles or the otic capsule (surrounding bone) is affected. If both types occur, the individual is said to have a mixed hearing loss.

Flashpoint

Otosclerosis is an inherited disorder.

Signs and Symptoms

Most people with otosclerosis are asymptomatic. When manifestations occur, they include progressive hearing loss, *tinnitus*, and, occasionally, dizziness. For some women, symptom onset occurs during pregnancy.

Diagnosis

Diagnosis of otosclerosis is made based upon a combination of data, including otoscopic-examination findings, audiometry and audiology test results, and family history. A CT may be done to differentiate otosclerosis from other disorders.

Treatment

The most effective form of treatment for otosclerosis is a surgical procedure called a stapedectomy. In this procedure, a surgeon removes the diseased stapes and replaces it with a metal, plastic, or ceramic prosthesis. This procedure is considered curative for conductive hearing loss but not for sensorineural loss. Another option is the use of a hearing aid, which may improve hearing but does not stop the progression of the disease.

Prognosis

The prognosis is very good if stapedectomy is done; approximately 90% of individuals experience a good return of hearing. A small percentage experience limited or no improvement. In 1% of cases, hearing loss occurs in the inner ear; therefore, surgery is performed on one ear at a time, the worst ear first. Other potential side effects include intolerance of loud noises, perforation of the TM, *vertigo* (sensation of moving around in space and extreme dizziness), and taste changes on the same side of the tongue as the surgical ear.

Cholesteatoma

ICD-9-CM: 385.35   [ICD-10: H71]

Cholesteatoma is a condition in which a cyst develops in the middle ear.

Incidence

Estimations of the incidence of cholesteatoma in the United States vary between 10,000 and 30,000 individuals. The incidence is higher in men than in women; it is also higher in individuals with a history of chronic ear infection or with dysfunction of the eustachian tubes, and it is significantly higher in those with cleft palate.

Etiology

Cholesteatoma is sometimes congenital. Acquired cholesteatoma can develop secondary to otitis media if the TM has been perforated and the skin of the TM then grows through the hole into the middle ear. As it grows, the cholesteatoma can destroy the ossicles. Chronic swelling of the eustachian tube leads to negative pressure within the middle ear, which pulls the TM in the wrong direction. This creates a cyst that fills with sloughed skin cells and debris. When the cyst becomes inflamed and infected, it may cause degeneration of the ossicles. In some cases, continued erosion can lead the infection to spread to the brain.

> **Flashpoint**
> Cholesteatoma may be congenital or may be related to otitis media with TM rupture.

Signs and Symptoms

Symptoms of cholesteatoma include pain or numbness around the ear, hearing loss in one ear, recurrent foul-smelling discharge from the ear, and dizziness. The individual usually has a history of ear infections after URI or after getting water into the ear canal.

Diagnosis

Diagnosis is based upon an otoscopic examination, which reveals a perforated TM, often with drainage. Testing may include electronystagmography, which is a test that evaluates the acoustic nerve, and a caloric stimulation test that uses differences in temperature to diagnose damage to the nerves of the ear. CT scan may be done to help the physician identify how far the cholesteatoma has spread into the middle ear and surrounding structures.

Treatment

Treatment includes systemic and topical antibiotics along with weekly cleaning of the ear under a surgical microscope. Once the infection is cleared, surgery is done to remove the cyst. Polyps are often present in the ear along with the cholesteatoma. If so, they may need to be surgically removed as well.

Prognosis

Cholesteatomas generally continue to grow unless they are removed. Surgery is usually successful but may need to be repeated if the cholesteatoma grows back. Possible complications include deafness in the affected ear, vertigo, persistent drainage, labyrinthitis, mastoiditis, meningitis, brain abscess, and erosion of the facial nerve, resulting in facial paralysis.

Labyrinthitis

ICD-9-CM: 386.30 (unspecified)   [ICD-10: H83.0]

Labyrinthitis, also called *otitis interna*, is inflammation of the labyrinth within the inner ear. The labyrinth is a tiny structure with a mazelike configuration of fluid-filled canals. It is instrumental in the maintenance of balance and sends messages to the brain regarding position and movement of the body. Labyrinthitis may be either viral or bacterial.

Incidence

The incidence of labyrinthitis is estimated at 30,000. Typical patients are adults between ages 30 and 60.

Etiology

Labyrinthitis typically follows a URI and is thought to be itself caused by viral or bacterial infection. It also often follows otitis media or meningitis, and it may be related to head trauma. Other factors associated with labyrinthitis include allergies, tumors of the middle ear, alcohol abuse, and the use of some medications. Episodes typically last up to 6 weeks but may occasionally last for years.

Signs and Symptoms

The most common symptom of labyrinthitis is *vertigo*, which often causes nausea and vomiting. In addition, some individuals experience tinnitus, hearing loss, fever, nystagmus, and headache. Symptoms are triggered or worsened by sudden head movement.

Diagnosis

Diagnosis is based upon the patient's description of symptoms and examination of the ears and nervous system. Hearing is evaluated, and occasionally a CT scan or MRI may be done.

Treatment

In many cases labyrinthitis resolves on its own after several weeks. Antiemetic (antinausea) medications and those used to treat motion sickness are sometimes prescribed to alleviate vertigo, nausea, and vomiting. Selective serotonin reuptake inhibitors may help relieve anxiety and promote functioning of the inner ear. Viral infections may respond to antiviral medications or corticosteroids. Antibiotics may be prescribed if infection is persistent. Dietary restrictions may be recommended, including reduction of salt, sugar, chocolate, caffeine, and alcohol. Smoking cessation is encouraged.

Prognosis

The prognosis for patients with labyrinthitis is generally good. Most cases resolve within a few weeks, although some individuals may experience symptoms for months. Periodic recurrences are possible.

Ménière Disease

ICD-9-CM: 386.00   [ICD-10: H81.0]

Ménière disease is a chronic noncontagious disorder affecting the structures of the inner ear.

Incidence

Ménière disease is estimated to affect as many as six million Americans, men and women equally. Most are between the ages of 30 and 60.

Etiology

The exact cause of Ménière disease is not fully understood. An excessive amount of endolymph in the inner ear is thought to be a factor. As fluid level increases, pressure is thought to be exerted against the delicate structures of the inner ear. Triggering factors for Ménière disease include viral infections, heredity, allergies, infections of the middle ear, head trauma, and the use of aspirin, alcohol, or cigarettes. Presence of the herpesvirus is also considered a risk factor.

Signs and Symptoms

Manifestations of Ménière disease are episodic, with attacks lasting from 20 minutes to several hours or even several days. A common symptom is vertigo that may become more frequent and more severe over time and can significantly impair the individual's ability to work, drive, or perform other activities. Other symptoms include tinnitus, intermittent hearing loss, nausea, vomiting, nystagmus, perspiration, a feeling of fullness or pressure in the ears, and periodic loss of balance. Hearing usually improves after an attack but may progressively worsen over time. Some individuals may experience brain fog, which is the onset of confusion and short-term memory loss. Women sometimes experience episodes premenstrually or during pregnancy, possibly due to fluid retention.

Diagnosis

Diagnosis of Ménière disease is established by ruling out other disorders. A physical examination is done and the patient's report of symptoms is gathered. Testing might include head MRI or CT scan, audiometry, and electronystagmography.

Treatment

There is no cure for Ménière disease. Treatment is focused on dietary modification, medications to reduce symptoms, and possible surgery. Recommended dietary changes include limiting salt and sugar intake and eliminating alcohol and caffeine. Some physicians also recommend avoiding foods and drinks containing aspartame (an artificial sweetener). Smoking cessation is encouraged. Bedrest may be advised for acute attacks. A variety of medications are used to relieve symptoms, including antihistamines, anticholinergics, sedatives, antiemetics, anticonvulsants, and corticosteroids. In extreme cases, surgery may be done to relieve pressure or even to destroy or remove part of the inner ear. A vestibular neurectomy (cutting the nerve) may also be done to relieve vertigo.

Prognosis

Ménière disease usually begins in one ear only, but after a number of years, half of all patients have bilateral disease. In most cases, progressive hearing loss develops and can become severe. Tinnitus may also worsen over time. However, in some individuals the attacks lessen in severity and frequency over time or even resolve spontaneously and completely—they may then never recur.

STOP HERE.
Select the flash cards for this chapter and run through them at least three times before moving on to the next chapter.

Student Resources

American Academy of Ophthalmology: http://www.aao.org
American Academy of Otolaryngology–Head and Neck Surgery: http://www.entnet.org
American Foundation for the Blind: http://www.afb.org
American Optometric Association: http://www.aoa.org
American Society for Deaf Children: http://www.deafchildren.org
Deafness Research Foundation: http://www.drf.org
The Ear Foundation: http://www.earfoundation.org.uk
Glaucoma Research Foundation: http://www.glaucoma.org
Kids Health: http://www.kidshealth.org

Chapter Activities

Learning Style Study Strategies

Try any or all of the following strategies as you study the content of this chapter:

All learners: Use washable sidewalk chalk and (with permission) draw a supersized illustration of the three parts of the ear or the structures of the eye. Label all parts accurately. Now take turns walking along the path of sound transmission or the visual-image pathway. Verbally name the parts and describe their functions as you do so. Use lots of color and make this fun.

All learners: With your study group, create a human representation of the structures of the ear. Members will be assigned to play the roles of auricle, external auditory canal, TM, ossicles, cochlea, oval window, and semicircular canals. If the group is small, members may take on dual roles. If the group is large, additional members can be assigned to play the roles of the separate ossicles, the eighth cranial nerve, and even the *sound* as it moves from member to member. Each member must verbally describe the function of the part being played and physically act it out. Try to be accurate, but make this fun.

Practice Exercises

Answers to practice exercises can be found in Appendix D.

Case Studies

CASE STUDY 1

Mrs. Martison has brought her 6-year-old daughter Melissa to the medical clinic for evaluation. Melissa's eyes are reddened and inflamed. She complains of itching, and her eyelashes were stuck together with dried drainage when she awoke this morning. After examination, the physician diagnoses Melissa with conjunctivitis.

1. What are the most common causes of conjunctivitis?

2. What important points should the health-care provider cover when teaching Mrs. Martison and Melissa about conjunctivitis?

3. Describe the typical signs and symptoms of conjunctivitis.

4. How is this disorder usually treated?

CASE STUDY 2

Hugo Montoya is a 32-year-old man who came to the medical clinic today complaining that shortly after he awoke this morning, he began seeing flashes of light and noticed small floating shapes in the visual field of his left eye. He has no pain or discomfort but does note a feeling of heaviness in his eye. After examination with a slit-lamp microscope and administration of an Amsler grid test, the physician diagnoses Hugo with retinal detachment.

1. What symptom might Hugo describe if the retinal detachment progresses?

2. Describe what happens when the retina detaches.

3. Describe common treatment measures for retinal detachment.

CASE STUDY 3

Howard Mueller is a 58-year-old man suffering from Ménière disease. His symptoms fluctuate as episodes recur and resolve. His most troublesome symptoms include vertigo and tinnitus.

1. Define vertigo and tinnitus.

2. Describe the usual treatment for Ménière disease.

3. Mr. Mueller states that he understands that there is no cure for this disorder, but he wants to know what the prognosis usually is. What might his health-care provider tell him?

Multiple Choice

1. Which of the following disorders is paired with the correct description?

   a. Conjunctivitis: loss of visual acuity caused by a defective curvature in the cornea

   b. Nystagmus: contagious eye infection

   c. Macular degeneration: opacity of the lens of the eye that develops as a gradual clouding

   d. Glaucoma: disorder in which increased intraocular pressure results in loss of peripheral vision and eventual blindness

2. Which of the following statements is true regarding otitis media?

   a. It involves the outer ear canal.

   b. It must always be treated with antibiotics.

   c. It is usually preceded by an upper respiratory infection.

   d. It most commonly affects the elderly.

3. Which of the following disorders involves the ears?

   a. Ectropion

   b. Labyrinthitis

   c. Keratitis

   d. Blepharitis

4. Which of the following disorders is paired with the correct description?

   a. Hyperopia: nearsightedness

   b. Myopia: farsightedness

   c. Presbyopia: age-related vision loss

   d. Presbycusis: hearing loss related to the formation of a cyst in the middle ear

5. Which of the following disorders involves the ears?

   a. Cholesteatoma

   b. Chalazion

   c. Entropion

   d. Uveitis

Short Answer

1. Describe how acquired cholesteatoma develops.

2. Describe the type of patients who most commonly present with foreign bodies in their ears.

3. Which type of ear infection is sometimes called swimmer's ear?

4. Explain the difference between entropion and ectropion.

5. Explain the difference between chalazion and hordeolum.

GENETIC AND CONGENITAL DISORDERS

16

Learning Outcomes

Upon completion of this chapter, the student will be able to:

- Define and spell key terms related to genetic and congenital disorders
- Identify characteristics of common genetic and congenital disorders, including:
  - description
  - incidence
  - etiology
  - signs and symptoms
  - diagnosis
  - treatment
  - prognosis

KEY TERMS	
anomaly	abnormality that develops in utero
autosomal dominant disorder	disorder that can be passed on when just one faulty gene is inherited from one parent
autosomal recessive disorder	disorder that can be passed on only when two faulty genes are inherited, one from each parent
autosome	any chromosome other than the sex chromosomes
birth defect	congenital anomaly
chromosome	linear strand of DNA that carries genetic information
congenital	present at birth
DNA	deoxyribonucleic acid; material inside cells that carries genetic instructions for the individual's development and survival
gene	basic, self-replicating unit of heredity, made up of pieces of DNA
genetic	inherited
genetic mutation	permanent change in genetic structure within the sperm or egg cell that causes a change in the offspring that is different from the parents; or a permanent change in an individual's DNA triggered by exposure to an environmental factor
karyotype	analysis based on a photomicrograph of the chromosomes of a single cell
spontaneous bleeding episodes	episodes of bleeding with no identifiable cause that are sometimes seen in individuals with hemophilia
tet spells	episodes in which an infant's arterial oxygen level drops, seen in infants with tetralogy of Fallot
X chromosome	one of two chromosomes that determine gender in humans; determines female gender

Continued

KEY TERMS—cont'd	
X-linked recessive disorder	disorder inherited by a man from his mother because the trait is attached to a gene error on the X chromosome
Y chromosome	One of two chromosomes that determine gender in humans; determines male gender

Abbreviations

Table 16-1 lists some of the most common abbreviations related to genetic and congenital disorders.

Errors in Human Development

Some conditions and disorders occur very early in human development—before infants are born. When these conditions and disorders are the result of some type of faulty information inherited from one or both parents, they are considered to be *genetic* (inherited) in nature. Some conditions have been clearly identified as genetic. In other cases, a specific genetic cause is not identified; rather, some other factor, such as a toxic exposure during gestation or a birth injury, may be the cause. In such cases, the condition is identified as *congenital* (present at birth). The specific cause of some disorders is not yet fully understood, and experts may suggest a variety of theories, falling into both of these categories. For this reason, both types of disorders are addressed in this chapter.

Congenital Conditions

There are numerous congenital conditions. While all are present at birth, some are not discovered until a later time. They can affect virtually any body system and may be very minor or severe enough to be fatal. Causes are numerous and may include genetic and nongenetic factors. Examples of nongenetic factors include exposure to toxic substances during gestation, maternal illness or infections during pregnancy, severe malnutrition, radiation exposure, fetal

TABLE 16-1
ABBREVIATIONS

Abbreviation	Meaning	Abbreviation	Meaning
ASD	atrial septal defect	DNA	deoxyribonucleic acid
BMD	Becker muscular dystrophy	FAS	fetal alcohol syndrome
CF	cystic fibrosis	HD	Huntington disease
CP	cerebral palsy	NTD	neural tube defect
CVS	chorionic villus sampling	OI	osteogenesis imperfecta
DDH	developmental dislocation of the hip	PDA	patent ductus arteriosus
DMD	Duchenne muscular dystrophy	VSD	ventricular septal defect

hypoxia (low oxygen), and other prenatal injury. Physical defects in newborn infants are sometimes called *anomalies* (abnormalities that develop in utero) or *birth defects* (congenital anomalies). In approximately two-thirds of those cases, the exact cause is not clear.

Genetic Conditions

Genetic conditions are congenital in that they are present at birth; however, they are caused by errors in development related to faulty instructions from the person's *genes.* Genes are basic, self-replicating units of heredity, made up of pieces of *DNA*—deoxyribonucleic acid, the material inside cells that carries genetic instructions for the individual's development and survival. Most DNA is located within the cell's nucleus (nuclear DNA), but a small amount is located within the cell's mitochondria (mitochondrial DNA). Mitochondria are structures that provide energy for cells to function. Normally, DNA is stored efficiently in the form of *chromosomes,* which are linear strands of DNA that carry genetic information (see Fig. 16-1). Each gene occupies a specific location on a chromosome and contains the instructions for making specific proteins. During cell division, chromosomes unwind to make copies of themselves, allowing all new cells to have the exact same DNA as the old ones.

Humans normally have 23 pairs of chromosomes, for a total number of 46. Half of the nuclear DNA is inherited from the father and half from the mother. During reproduction, the ovum (egg from the mother) and sperm each contribute 23 chromosomes. Twenty-two of these are *autosomes* (any chromosome other than the sex chromosomes). The other chromosome is the one that determines gender in humans. The two variations are labeled X for female an Y for male. Females normally have two *X chromosomes* and males normally have one X and one *Y chromosome.* The ovum always contributes an X chromosome; therefore, the sperm determines the gender of the offspring. If the sperm contributes an X chromosome, the offspring is female, and if the sperm contributes a Y chromosome, the offspring is male.

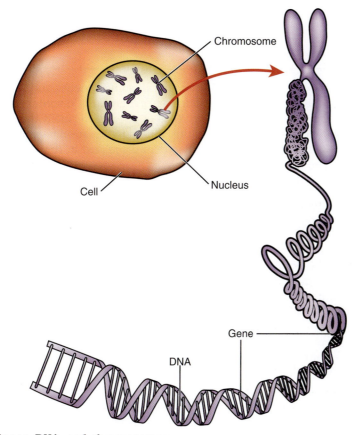

Chromosome

Cell

Nucleus

Gene

DNA

FIGURE 16-1 Genes, DNA, and chromosomes

Inheritance Patterns

Genetic conditions are categorized according to whether they are passed on by autosomes or by sex chromosomes and whether the inheritance pattern is dominant or recessive. An **autosomal dominant disorder** can be passed on when just one faulty gene is inherited from one parent. For an **autosomal recessive disorder** to be passed on, two faulty genes must be inherited, one from each parent. However, with an **X-linked recessive disorder** this is not the case. Because men inherit only one X chromosome, the one from the mother, a gene error on that chromosome will cause a disorder. In contrast, women inherit two X chromosomes—one from each parent—so a normal one can usually compensate if an abnormal one is inherited. Consequently, the woman usually remains healthy but may be a carrier with the potential to pass the faulty gene on to her children.

Genetic Mutations

Some disorders are thought to be caused by **genetic mutations.** Mutation may occur when a permanent change in genetic structure within the sperm or egg cell causes a change within the offspring that is different from the parents. It may involve a single piece of DNA or a large portion of a chromosome. Because the change occurs in the DNA, it may then be passed on to future generations. Mutation may also be acquired when an individual is exposed to a toxic substance or some other environmental factor. This type of mutation is usually not passed on to offspring, unless it involves the egg cells or sperm.

Common Congenital and Genetic Disorders

There are numerous congenital and genetic disorders, affecting every body system. Each year in the United States, approximately 150,000 infants are born with birth defects. In approximately two-thirds of those cases, the exact cause is not clear.

Nervous System Disorders

There are many nervous system disorders, some congenital, some genetic, and some possibly caused by a combination of factors. Neural tube defects are a group of disorders in which the neural tube that contains the brain and spinal cord fails to develop normally during early fetal development. This group includes spina bifida occulta, meningocele, myelomeningocele, anencephaly, and iniencephaly. Other nervous system disorders discussed in this chapter are hydrocephalus, Huntington disease, cerebral palsy, and epilepsy.

Neural Tube Defects

Neural tube defects (NTDs) are a group of defects involving malformation of the spinal cord and surrounding structures. The neural tube is the name given to the embryonic structure that eventually develops into the brain, spinal cord, and enclosing tissue. Neural tube defects occur when part of the neural tube fails to close during the first 3 or 4 weeks of development.

Normally the brain and the spinal cord are covered by three membranes called the *meninges,* which continue beyond the end of the spinal cord to the distal end of the sacrum. The meninges provide a supportive structure for many small blood vessels on the brain's surface. They also house the cerebrospinal fluid (CSF), which continuously circulates around the brain and spinal cord and provides a cushion to protect against injury from impact and sudden movement. An NTD creates a gap in these protective structures and leaves the delicate spinal cord vulnerable to injury. There are several types of NTD, including spina bifida occulta, meningocele, myelomeningocele, anencephaly, and iniencephaly (see Fig. 16-2).

Flashpoint

The meninges protect the brain and spinal cord.

Spina Bifida Occulta
ICD-9-CM: 756.17   [ICD-10: Q76.0]

Spina bifida occulta, also called *hidden spina bifida,* is a condition in which the individual has a small gap in one or more vertebrae but other tissues are normal. These individuals may be completely symptom free and may not know they have the condition unless it is discovered

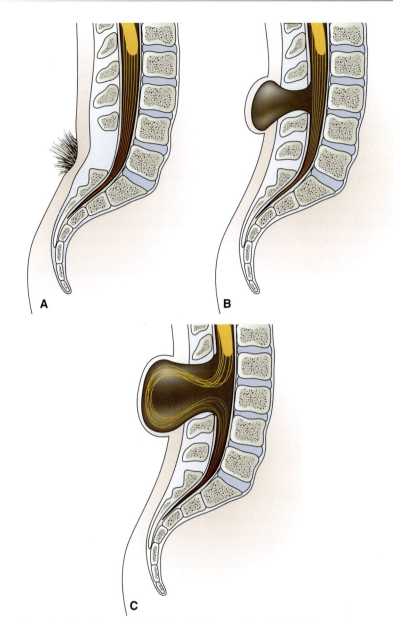

FIGURE 16-2 Neural tube defects: (A) Spina bifida occulta; (B) Meningocele; (C) Myelomeningocele

when tests are done for other purposes. Closed neural tube defects are usually categorized along with hidden spina bifida. They include a variety of malformations involving bone, fat, and other tissues. There may be a visible external indicator at the site, such as a small opening in the skin, lump, dimple, tuft of hair, or birthmark.

Meningocele
ICD-9-CM: 741.90   [ICD-10: Q05.9] (unspecified level for both codes)
Meningocele is an open NTD in which a portion of the meninges and some CSF are protruding out of the abnormal spinal opening. However, the spinal cord itself remains in its normal position and is usually not damaged. The bulging tissue caused by the herniation is sometimes covered by a skin layer.

Myelomeningocele
ICD-9-CM: 741.90   [ICD-10: Q05.9] (unspecified level for both codes)
Myelomeningocele is an open NTD in which a portion of the meninges, some CSF, and a portion of the spinal cord have herniated and are protruding out of the abnormal spinal opening. As a result, the delicate spinal cord is often damaged.

Anencephaly
ICD-9-CM: 741.90   [ICD-10: Q00.0]

Anencephaly is a very severe form of NTD in which a significant portion of the brain and skull fail to form properly. This is caused by failure of the neural tube to develop and close at the head. This condition is incompatible with life and affects 1,000 to 2,000 infants each year.

Iniencephaly
ICD-9-CM: 740.2   [ICD-10: Q00.2]

Iniencephaly is a rare NTD in which the infant does not have a neck and the head is severely retroflexed (bent backward). The body is usually short and the head may be abnormally large. Other severe anomalies are usually present as well. Infants with iniencephaly rarely survive.

Incidence

Estimates regarding the incidence of NTD vary widely and depend upon the type of NTD. In 1995 there were nearly 90,000 infants born in the United States with any type of neural tube defect. Since that time, the annual incidence has dropped to approximately 57,000. There are an estimated 16 million infants globally born with NTD annually. Each year, approximately 2,000 infants are born with spina bifida or closed NTD. Female infants are affected more often than males. Hispanics and Caucasians of northern European descent are affected more often than other groups.

Etiology

The cause of NTD is not fully understood. Contributors are thought to include genetic, nutritional, and environmental factors. Some antiseizure medications, such as valproic acid, and certain maternal diseases, such as diabetes and obesity, have been identified as increasing the risk of an NTD. Maternal malnutrition plays a role as well, specifically a lack of folic acid in the diet. This theory has been strengthened by the reduction of NTDs among children of women who ingest adequate amounts of folic acid and folate around the time of conception and during the early weeks of pregnancy. Other risk factors include a parent who was born with NTD, having previously had a baby with an NTD, and elevated maternal body temperature during early pregnancy (from fever or the use of saunas or hot tubs).

Flashpoint

There is a connection between folic-acid deficiency and neural tube defects.

Signs and Symptoms

Signs and symptoms of NTDs vary by type and between individuals:

- Spina bifida occulta: These individuals may be symptom free or may suffer from some nerve impairment that affects lower-body functioning as well as functioning of the bowel and bladder.
- Meningocele: A rounded sac containing fluid and meninges is present at the site. The individual is otherwise usually symptom free.
- Myelomeningocele: A rounded sac is present at the site, containing fluid, meningeal tissue, and portions of the spinal cord or nerve roots. It may be covered by a layer of skin, or the nerve tissue may be fully exposed. The individual usually suffers paralysis below the level of the herniation, as well as bowel and bladder dysfunction. The individual may also experience seizure disorders.
- Anencephaly: The infant has a very small head containing very little brain tissue. The head, face, and other parts of the body are malformed. The infant usually dies before or during birth, but may survive a very short time.
- Iniencephaly: The infant has no neck; the head is disproportionately large, compared with the body, and is severely retroflexed. The body is short, and other severe anomalies are usually present. The infant rarely survives.

Diagnosis

Neural tube defects may be detected with prenatal screening and testing; however, the results are not infallible. The maternal serum alpha-fetoprotein test is the most common means of testing for myelomeningocele. It measures the level of alpha-fetoprotein that has crossed the placenta and entered the mother's blood. Abnormally high levels may indicate that the fetus has an NTD. However, false positives do occur about 5% of the time; therefore, follow-up testing is needed. Ultrasound is most commonly done and is safe for both fetus and mother. Amniocentesis may also be done to check for elevated alpha-fetoprotein in the amniotic fluid (see Box 16-1). Detecting an NTD before birth allows parents and health-care providers to prepare for delivery so that

Box 16-1 Diagnostic Spotlight

AMNIOCENTESIS

Amniocentesis is performed at 16 to 18 weeks' gestation. The physician inserts a hypodermic needle into the amniotic sac and extracts a sample of 10 to 20 milliliters of amniotic fluid. The laboratory examines the chromosomes of fetal cells present in the fluid to identify possible chromosomal abnormalities, such as Down syndrome. Because the risk of having a child with Down syndrome increases with maternal age, many physicians routinely order amniocentesis for patients over age 35.

necessary equipment and supplies are on hand and corrective surgery, if needed, can take place in a timely fashion. It also allows for planning the most appropriate type of delivery, since some infants with NTDs should be delivered by cesarean section.

Diagnosis after birth is generally based upon physical-examination findings. Additional testing may be done as needed to identify which type of NTD the infant has and any complications. Radiological imaging, such as x-ray, magnetic resonance imaging (MRI), and computed tomography (CT), may be done to carefully examine the infant's spine and head and determine the best course of treatment.

Flashpoint
Identifying an NTD before birth allows better preparation for delivery.

Treatment

It is recommended that all women of childbearing age eat a well-balanced diet rich in folic acid (see Box 16-2). This has been found to help prevent NTDs. Treatment for infants with an NTD depends upon the type and severity. Most with spina bifida occulta require no treatment. Those with meningocele undergo surgical removal of the herniated tissue. Infants with myelomeningocele are at risk of infection if nervous tissue is exposed; they are treated with antibiotics, and surgical correction is usually done within 48 hours of delivery. This involves placing the exposed nervous tissue back inside the spinal canal and covering it with muscle and skin. This does not cure damage that has already occurred but does help to prevent further damage. Physical therapy begins as soon as the infant has recovered from surgery. Braces for walking, a wheelchair, or other mobility devices may eventually be needed.

Prognosis

Prognosis for infants with NTDs is quite variable and depends upon the type of NTD and the initiation of appropriate treatment:

- Spina bifida occulta: Individuals with this condition generally lead very normal lives and may never know they have the condition.
- Meningocele: If the condition is surgically repaired, individuals usually lead healthy lives without complications. However, a small percentage may have tethered cord syndrome. This is a condition in which the spinal cord is attached to another structure, such as skin or bone. This impedes its mobility and flexibility and can lead to nerve damage.

Flashpoint
The prognosis for patients with NTDs is quite variable and depends upon the type of NTD and the initiation of appropriate treatment.

Box 16-2 Wellness Promotion

PREVENT BIRTH DEFECTS BY EATING A HEALTHY DIET

The risk of birth defects like neural tube defects, cleft lip, and cleft palate can be reduced by as much as 70% if the mother eats a healthy diet. This should begin before pregnancy occurs. General recommendations include eating foods high in folic acid, such as grains and cereals, leafy green vegetables, dried beans and legumes, and oranges. Some individuals may consider taking a supplement of 400 micrograms of folic acid every day.

- Myelomeningocele: Individuals with this condition can lead productive lives but may suffer a variety of complications, including paralysis and bowel and bladder dysfunction. They have a high incidence of tethered cord syndrome, hydrocephalus, and Chiari deformity. They are also at risk of meningitis and, later on, latex allergies, gastrointestinal disorders, and learning disabilities.
- Anencephaly and iniencephaly: These conditions are nearly always fatal.

Hydrocephalus

ICD-9-CM: 741.0 (with spina bifida only), 331.3 (communicating), 331.4 (obstructive)   **[ICD-10: Q03.9 (with spina bifida only), G91.0 (communicating), G91.1 (obstructive)]**

Hydrocephalus, known at one time as *water on the brain,* is a condition in which an excessive amount of CSF builds up within the ventricles of the brain. This can cause an enlarged head as well as brain damage, as pressure is exerted against brain tissue (see Fig. 16-3). The two most common types of hydrocephalus are communicating and noncommunicating. In communicating hydrocephalus, CSF continues to flow between ventricles but is impeded after leaving the ventricles. In noncommunicating or *obstructive* hydrocephalus, the normal flow of CSF is blocked between ventricles.

> **Flashpoint**
>
> *Hydro-* means *water.* In hydrocephalus, fluid builds up within the ventricles of the brain.

Incidence

The incidence of hydrocephalus is about two per 1,000 infants born.

Etiology

CSF is contained between layers of the meninges and circulates through the brain ventricles and around the brain and spinal cord. It is a colorless, clear fluid similar to blood plasma. It provides a cushion to protect against injury from impact and sudden movement. CSF normally flows deep within the brain, between four ventricles that are connected by narrow channels. It then flows to an area between the brain and skull, where it is absorbed into the bloodstream. Anything that disrupts the normal flow or absorption of CSF causes hydrocephalus. As the fluid builds up, brain tissue is damaged from compression and the head may enlarge. This condition may be congenital and is frequently associated with neural tube defects and genetic problems. It may also develop because of brain injury from tumors, trauma, or infection. Prematurity is also a risk factor.

Signs and Symptoms

The signs and symptoms of hydrocephalus are numerous, and individuals may exhibit any or all of them. Signs and symptoms in infants may include seizures, dyspnea, poor sucking or feeding, high-pitched crying, vomiting, irritability, unusual sleepiness, developmental delays, prominent scalp veins, reluctance to move or bend the neck, bulging fontanels (soft spots), downward-fixed eyes, and rapidly increasing head size.

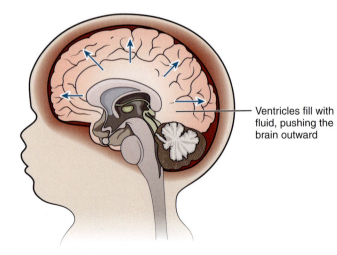

Ventricles fill with fluid, pushing the brain outward

FIGURE 16-3 Hydrocephalus

Signs and symptoms of hydrocephalus in older patients include disturbances in gait (manner of walking), headache, lethargy, papilledema (swelling of the optic disk), vision problems, nausea, vomiting, downward-fixed eyes, irritability, memory deficits, confusion, personality changes, mental slowing, and bladder incontinence.

Diagnosis

Prenatal ultrasound may aid in the diagnosis of hydrocephalus. After infants are born, routine well-child health screening includes growth monitoring. Measurements of the infant's height, weight, length, and head circumference are plotted on growth charts; if the infant displays abnormally rapid growth of the head circumference, further diagnostic testing is done. Diagnosis of older individuals may be suspected based upon the patient's physical changes and description of symptoms. Radiological tests used to confirm diagnosis in patients of all ages include CT and MRI, to measure structures within the brain. Other tests may include lumbar puncture (to obtain a sample of CSF), intracranial pressure monitoring, and ultrasonography.

Flashpoint

Prenatal ultrasound may be used to diagnose hydrocephalus.

Treatment

Hydrocephalus is commonly treated with the placement of a shunt (long, flexible, synthetic tube) beneath the skin to drain the CSF to another area in the body, such as the abdomen or a heart chamber. A valve within the shunt ensures one-way flow and regulation of the CSF. Some patients may also undergo a ventriculostomy. In this procedure, a tiny hole is created in the floor of the third ventricle of the brain to allow CSF to flow toward the base of the brain and be absorbed.

Prognosis

Prognosis for patients with hydrocephalus depends upon the underlying cause, any associated disorders, and the earliness of diagnosis and treatment. Untreated hydrocephalus leads to severe brain damage, physical disability, and possibly death; however, patients who receive early, effective treatment can lead reasonably normal, productive lives. Potential complications of shunt systems include infection, obstruction, and mechanical failure. For these reasons, patients may need to undergo shunt revision or replacement a number of times throughout their lives.

Huntington Disease
ICD-9-CM: 333.4   [ICD-10: G10]

Huntington disease, also called *Huntington chorea*, is an inherited progressive degenerative neurological disease that results in physical and mental decline. It was first studied in the late 1800s by a physician named George Huntington, who used the Greek term *chorea*, which means "dance," to refer to the typical involuntary, jerky movements made by individuals with this disease. See Chapter 6 for a detailed description of Huntington disease.

Cerebral Palsy
ICD-9-CM: 343.9   [ICD-10: G80.9] (unspecified for both codes)

Cerebral palsy (CP) is a disorder of the brain that affects posture, balance, and movement.

Incidence

An estimated 8,000 to 16,000 American children are born each year with cerebral palsy. Boys have a higher risk than girls. Also at higher risk are African Americans and children from low- or middle-income families.

Etiology

The cause of CP is a defect in, or injury to, areas of the brain that control posture, balance, and movement. Congenital causes include a genetic disorder, a maternal infection during pregnancy, such as meningitis, and Rh incompatibility of the blood between mother and fetus. Acquired causes include brain injury and any circumstances that cause cerebral hypoxia during fetal development, birth, infancy, or early childhood.

Flashpoint

Children with cerebral palsy experience poor muscle control, muscle weakness and spasticity, developmental delays, mental deficits, and sensory deficits.

Signs and Symptoms

CP is characterized by a wide variety of symptoms, including lack of muscle control, muscle weakness, spastic muscles, delayed development, mental deficits, and hearing and vision problems. The disorder appears within the first few years of the patient's life and does not worsen over time.

Diagnosis

The pediatrician can diagnose the patient with CP based on physical-examination findings. Lack of muscle tone, or *floppy baby syndrome,* is an indication of CP. The pediatrician can refer patients to physical, speech, and occupational therapists to maximize functioning. The pediatrician still provides routine care for the patient.

Treatment

There is no cure for CP. However, various treatments can improve the child's ability to function with increased independence and improved quality of life. Treatment often includes physical and occupational therapy, which can help increase strength and functioning and reduce spasticity. Speech therapy can help improve difficulties in speech and swallowing. Medications can be given to relieve pain, minimize muscle spasms, and manage seizures. Mobility devices can be used as needed to provide for safe mobility and increased independence; these may include orthotics, braces, splints, walkers, and wheelchairs. Computers and other forms of technology can be used to aid communication. Surgical procedures are sometimes helpful in reducing or resolving contractures and deformities. Children and their parents often find that support groups help provide information, socialization, and emotional support.

Prognosis

The prognosis for patients with CP is very individualized. With supportive treatments, such as medications, surgery, and assistive devices, patients with CP can reach their individual potentials. Fifty percent of children with CP suffer from seizure disorders. Other complications include intellectual disability, learning disabilities, and attention-deficit hyperactivity disorder.

Epilepsy

ICD-9-CM: 345.90   [ICD-10: G40.9] (unspecified for both codes)

Epilepsy is a chronic disorder of the brain marked by recurrent seizures, which are repetitive abnormal electrical discharges within the brain. Epilepsy seizure types are categorized as *partial, generalized,* and *unclassified.* In generalized seizures, the excessive electrical activity affects both sides of the brain. In partial seizures, also called *focal* or *local* seizures, activity begins in one part of the brain, but these seizures may occasionally evolve into generalized ones. See Chapter 6 for a detailed description of epilepsy.

Cardiovascular System Disorders

Among the most significant congenital disorders of the cardiovascular system are those affecting the heart. To understand these disorders, one must first understand the structure and function of the fetal heart.

The fetus does not need its lungs to breathe, because the placenta provides for the exchange of oxygen and carbon dioxide, as well as nutrients and wastes, through maternal circulation. Therefore, most fetal blood is not circulated through the lungs. The route that blood takes as it flows though the heart of a fetus is different from the route it takes in an individual after birth. In a fetus, blood returns to the heart by entering the right atrium. Nearly two-thirds of it then flows into the left atrium through an opening called the foramen ovale. From there, blood flows into the left ventricle and out through the aorta. Only about one-third of the blood that enters the right atrium flows down into the right ventricle and then out through the pulmonary artery. Instead of going to the lungs, most of it is shunted through the ductus arteriosus into the aorta.

Shortly after birth, the umbilical cord is clamped and the infant is separated from the placenta. This is also when the infant's first breaths are taken. These things bring about a change in circulation. A greater amount of blood now flows to the lungs, where it picks up oxygen. The ductus arteriosus no longer serves a purpose, and it begins to constrict and seal shut. As larger amounts of blood flow into the left atrium from the lungs, the increased pressure causes the septum primum, a one-way flap, to close over the foramen ovale. This in turn causes all blood returning to the right atrium to flow down to the right ventricle and on to the lungs through the pulmonary artery. If any of these processes fails to occur, the infant will develop congenital heart disease. Common forms include atrial septal defect, ventricular septal defect, patent ductus arteriosus, tetralogy of Fallot, and hemophilia.

Flashpoint

Fetal circulation is quite different from that of other individuals; most of the blood bypasses the lungs.

Atrial Septal Defect

ICD-9-CM: 745.5   [ICD-10: Q21.1]

An atrial septal defect (ASD) is a condition in which there is a hole between the right and left atria that allows blood flow between the two chambers (see Fig. 16-4). Mostly, oxygenated blood that has just returned to the left atrium from the lungs flows into the right atrium.

Incidence

As many as one in 1,500 infants are born with some degree of ASD. However, many individuals are not symptomatic.

Etiology

Atrial septal defects are caused by an absence of atrial septal tissue that leaves a hole between the right and left atria. ASDs are present from birth and often have no identifiable cause. Because of the additional blood flow back to the right atrium, the right side of the heart becomes overworked and gradually enlarges in an attempt to manage the extra volume. However, it was never meant to do so; the hypertrophy (excessive growth) causes it to eventually weaken. In addition, the extra blood flow from the right side of the heart back through the lungs can cause pulmonary hypertension.

Patent foramen ovale is a type of ASD in which the foramen ovale fails to close normally when the individual first breathes shortly after birth. When the patient has a large ASD, the increased blood flow to the right side of the heart and the right-sided heart enlargement that occurs will eventually cause pressure within the right side of the heart to exceed pressure within the left side of the heart. If this occurs, the direction of blood flow through the ASD reverses and blood is shunted from the right atrium into the left atrium. This phenomenon causes low-oxygen blood to bypass the lungs and move directly to the left side of the heart, from where it is pumped out to the body. Because this blood is low in oxygen, the individual begins to show signs and symptoms of hypoxemia (low blood oxygen).

Some conditions are known to be associated with, or contribute to, ASD. Down syndrome is an example. Other risk factors include maternal rubella (German measles) during pregnancy, poorly managed maternal diabetes, and maternal abuse of alcohol or other substances.

> **Flashpoint**
>
> Atrial septal defects are caused by an absence of atrial septal tissue that leaves a hole between the right and left atria.

Signs and Symptoms

Individuals with very small atrial septal defects may never have any symptoms. Others may be symptom free during infancy but begin showing signs and symptoms during adulthood. Infants who are symptomatic may feed poorly, fail to grow normally, or show signs of heart failure. Individuals with severe or worsening conditions may have dyspnea, fatigue, edema of the abdomen or lower extremities, frequent respiratory infections, and heart palpitations.

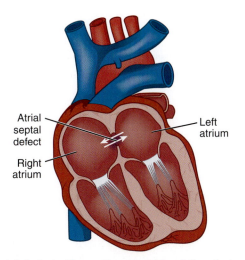

FIGURE 16-4 An atrial septal defect allows abnormal blood flow between the upper chambers of the heart.

Diagnosis

Diagnosis is sometimes possible prenatally through ultrasonography. Otherwise, it may be first suspected at a later time, when the health-care provider notes a heart murmur upon auscultation of the patient's heart with a stethoscope. A variety of radiological tests may be done to confirm diagnosis; the most common is an echocardiogram (see Box 16-3). Other tests may include chest x-ray, electrocardiography (ECG), coronary angiography, Doppler studies, MRI, and cardiac catheterization. In the latter test, a long, flexible catheter (tube) is inserted into the heart through a large artery near the groin or in the arm. Combining this procedure with radiological imaging allows the physician to visualize moving heart structures, including the chambers, valves, and coronary vessels. It also allows the physician to measure blood pressure within the heart and lungs.

Treatment

Approximately 50% of ASDs will close on their own. Therefore, health-care providers may opt to monitor infants with ASD who are asymptomatic or whose symptoms are mild. During this time, medication may be used to manage symptoms, including beta blockers and inotropics to keep the heartbeat strong and regular, diuretics to minimize fluid overload, and anticoagulants to reduce the risk of complications from formation of blood clots. If the ASD has not closed by early childhood, and especially if the patient is symptomatic, surgical correction is done. This may be done through cardiac catheterization or open heart surgery. In either case, some technique such as the placement of a patch or sutures (stitches) is done to close the hole in the atrial septum.

Flashpoint

Approximately half of ASDs will close on their own.

Prognosis

Prognosis for individuals with an ASD varies according to the severity of the condition and the timeliness of intervention. Complications associated with ASDs include heart failure, abnormal heart rhythms, stroke, pulmonary hypertension, and permanent lung damage. For those who require surgical correction, prognosis is best when intervention occurs before age 25, before permanent damage has occurred. Later correction may still be beneficial, but it is controversial because of a much higher incidence of complications. Having ASD or heart and lung damage caused by ASD increases risks for some women during pregnancy.

Ventricular Septal Defect
ICD-9-CM: 745.4   [ICD-10: Q21.0]

A ventricular septal defect (VSD), also called an *interventricular septal defect* and sometimes called a *hole in the heart*, is a condition in which there are one or more holes in the septal wall that separates the right and left ventricles (see Fig. 16-5).

Flashpoint

VSDs are among the most common congenital heart defects.

Incidence

VSDs are among the most common congenital heart defects and are estimated to account for up to 30% of all congenital heart problems.

Box 16-3 Diagnostic Spotlight

ECHOCARDIOGRAM

An echocardiogram is a test that employs sound waves to create a video image of the heart. It can also create cross-sectional slices of the heart, which allows close inspection of valves, chambers, and blood vessels. The test can be done in a hospital or clinic. Patient preparation is simple and generally requires only undressing the upper half of the body, although the patient can wear a gown or drape for privacy. Electrodes are applied to the patient's chest and shoulders. This allows an electrocardiogram to be recorded during the test. A clear gel is applied to the chest and the transducer is placed over it. The technician then makes several recordings from different views. The patient may be instructed to change positions and to hold the breath at various times. The video that is created is then examined by the physician.

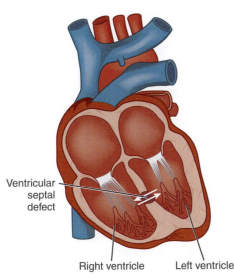

Ventricular septal defect

Right ventricle   **Left ventricle**

FIGURE 16-5 A ventricular septal defect allows abnormal blood flow between the right and left ventricles.

Etiology

Early in its development, the lower portion of the fetal heart is comprised of just one chamber. As it develops further, the septal wall forms, separating the right and left ventricles. In infants born with a VSD, the septal wall fails to completely develop, leaving a hole between the chambers. The exact reason this happens is not clear but genetic factors are thought to play a role, since women with VSDs have an increased chance of having an infant with a VSD. This condition causes shunting of oxygenated blood from the left ventricle into the right ventricle, from where it passes out through the pulmonary artery to the lungs and back to the left ventricle. As a result, the heart is overworked and the lungs become congested with too much blood flow, causing pulmonary hypertension and heart failure. Some conditions are known to be associated with, or contribute to, VSDs, such as Down syndrome. Other risk factors include maternal rubella (German measles) during pregnancy, poorly managed maternal diabetes, and maternal abuse of alcohol or other substances.

Signs and Symptoms

Infants with very small VSDs may be completely symptom free. Infants with larger VSDs may appear cyanotic (bluish) due to hypoxemia and may have other symptoms, including dyspnea, tachycardia, pallor (pale color), fatigue, edema of the abdomen or lower extremities, poor feeding, failure to gain weight, and frequent respiratory infections. Older children with VSDs may exhibit decreased energy and may tire quickly with physical exertion.

Diagnosis

Diagnosis of a VSD is often suspected when the health-care provider notes the infant's heart murmur. Diagnosis is confirmed with echocardiogram. Other tests may include chest x-ray, ECG, and MRI. Rarely, cardiac catheterization may be done to help determine whether the infant needs surgery.

Treatment

Infants with small VSDs may require no treatment, since the VSD often closes on its own. Mild symptoms may be managed with medications to increase the pumping strength of the heart and reduce fluid volume. Infants may also benefit from supplemental feeding with high-calorie formula or feeding through a nasogastric tube. This is especially beneficial in infants who feed poorly due to fatigue. If symptoms are severe, or if the septal opening fails to close, surgical correction is indicated. Open heart surgery is usually done to close the hole with a patch or sutures.

Prognosis

Individuals with very small VSDs may lead normal, symptom-free lives. Patients with moderate or large VSDs may suffer complications related to heart failure. These include

Flashpoint
A VSD often closes on its own.

poor physical growth and development, increased incidence of lung infections, bacterial heart infection, pulmonary hypertension, stroke, and hypoxemia. Women with untreated VSDs may be advised to avoid pregnancy, as it increases the risk of these complications.

Patent Ductus Arteriosus
ICD-9-CM: 747.0   [ICD-10 : Q25.0]

Patent ductus arteriosus (PDA) is a condition in which the ductus arteriosus, normally present in the fetus, fails to close within 10 days after birth. As a result, blood continues to flow abnormally between the pulmonary artery and the aorta (see Fig. 16-6).

Incidence

PDAs are present in 20% to 60% of premature infants but are much less common in full-term newborns.

Etiology

The ductus arteriosus serves a useful purpose in the fetus by shunting blood from the pulmonary artery directly into the aorta, thereby allowing most blood to bypass the lungs. Shortly after birth, this connection normally closes so that blood can circulate through the lungs to eliminate carbon dioxide and pick up oxygen. In patent ductus arteriosus, the connection between these two vessels remains patent (open and functioning), and because pressure is much higher in the aorta after birth, blood flow through the connection is now reversed. Already-oxygenated blood flows from the aorta back into the pulmonary artery and back again to the lungs.

Exactly what causes a PDA is not clear. However, it is known to occur more commonly among premature infants and those with low birth weight. Other potential contributors include maternal rubella (German measles) during pregnancy, high altitude, and other genetic disorders, such as Down syndrome. Infants of a parent with a congenital heart defect have up to a 20% chance of being born with a heart defect. Increased pressure from too much blood circulating through the lungs causes pulmonary hypertension.

Signs and Symptoms

Infants with a small PDA may be free of symptoms. Those with large PDAs experience fatigue, poor feeding and poor weight gain, tachycardia, dyspnea, cyanosis, and frequent lung infections. Over time they develop finger clubbing. They also have a murmur that is heard when the physician auscultates the infant's heart.

Diagnosis

Infants with a PDA often have a specific type of heart murmur that may lead the physician to suspect the diagnosis. It is confirmed with an echocardiogram. Other tests may include chest x-ray and ECG.

Flashpoint

PDAs are common in premature infants.

Flashpoint

Patients with a PDA may develop finger clubbing and a heart murmur.

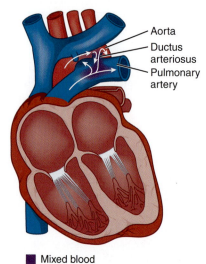

■ Mixed blood

FIGURE 16-6 Patent ductus arteriosus allows abnormal blood flow between the pulmonary artery and the aorta.

Treatment

In newborns with a PDA, the condition usually resolves on its own as the ductus arteriosus closes within several weeks of birth. This is also true for most premature infants, although closure may take longer. When treatment is required, NSAIDs may be used. They act by impeding the action of prostaglandin, a hormonelike substance produced by the body that acts to keep the ductus arteriosus open. If medication does not work or is not a good option for the patient, surgical repair may be done, either through a long catheter device inserted into the PDA site through a vessel near the groin or as an open surgery. The latter involves an incision between the ribs near the PDA site. In either case, the PDA is then closed with one of several techniques, such as sutures or a metal clip.

Prognosis

Prognosis for patients with a PDA is variable and depends upon the size of the PDA and the initiation of treatment. Individuals with a small PDA may never become symptomatic and may do fine without treatment. However, those with moderate to large PDAs will develop heart problems without treatment, including heart failure, bacterial endocarditis (infection of the inner lining of the heart), defective lung development, pulmonary hypertension, and heart arrhythmias. The mortality rate is high for these people: 20% by age 20, with increasing incidence as individuals continue to age. Women with a PDA may be advised to avoid pregnancy because of the increased risk of complications.

Tetralogy of Fallot
ICD-9-CM: 745.2   [ICD-10: Q21.3]

Tetralogy of Fallot is a condition in which an infant is born with a group of four different heart defects: a large ventricular septal defect, an overriding aorta (aorta arises from both ventricles), pulmonic stenosis that causes obstruction of outflow from the right ventricle, and hypertrophy of the right ventricle (see Fig. 16-7). Other abnormalities are also frequently present. As a result of these defects, the infant has bluish coloring from poor oxygen delivery to the body.

Incidence

Tetralogy of Fallot is uncommon, occurring in five of every 10,000 infants born. It accounts for up to 10% of all congenital heart defects.

Etiology

Tetralogy of Fallot includes the following four structural defects:

- ***Ventricular septal defect***: a condition in which there are one or more holes in the septal wall that separates the right and left ventricles. This allows a right-to-left shunt, in which oxygen-poor blood from the right ventricle flows into the left ventricle and mixes with

Flashpoint
The mortality rate is high for individuals with a large PDA.

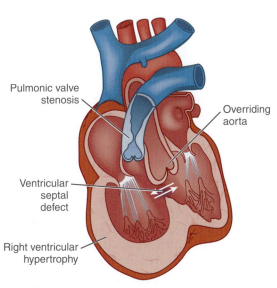
Flashpoint
Tetralogy of Fallot includes four different structural defects.

Pulmonic valve stenosis

Overriding aorta

Ventricular septal defect

Right ventricular hypertrophy

FIGURE 16-7 Tetralogy of Fallot

oxygen-rich blood. This diminishes the supply of oxygen delivered to the body. The condition may also allow a left-to-right shunt, in which blood from the left ventricle flows into the right ventricle. This blood, which has already circulated through the lungs, does so again, causing an inefficient increase in the heart's workload.

- **Pulmonic stenosis**: a condition in which the pulmonic valve, which serves as the exit point between the right ventricle and the lungs, is thickened and narrowed. This condition decreases blood flow to the lungs.
- **Overriding aorta**: a condition in which a malpositioned aorta is connected to both ventricles rather than just the left ventricle. This allows oxygen-poor blood to mix with oxygenated blood and flow out to the body.
- **Right ventricular hypertrophy**: a condition in which the right ventricular walls become thicker than normal as a result of higher blood pressure than normal within the chamber. Eventually this causes the heart walls to stiffen and weaken.

The exact cause of these defects is not known. However, multiple risk factors have been identified. They include maternal viral illness during pregnancy, such as rubella; prenatal malnutrition; and maternal alcohol abuse, diabetes, or advanced age (over 40). Genetics also are a factor, as indicated by the increased incidence of infants with congenital heart defects born to parents with congenital heart defects, as well as a high incidence of chromosomal disorders among these infants. Examples include DiGeorge syndrome and Down syndrome. The ultimate result of these defects is that less oxygen-rich blood is delivered to the body.

Signs and Symptoms

Infants born with tetralogy of Fallot may initially be symptom free. However, as symptoms begin to appear, infants will demonstrate poor feeding, poor growth and development, irritability, and easy fatigue. These infants have a harsh heart murmur and over time will develop fingernail clubbing. Physical stress from simple activities such as crying, defecating, kicking the legs, or playing may trigger **tet spells.** These are episodes in which the infant's arterial oxygen level drops, stimulating the respiratory center to increase the rate and depth of respirations. Unfortunately, this increases blood return to the right ventricle, which increases the heart's workload. Resistance to blood flow to the lungs, caused by pulmonic stenosis, causes even more oxygen-poor blood to flow out to the body through the overriding aorta; a vicious cycle ensues. Symptoms of tet spells include sudden, severe cyanosis; dyspnea; prolonged crying; and irritability. Severe spells can lead to seizures, stroke, and death. These spells are most common in young infants but can occur in older children, who may be observed assuming a squatting position to improve circulation to the lungs.

Flashpoint

During tet spells the infant's arterial oxygen level drops.

Diagnosis

Diagnosis of tetralogy of Fallot may be suspected based upon the infant's symptoms and the presence of a heart murmur. It is confirmed by echocardiography, although other tests, such as chest x-ray, cardiac catheterization, and ECG, may also be done. Blood tests may identify erythrocytosis, an abnormal increase in the number of red blood cells, as the body attempts to increase the oxygen-carrying capacity of the blood.

Treatment

Treatment of tet spells includes positioning the infant in a knee-chest position and administering morphine. If needed, medication may also be given to increase blood pressure. One or more surgeries are usually done within the first year to correct the heart defects. These include procedures to close the VSD and widen or replace the stenosed pulmonic valve. Preventive treatment with antimicrobial medications may also be recommended before any dental or surgical procedures, to reduce the risk of endocarditis.

Prognosis

Prognosis for infants born with tetralogy of Fallot depends upon the severity of the heart defects and the timeliness of treatment. Those who receive treatment have a 90% to 97% rate of surviving to adulthood and leading healthy, active lives. Those who do not receive treatment are at high risk of serious complications, including heart arrhythmias, delayed development, stroke, seizures, endocarditis, disability, and death. Their mortality rate is 45% by 5 years of age and 70% by 10 years of age. Few survive to age 20.

Hemophilia

ICD-9-CM: 286.0 (hemophilia A, factor VIII disorder), 286.1 (hemophilia B, factor IX disorder)

[ICD-10: D66 (hemophilia A, factor VIII disorder), D67 (hemophilia B, factor IX disorder)]

Hemophilia is a group of hereditary disorders characterized by easy or prolonged bleeding. The most common types are A and B. Hemophilia A, sometimes called *classical hemophilia* or *factor VIII deficiency*, is the most common type. It may be mild, moderate, or severe. Hemophilia B is sometimes called *Christmas disease* or *factor IX deficiency*.

Incidence

Hemophilia is uncommon and affects approximately 15,000 to 30,000 Americans. Type A is about five times more common than type B. Both types affect males of all races.

Etiology

Hemophilia A and B are usually inherited and are passed from parent to child as an X-linked recessive disorder. This means that it is attached to the X chromosome and is passed from a female carrier to her son (see Fig. 16-8). In some cases there is no family history of hemophilia, and the disease is thought to result from a genetic mutation. The normal blood-clotting process involves platelets and a number of plasma proteins called clotting factors. Patients with hemophilia A are deficient in factor VIII, while those with hemophilia B are deficient in factor IX.

Signs and Symptoms

Patients with hemophilia experience bruising and bleeding that is more prolonged than normal. If the condition is mild, excessive bleeding may only be noticed after the individual suffers a serious injury or has surgery. Those with moderate or severe hemophilia may also experience ***spontaneous bleeding episodes*** that have no identifiable cause. These episodes, which occur most frequently in those with severe hemophilia, often affect joints such as the knees, ankles, and elbows, as well as muscles. Patients may complain of tightness in joints and may also notice blood in their urine or feces.

> **Flashpoint**
> Hemophilia is a group of hereditary bleeding disorders.

> **Flashpoint**
> Spontaneous bleeding, often into the joints and muscles, may occur for no identifiable reason.

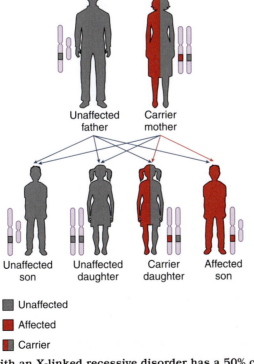

Unaffected father Carrier mother

Unaffected son Unaffected daughter Carrier daughter Affected son

■ Unaffected
■ Affected
■ Carrier

FIGURE 16-8 A woman with an X-linked recessive disorder has a 50% chance of having affected sons and a 50% chance of having daughters who are unaffected carriers.

Diagnosis

Prenatal testing can be done on the fetus if there is a known family history of hemophilia. Chorionic villus sampling can be done at 9 to 11 weeks' gestation (see Box 16-4). Fetal blood sampling can be done at 18 weeks or later. Testing of a blood sample from any individual allows the measurement of various clotting factors.

Treatment

Treatment of minor injuries, such as scrapes and small lacerations, is the same for patients with hemophilia as for other individuals. The wound is cleaned and an adhesive bandage or dressing is applied. Pressure is applied as needed until the bleeding stops. Patients with more severe injuries are given a replacement of the deficient clotting factor. Some individuals are advised to receive regular factor replacement, to prevent hemorrhage from trauma and spontaneous bleeding. Patients with hemophilia A may also use a synthetic hormone called desmopressin acetate that stimulates the release of factor VIII. Some patients may benefit from physical therapy to preserve or improve joint mobility. Education for patients with hemophilia should focus on strategies to prevent injury and control bleeding (see Box 16-5).

Prognosis

There is no cure for hemophilia. Prognosis and life expectancy depend upon the type and severity of the condition and upon the quality of the patient's self-care and medical care. With good care, most individuals can lead productive, active lives. Complications are possible, however, and include bleeding into the joints (leading to arthritis) and bleeding in the brain (hemorrhagic

---

Box 16-4 Diagnostic Spotlight

CHORIONIC VILLUS SAMPLING

Chorionic villus sampling (CVS) is a procedure in which the physician inserts a biopsy catheter through the vagina and cervix to collect a small portion of the chorionic villi, the vascular projections from the chorion that form the fetal portion of the placenta. Microscopic and chemical examination of the sample evaluates the chromosomal, enzymatic, and DNA status of the fetus. If it is necessary, the physician performs this procedure at 8 to 12 weeks' gestation. CVS is not a routine procedure, because it is more invasive than amniocentesis. A woman who has previously experienced miscarriage or given birth to a baby with chromosomal abnormalities is considered at high risk and therefore may require CVS.

Box 16-5 Wellness Promotion

PREVENTIVE CARE FOR PATIENTS WITH HEMOPHILIA

Patients with hemophilia can reduce the risk of bruising and bleeding by following these guidelines:

- Exercise regularly with low-impact, noncontact activities, such as swimming and walking.
- Wear helmets, safety belts, and padding appropriate to selected activities.
- Avoid medications that prolong bleeding time unless they are specifically prescribed by a physician. Examples include aspirin, NSAIDs, anticoagulants, antiplatelet medications, and some herbal supplements.
- Practice regular dental hygiene using a soft-bristle toothbrush.
- Inspect the home for potential injury hazards (loose rugs, cords, etc.).
- Install safety items in the home and workplace to reduce injury risk. Examples include adequate lighting, handrails, and safety bars.

stroke). Those with severe hemophilia may experience spontaneous bleeding as often as once or twice a week.

Musculoskeletal System Disorders

Many disorders of the musculoskeletal system are congenital. Their causes are not always clear. In some cases a genetic cause is implicated, while in others, toxic exposures or injury before or during birth may contribute.

Duchenne Muscular Dystrophy and Becker Muscular Dystrophy
ICD-9-CM: 359.1   [ICD-10: G71.0] (hereditary progressive for both codes)

Muscular dystrophy is a group of genetic disorders that cause progressive muscle weakness. Duchenne muscular dystrophy (DMD) is also called *pseudohypertrophic muscular dystrophy*. Becker muscular dystrophy (BMD) is a less severe form that affects older individuals. Both are named after the physicians who first described them.

Incidence

DMD and BMD nearly always affect boys. DMD is the most common type in children and affects very young boys, around ages 2 to 6. BMD affects boys in their adolescence or early adulthood.

Etiology

Duchenne muscular dystrophy is caused by an absence of dystrophin, which is an important protein for muscle structure and functioning. Individuals with Becker muscular dystrophy produce some of this protein, but it is either too little or of poor quality. DMD and BMD are X-linked genetic disorders passed from female carriers to their sons.

Signs and Symptoms

The symptoms of Duchenne and Becker muscular dystrophy are similar. With DMD, symptoms occur as early as age 2. Walking may be delayed and children appear clumsy, fall frequently, and have difficulty rising from lying or sitting. Generalized muscle wasting and weakness first affects voluntary muscles of the shoulders, pelvis, and thighs. The calves may appear enlarged. This can be misleading, because it is caused by fat accumulation rather than muscle development. The child walks with an odd, waddling gait and may walk on his toes or the balls of his feet, with the belly stuck out and shoulders held back (see Fig. 16-9). This is an attempt to maintain balance. He may struggle to raise his arms and will lose the ability to walk around age 7 to 12. Eventually, respiratory and cardiac muscles are affected; patients typically enter the final stages of the disorder in their late teens or early 20s. Approximately one-third of individuals with muscular dystrophy also have learning disabilities.

The course of BMD is similar but slower and less predictable. Consequently, diagnosis may not occur until the patient's late teens or adulthood. The pattern of muscle wasting and loss of functioning is similar to that in DMD, though more variable. These individuals may not lose the ability to walk until their middle or late 30s.

Diagnosis

Diagnosis of muscular dystrophy may be suspected based upon information obtained through an interview of the patient or the patient's parents and through physical examination. Diagnosis is confirmed though a number of tests. Elevated levels of creatine kinase indicate muscle damage. Genetic testing can determine whether individuals are carriers of the disease. Muscle biopsy can identify the presence or absence of dystrophin and help differentiate between various types of dystrophy.

Treatment

There is no cure for muscular dystrophy. However, many forms of treatment are available to prolong life, maximize functioning, and improve comfort. Contractures (tightened ligaments, tendons, muscles, and other tissues around a joint that impede normal motion) are minimized with range-of-motion exercises, physical therapy, occupational therapy, and the use of braces. Severe contractures can be relieved with a surgical procedure to release tendons. Abnormal spinal curvatures, including scoliosis, lordosis, and kyphosis, can be minimized through exercises, positioning, and physical therapy. Spine-straightening surgery may also be done. Corticosteroid medication may

Flashpoint
Muscular dystrophy is a group of genetic disorders that cause progressive muscle weakness.

Flashpoint
Children with muscular dystrophy may appear clumsy and fall frequently.

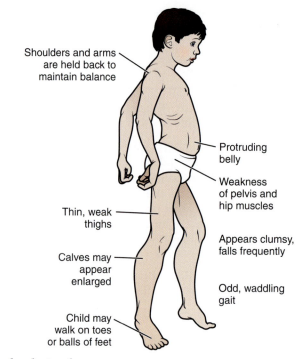

Shoulders and arms are held back to maintain balance

Protruding belly

Weakness of pelvis and hip muscles

Thin, weak thighs

Appears clumsy, falls frequently

Calves may appear enlarged

Odd, waddling gait

Child may walk on toes or balls of feet

FIGURE 16-9 Muscular dystrophy

help to slow the progression of the disorder; side effects of osteoporosis, weight gain, and fluid retention caused by corticosteroids may be minimized with the use of calcium and vitamin D supplements and a low-sodium, low-calorie diet. Braces to support the knees and ankles aid with walking and gait stability. Devices such as wheelchairs, mechanical lifts, and electronic beds are eventually needed. Cardiomyopathy may be treated with angiotensin-converting enzyme inhibitors and beta blockers. Patients who develop severe respiratory compromise may eventually require mechanical ventilation.

Prognosis

Flashpoint

Life expectancy for patients with DMD is low.

The prognosis for patients with muscular dystrophy depends upon the type and severity of the condition and on the patient's access to medical care. Those with DMD often die before the age of 20 and rarely survive past 30. Life expectancy is better for those with BMD; they often survive into their middle or late adult years.

Osteogenesis Imperfecta
ICD-9-CM: 756.51   [ICD-10: Q78.0]

Osteogenesis imperfecta (OI), sometimes called *brittle bone disease*, is a condition in which defective bone development results in bones that are fragile and easily broken. There are many types. Type 1 is the most common and mildest form; type 2 is the most severe.

Flashpoint

Osteogenesis imperfecta literally means imperfect bone formation.

Incidence

OI is estimated to affect 25,000 to 50,000 Americans. Those with milder forms of the disease may not know they have it. OI affects men and women equally and affects members of all racial groups.

Etiology

OI is usually caused by a genetic disease that affects the production of collagen in bones. It is an autosomal dominant disease, which means that only one affected gene, inherited from either parent, will cause the child to have OI. Children of affected parents have a 50% chance of inheriting the disease (see Fig. 16-10). Collagen is a substance that provides strength to many body structures, including bones. In people with OI, the body produces too little collagen or poor-quality collagen. It is also possible for an individual to have a spontaneous mutation and develop OI that was not inherited. In this case, the disease can still be passed on to the person's children.

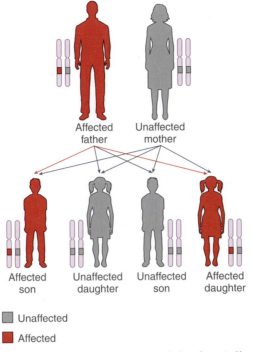

Affected
father

Unaffected
mother

Affected
son

Unaffected
daughter

Unaffected
son

Affected
daughter

☐ Unaffected

■ Affected

FIGURE 16-10 Osteogenesis imperfecta is an autosomal dominant disease, which means that each child of a parent with the disorder has a 50% chance of inheriting the disorder.

Signs and Symptoms

OI is best known for causing brittle, fragile bones that are easily fractured. In the most severe form of OI, type 2, individuals may suffer hundreds of fractures, sometimes even before or during birth. OI also affects other structures within the body; patients may be short in height, with lax joints, blue sclerae (whites of the eyes), scoliosis, brittle teeth, hearing loss, and fragile skin that bruises easily. They may complain of fatigue, muscle weakness, difficulty breathing, and frequent nosebleeds. In some individuals the frequency of bone fracture decreases with maturation during childhood, but it may increase again after menopause in women or age 60 in men.

Diagnosis

OI is occasionally detected prenatally by ultrasound. If the parents are known to have the disorder, genetic testing may be done on the infant before or after birth. In cases where no family history of OI is known, the diagnosis may be made after the young child suffers numerous fractures. Collagen testing or genetic testing is done on skin or blood specimens to confirm the diagnosis.

Flashpoint

Patients with severe OI may suffer hundreds of fractures.

Treatment

There is no cure for OI. Therefore, treatment is focused on preventing complications and minimizing symptoms (see Box 16-6). Fractures are immobilized with splints, braces, casts, traction, or surgical fusion. Pain is treated by application of heat or cold, analgesic medications, nerve blocks (injection of medication into tissue around a nerve), physical therapy, and low-impact exercise such as swimming. Attention to diet, including optimal intake of calcium and vitamin D, helps prevent complications caused by osteoporosis. Some individuals benefit from bisphosphonate medication, which helps increase bone mineralization. Devices such as walkers, canes, and wheelchairs may be used to aid with mobility.

Prognosis

The prognosis for patients with OI depends upon the type and severity of the condition. Those with mild or moderate forms may lead reasonably normal lives; those with severe forms may not. The most severe form of OI often causes death due to respiratory failure or trauma at birth or during infancy.

Box 16-6 Wellness Promotion

HOME CARE OF THE PATIENT WITH OSTEOGENESIS IMPERFECTA

Patients with OI are at very high risk of injury. These guidelines will help to reduce injury and improve quality of life for these patients:

- Don't be afraid to touch the infant with OI, but do so gently.
- Do not lift the patient by grasping the arms, legs, or ankles. Instead, spread your fingers apart and place one hand between the legs and under the buttocks and place the other hand behind the shoulders, neck, and head. This helps to hold the patient securely while spreading the pressure exerted by the hands and fingers.
- Understand that fractures occur very easily; try not to feel guilty when this happens.
- Use an infant car seat that reclines. Add extra foam padding if possible.
- Use a good-quality stroller that is large enough to allow for casts.
- Encourage the patient to participate in physician-approved, safe exercise, such as walking and swimming.
- Avoid the use of tobacco, alcohol, and corticosteroid medications, because they can decrease bone density.
- Keep a copy of the patient's medical records on hand, along with a letter from the primary health-care provider describing the patient's diagnosis.
- If possible, live in a one-level home with no stairs.
- Install handrails in stairwells, around bathtubs and showers, and in any other high-risk areas.
- Install carpeting on all floors.

Flashpoint

The name clubfoot is taken from the sharp angle of the turned foot.

Clubfoot

**ICD-9-CM: 754.70 (unspecified; code [ICD-10: Q66.8]
by affected part of the foot)**

Clubfoot, also known as *talipes*, is a congenital condition in which an otherwise healthy infant is born with one or both feet turned in and downward (see Fig. 16-11). The name is taken from the sharp angle of the turned foot, similar to a golf club.

Incidence

Clubfoot is the most common congenital disorder of the lower extremities. It occurs in approximately one of every 1,000 Americans born. Approximately 50% of cases involve both feet.

Flashpoint

Clubfoot is the most common congenital disorder of the lower extremities.

Etiology

The exact cause of clubfoot is not known. During fetal development, the tendons and ligaments on the back and inside of the foot fail to grow at the same rate as the others.

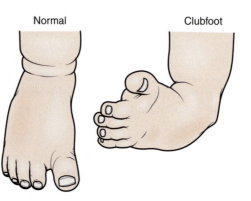

Normal   Clubfoot

FIGURE 16-11 Clubfoot

Consequently, they pull the foot down and inwards. The condition tends to run in families, which indicates a hereditary factor.

Signs and Symptoms
If clubfoot is not corrected, the defect will worsen with time and cause bony changes within the feet. Walking on the outsides of the feet leads to skin breakdown and infection.

Diagnosis
Clubfoot is identified at birth by visual inspection. X-rays may be done to determine the severity. In some cases it may be diagnosed prenatally, based upon ultrasound results.

Treatment
Clubfoot may be corrected through stretching and casting, surgery, or a combination of the two. Correction should occur soon after birth, when reshaping of the foot is most likely to be successful. Braces may also need to be worn full-time for a matter of months, and during sleep for several years.

Prognosis
Prognosis for infants with clubfoot is usually very good if appropriate treatment occurs. There is approximately a 25% chance of recurrence within the first year. If this happens, treatment is needed again. Untreated, the condition impairs mobility and may impair normal development of the calf muscles.

Congenital Hip Dysplasia
ICD-9-CM: 754.3   [ICD-10: Q65.2]
Congenital hip dysplasia is also called *congenital dislocation of the hip* and *developmental dislocation of the hip (DDH)*. It is a condition in which an infant is born with an abnormally developed hip that is unstable and partially or totally dislocated (see Fig. 16-12).

Incidence
Congenital hip dysplasia occurs in about one of every 1,000 infants born. A much larger number of newborns may have some initial hip instability, but it usually corrects itself within 1 or 2 weeks. The condition is more common among Native Americans, Sami, and Caucasians than other racial groups.

Etiology
The hip joint comprises the rounded head, or top, of the femur sitting within the socket, a rounded pocket formed by bones of the pelvic girdle. In congenital hip dysplasia, the socket is usually shallower than normal and the ligaments that help to provide joint stability are laxer (looser) than normal. The exact cause of this disorder is not known, but genetics appear to play a role. Other risk factors include female gender, first born, and breech delivery, in which the infant is born with the feet or buttocks first.

> **Flashpoint**
> Congenital hip dysplasia is a condition in which an infant is born with a partially or totally dislocated hip.

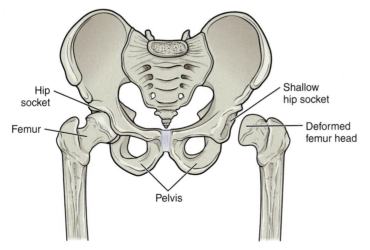

FIGURE 16-12 **Congenital hip dysplasia**

Signs and Symptoms

An infant with congenital hip dysplasia may exhibit no symptoms. However, examination reveals that the affected leg appears shorter, may be more externally rotated (turned outward), and has uneven fat folds, compared with the other leg.

Diagnosis

Diagnosis of congenital hip dysplasia commonly occurs when the newborn undergoes physical examination. The physician routinely maneuvers the infant's hips and notes the presence of any abnormal "pops" or "clunks," as well as whether the hip is easily dislocated. This is usually done by applying gentle pressure while moving the hips in the Barlow and Ortolani maneuvers (see Box 16-7). Diagnosis may be confirmed with hip x-rays.

Treatment

Congenital hip dysplasia is treated by the application of splints or casts to keep the legs abducted (apart) and turned outward, in a "frog-leg" position. As the infant grows, the joint further develops and stabilizes. If this form of treatment is not successful, surgery may be performed.

Prognosis

Prognosis for infants with congenital hip dysplasia is very good if the condition is noted and treated early. The later that diagnosis and treatment occur, the more likely it is that surgery will be needed. Without treatment, the patient is at risk of arthritis and disabling deterioration of the hip.

Box 16-7 Diagnostic Spotlight

BARLOW AND ORTOLANI MANEUVERS

The Barlow and Ortolani maneuvers are standard examination techniques used together for identifying hip dysplasia in newborns. For them to be successfully performed, the infant must be relaxed. The examiner holds the infant's hips flexed at 90 degrees, with thumbs on the inner upper thigh and fingers over the greater trochanter.

Barlow Maneuver

The examiner adducts the hip and pushes the thigh posteriorly (backwards). If the hip easily dislocates, the test is positive. The Ortolani maneuver is then performed to relocate the hip.

Ortolani Maneuver

The examiner holds the infant's opposite hip still and gently abducts and pulls anteriorly (forward) on the hip being tested. If the hip is unstable, it may cause a palpable or audible clunk as the head of the femur relocates into the hip socket.

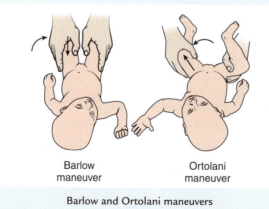

Barlow
maneuver

Ortolani
maneuver

Barlow and Ortolani maneuvers

Urinary System Disorders

Many disorders of the urinary system are congenital. The causes are not always clear. In some cases a genetic cause is implicated, while in others, toxic exposures or injury before or during birth may contribute.

Wilms Tumor
ICD-9-CM: 189.0   [ICD-10: C64]

A Wilms tumor, also known as a *nephroblastoma*, is a rapidly growing type of kidney cancer that most commonly affects children. Usually only one kidney is cancerous. See Chapter 17 for a detailed description of a Wilms tumor.

Reproductive System Disorders

Some disorders of the reproductive system are congenital. The causes are not always clear. However, a genetic cause is sometimes implicated. Other causes include toxic exposures or injury before or during birth.

Cryptorchidism
ICD-9-CM: 752.51   [ICD-10: Q53.9]

Cryptorchidism is a condition in which one or both testicles have not descended into the scrotum prior to birth (see Fig. 16-13).

Incidence

Approximately 3% to 4% of American males are born with cryptorchidism. The incidence increases to 30% among premature infants. It is also increased among individuals who have an immediate family member with this disorder, babies with low birth weight, and twins.

Etiology

The testicles develop within the abdomen of the male fetus. Between 28 and 40 weeks' gestation, they normally descend through the inguinal canal into the scrotum. This provides an environment that is slightly cooler than normal body temperature and is more conducive to sperm

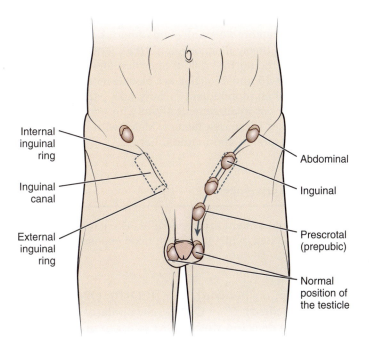

FIGURE 16-13 Cryptorchidism

production. The mechanisms that cause testicular descent are not fully understood but are thought to include maturation and development of the epididymis, hormonal influences, and pressure within the abdomen. The cause of cryptorchidism is not clearly understood but is thought to be related to some interference with these normal mechanisms. Risk factors associated with this condition include abnormalities of the abdominal wall, maternal alcohol abuse, maternal diabetes, and maternal exposure to cigarette smoke or pesticides. Maternal caffeine exposure (more than three cups of coffee per day) has also been implicated.

A condition that may be confused with cryptorchidism is testicular retraction. In this condition, the cremaster muscle reflexively contracts and withdraws the testis (or testes) from the scrotum. This condition usually resolves by puberty and rarely requires treatment. Other uncommon conditions that may be confused with cryptorchidism are anorchism (completely absent testicle) and ectopic testicle, which is malposition of a testicle in an area outside the normal descent pathway, such as the suprapubic area or femoral canal.

Signs and Symptoms

The primary defining indicator that an infant has cryptorchidism is the absence of one or both testicles within the scrotal sac.

Diagnosis

Diagnosis of cryptorchidism is based upon physical-examination findings that reveal an absent testicle. Further examination may reveal the testicle within the inguinal canal. However, in some cases the testicle is nonpalpable, and further diagnostic testing may be necessary to determine its exact location. This may include pelvic ultrasound or MRI, both of which are generally safe, noninvasive procedures. In some cases genetic testing is necessary to identify or rule out other genetic disorders.

Treatment

Most infants with cryptorchidism do not require treatment, since the condition often corrects itself within several months. However, if the testicle has not properly descended by the time the infant is 4 to 6 months old, treatment is needed. Hormonal therapy may include injections of human chorionic gonadotropin over a 5-week period. This causes testicular descent in up to 50% of children but is rarely effective after the child is 2 years old. Orchidopexy (surgical fixation of a testicle) is done to correctly place and anchor the testicle within the scrotum and close the inguinal canal. In some cases, laparoscopy is first needed to locate the testicle hidden within the abdomen.

Flashpoint

Most infants with cryptorchidism do not require treatment.

Prognosis

The prognosis for boys with cryptorchidism depends upon the underlying cause. In most cases the prognosis is good, if timely diagnosis and treatment occur. Males with cryptorchidism have eleven times the normal risk of later developing testicular cancer, which generally occurs between the ages of 15 and 45. They are also at increased risk of impaired fertility. Risk is greater with bilateral cryptorchidism—nearly 40%—than with unilateral cryptorchidism, at 10%. Experts are not in agreement about whether corrective treatment of the disorder during infancy reduces these risk factors. Males with cryptorchidism also have an increased incidence of testicular torsion and inguinal hernia.

Gastrointestinal System Disorders

Many disorders of the gastrointestinal system are congenital. The causes are not always clear: In some cases a genetic cause is implicated, while in others, toxic exposures or injury before or during birth may contribute.

Cleft Lip and Cleft Palate

ICD-9-CM: 749.10 (cleft lip, unspecified),   [ICD-10: Q36.1 (cleft lip, median),
749.00 (cleft palate, unspecified)   Q35.9 (cleft palate, unspecified)]

Flashpoint

Cleft lip and cleft palate often occur together.

Cleft lip is a congenital birth defect in which there is a gap in the upper lip (see Fig. 16-14). Cleft palate is a congenital birth defect in which there is a gap in the roof of the mouth (see Fig. 16-15). Some infants have only one or the other, while some have a combination of cleft lip and cleft palate.

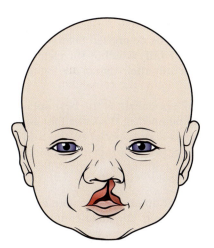

FIGURE 16-14 Cleft lip

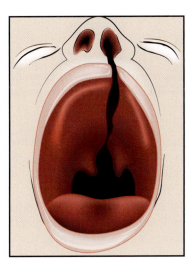

FIGURE 16-15 Cleft palate

Incidence

It is estimated that nearly 7,000 infants are born each year in the United States with oral clefts. Approximately 60% of these have a combination of cleft lip and cleft palate; the other 40% have one or the other. The incidence among Asians is twice that of Caucasians. Males are affected more often than females.

Etiology

The cleft, or opening, results when the tissues that comprise the upper lip and the roof of the mouth fail to fuse during the seventh to 12th week of fetal development. The opening can range in size from a small notch to a cleft that extends into the base of the nostril. The risk of an infant being born with either cleft lip or cleft palate increases with the number of affected relatives and the severity of those relatives' clefts. Environmental factors that increase risk of both disorders include maternal cigarette smoking, alcohol use, antiseizure medication, and deficiencies of folate and folic acid.

Signs and Symptoms

Cleft lip can appear as a small notch or a vertical groove, with varying degrees of lip deformation. Clefts may be bilateral or unilateral. Infants with cleft lip or cleft palate have difficulty feeding due to a lack of ability to create the pressure in the mouth that is necessary for swallowing. Infants with cleft palate may regurgitate milk through their noses when feeding. They are also prone to frequent ear infections, deficits in speech development, and dental problems.

Diagnosis

Many cases of cleft lip and cleft palate can be diagnosed before birth by ultrasound; others are diagnosed at birth. Genetic testing may identify whether the cleft is associated with other genetic conditions and can also help parents identify their risk of having other children with a cleft defect.

Treatment

Plastic surgery coordinated by a team of specialists is the best option for correcting both types of facial cleft. More than one surgery may be needed; if so, the first is done when the infant is around 3 months old. Parents are advised about special bottles and nipples that can be used to aid in feeding before the surgery. Speech therapy is commonly needed later in life, as is orthodontic care.

Flashpoint

Bottles with special nipples can be used until the infant undergoes surgery.

Prognosis

The prognosis for patients with cleft lip and cleft palate depends upon the severity of the defects and the timeliness of treatment. The most common complication that occurs before surgical correction is feeding problems, because the lips cannot completely close around a nipple to create suction. Other problems include frequent ear infections, hearing loss, impaired tooth development, deficits in speech and language, and emotional and behavioral problems.

Pyloric Stenosis
ICD-9-CM: 750.5   [ICD-10: Q40.0]

Pyloric stenosis is also known as *congenital hypertrophic pyloric stenosis* and *gastric outlet obstruction*. It is a condition in which the walls of the pyloric sphincter (exit of the stomach) are thickened and the opening is narrowed (see Fig. 16-16). This impedes the passing of food from the stomach into the duodenum.

Incidence

The incidence of pyloric stenosis is estimated at three per 1,000 live births. This condition is more common among Caucasians than other racial groups and is four times more common in males than in females. Patients with pyloric stenosis are usually infants under 3 weeks of age.

Etiology

Pyloric stenosis occurs when the muscle layers of the pylorus, the structure that serves as the exit from the stomach, become hypertrophied (thickened) and lengthened. The stomach may also become dilated. The exact cause of pyloric stenosis is not fully understood; however, heredity and environment are thought to play a role.

Flashpoint

Infants with pyloric stenosis often have projectile vomiting.

Signs and Symptoms

Signs and symptoms common to patients with pyloric stenosis include projectile (forceful) vomiting after feeding, belching, abdominal pain, hunger, dehydration, weight loss, malnutrition, diarrhea, lethargy, and wavelike motion of the abdomen before vomiting.

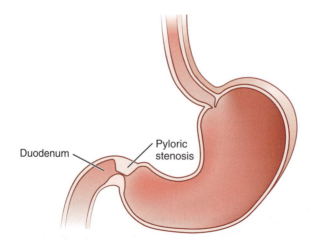

Duodenum

Pyloric stenosis

FIGURE 16-16 Pyloric stenosis

Diagnosis

Diagnosis is suspected from the pattern of vomiting and other signs, as well as physical-assessment findings. When palpating (feeling) the infant's abdomen, the physician may note an olive-shaped lump caused by the enlarged pylorus. Blood tests may reveal electrolyte abnormalities. Radiological testing may include ultrasonography and barium x-ray. Occasionally, an upper endoscopy is done.

Treatment

Treatment of patients with pyloric stenosis involves IV replacement of fluids and electrolytes, if dehydration is severe. If the infant's parents refuse consent for surgery or if the infant is a poor surgical candidate, medical management may be offered with either oral or IV atropine. This intervention will sometimes cause the pyloric hypertrophy to diminish. In most cases, however, surgery is considered the best form of treatment. A pyloromyotomy is a procedure in which the physician splits the overdeveloped muscles of the pyloric sphincter; it can be done either laparoscopically or through open surgery. Occasionally dilation is done with a balloon, but this is not usually as effective.

Prognosis

Prognosis for patients with pyloric stenosis is generally very good, since surgery is curative. Most infants can be taken home after 2 days. Untreated pyloric stenosis can lead to jaundice, severe dehydration, malnutrition, and possibly death. Complications of surgery can include infection and bleeding.

Meckel Diverticulum
ICD-9-CM: 751.0   [ICD-10: Q43.0]

Meckel diverticulum is a congenital condition in which there is a small sac or pouch, called a diverticulum, in the wall of the distal portion of the small intestine. It contains remnants of pancreatic or gastric (stomach) tissue.

Flashpoint

Memory tip: Meckel diverticulum involves two types of tissue, in 2% of people, around 2 years of age, males two times more than females.

Incidence

Meckel diverticulum occurs in 2% to 3% of the population, affecting males more often than females.

Etiology

Meckel diverticulum is caused by remnants of fetal gastric or pancreatic tissue that was misplaced within the distal ileum during development. This tissue may produce gastric acids or pancreatic enzymes that begin to erode the nearby intestinal wall, causing symptoms.

Signs and Symptoms

Many individuals with Meckel diverticulum have no symptoms. When signs and symptoms occur, they include gastrointestinal obstruction, rectal bleeding, diverticulitis, and the development of tumors. Symptoms usually occur during the first several years of life but may also occur later.

Diagnosis

A radiological scan called a technetium-99m pertechnetate scan, also called a Meckel scan, may be done. It involves intravenous injection of a radioactive substance that shows up under radiological imaging and identifies the presence of gastric tissue within the diverticulum. Other tests may include radionuclide scan, CT with oral contrast, flat and upright abdominal x-rays, and colonoscopy. If rectal bleeding is evident, a complete blood count may be done to determine the extent of blood loss.

Treatment

The most curative form of treatment for patients with Meckel diverticulum is surgical removal of the affected portion of the intestine. If anemia is a problem, blood transfusion or iron supplementation may also be administered.

Flashpoint

The most curative form of treatment is surgical removal.

Prognosis

Patients with Meckel diverticulum can expect a full recovery and resolution of symptoms after surgery. Potential complications without treatment include bleeding, obstruction, infection, and perforation.

Hirschsprung Disease
ICD-9-CM: 751.3   [ICD-10: Q43.1]

Hirschsprung disease, also called *congenital megacolon*, is a congenital absence of peristalsis in a portion of the large intestine due to lack of muscle innervation (see Fig. 16-17). This results in partial or complete obstruction of the bowel.

Incidence

Hirschsprung disease is present in approximately one per 5,000 live births. This disorder is four to five times more common in males than in females and accounts for 25% of all cases of intestinal obstruction in newborns.

Etiology

In infants with Hirschsprung disease, nerves are missing from a portion of the smooth-muscle layer of the large intestine. Without innervation, peristalsis does not occur. Consequently, stool is not propelled normally through the bowel and eliminated. When stool builds up, the bowel becomes distended (enlarged) and swollen. Infection may develop and bowel perforation (rupture) is possible. If this occurs, the infant will develop sepsis and become gravely ill.

Exact causes of Hirschsprung disease are unknown. However, genetics are known to be a contributing factor. Children of parents (especially mothers) with Hirschsprung disease have a much higher chance of having the disorder than other infants have. Children with Down syndrome also have eleven times the risk that other children have.

Flashpoint

Without innervation, normal peristalsis does not occur.

Signs and Symptoms

Most infants with Hirschsprung disease become symptomatic within the first several weeks. They may not pass a bowel movement during the first 48 hours after birth. They also develop abdominal swelling, vomiting, fever, and poor appetite. Children with less severe forms may not be diagnosed for several years but may display problems with constipation or watery diarrhea and poor nutrient absorption. The latter condition results in delayed growth and development. A complication of Hirschsprung disease is enterocolitis, a severe infection that causes vomiting, diarrhea, fever, and severe distention of the colon.

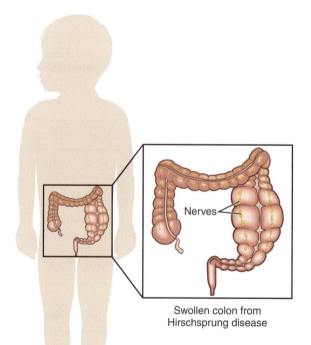

Nerves

Swollen colon from
Hirschsprung disease

FIGURE 16-17 Hirschsprung disease

Diagnosis

Most patients with Hirschsprung disease are diagnosed in the first several weeks of life. However, those with less severe symptoms may not be diagnosed for many months or years. In addition to physical examination, the patient will undergo a variety of testing, including abdominal x-ray, contrast enema, rectal biopsy, and anorectal manometry. The latter test measures pressure in these structures and determines whether normal reflexes are intact.

Treatment

Treatment for patients with Hirschsprung disease involves surgical correction. If infection is present, surgery occurs in two steps. The first step involves removal of the portion of the colon without proper innervation and creation of an ostomy (artificial mouthlike opening) in the distal end of the healthy intestine. This may be an ileostomy (opening in the ileum) or a colostomy (opening in the colon), depending upon how much of the large bowel is removed. After the infection has resolved, usually several months later, a second surgery is done to remove the ostomy and attach the distal end of the healthy intestine to the anus. In some cases this can all be done in one operation.

Prognosis

Prognosis is very good for most patients who undergo surgery; 90% to 95% of them develop normal patterns of bowel elimination and are able to eat and grow normally. A small percentage experience ongoing complications in the form of constipation, enterocolitis, incontinence, bowel perforation, and short bowel syndrome (malabsorption and malnutrition due to the loss of a significant portion of functioning bowel).

Flashpoint
Treatment involves surgical removal of the affected part of the colon.

Endocrine System Disorders

Many disorders of the endocrine system are congenital. The causes are not always clear; in some cases a genetic cause is implicated, while in other cases toxic exposures or injury before or during birth may contribute.

Hypopituitarism
ICD-9-CM: 253.2; 253.3 (dwarfism)   [ICD-10: E23.0]

Hypopituitarism, also called *underactive pituitary gland*, is a condition of diminished secretion of pituitary hormones. Panhypopituitarism results from diminished secretion of all hormones secreted by the anterior pituitary gland. Pituitary dwarfism is a condition of reduced growth and development due to deficiency of growth hormone in childhood. See Chapter 13 for a detailed description of hypopituitarism.

Klinefelter Syndrome
ICD-9-CM: 758.7   [ICD-10: Q98.0]

Klinefelter syndrome is a chromosomal disorder marked by primary testicular failure and infertility.

Incidence

Klinefelter syndrome affects only males and is the most common genetically caused type of hypogonadism in men. It is estimated that approximately 3,000 males are born each year with Klinefelter syndrome and that approximately 250,000 men in the United States currently have the condition. It affects males of all races.

Etiology

Two of the 46 chromosomes in each individual determine gender. If both are X chromosomes—written as XX—the person is female; if one is X and one is Y—written as XY—the person is male. Both chromosomes provide important genetic information that determines sexual features and fertility. Individuals with Klinefelter syndrome usually have one extra X chromosome, written as XXY, although other variations can occur. A risk factor for this syndrome is maternal age of 35 or above during pregnancy.

Flashpoint
Klinefelter syndrome only affects males.

Signs and Symptoms

Individuals with Klinefelter syndrome are often tall, with long arms and legs and a short trunk. They usually have decreased muscle mass and strength; gynecomastia (enlarged breasts); female distribution of fat; small, firm testes; a small penis; decreased libido; and absent or minimal amounts of axillary, facial, or body hair (see Fig. 16-18). They have low testosterone levels and high levels of female sex hormones. Sperm production is often low or absent, causing infertility.

Diagnosis

Concerns about infertility and gynecomastia are often what prompts patients to seek evaluation. The diagnosis is confirmed by **_karyotype,_** which is an analysis based on a photomicrograph of the chromosomes of a single cell (see Box 16-8).

Treatment

Treatment of Klinefelter syndrome includes testosterone replacement, education, and speech therapy, physical therapy, or occupational therapy as needed.

Prognosis

Prognosis for individuals with Klinefelter syndrome depends upon whether they are diagnosed with the classic type or a variant type, and on how early treatment begins. Most individuals are able to lead normal lives and have an active sex life. However, they are at increased risk of breast cancer, certain types of gonadal tumors, and many other problems, which can include varicose veins, venous ulcers, osteoporosis, cardiac problems, and autoimmune diseases such as rheumatoid arthritis, diabetes, and systemic lupus erythematosus. Furthermore, these individuals may suffer behavioral problems due to low self-esteem, language impairment, and learning disabilities.

Turner Syndrome
ICD-9-CM: 758.6   [ICD-10: Q96.9]

Turner syndrome is a chromosomal disorder in females marked by delayed puberty and infertility, due to a missing or incomplete X chromosome.

Flashpoint

Turner syndrome affects only girls.

Incidence

Turner syndrome affects approximately one in 2,500 to 5,000 infant girls born. However, it occurs more frequently among stillbirths and miscarriages.

Etiology

Individuals with Turner syndrome are born with a partial or completely missing X chromosome. This is thought to result from a spontaneously occurring mutation and is not considered hereditary. The missing genetic material accounts for the features of Turner syndrome.

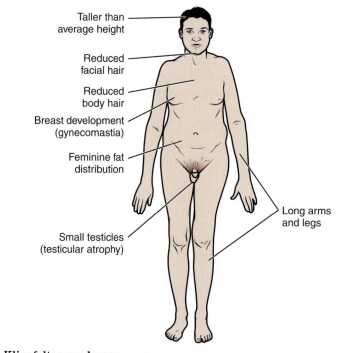

Taller than average height

Reduced facial hair

Reduced body hair

Breast development (gynecomastia)

Feminine fat distribution

Long arms and legs

Small testicles (testicular atrophy)

FIGURE 16-18 Klinefelter syndrome

Box 16-8 Diagnostic Spotlight

KARYOTYPE TEST

The karyotype test is used to evaluate the chromosomes in a cell sample. Specimens tested usually include blood cells, fetal skin cells obtained via amniocentesis, and bone marrow cells. The number, shape, and size of chromosomes are noted. Extra chromosomes or ones that that are missing or abnormally positioned may reveal genetic abnormalities, aid in diagnosis, and provide information for genetic counseling.

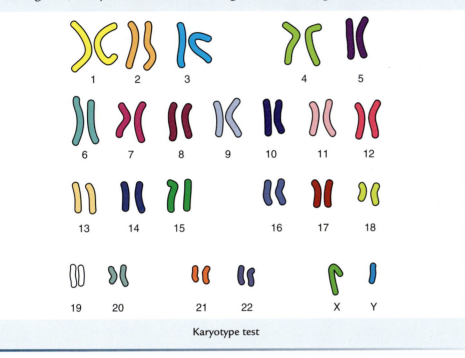

Karyotype test

Signs and Symptoms

Girls with Turner syndrome are short in stature and usually experience early ovarian failure, with infertility. Consequently, they may fail to enter puberty without hormonal supplementation. Many will fail to begin menstruation or will have irregular cycles. Approximately 30% of girls with Turner syndrome have extra skin folds on the neck (webbed neck), a low hairline along the back of the neck, receding jaw, lymphedema (swelling) of the feet and hands, low-set ears, drooping eyes, and broad chest. Skeletal problems may cause outwardly turned arms, scoliosis, and flat feet (see Fig. 16-19).

Diagnosis

Turner syndrome may be suspected based upon the physical characteristics described. Blood or urine testing may indicate abnormally low hormone levels. Diagnosis is confirmed based upon karyotype testing.

Treatment

There is no cure for Turner syndrome. However, certain treatments may minimize its impact on the individual. If administered during early childhood, growth hormone may increase the girl's adult height by several inches. Estrogen therapy can help the girl enter puberty, develop normal sexual characteristics, increase fertility, and prevent osteoporosis. If needed, reproductive technology may help women achieve pregnancy.

Prognosis

Prognosis for girls with Turner syndrome is very good, with early diagnosis and treatment. They are at risk for hypertension, type 2 diabetes, osteoporosis, ear infections, and thyroid

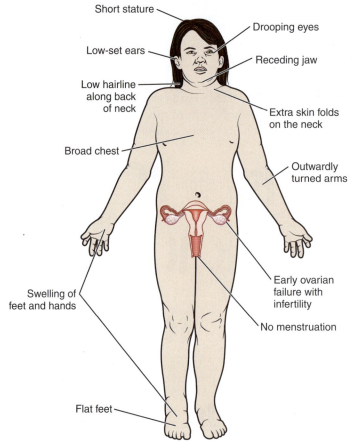

Short stature

Drooping eyes

Low-set ears

Receding jaw

Low hairline along back of neck

Extra skin folds on the neck

Broad chest

Outwardly turned arms

Swelling of feet and hands

Early ovarian failure with infertility

No menstruation

Flat feet

FIGURE 16-19 Turner syndrome

problems. Many also have defects of the aorta or aortic valve. Most are of normal intelligence, although learning disabilities, developmental delays, and delayed social development are possible.

Miscellaneous Disorders

There are a number of other genetic or congenital disorders that do not fit clearly into any specific body system. For example, albinism affects the integumentary system and the sensory system. Marfan syndrome, a disorder of the connective tissue, affects numerous body systems, including the integumentary, skeletal, cardiovascular, and sensory systems. Cystic fibrosis affects many body structures, especially the respiratory and gastrointestinal systems. Phenylketonuria is a condition in which defective protein metabolism leads to neurological damage. Fetal alcohol syndrome and Down syndrome, each with different causes, have significant effects on multiple body systems.

Albinism
ICD-9-CM: 270.2   [ICD-10: E70.3]

Albinism is a group of conditions in which the individual lacks pigment in the eyes (ocular albinism) or both the skin and eyes (oculocutaneous albinism).

Incidence

The exact incidence of albinism has not been established. However, it is listed as a "rare disease" by the Office of Rare Diseases Research of the National Institutes of Health, which means that it affects fewer than 200,000 Americans.

Flashpoint

Individuals with albinism lack pigment in the eyes and sometimes the skin.

Etiology

Albinism is inherited. There are several different types, and the inheritance pattern differs with each. Most types occur when individuals receive the albinism gene from both parents; however, one type of ocular albinism is passed from mothers to sons.

Signs and Symptoms

The appearance of individuals with albinism depends upon which type they have. Most, but not all, have very light skin and hair (see Fig. 16-20). Some have slight pigmentation, which results in hair that is more yellow or reddish. Those with ocular albinism have a relatively normal appearance. Most have blue eyes but some have hazel, brown, or even pink eyes.

Individuals with albinism commonly have eye problems. Some include nystagmus (rapid irregular movement of the eyes in circular or back-and-forth patterns), strabismus (crossed eyes), myopia (nearsightedness), hyperopia (farsightedness), astigmatism (irregular curvature of the cornea and lens that causes refractive error), and photophobia (sensitivity to light). The lack of skin pigment makes individuals especially vulnerable to sunburn.

Diagnosis

Diagnosis of albinism may require only physical examination. However, genetic testing may be done to confirm the diagnosis. Other testing can also be done on a hair from the patient's head to determine whether melanin synthesis is present.

Treatment

Albinism is not curable. However, there are many things individuals with albinism can do to protect themselves and enhance their quality of life. Treatment for eye conditions and visual deficits is tailored to the individual and may include surgery of the ocular muscles and the use of vision aids, such as glasses and contact lenses. Individuals may also benefit from the use of large-print reading materials and closed captioning. Skin protection is very important, since there is little or no melanin in the skin to protect the patient from ultraviolet rays (see Box 16-9). Individuals with albinism also tolerate light bulbs that are yellowish in color better than those that are bluish.

Prognosis

There is no cure for albinism. However, many of the associated eye problems can be treated. Avoidance of the sun is important in preventing damage to the eyes and skin.

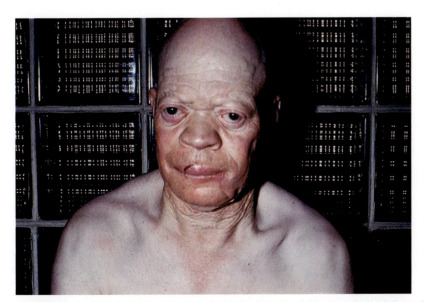

FIGURE 16-20 Albinism (From Goldsmith, LA, Lazarus, GS, and Tharp, MD. *Adult and Pediatric Dermatology: A Color Guide to Diagnosis and Treatment.* 1997. Philadelphia: F.A. Davis Company, with permission.)

Box 16-9 Wellness Promotion

SKIN PROTECTION FOR THE PATIENT WITH ALBINISM

Protection from harmful ultraviolet rays is very important for patients with albinism, because they are at high risk of skin cancer. Strategies include the following:

- Apply good sunscreen each day (SPF 30 or higher) before leaving the house and reapply as needed throughout the day.
- Select and wear makeup with sunscreen.
- Wear sunglasses to protect the eyes.
- Wear a wide-brimmed hat when walking, gardening, or participating in other outdoor activities.
- Seek shady areas when spending time outdoors.
- When buying, leasing, or renting a car, get one with tinted windows.
- When buying or building a house, consider the value of an enclosed or covered porch.
- Select clothing that provides maximal coverage.

Marfan Syndrome
ICD-9-CM: 759.82   [ICD-10: Q87.4]

Marfan syndrome is a genetic condition that affects connective tissue in the body. Consequently, it affects structures of the skin, skeletal system, heart, blood vessels, and eyes.

Incidence
Marfan syndrome affects an estimated 60,000 to 200,000 Americans, men and women equally.

Etiology
Marfan syndrome is usually inherited as an autosomal dominant disorder. This means that individuals who inherit one affected gene from either parent will have the disorder. Their children will then have a 50% chance of inheriting the disorder. However, 25% to 30% of cases are thought to be the result of genetic mutations, since some patients have no family history of the disease. Individuals with Marfan syndrome have defects in a gene that is important to the development of elastic tissues within the body. It also causes excessive length in long bones.

Signs and Symptoms
Individuals with Marfan syndrome may have no symptoms during their early years. Features can begin appearing at any age but tend to worsen with age. There are many possible physical features of the disorder. Some of the more typical include tallness with long, thin limbs and fingers; a protruding or indented chest; scoliosis; small wrists; and flat feet. Others include hammertoes, stooped shoulders, narrow face, crowded teeth, joint laxity, nearsightedness, and a small lower jaw (see Fig. 16-21). Less visible, but perhaps more serious, are inflammatory changes to the heart valves, aorta, lungs, and eyes. Aortic enlargement, aneurysm, or dissection (tearing) may occur. The mitral valve within the heart may become prolapsed. Eye changes may include myopia, lens dislocation, retinal detachment, glaucoma, and formation of cataracts. Other effects may include spontaneous pneumothorax (collapsed lung) and striae (stretch marks) on the skin.

Patients with Marfan syndrome may complain of fatigue, heart palpitations, chest pain, cold extremities, and joint and muscle pain.

Flashpoint

Individuals with Marfan syndrome typically have unusually long arms, legs, and fingers.

Diagnosis
There is no specific test that conclusively confirms the diagnosis of Marfan syndrome. Therefore, data are gathered through physical examination and tests such as echocardiogram, which may reveal some of the complications associated with the disorder. In some cases, testing may be done to identify mutation of the gene that is associated with the condition.

Treatment
There is no cure for Marfan syndrome. It is treated through the provision of good health care with the goal of preventing or minimizing complications. Consultation with a team of medical

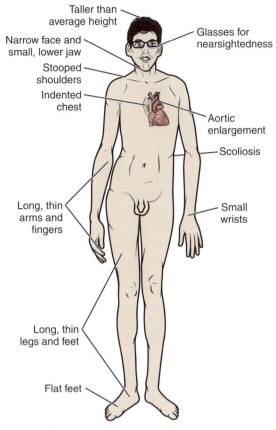

Taller than average height

Narrow face and small, lower jaw

Stooped shoulders

Indented chest

Glasses for nearsightedness

Aortic enlargement

Scoliosis

Long, thin arms and fingers

Small wrists

Long, thin legs and feet

Flat feet

FIGURE 16-21 The features of Marfan syndrome

specialists may be needed, especially during periods of rapid growth, such as adolescence. Regular evaluation from a cardiologist, management of blood pressure, and annual echocardiography testing help to minimize or detect aortic enlargement. When needed, vascular repair and grafting are done to prevent aortic rupture. Regular evaluation by an orthopedist helps to identify and treat skeletal problems. If sunken or protruding chest are severe, surgical correction may be done. Regular vision care is recommended; vision problems are treated as appropriate. Antibiotics may be recommended before dental procedures to prevent endocarditis. Analgesics and muscle relaxants may ease musculoskeletal pain. Physical therapy may also be beneficial. Patients may be advised to avoid contact sports and strenuous activities.

Prognosis

Prognosis for patients with Marfan syndrome has improved significantly in recent decades, and many individuals are surviving into their 50s. Women must be monitored carefully during pregnancy because pregnancy increases stress on the heart and aorta. Echocardiography is done every 6 to 10 weeks. There are many potential complications, the most serious being aortic rupture, which is nearly always fatal.

Cystic Fibrosis
ICD-9-CM: 277.0　　[ICD-10: E84.9]

Cystic fibrosis (CF) is a genetic condition that causes severe damage to the lungs and other organs, and nutritional problems.

Incidence

An estimated 10 million Americans are carriers of the CF gene, and approximately 30,000 individuals currently have CF. One thousand more are diagnosed each year. The incidence is highest among Caucasians, but the condition can affect individuals of all races.

Etiology

Cystic fibrosis is an inherited disorder caused by a defective gene that changes the distribution of sodium chloride in the body and affects the composition of the mucus produced by the lungs, salivary glands, pancreas, and intestines. CF is an autosomal recessive disorder; therefore, a person may be a carrier but not have the disorder. However, if a child inherits two copies of the defective gene, one from each parent, then the child will have CF (see Fig. 16-22). The defective gene alters the movement of sodium chloride in and out of body cells. As a result, mucous secretions that should be thin and slippery are thick and tenacious. Thus, instead of acting as a lubricant, it clogs up various passageways, tubes, and vessels in the lungs, pancreas, and intestines. Nutritional deficiencies also occur as mucus blocks pancreatic enzymes from contributing to the digestive process. Consequently, key vitamins are not well absorbed.

Thick respiratory secretions clog small airways of the lungs and create a hospitable environment for bacterial growth. As a result, respiratory infections are common.

Flashpoint

CF is an autosomal recessive inherited disorder.

Signs and Symptoms

There are many mutations of the CF gene, such that signs and symptoms of CF vary somewhat from one individual to the next. Some patients suffer more from respiratory problems, while others suffer more from pancreatic and gastrointestinal problems (see Fig. 16-23). The first sign of CF in a newborn infant may be meconium ileus, a condition in which the infant is not able to pass the normal meconium stool (green-black stool normal to newborns). Infants with CF also exhibit steatorrhea (greasy stools), frequent respiratory infections, and delayed growth and development. In children and young adults, common respiratory symptoms include coughing with thick sputum, frequent sinus and respiratory infections (such as bronchitis and pneumonia), and the formation of nasal polyps. A long-term change caused by respiratory compromise is clubbing of the fingertips and toes. Gastrointestinal signs and symptoms include steatorrhea, diarrhea, vomiting, bowel obstruction, and cirrhosis of the liver due to obstruction of the bile duct. These individuals also have an extra salty taste to their skin, and delayed growth and development.

Flashpoint

Some patients with CF suffer severe respiratory problems; others suffer severe gastrointestinal problems.

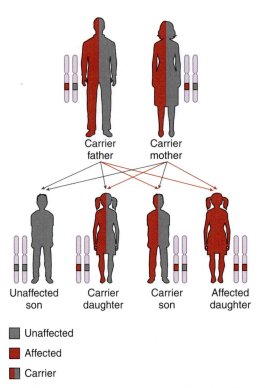

Carrier father

Carrier mother

Unaffected son

Carrier daughter

Carrier son

Affected daughter

■ Unaffected

■ Affected

■ Carrier

FIGURE 16-22 Cystic fibrosis is an autosomal recessive disorder; therefore, two carriers have a 25% chance of having a child with CF, a 50% chance of having a child who is a carrier, and a 25% chance of having a child who is normal.

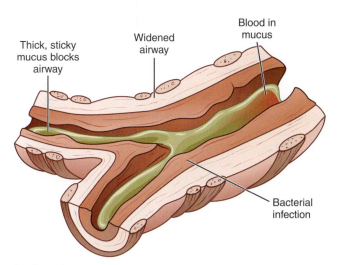

Thick, sticky
mucus blocks
airway

Widened
airway

Blood in
mucus

Bacterial
infection

FIGURE 16-23 **Cystic fibrosis**

Diagnosis

Prenatal screening can be used to help identify a fetus with CF. After birth, diagnosis may be suspected based upon the parent's genetic history and the infant's signs and symptoms. Over 70% of patients are diagnosed before their second birthday. Because people with CF have an abnormally high amount of sodium in their sweat, diagnosis is usually confirmed with a sweat test (see Box 16-10). In some cases genetic testing may also be done.

Box 16-10 Diagnostic Spotlight

THE SWEAT TEST

The sweat test is commonly done to diagnose cystic fibrosis. In this noninvasive, painless test, an electrode is placed on the skin to stimulate the sweat glands. After a few minutes, sweat is collected from the area and sent to a laboratory to be analyzed. Two samples are usually collected from two areas of the skin. An abnormally high sodium level indicates that the patient has cystic fibrosis. Because newborns may not produce an adequate amount of sweat for reliable test results, the physician may choose to wait until a baby is several months old.

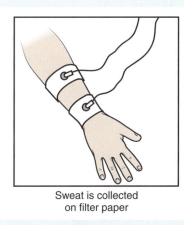

Sweat is collected
on filter paper

Sweat test

Treatment

The treatment plan for CF varies with each individual. Patients often require enzyme replacement to aid in digesting food and absorbing nutrients. They also need a high-sodium, high-calorie, nutrient-dense diet and a liberal amount of fluids.

Respiratory care becomes a significant part of most patients' treatment routine. Medications may include mucolytics to thin secretions, antibiotics to clear infection, NSAIDs to reduce inflammation, and bronchodilators to help open the airways. Chest physiotherapy includes the application of physical vibration to help dislodge secretions. This is done by a second person, who claps the patient's chest and back with cupped hands while the patient is positioned with the head and shoulders lower than the rest of the body. This treatment can also be applied with a handheld device called a mechanical percussor or with a vibrating inflatable vest. Regardless of the type of physiotherapy applied, it is generally done twice each day for 30 minutes. This therapy, combined with the use of medications, significantly improves the patient's ability to breathe and reduces the incidence of respiratory infections. Lung transplantation may be considered for individuals with life-threatening lung problems.

Prognosis

Aggressive medical care and good self-care can lengthen life and improve its quality for individuals with CF. Predicting longevity is difficult, since each patient's experience varies. Currently, over 45% of Americans with CF are over 18 years old; the predicted average survival age is over 37. While this is not where patients or health-care providers would wish, it does show a significant improvement since the 1950s, when children with CF rarely lived long enough to begin grade school. Complications of CF, in addition to those already mentioned, include hemoptysis (coughing up blood), pneumothorax, respiratory failure, diabetes, cirrhosis, fertility problems, and death.

> **Flashpoint**
>
> The life expectancy for patients with CF has improved significantly in the past 60 years.

Phenylketonuria

ICD-9-CM: 270.1   [ICD-10: E70.0]

Phenylketonuria is a genetic disorder in which infants are born with a lack of the enzyme phenylalanine hydroxylase. As a result, they are unable to properly utilize protein, specifically the amino acid called *phenylalanine*. See Chapter 4 for a detailed description of phenylketonuria.

Fetal Alcohol Syndrome

ICD-9-CM: 760.71   [ICD-10: Q86.0]

Fetal alcohol syndrome (FAS) is among the most severe disorders included in a larger group of disorders known as fetal alcohol spectrum disorders. FAS is a condition of permanent physical, behavioral, or mental impairment that is caused by prenatal exposure to alcohol. It is a leading cause of preventable mental and physical birth defects.

Incidence

Estimates of the number of babies born each year with FAS vary but run as high as 6,500. As many as 40,000 infants are thought to be born each year with some type of alcohol-related impairment.

Etiology

FAS develops when a woman drinks alcohol during pregnancy. Alcohol readily crosses the placenta to the fetus; therefore, when the pregnant woman drinks alcohol, so does her fetus. However, the fetus is not able to metabolize the alcohol as efficiently as the mother, so its blood alcohol rises to a much higher level.

> **Flashpoint**
>
> When a pregnant woman drinks alcohol, her fetus drinks even more.

Signs and Symptoms

Alcohol exposure harms the unborn fetus in numerous ways. It impedes normal delivery of oxygen and nutrients to the fetus's brain and causes damage to the central nervous system. It affects other organs and tissues in the body as well. Physical defects of FAS include heart defects, growth deficits, malformed facial features (see Fig. 16-24), malformed extremities, poor muscle tone, and decreased physical coordination. Learning and behavioral disorders are common. Children with FAS frequently struggle with impaired attention span, memory deficits, hyperactivity, faulty judgment, poor impulse control, and sensory (hearing, vision) and communication problems. Infants with FAS also struggle with sleep and sucking and feeding.

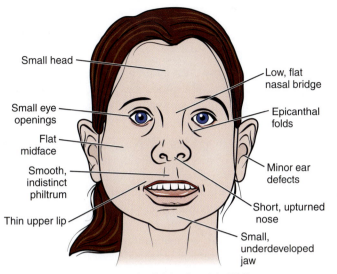

Small head

Low, flat
nasal bridge

Small eye
openings

Epicanthal
folds

Flat
midface

Smooth,
indistinct
philtrum

Minor ear
defects

Thin upper lip

Short, upturned
nose

Small,
underdeveloped
jaw

FIGURE 16-24 Facial features common to individuals with FAS

Diagnosis

FAS cannot be diagnosed before birth, although an ultrasound may reveal slowed fetal growth (see Box 16-11). After the infant is born, diagnosis is based upon an evaluation of physical features and observation of the infant's developmental delays and behavioral problems. Heart defects may cause a heart murmur, which will be audible upon auscultation. MRI or CT testing may indicate abnormal development of the brain.

Treatment

FAS is a preventable disorder but not a curable one. Therefore, emphasis is placed upon education and prenatal health care. Women who are pregnant or might become pregnant must be informed about the risks of FAS and counseled to avoid drinking alcohol (see Box 16-12). Appropriate referrals to treatment programs for drug and alcohol abuse should be made when necessary.

Infants and children identified as having FAS or fetal alcohol spectrum disorders should be referred to resources within the community and school system for help with emotional, behavioral, and learning problems. Parents of children with FAS also benefit from educational and emotional support.

Flashpoint

There is no amount of alcohol that is safe for a pregnant woman to drink.

Prognosis

The prognosis for individuals with FAS depends upon the severity of their symptoms and the provision of appropriate education and support. Those who do receive the help they need have a

---

Box 16-11 Diagnostic Spotlight

FETAL ULTRASOUND

During the course of a woman's pregnancy, the physician may order a fetal ultrasound for various reasons. It may be used to confirm multiple pregnancies and to determine fetal age, position, and sex. It can also detect such fetal abnormalities as defects in the heart or other organs.

A fetal ultrasound may be vaginal or abdominal. The patient is usually instructed to drink at least 32 ounces of water 1 hour before the test, because a full bladder enhances visualization of the fetus. If the ultrasound is performed at 12 weeks' gestation or later, the physician can determine the sex of the fetus. The patient may choose to know the sex of the fetus or may elect to be surprised when the baby is born. If the patient does not want to know the sex of the baby, this should be noted in the patient's medical record.

Box 16-12 Wellness Promotion

PREVENTING FETAL ALCOHOL SYNDROME

The sad news about FAS is that it is one of the most common causes of birth defects, learning disabilities, and behavioral problems. The good news is that it is totally preventable. Here are some helpful facts that must be shared with everyone, especially women who are or may become pregnant:

- It is never too late to stop drinking, even in advanced pregnancy.
- Alcohol use during the first 3 months of pregnancy and binge drinking during pregnancy causes the greatest damage, but any amount of alcohol puts the fetus at risk.
- Any woman who is sexually active and not using a reliable means of birth control should not drink alcohol, since pregnancy may occur but not be detected for some time.
- Spouses, partners, and friends of pregnant women can help by sharing information about the risks of FAS, avoid offering or serving alcoholic beverages to pregnant women, and encouraging any pregnant women who do drink to stop and get help if needed.
- Women who are unable to stop drinking for the sake of their unborn baby clearly have a problem and need to receive treatment; contact Alcoholics Anonymous or the Substance Abuse and Mental Health Services Administration for help.

good prognosis for a productive and rewarding life. Those who do not are at high risk of dropping out of school, substance abuse, psychiatric problems, criminal behaviors, unemployment, and relationship difficulties.

Down Syndrome

ICD-9-CM: 758.0   **[ICD-10: Q90.9]**

Down syndrome, also called *trisomy 21*, is a genetic condition caused by an extra copy of chromosome 21 that affects the development of the brain and body.

Flashpoint

Down syndrome is caused by an extra copy of chromosome 21.

Incidence

Down syndrome is one of the most common causes of birth defects. An estimated 350,000 to 400,000 Americans are currently living with this disorder, and 5,000 more infants are diagnosed with it in the United States each year. Down syndrome occurs in all populations, regardless of race, sex, or socioeconomic status.

Etiology

People are normally born with 23 pairs of chromosomes, for a total of 46. Half are contributed by the mother's egg and half by the father's sperm. Down syndrome occurs when a whole or partial extra copy of chromosome 21 is present. Because chromosomes contain critical genetic material that determines the individual's development, this extra material affects that development. If an egg or sperm develops incorrectly prior to fertilization and creates an extra chromosome 21, then the excess genetic material is incorporated into the forming individual after conception. Risk factors have been identified that lend support to genetics as a cause. For instance, parents of a child with Down syndrome have a greater chance of having another child with Down syndrome, and parents whose own chromosome 21 is abnormal are also at risk of having an infant with Down syndrome. Age is also a risk factor, with women over age 40 having a one in 100 chance of conceiving a child with Down syndrome, compared to a risk of less than one in 10,000 for women age 25. Even so, most babies with Down syndrome are born to younger women, simply because younger women have babies much more frequently than do older women.

Signs and Symptoms

Individuals with Down syndrome have distinguishing physical characteristics, including a somewhat flattened face and back of the head; small, low-set, oddly shaped ears; a small, flattened nose; and eyes that slant upward. A small mouth that tends to hang open gives the appearance of a large, protruding tongue. Other possible features include a short neck, small feet with a gap between the great toe and smaller toes, and small hands with a deep palmar crease and short fingers (see Fig. 16-25). These individuals also tend to have loose ligaments and poor muscle tone. They have some degree of mental disability and demonstrate slowed development of motor skills and language. Individuals with Down syndrome often have other health problems, including: hearing deficits, eye problems, congenital heart defects, thyroid problems, skeletal conditions, dementia, and intestinal problems, such as bowel obstruction or celiac disease.

Diagnosis

In many cases, diagnosis is made after the infant is born. Screening tests may be done before or during pregnancy to identify women who are at risk of having an infant with Down syndrome, but further testing is needed to confirm the diagnosis in an infant. A maternal blood test may be done between weeks 11 and 20. Other testing includes fetal ultrasound, amniocentesis, and chorionic villus sampling.

Treatment

There is no cure for Down syndrome, but individuals with the disorder can usually lead healthy, fulfilling lives if they receive appropriate health care, therapy, and education. With good health care, life expectancy is into the 50s. Therapies that generally benefit these individuals include speech therapy and occupational therapy. Individuals with Down syndrome may benefit from special-education classes or may do well integrated into regular classes. The key is for their parents or care providers to communicate clearly and proactively with teachers and school officials so that everyone understands the child's needs and works together to achieve the best outcome possible. Patients with Down syndrome should receive standard childhood vaccinations, because they are more susceptible to infection.

Prognosis

The prognosis for most individuals with Down syndrome is quite good if they live in a supportive environment and receive the care and education they need. Average life expectancy is in the 50s. However, these individuals are at increased risk for certain physical problems. These include heart defects, intestinal defects, eye and vision problems, hearing loss, thyroid problems, onset of dementia after age 35, seizure disorders, and leukemia.

Flashpoint
Individuals with Down syndrome have distinguishing physical characteristics.

Flashpoint
Prenatal testing can diagnose Down syndrome.

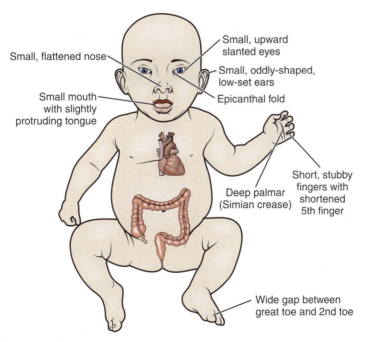

FIGURE 16-25 **Down syndrome**

STOP HERE.
Select the flash cards for this chapter and run through them at least three times before moving on to the next chapter.

Student Resources

Centers for Disease Control and Prevention: http://www.cdc.gov
Cleft Palate Foundation: http://www.cleftline.org
Cystic Fibrosis Foundation: http://www.cff.org
Genetic.org: http://www.genetic.org
Hydrocephalus Association: http://www.hydroassoc.org
March of Dimes: http://www.marchofdimes.com
Muscular Dystrophy Association: http://www.mda.org
National Down Syndrome Society: http://www.ndss.org
National Hemophilia Foundation: http://www.hemophilia.org
National Marfan Foundation: http://www.marfan.org
National Organization for Albinism and Hypopigmentation: http://www.albinism.org
National Organization on Fetal Alcohol Syndrome: http://www.nofas.org
Osteogenesis Imperfecta Foundation: http://www.oif.org
Turner Syndrome Society of the United States: http://www.turnersyndrome.org

Chapter Activities

Learning Style Study Strategies

Try the following strategy as you study the content of this chapter:

All learners: If you are unable to meet in person with your study buddy, try having webcam conversations. You can exchange study tips, quiz one another, and even visit websites to research diseases or locate visual images together.

Practice Exercises

Answers to practice exercises can be found in Appendix D.

Case Studies

CASE STUDY 1

Claire Fellows has just been hired to work in the obstetrics and gynecology department at Valley Medical Clinic. She has worked as a CMA for 5 years in the gastrointestinal department. Working with obstetric patients will be a new experience for her. She is very excited about her new position but realizes that since she has been out of school for 5 years, she needs to study and review information about the obstetric patient population. Today she is reading about physical development in the fetus and newborn.

1. As Claire reviews fetal development, what will she learn about blood flow through fetal lungs?

2. What will she learn about the circulation of blood through the fetal heart?

3. As Claire reviews information about changes in the infant at birth, what will she note about the circulation through the heart and lungs?

4. Claire learns about four types of congenital heart conditions that can occur when expected changes in circulation do not occur shortly after birth. What are their names and descriptions?

CASE STUDY 2

Edelia is an LPN at Valley Medical Center. She has become well acquainted with two regular patients, Larry and Gary. They were both diagnosed with muscular dystrophy approximately 1 year ago. Larry has DMD and Gary has BMD. In helping provide care for these two patients, Edelia has learned a great deal about this disorder. How might she answer the following questions?

1. What do the abbreviations DMD and BMD stand for?

2. What effect do both forms of muscular dystrophy have on the patient's muscles?

3. Which of the two forms of muscular dystrophy is more severe?

4. What types of patients typically develop DMD and BMD?

5. What is the main cause of these disorders?

6. What are the expected signs and symptoms of DMD and BMD?

7. Describe the prognosis for patients with muscular dystrophy.

CASE STUDY 3

Mr. and Mrs. Jackson have brought their 2-day-old son to the clinic today. He was delivered at home by his father; both parents wanted a natural delivery in their home environment. They state that the delivery went fine and the baby seems healthy and content. However, they have one serious concern that they wish to discuss with their son's pediatrician. They've noticed that the infant has no testicles in his scrotum, and they are extremely concerned about whether he will be a normal male with normal fertility. How might their questions be answered?

1. What could have caused this problem?

2. How will you find out if he has testicles?

3. Can anything be done to fix this problem?

Multiple Choice

1. All of the following terms are matched with the correct definition **except:**

    a. Anomaly: abnormality that develops in utero

    b. Congenital: present at birth

    c. Karyotype: analysis based on a photomicrograph of the chromosomes of a single cell

    d. Y chromosome: one of two chromosomes that determine gender in humans; determines female gender

2. An X-linked recessive disorder is one that:

    a. Is passed on when two faulty genes are inherited, one from each parent

    b. Is inherited by a man from his mother

    c. Is triggered by exposure to an environmental factor

    d. Is caused by any chromosome other than the sex chromosomes

3. Which of the following statements is true regarding Down syndrome?

    a. It is caused by a missing chromosome.

    b. It only occurs in the Caucasian population.

    c. It can be diagnosed prenatally.

    d. Most babies with Down syndrome are born to women who are over age 40.

4. The sweat test is used to diagnose:

    a. Marfan syndrome

    b. Cystic fibrosis

    c. Turner syndrome

    d. Duchenne muscular dystrophy

5. Which of the following disorders is most likely to result in malnutrition?

    a. Pyloric stenosis

    b. Myelomeningocele

    c. Wilms tumor

    d. Tetralogy of Fallot

Short Answer

1. Which disorders share maternal deficiencies of folate and folic acid as potential contributing causes?

2. Describe the similarities between Klinefelter syndrome and Turner syndrome.

3. Describe the signs and symptoms of FAS.

17 MALIGNANCY

Learning Outcomes

Upon completion of this chapter, the student will be able to:

- Define and spell key terms related to cancer
- Describe the general incidence of cancer
- Describe the general etiology of cancer
- Explain how cancer is diagnosed
- List and describe common forms of treatment for cancer
- Identify characteristics of cancers of the various body systems, including:
  - description
  - incidence
  - etiology
  - signs and symptoms
  - diagnosis
  - treatment
  - prognosis

KEY TERMS	
benign	noncancerous
biopsy	removal of a tissue sample from the body for microscopic examination
carcinogen	cancer-causing substance
carcinoma	cancer arising from epithelial tissue
glioma	cancer arising from glial cells
grading	standardized process of describing differentiation of cancer cells, from grade I to grade IV
in situ	confined to the original site
leukemia	cancer arising from blood-forming cells
leukocoria	white pupil caused by retinoblastoma; also called *cat's eye reflex*
lymphoma	cancer arising from lymphatic cells
malignant	cancerous
melanoma	cancer arising from pigmented skin cells
melena	tarry black stool caused by the presence of digested blood
metastasize	to spread to distant sites
myeloma	cancer arising from cells that comprise the blood-forming part of the bone marrow
palliative surgery	surgery done to ease pain and improve quality of life
primary eye cancer	cancer that originates within the eyes

KEY TERMS—cont'd	
reconstructive surgery	surgery done to restore the body as close as possible to its original appearance and function
staging	identifying the extent of dissemination of cancer, including tumor size and regional and distant metastasis
staging surgery	surgery done to identify the extent of cancer
supportive surgery	surgery done to aid in the delivery of other therapies

Abbreviations

Table 17-1 lists some of the most common abbreviations related to malignancy.

Coding for Cancer Pathologies

Note: This chapter includes ICD-9-CM and ICD-10 codes for specific cancer pathologies. The ICD-9-CM and ICD-10 codes indicate a specific location on the body (topography code) but do not describe the structure or behavior of the cancer. For treatment and payment, either ICD-9-CM or ICD-10 is required.

The International Classification of Diseases for Oncology (ICD-O) is a domain-specific extension of the International Statistical Classification of Diseases and Related Health Problems for tumor diseases. This classification is widely used by cancer registries and describes the morphology (structure and form) of the tumor. It is currently in its third revision (ICD-O-3). ICD-O-3 codes are listed where possible.

TABLE 17-1
ABBREVIATIONS

Abbreviation	Meaning	Abbreviation	Meaning
AFP	alpha-fetoprotein	HPV	human papillomavirus
BSE	breast self-examination	PAP, Pap	Papanicolau test
Bx, bx	biopsy	PSA	prostate-specific antigen
CA	cancer	SCC	squamous cell carcinoma
CIS	carcinoma in situ	TNM	tumor, node, metastasis
DRE	digital rectal examination	TSE	testicular self-examination
HCG, hCG	human chorionic gonadotropin		

Malignancy

Cancer is defined as a **malignant** (cancerous) neoplasia (new tissue growth), marked by uncontrolled growth of abnormal cells, that often spreads to other parts of the body. General categories of cancer include:

Carcinoma: cancer arising from epithelial tissue (epidermis of the skin or mucous membrane)

Sarcoma: malignant tumors that develop in tissues which connect, support, or surround other structures and organs of the body

Glioma: cancer arising from glial cells (cells that comprise the non-nervous supporting structure for the brain and spinal cord)

Lymphoma: cancer arising from lymphatic cells (cells that comprise the tissues of the lymphatic system)

Leukemia: cancer arising from blood-forming cells

Melanoma: cancer arising from pigmented skin cells

Myeloma: cancer arising from cells that comprise the blood-forming part of the bone marrow

Incidence

Cancer is the second-most common cause of death in the United States, following cardiovascular disease. Well over one million Americans are diagnosed each year, and more than half a million die. There are more than 200 kinds of cancer but the most common are cancers of the lung, breast, colon, prostate, and skin. Cancer is most common in elderly individuals over age 65.

Etiology

The cause of most forms of cancer is still not well understood. It is believed that oncogenes (genes that cause cells to mutate and become cancerous) commonly occur in the body and that *suppressor cells* from the immune system normally destroy them. Therefore, it is possible that the development of cancer is due to some type of immune system failure. Genetics is also known to play a role, but its exact influence is often not clear. In a few cases, specific genes have been identified that directly contribute to the development of some forms of cancer (see Table 17-2). For example, individuals with the *BRCA1* and *BRCA2* genes are known to have an extremely high risk of developing breast cancer. In other cases, a familial tendency is apparent but no specific genetic cause is identified. In yet other instances, the occurrence of cancer appears random. Viruses are suspected to cause some forms of cancer; for example, the human

TABLE 17-2			
ONCOGENES RESPONSIBLE FOR SOME INHERITED FORMS OF CANCER			
Cancer	Gene	Cancer	Gene
Retinoblastoma	RB1	Wilms tumor	WT1
Melanoma	INK4A	Some types of kidney cancer	VHL
Colorectal cancer from familial polyposis	APC	Breast cancer	BRCA1, BRCA2
Colorectal cancer without polyposis	MLH1, MSH2, MSH6		

papillomavirus has been connected to some forms of cervical cancer in women. Other risk factors for cancer include exposure to a long list of environmental agents: tobacco products, ultraviolet rays, radiation, pesticides, asbestos, industrial pollutants such as coal or silica dust, and more.

Diagnosis

Diagnosis is often suspected based upon defining physical characteristics or common signs and symptoms. However, the most reliable means of diagnosing malignancy is through *biopsy,* the removal of a tissue sample from the body for microscopic study (see Box 17-1). In this process the pathologist determines whether the tissue is malignant or *benign* (noncancerous) and identifies the type of cancer cells. If the tissue is malignant, the next step is to determine whether the patient's cancer is *in situ* (confined to the original site), has spread regionally, or has *metastasized* (spread to distant sites—see Fig. 17-1). As part of this process, regional lymph nodes may be removed and studied. The presence of cancer within one or more lymph nodes indicates involvement of the lymphatic system and the possibility that the cancer may have spread to other, more distant sites.

In addition to biopsy, or occasionally in its place, other tests may be done. These may help to diagnose the specific type of cancer and to identify whether it has metastasized to surrounding structures.

Once diagnosis has occurred, the cancer must be graded and staged. *Grading* refers to a standardized process of describing differentiation of cancer cells, where Grade 1 tumors

Flashpoint

Oncogenes cause cells to mutate and become cancerous.

Flashpoint

To determine whether a growth is cancerous, it must usually be studied under a microscope.

Box 17-1 Diagnostic Spotlight

BIOPSY

Biopsy is a procedure in which a tissue specimen is removed for study. Removal is performed in a variety of ways, depending upon the location of the suspected cancer. Common methods include surgery; syringe and needle; a hollow, round cutting tool called a punch; suction; and a tiny brush. Retrieval may be aided by use of ultrasonography or radiological means.

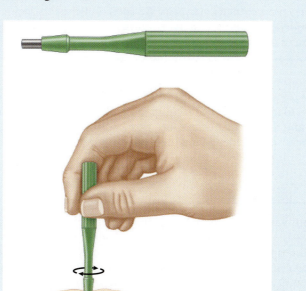

A

Continued

Box 17-1 Diagnostic Spotlight—cont'd

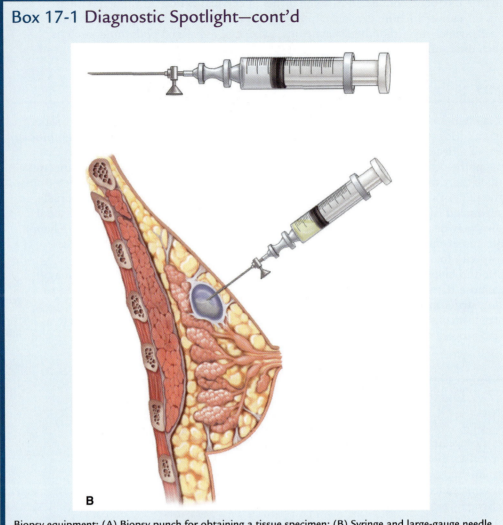

B

Biopsy equipment: (A) Biopsy punch for obtaining a tissue specimen; (B) Syringe and large-gauge needle for aspirating a fluid specimen (From Eagle, S, et al. *The Professional Medical Assistant: An Integrative Teamwork-Based Approach.* 2009. Philadelphia: F.A. Davis Company, with permission.)

indicate cells that closely resemble normal cells, while Grade 4 tumors indicate cells that are very abnormal. **Staging** refers to identifying the extent of dissemination of the cancer, including tumor size and regional and distant metastasis (see Box 17-2). This information is crucial in helping determine the prognosis and identifying the most effective treatment plan.

> **Flashpoint**
>
> Grading and staging comprise a system for determining the extent to which the cancer has advanced.

Treatment

Forms of treatment vary widely, depending upon the type, location, and progress of the cancer. When possible, the primary tumor is surgically removed. If the cancer has already metastasized at the time of treatment, then surgery may or may not be helpful. In some cases the tumors may be removed to improve comfort and quality of life. Additional treatment is needed to eradicate the cancer, which may include a wide array of therapies; the most common are chemotherapy, radiation therapy, and immunotherapy.

Surgery
Approximately 60% of cancer patients have surgery as a part of their treatment plan, often combined with other forms of treatment. Surgery may be considered curative if it removes all

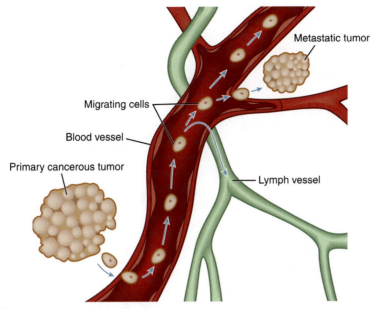

FIGURE 17-1 Cancer metastasis

Box 17-2 Diagnostic Spotlight

TNM SYSTEM OF CANCER STAGING

Staging indicates the extent of the spread of cancerous tumors and provides standardized descriptions of tumors, treatment recommendations, and outcomes. It is used to create criteria for including patients in clinical trials and to determine a treatment regimen and prognosis.

The universally used tumor, node, metastasis (TNM) staging system is based on three factors:

- tumor (T)—the size or extent of local spreading of a primary tumor
- node (N)—the presence or absence and extent of regional or distal metastasis to the lymph nodes
- metastasis (M)—the presence or absence of distant metastasis (cancer in other organs)

of the cancerous tissue before it has a chance to spread; it may be considered preventive if the purpose is to keep cancer from developing. An example of preventive surgery is the removal of colon polyps, which are known to sometimes become malignant. Surgery may be diagnostic if it is performed to remove tissue for further study. The most common example of this is tissue biopsy performed by needle aspiration or through an incision. *Staging surgery* may be performed to identify the extent of the cancer. This may be done through a surgical incision or through the use of an endoscope into the upper or lower gastrointestinal tract. *Supportive surgery* is sometimes performed to aid in the delivery of other therapies. An example is the surgical insertion of a special port or catheter into a large vein beneath the patient's skin (see Fig. 17-2). The port is then used for the infusion of chemotherapy. *Reconstructive surgery* may be performed to restore the body as close as possible to its original appearance and function, such as breast reconstruction after a mastectomy. *Palliative surgery* is not curative but may be performed to ease pain and improve quality of life for whatever time the patient has left.

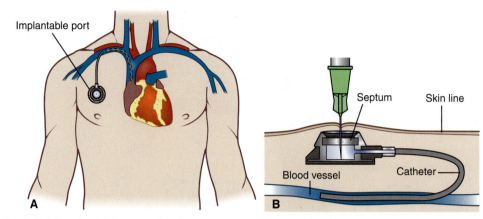

Implantable port

Septum   Skin line

Blood vessel   Catheter

A   **B**

FIGURE 17-2 **Implantable central vein port**

Chemotherapy

Chemotherapy is the use of potent medications to control or kill malignant cells. Chemotherapy may involve the use of one or several different chemical agents and may be used alone or in combination with other therapies, such as surgery or radiation. Some forms of chemotherapy can be administered orally in the form of liquid or pills, and others may be injected into muscle tissue; however, it is most commonly given as an IV infusion. Because a series of infusions is often needed, some patients may have a special IV catheter inserted and left in place for the duration of their treatment. This reduces the number of times they must undergo needlesticks for chemotherapy infusion and blood draws for laboratory tests.

Side effects of chemotherapy vary widely, depending upon the patient and on the agents used. Side effects may be mild and barely noticeable, such as mild fatigue. In other cases they may be more severe, such as nausea, vomiting, moderate to severe fatigue, numbness of the hands and feet, photophobia (sensitivity to light or the sun), hair loss, and vulnerability to infection. Side effects generally lessen between treatments and subside after therapy has ended. Hair grows back, although in some cases it may be of a different texture or color.

Flashpoint

Chemotherapy is the use of potent medications to control or kill cancer cells.

Radiation Therapy

Radiation therapy, sometimes called *radiotherapy,* involves the use of high-energy beams aimed at specific areas of the body. Radiation therapy inhibits the growth of cancer cells by damaging their chemical structure. It is most often used on cancers of the blood and lymphatic system, such as lymphoma and leukemia, and on solid tumors. Radiation may be the only treatment that some people need; others will undergo radiation therapy to shrink their tumor in order to increase the effectiveness of chemotherapy or surgery. Radiation therapy may also be used after surgery, with the goal of destroying any remaining malignant cells. The two types of radiation therapy are external beam radiation and internal radiation. During external beam radiation, a high dose of radiation is delivered directly to the cancerous tissue and a small margin of healthy tissue. During internal radiation, also called *brachytherapy,* tiny capsules, seeds, or tubes filled with a radioactive substance are implanted at the cancer site. Side effects are mostly limited to the radiation site and include skin irritation, sensitivity, and color change. Some patients may also complain of general fatigue and, if the site is in the abdomen, nausea or diarrhea.

Immunotherapy

Immunotherapy is also called *biotherapy* or *use of biological response modifiers.* It uses the body's immune system by stimulating white blood cells to fight the cancer. Immunotherapy is administered by injection. The most common side effects are nausea, diarrhea, fever, fatigue, and swelling or a rash at the injection site. Biological response modifiers are available in five forms: interferons, interleukins, monoclonal antibodies, vaccines, and colony-stimulating factors.

Flashpoint

Immunotherapy uses the body's immune system to fight cancer.

Malignancies of Body Systems

Cancer is a significant and growing concern in the United States. It causes untold pain and grief, not to mention the astronomical monetary costs of treatment and lost wages and productivity.

Cancer of the Integumentary System

Cancerous neoplasms of the skin are classified as basal cell carcinoma, squamous cell carcinoma, and malignant melanoma; together they make up the most common form of cancer.

Basal Cell Carcinoma

ICD-9-CM: 173.0–173.9	[ICD-O-3 M8090/3	[ICD-10: C44.0–C44.9
(unspecified site)	(unspecified site)]	(code by site)]

Basal cell carcinoma (BCC) is the most common type of skin cancer. It grows slowly and rarely metastasizes. It arises from basal cells, which are small round cells found in the lower layer of the epidermis (see Fig. 17-3).

Incidence

BCC is the most common form of skin cancer and is more common in men than women. It accounts for 80% of all skin cancers with 2.8 million diagnosed in the United States each year.

Etiology

BCC develops when DNA of skin cells develop cumulative damage from repeated exposure to harmful elements and begin growing in an abnormal and uncontrolled fashion. Harmful elements include sunlight, ultraviolet light (including tanning beds), x-rays, and arsenic or chemical exposure. The latter occurs through exposure to contaminated foods such as seafood, rice, mushrooms, and chicken, as well as exposure to contaminated soil and groundwater. Risk factors include having fair skin; having blue, gray, or green eyes; having light or red hair; having previous burn injuries or inflammatory skin conditions; tobacco use; and immune suppression.

Signs and Symptoms

The appearance of BCC varies and is sometimes easily confused with squamous cell carcinoma (SCC). It may appear as an open, persistent, non-healing sore that bleeds easily. It may appear as an irritated, reddened area that may itch, hurt, or feel normal. It may appear as a shiny bump that varies in color (pink, red, white, tan, black, or brown) and may be confused with a mole. It may appear as a slightly elevated lesion with an indented, crusty center, visible blood vessels, and rolled border. It may also appear as a scar-like, yellow, white, or waxy area. Additionally, it may resemble noncancerous skin conditions such as psoriasis or eczema.

Diagnosis

Skin cancer may be suspected based upon its physical appearance. However, a biopsied specimen must be studied under a microscope to confirm the type of skin cancer and confirm the diagnosis.

> **Flashpoint**
>
> A sore that does not heal or a change in an existing wart, mole, or other skin lesion may be a sign of cancer.

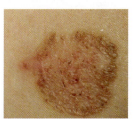

FIGURE 17-3 Basal cell carcinoma (From Barankin, B, and Freiman, A. *Derm Notes: Clinical Dermatology Pocket Guide.* 2006. Philadelphia: F.A. Davis Company, with permission.)

Treatment

Treatment of BCC varies depending upon the size, location, and whether the lesions have spread. Small lesions may be surgically removed or treated with electrodesiccation (electrosurgery), which scrapes tissue away and uses electricity to kill remaining cancer cells and control bleeding. Mohs surgery is often used to ensure removal of all cancerous cells. It involves methodical removal of tissue, followed by immediate inspection of the removed tissue under a microscope. The procedure is repeated until only healthy tissue is seen. This procedure has a high cure rate, yet preserves the healthiest tissue. It is often used for cancers of the head and face. Cryosurgery involves application of a cold substance such as liquid nitrogen to kill cancer cells by freezing. It is effective on small lesions but is not recommended for large ones or those located on the ears, nose, or eyelids. Topical medications may be used on tissue that is determined to be in a precancerous stage. Photodynamic therapy (a type of light treatment) may be used to treat Bowen disease. It involves application of a photosensitizing agent one day, followed by targeting the tissue with a strong light the next day. Laser surgery may also be used to remove tissue.

Prognosis

Prognosis is quite good for patients treated for BCC, although recurrence is common. Rarely, an aggressive form may invade and destroy nearby structures or more rarely, may spread to distant sites. It is rarely fatal.

Squamous Cell Carcinoma

ICD-9-CM: 173.0–173.9   **[ICD-O-3: M8070/3]**   **[ICD-10: C44.0–C44.9**
(code by site)   **(code by site)]**

SCC grows more rapidly than basal cell carcinoma and spreads more easily. It develops in squamous tissue, found on or in the mouth, esophagus, bronchi, lungs, or cervix. It may appear as a firm, red nodule, have a scaly appearance, and ulcerate (see Fig. 17-4 and Box 17-3).

Flashpoint

Squamous cell carcinoma grows on or in the mouth, esophagus, bronchi, lungs, or cervix.

Incidence

SCC is the second most common form of skin cancer, with more than 700,000 cases diagnosed in the United States each year. It causes approximately 2,500 deaths in the United States each year. It is most common among those over age 50—men more than women.

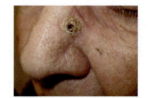

FIGURE 17-4 **Squamous cell carcinoma** (From Barankin, B, and Freiman, A. *Derm Notes: Clinical Dermatology Pocket Guide.* 2006. Philadelphia: F.A. Davis Company, with permission.)

Box 17-3 Wellness Promotion

THE SEVEN WARNING SIGNS OF CANCER

Health-care providers should teach patients about CAUTION—the seven warning signs of cancer:

- **C**hange in bowel or bladder habits
- **A** sore throat that does not heal
- **U**nusual bleeding or discharge
- **T**hickening or a lump in the breast or other area
- **I**ndigestion or difficulty swallowing
- **O**bvious change in a mole or wart
- **N**agging cough or hoarseness

Etiology

Like BCC, SCC develops when DNA of skin cells develop cumulative damage from repeated exposure to harmful elements and begin growing in an abnormal and uncontrolled fashion. Harmful elements include sunlight, ultraviolet light (including tanning beds), x-rays, and arsenic or chemical exposure. The latter occurs through exposure to contaminated foods such as seafood, rice, mushrooms, and chicken, as well as exposure to contaminated soil and groundwater. Infection with the human Papillomavirus (HPV) may also lead to SCC of the genitals. Risk factors include having fair skin; having blue, gray, or green eyes; having light or red hair; having previous burn injuries or inflammatory skin conditions; tobacco use; and immune suppression.

Diagnosis

Skin cancer may be suspected based upon its physical appearance. However, a biopsied specimen must be studied under a microscope to confirm the type of skin cancer and confirm the diagnosis.

Treatment

Treatment for SCC is generally the same as BCC. Small lesions may be surgically removed or treated with electrodesiccation. Mohs surgery and cryosurgery are frequently used. However, cryosurgery is not recommended for large lesions or those located on the ears, nose, or eyelids. Topical medications may be used on tissue that is determined to be in a precancerous stage. Photodynamic therapy (a type of light treatment) may be used to treat Bowen disease. It involves application of a photosensitizing agent one day, followed by targeting tissue with a strong light the next day. Laser surgery may also be used to remove tissue.

Prognosis

Prognosis is generally very good for patients with SCC. Those treated with Mohs surgery experience a cure rate of 94% to 99%. However, the cure rate drops to 77% for those with recurrent lesions. SCC usually affects the epidermis, but left untreated, it can spread to deeper tissues, leading to disfigurement. In up to 10% of cases, SCC spreads to distant tissues and organs.

Malignant Melanoma

ICD-9-CM: 172.0–172.9   **[ICD-O-3: M8720/3]**   **[ICD-10: C43.0–C43.9**
(code by site)   **(code by site)]**

Malignant melanoma is the most lethal form of skin cancer. It develops in melanin-producing skin cells. It commonly arises from a brown or black mole and has a tendency to spread aggressively to distant sites.

Incidence

Malignant melanoma is not the most common form of skin cancer, but it accounts for the most deaths, because of its aggressive nature. Its incidence has tripled among Caucasians in the United States in the past two decades. Approximately 65,000 Americans are diagnosed each year, men more often than women. Each year, approximately 8,500 Americans and more than 40,000 people worldwide die from this form of cancer. The highest incidence of malignant melanoma is in Queensland, Australia, where it is three to four times that of the rate in the United States.

Flashpoint
Malignant melanoma has a tendency to spread aggressively.

Etiology

The exact cause of melanoma is not fully understood. Something triggers melanocytes, which produce the melanin that gives skin its color, to proliferate in a rapid and uncontrolled manner. A variety of environmental and genetic factors are thought to contribute to this, including ultraviolet exposure from sunlight or tanning beds, childhood sunburns, fair skin, red hair, and family history.

Flashpoint
The most common cause of skin cancer is repeated sun or UV exposure. This includes tanning beds!

Signs and Symptoms

The initial appearance of malignant melanoma lesions is variable but includes pigmented color (tan, brown, blue, red, black, or white), asymmetry (lack of balanced proportions), and irregular borders (see Fig. 17-5). Lesions are generally larger than 6 millimeters and often metastasize. They can recur, so patients should be reevaluated on a regular basis after the malignant tissue has been surgically removed (see Box 17-4).

Diagnosis

Skin cancer may be suspected based upon its physical appearance. However, a biopsied specimen must be studied under a microscope to confirm the type of skin cancer and confirm the diagnosis.

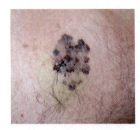

FIGURE 17-5 **Malignant melanoma** (From Barankin, B, and Freiman, A. *Derm Notes: Clinical Dermatology Pocket Guide.* 2006. Philadelphia: F.A. Davis Company, with permission.)

Box 17-4 Wellness Promotion

WARNING SIGNS OF MALIGNANT MELANOMA: THE ABCDE SYSTEM
A helpful way to remember and identify the warning signs of malignant melanoma is the ABCDE system:

- **A**symmetry: The mole is irregular in shape; one half does not match the other half.
- **B**order: The edges of the mole are irregular, notched, scalloped, or blurred.
- **C**olor: Varying shades of color appear throughout, including tan, brown, black, blue, red, and white.
- **D**iameter: The mole is larger than 6 millimeters, or it displays new growth.
- **E**volution: The appearance of the mole changes over time, or symptoms of bleeding or itching develop.

Treatment

Treatment for patients with malignant melanoma depends upon the stage of the cancer and the patient's age, health, and personal preferences. Simple excision (surgical removal) may be all that is needed for some lesions. Treatment of melanoma that has spread is more challenging and may include chemotherapy, radiation therapy, and immunotherapy. Surgery is not curative for melanoma that has spread, but it may occasionally be done to improve comfort or appearance.

Flashpoint

Malignant melanoma is responsible for 75% of all deaths from skin cancer.

Prognosis

Malignant melanoma accounts for a small percentage of skin cancers but is responsible for 75% of deaths from skin cancer. The prognosis is best for individuals whose cancer is diagnosed and treated early, before metastasis has occurred.

Cancer of the Neurological System

Tumor is a vague term used to describe any type of abnormal mass or growth of tissue that is different from neighboring tissue. A brain tumor is any type of abnormal mass growing within the cranium (see Fig. 17-6) and may be benign or malignant.

Flashpoint

A brain tumor is any abnormally growing mass or tissue in the brain. It may or may not be cancerous.

Brain Cancer

| ICD-9-CM: 191.0–191.9 (code by site) | [ICD-O-3: M9440/3 (glioblastoma multiforme), M9400/3 (astrocytoma)] | [ICD-10: C71.0–C71.9 (code by site)] |

Brain cancer is the proliferation of malignant cells within the brain or other tissue of the central nervous system. Nine categories of primary malignant brain tumors have been identified. The two most common, glioblastoma multiforme and astrocytoma, account for the vast majority of cases.

Incidence

Approximately 22,000 Americans are diagnosed with brain cancer each year, and about 13,000 die.

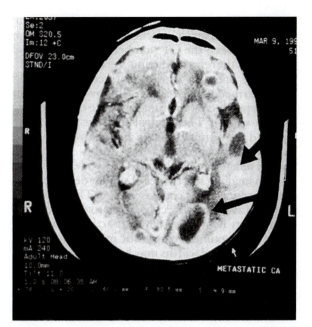

FIGURE 17-6 **Brain tumor** (From Tortorici, MR, and Apfel, PJ. *Advanced Radiographic and Angiographic Procedures.* 1995. Philadelphia: F.A. Davis Company, with permission.)

Etiology

Cancerous brain tumors may be primary, meaning they originated within the brain and are composed of brain tissue, or metastatic (secondary), meaning they originally developed elsewhere in the body and spread to the brain. About half of malignant brain tumors are primary and half are metastatic. Astrocytomas usually grow within the brainstem, spinal cord, cerebellum, or white matter of the cerebrum. Glioblastoma multiforme cancers are composed of glial cells within the cerebrum.

The cause of brain cancer is not fully understood. An identified risk factor is exposure to vinyl chloride, which is a *carcinogen* (cancer-causing substance) present in certain chemicals used for the production of rubber, oil-based products, embalming fluids, pipes, wire coatings, car parts, and some types of housewares. It is also present in tobacco smoke.

Signs and Symptoms

Many of the signs and symptoms of brain cancer are related to the pressure exerted on surrounding structures by the tumor and the increased intracranial pressure it causes. Such signs and symptoms include headaches, seizures, nausea, vomiting, changes in mental status, memory problems, personality changes, muscle weakness, sensory loss, speech difficulties, alterations in gait and balance, and visual disturbances.

Diagnosis

Diagnosis of brain cancer is based on a description of signs and symptoms, a thorough neurological evaluation, a medical history, and results of magnetic resonance imaging (MRI) or a computed tomography (CT) scan. Examination of cerebrospinal fluid may reveal cancerous cells, indicating spread of the cancer to the spinal cord. Edema of the optic nerve may be apparent on ophthalmic examination. Study of biopsied tissue confirms whether the growth is cancerous or benign.

Treatment

Treatment for brain cancer depends on the type and location of the tumor. When possible, the tumor is surgically removed. This is followed by chemotherapy or radiation. Additional measures may be taken to relieve intracranial pressure and associated symptoms. Antiseizure medication is given to treat or prevent seizures, and corticosteroids may be given to decrease inflammation, thereby decreasing intracranial pressure.

Flashpoint
Exposure to vinyl chloride is a risk factor for brain cancer.

Flashpoint
Treatment for brain cancer usually includes surgery and chemotherapy, or radiation.

Prognosis

Prognosis is generally poor, because of the invasive and aggressive nature of brain cancers. Specific outcomes depend on the type and location of the tumor and on the age and underlying health of the patient. The general 5-year survival rate is under 10%.

Cancer of the Urinary System

Cancers of the urinary system can involve any of the structures within the system, including the kidneys, ureters, and bladder. Most common are those affecting the kidneys and the bladder.

Renal Cancer

ICD-9-CM: 189.0   [ICD-O-3: M8312/3]   [ICD-10: C64]

Renal cancer is cancer of the kidneys (see Fig. 17-7). It includes renal cell carcinoma and renal pelvis carcinoma. It also includes Wilms tumor, which usually develops in young children.

Incidence

An estimated 54,000 Americans are diagnosed with renal cancer each year, and an estimated 13,000 people die from it. It most commonly affects elderly individuals between ages 50 and 70, men more often than women.

Etiology

The specific cause of renal cancer is not clear. However, there are a number of known risk factors, including age of at least 60, male gender, African American descent, tobacco use (especially pipes and cigars), obesity, hypertension, and exposure to toxins such as solvents, asbestos, and radiation. Individuals with a history of bladder cancer and those who undergo long-term dialysis are also at increased risk.

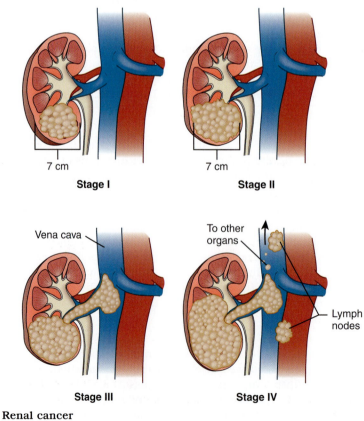

FIGURE 17-7 Renal cancer

Signs and Symptoms

Patients with renal cancer are commonly symptom free in the early stages. In later stages, they may experience hematuria, back pain, weight loss, fatigue, and intermittent fever.

Diagnosis

The diagnostic process begins with routine blood and urine tests. These help the physician determine current kidney functioning and provide baseline data to help measure the patient's response to therapy. A complete health history and physical examination reveal signs and symptoms associated with renal cancer. Radiological studies such as intravenous pyelogram, ultrasound, CT, and MRI can create detailed images of the kidneys and bladder and may detect unusual masses. Tissue biopsy, sometimes required for definitive diagnosis, reveals cancer cells.

> **Flashpoint**
> Patients with renal cancer are usually symptom free in the early stages.

Treatment

Treatment of renal cancer includes partial or total nephrectomy (surgical removal of the kidney). When surgery is not possible, another treatment option is arterial embolization, in which the surgeon injects material to clog the main vessel leading to the kidney. This robs the tumor of nutrients and oxygen and relieves pain and bleeding. Radiation therapy may target and kill cancer cells and relieve the pain of metastatic cancer. Other forms of treatment include immunotherapy and chemotherapy.

Prognosis

The general 5-year survival rate for patients with renal cancer is 55%. However, prognosis is variable and depends on the stage at the time of diagnosis. The 5-year survival rate for those with stage I is 95%, stage II is 65% to 75%, stage III is 40% to 70%, and stage IV is only 10%.

Wilms Tumor
ICD-9-CM: 189.0   [ICD-O-3: M8960/3]   [ICD-10: C64]

Wilms tumor, also known as *nephroblastoma*, is a rapidly growing type of kidney cancer that most commonly affects children. Usually only one kidney is cancerous.

Incidence

Wilms tumor most commonly affects children between the ages of 1 and 5.

Etiology

Wilms tumor develops from immature kidney cells that multiply and grow in an abnormal manner. There is a genetic component in some cases, and the condition is commonly associated with other genetic abnormalities.

Signs and Symptoms

Patients with Wilms tumor may be asymptomatic in the early stages. An abdominal mass is a common finding that may be detected by the parent when bathing or dressing the child or by the physician upon physical examination. Signs and symptoms include hematuria, weight loss, constipation, nausea, vomiting, abdominal pain, fever, anorexia, and malaise.

> **Flashpoint**
> The parent may notice an abdominal mass when bathing or dressing the child.

Diagnosis

Diagnosis is based on physical examination, family medical history, tests of urine and blood, and diagnostic imaging. MRI, CT scan, and ultrasound are used to locate and visualize the tumor.

Treatment

Treatment of Wilms tumor includes surgery, chemotherapy, bone-marrow transplant, and radiation therapy. As with most types of cancer, the physician will order an analysis of tissue cells for staging in order to determine the most appropriate course of treatment. Surgery usually includes partial or complete nephrectomy and may include removal of local lymph nodes and other surrounding tissue as well.

Prognosis

The prognosis for patients with Wilms tumor has improved substantially in recent decades; the survival rate is currently around 90%. The outcome is best when only one kidney is involved.

Bladder Cancer
ICD-9-CM: 239.4   [ICD-O-3: M8070 /3]   [ICD-10: C67.0–C67.9 (code by site)]

Bladder cancer includes a variety of malignancies of the bladder. Most involve the lining of the bladder (see Fig. 17-8).

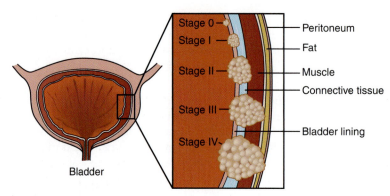

Stage 0 —
Stage I —
Stage II —
Stage III —
Stage IV —

— Peritoneum
— Fat
— Muscle
— Connective tissue
— Bladder lining

Bladder

FIGURE 17-8 Bladder cancer

Incidence

Bladder cancer is the most common form of cancer of the urinary tract. Most tumors develop in the bladder lining, while more invasive tumors develop in the muscle. Transitional cell carcinoma is most common in industrialized countries; squamous cell carcinomas caused by parasitic infestations are most common in developing countries. Bladder cancer is most common in industrialized countries, such as the United States, Canada, and France. Nearly 40,000 Americans are diagnosed with it each year, and more than 14,000 die. The incidence increases with age, especially over age 55. Bladder cancer is three times more common in men than in women and is more common in the Caucasian population.

Flashpoint

Bladder cancer is the most common form of cancer of the urinary tract.

Etiology

The cause of bladder cancer is unknown. However, there are many contributors and risk factors, including exposure to tobacco smoke, radiation, arsenic, and other carcinogens; advanced age; chronic bladder inflammation; high-fat diet; genetics; male gender; and a history of parasitic infection with *Schistosoma haematobium*. Persons at increased risk due to workplace exposures include truck drivers, machinists, printers, painters, hairdressers, and those working in the rubber, metal, leather, textile, and chemical industries.

Signs and Symptoms

Flashpoint

Hematuria is the most common symptom of bladder cancer.

Bladder cancer is generally painless and may not be obvious in early stages. The most common symptom is hematuria; other symptoms may include urinary frequency and dysuria.

Diagnosis

Diagnosis of bladder cancer is based on urinalysis and diagnostic imaging. Urinalysis rules out infection and identifies the presence of blood and abnormal cells. Intravenous pyelogram enables better examination of all structures within the urinary tract. Cystoscopy allows visual examination of the inner bladder wall and provides opportunity to take a tissue sample for biopsy, which is used to confirm the diagnosis. The physician will stage the cancer according to the tumor, node, metastasis system. Other diagnostic tests used to determine the extent or stage of the cancer may include CT scan, MRI, bone scan, and ultrasound. Newer tests may be used to identify tumor markers, which are substances released by tumors.

Treatment

Treatment varies for each patient, depending on the type and stage of the cancer and other health factors. Interventions include surgery, radiation, chemotherapy, and immunotherapy. Surgery may be as simple as transurethral (through the urethra) excision of a small lesion or as complex as the surgical removal of the entire bladder, nearby lymph nodes, some of the reproductive organs or structures, and surrounding tissue.

Prognosis

The prognosis for patients with bladder cancer is guarded. The 5-year survival rate for those with superficial (affecting the surface) bladder cancer is 85%; those with more invasive forms have a poorer prognosis, and those with identified metastasis have a 5-year survival rate of just 5%. Because there is a high rate of recurrence, regular follow-up examinations, including cytology (study of tissue cells) and cystoscopy, are recommended. Complications of bladder cancer and its treatment include anemia, urinary incontinence, and metastasis to other organs.

Cancer of the Reproductive System

Flashpoint
Follow-up evaluation is important because bladder cancer has a high rate of recurrence.

Cancers of the reproductive system account for a large percentage of the total cancer cases in the United States. Among the most common types affecting the male reproductive system are prostate cancer and testicular cancer. The most common forms of cancer affecting the female reproductive system are breast cancer, cervical cancer, uterine cancer, and ovarian cancer.

Prostate Cancer
ICD-9-CM: 185   [ICD-O-3: M8140/3]   [ICD-10: C61]
Prostate cancer is a malignant tumor of the prostate gland that develops when prostate cells grow abnormally and uncontrollably (see Fig. 17-9).

Incidence
Prostate cancer is one of the most common forms of cancer in America. It affects one in six men, with nearly 190,000 diagnoses each year and nearly 30,000 deaths. It is rare in young men but much more common in older age-groups, with over 65% of prostate cancer diagnosed in those over age 65.

Etiology
The specific cause of prostate cancer is not clear; hormones such as testosterone are thought to play a role. Risk factors include advanced age, family history, genetics, and dietary factors. African American men are more likely than those in other ethnic groups to develop prostate cancer; however, Caucasian men are twice as likely to die from it.

Flashpoint
Prostate cancer affects 17% of all men.

Signs and Symptoms
Patients are commonly asymptomatic in the early stages of prostate cancer. As symptoms develop, the patient may notice urinary frequency, urgency, and hesitancy; nocturia; dysuria; erectile dysfunction; painful ejaculation; hematuria; and blood in the semen. As the cancer spreads to bones and

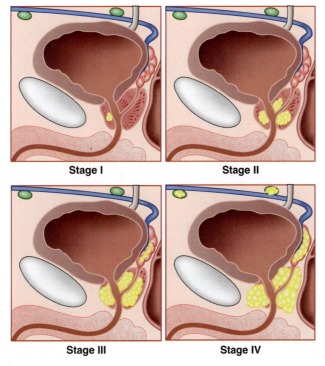

Stage I   Stage II

Stage III   Stage IV

FIGURE 17-9 Prostate cancer

surrounding structures, the patient may complain of pain or stiffness in the lower back, hips, or upper thighs.

Diagnosis

There is some controversy regarding the necessity of screening for prostate cancer. The American Cancer Society recommends that men over age 45 or 50 (depending on risk factors) undergo annual screening. Two common screening methods are digital rectal examination and prostate-specific antigen (PSA) testing (see Box 17-5). To perform a digital rectal examination, the health-care provider palpates the prostate gland with a gloved, lubricated finger inserted rectally and notes any irregularities in its shape, size, or texture. If the results of either test are abnormal, the physician will order a biopsy of prostate tissue, which confirms the diagnosis if cancer cells are detected.

Treatment

The treatment of prostate cancer depends on the age of the patient, the aggressiveness of the cancer, and the patient's personal preference. The healthcare team, comprised of a urologist and radiation oncologist and/or medical oncologist, will design a treatment plan which may include surgery, radiation, and chemotherapy. Orchiectomy (surgical removal of one or both testes) and drug therapy may reduce testosterone levels, which in turn reduces the risk of metastasis and the aggressiveness of the cancer.

Flashpoint

Orchiectomy and drug therapy may be used to reduce testosterone levels.

Prognosis

The prognosis for men with prostate cancer is variable, depending on the cancer stage, Gleason score (microscopic appearance of cells), and PSA level. Overall, the 5-year survival rate for patients with all types of prostate cancer is just over 70%, and the 10-year survival rate is around 55%. For those with metastatic cancer, the 5-year survival rate is only 30%.

Testicular Cancer
ICD-9-CM: 186.9   [ICD-10: C62.0–C62.9]

Testicular cancer is a malignancy that occurs when cells within the testicle grow abnormally and uncontrollably.

Incidence

Testicular cancer usually affects only one testicle and is the most common form of cancer in men between the ages of 18 and 32. Approximately 7,600 American men are diagnosed with this form of cancer each year, and 400 die. Incidence is higher in Caucasians than in other racial groups.

Flashpoint

Testicular cancer most often affects young men between the ages of 18 and 32.

Etiology

The specific cause of testicular cancer is unclear. Risk factors include a history of cryptorchidism (undescended testicle), HIV infection or AIDS, age between 15 and 34, Caucasian race, and a family history of testicular cancer.

Signs and Symptoms

Patients with testicular cancer may be asymptomatic in the early stages. The patient often first notices a lump or enlargement in the testicle, which may or may not be painful. Other signs and

Box 17-5 Diagnostic Spotlight

PROSTATE-SPECIFIC ANTIGEN (PSA)

The PSA test detects the presence of a specific protein in the blood that is commonly elevated in the presence of prostate cancer, benign prostatic hyperplasia, and prostatitis. Although results of this test are not always conclusive, it is currently the most effective test available for detecting prostate cancer in its early stages.

The level of PSA in a man's blood increases as he ages and his prostate enlarges. In general, a value below 4 nanograms per milliliter is considered normal. Levels between 4 and 10 nanograms per milliliter are considered borderline, and any level above 10 nanograms per milliliter is high. A high level does not necessarily mean a man has cancer; however, it does mean that further evaluation is necessary, because he *might* have cancer.

symptoms include a dull ache within the groin or abdomen, a feeling of heaviness within the scrotum, scrotal edema, breast enlargement, fatigue, and malaise.

Diagnosis

Diagnosis is generally made after the patient has noticed a lump or other abnormality and then seeks medical care. A physician may also note a lump during a regular health examination. Testicular ultrasound is highly effective in identifying testicular cancer. It helps the physician examine the shape, size, and density of the testicles as well as any other masses. A solid mass is a sign of a malignant tumor, because most other testicular conditions involve the presence of fluid. If findings are suspicious, tissue biopsy confirms the diagnosis. Blood tests may be done to detect the tumor markers alpha-fetoprotein and human chorionic gonadotropin. A CT scan may be done to help stage the cancer and identify whether it has spread to other organs.

Treatment

Treatment for testicular cancer depends on the type of cancer and whether it has spread. Surgical intervention usually includes orchiectomy and removal of local lymph nodes. Treatment also includes radiation therapy, chemotherapy, and, sometimes, bone-marrow transplantation.

Prognosis

The prognosis for men with testicular cancer is good when it is diagnosed early but declines as the cancer becomes more advanced. Therefore, all young men should be educated about how to perform regular testicular self-examinations (see Box 17-6). Overall, there is a 95% rate of successful treatment. Because cancer is usually limited to one testicle, men are usually able to retain normal sexual functioning and fertility.

> ### Flashpoint
> Testicular cancer is usually diagnosed after the patient has noticed an abnormal lump.

Box 17-6 Wellness Promotion

TESTICULAR SELF-EXAMINATION

The health-care provider should encourage male patients to perform monthly testicular self-examinations (TSE). Performing a monthly TSE familiarizes the patient with how these tissues normally feel and increases the odds that he will notice changes early. He should be instructed to report changes that persist for more than 2 weeks. He should also be reassured that other disorders besides cancer may explain testicular changes. Performing a TSE is easiest during a warm bath or shower. The basic steps are:

1. Hold the scrotum in the palms of the hands and feel one testicle.
2. Apply gentle pressure while rolling the testicle between the fingers, noting any hard, painless lumps.
3. Locate the circular cord behind the testicle and feel for any hard lumps.
4. Locate the firm, movable, smooth tube that runs upward from the epididymis and feel for any hard lumps.
5. Repeat the examination on the other side.

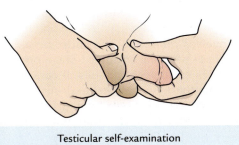

Testicular self-examination

Breast Cancer

ICD-9-CM: 174.9 (primary)   **[ICD-10: C50.0–C50.8 (code by site)]**

Breast cancer is the growth of abnormal cells in the tissue of the breast. It usually forms in the lactiferous ducts (the tubes that carry milk to the nipple) and the lobules (the glands that produce the milk).

Incidence

More than 180,000 women and 2,000 men develop breast cancer each year in the United States. More than 40,000 women and more than 400 men die from the disease each year. Breast cancer occurs most commonly in women over age 35 and is the leading cause of death in American women ages 40 to 55.

Flashpoint

Breast cancer is the second leading cause of death among American women.

Etiology

The exact cause of breast cancer is unknown. Scientists have discovered a link between breast cancer and the genes BRCA1 and BRCA2. The discovery of these genes shows that breast cancer has a link to genetic predisposition; however, it does not indicate that breast cancer's only cause is genetic. Women who are at risk of breast cancer include those with family history of breast cancer; those with early onset of menses (age 12 or earlier) or late menopause (age 55 or later); and those who have never had children or had their first child after age 35. Other risk factors include high-fat diet, obesity, history of endometrial or ovarian cancer, use of estrogen replacement therapy or oral contraceptives, and history of fibrocystic breast disease.

Signs and Symptoms

Signs and symptoms of breast cancer include a breast mass, bloody or brown discharge from the nipple, and breast nodules or irregularities. The breast mass is usually painless and freely movable in the early stage but later becomes fixed.

Diagnosis

Regular breast self-examination can help in the early detection of breast cancer (see Box 17-7). If the patient palpates a painless lump in her breast during a self-examination, the physician will conduct a breast examination and further testing to confirm the diagnosis. A mammogram can confirm the presence of a breast mass and can detect tumors that are too small to palpate (see Box 17-8). About 70% of masses found by mammography are benign. If a mass is found, a fine needle aspiration can be used to determine whether the mass is solid or a fluid-filled cyst. A tissue biopsy confirms malignancy.

Flashpoint

Mammography can detect tumors that are too small to be felt.

Treatment

The treatment plan depends upon the stage of the disease, the patient's age, gender, and whether the patient is currently menstruating or in menopause. A combination of therapies is used, including one of the following surgical options:

- *Lumpectomy* involves removal of the tumor, the surrounding tissue, and possibly the adjacent lymph nodes (for testing) through a small incision. This treatment is effective for early-stage breast cancer with small, well-defined lesions.
- *Partial mastectomy* involves removal of the tumor and a wedge of surrounding normal tissue, skin, fascia, and possibly axillary lymph nodes. This procedure is used for early-stage breast cancer with small, well-defined lesions. Radiation or chemotherapy is common after surgery to destroy undetected diseased tissue in the breast.
- *Total mastectomy* involves surgical removal of the entire breast and is used when the cancer is confined to the breast tissue with no involvement of the lymph nodes. If the patient does not have advanced disease, surgery can be used for cosmetic reconstruction.
- *Modified radical mastectomy* involves removal of the entire breast, axillary lymph nodes, and chest fascia. This procedure is used for advanced-stage breast cancer that may include metastasis to lymph nodes or adjacent tissues. If cancer has spread to the lymph tissue, radiation and chemotherapy are used to destroy more cancer cells. This newer procedure replaces the older radical mastectomy procedure, where chest muscles were also removed; it allows the patient more function and upper-body strength after surgery.

Box 17-7 Wellness Promotion

BREAST SELF-EXAMINATION

Breast self-examination is most effective if performed regularly. This allows the woman to become familiar with how her breast tissue normally feels and to detect changes. Steps of the breast self-examination are:

1. Remove clothing from the waist up, press the hands firmly on the hips, and observe the breasts in a mirror. Note changes in shape, contour, size, or scaliness of the breasts and nipples. Also note any areas where the skin is dimpled or reddened.
2. Feel the tissue of the underarm with that arm held slightly away from the body but relaxed. Note any changes or new lumps.
3. Perform the same examination on the underarm of the other side.
4. Lie down and place one arm behind the head. Using the pads of the three middle fingers of the opposite hand, feel the tissue of the breast on the same side as the raised arm with light and deep pressure. Follow a pattern than ensures that all breast tissue is examined.
5. Place the other arm behind the head and examine the breast on that side, following the same procedure.

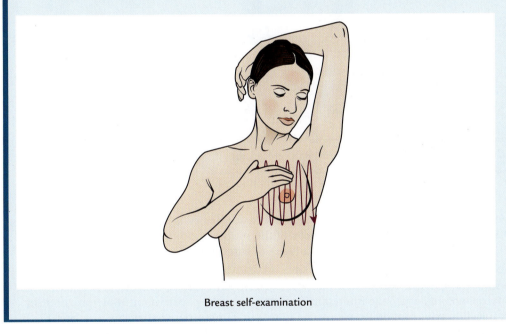

Breast self-examination

Prognosis

The prognosis for women with breast cancer is based primarily on the tumor's stage. Patients with large tumors that have metastasized to lymph nodes, the chest wall, or distal organs have a poor prognosis. Patients with smaller tumors with no metastasis have better outcomes.

Cervical Cancer

ICD-9-CM: 180.9 (primary)   [ICD-10: C53]

Cervical cancer is an abnormal growth and development of the cells of the cervix.

Incidence

Cervical cancer is the third-most common cancer of the female reproductive tract, causing 5% of all cancer deaths in women. It most often strikes women in their 50s. About 80% of all cervical

Box 17-8 Diagnostic Spotlight

MAMMOGRAPHY

Mammography, the x-ray examination of the breast, is considered one of the most effective methods of detecting breast cancer early (along with regular breast self-examinations). Women should receive their first mammogram at age 40 and have follow-up mammograms yearly or as directed by a physician. Males may also undergo a mammogram if abnormalities are detected in their breast tissue. To undergo a mammogram, the patient must stand facing the mammogram machine. The radiological technologist or technician will then position the patient's breast on a flat plate on the machine. The machine applies pressure from the top and bottom of the breast to compress the tissue and take an x-ray image of it. The process is then repeated with lateral compression applied from both sides.

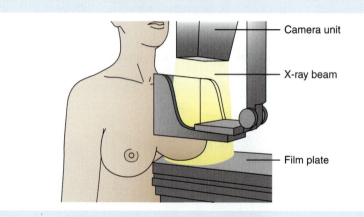

Mammography (From Eagle, S, et al. *The Professional Medical Assistant: An Integrative Teamwork-Based Approach.* 2009. Philadelphia: F.A. Davis Company, with permission.)

cancers are squamous cell carcinomas (changes in the surface cells of the cervix); the remaining 20% are adenocarcinomas (changes in the cells of the mucus-producing glands of the cervix). Very few cases of cervical cancer involve both types of carcinoma.

Etiology

The cause of cervical cancer is unknown. Factors contributing to cervical cancer include tobacco smoking, early-age intercourse, multiple sexual partners, multiple pregnancies, and infection with herpes simplex virus type 2 or human papillomavirus (see Box 17-9).

Flashpoint

Herpes simplex virus type 2 and human papillomavirus are both known risk factors for cervical cancer.

Signs and Symptoms

Women with early cervical cancer are asymptomatic. Signs and symptoms of later-stage cervical cancer include abnormal vaginal bleeding, persistent discharge, and pain and bleeding after intercourse.

Diagnosis

Papanicolaou (Pap) test screening enables a diagnosis before symptoms appear, so that treatment can begin early. The Pap test detects abnormal cellular changes with 95% accuracy (see Box 17-10).

Flashpoint

The Pap test is 95% accurate in detecting cellular changes.

Treatment

Treatment options for cervical cancer include cryosurgery and laser treatments to eliminate cancer cells. Surgical procedures include conization (removal of a cone-shaped section of cells from the mucous membrane) and removal of the cervix. Other therapies include radiation and chemotherapy, for cancer that has grown deeper into the cervix. Hysterectomy is a treatment option for women with preinvasive cervical cancer who do not wish to preserve fertility.

Box 17-9 Wellness Promotion

PREVENTING CERVICAL CANCER

Although a direct cause-and-effect relationship has not been proven, there are significant data indicating a link between the human papillomavirus (HPV) and cervical cancer. Therefore, the federal government issued a policy recommending immunization against HPV for all sexually active females. The immunization, a three-shot series, can be given to girls as young as 8 to establish immunity prior to sexual activity. Other measures that can be taken to reduce the risk of developing cervical cancer include:

- avoiding tobacco use
- avoiding early-age sexual intercourse
- practicing monogamy and limiting the number of sexual partners over time
- practicing safer sex by using barrier precautions to avoid contracting HPV or herpes simplex virus type 2

Box 17-10 Diagnostic Spotlight

THE PAP TEST

The Papanicolaou (Pap) test, also called *Pap smear*, is used to detect cancer cells in the cervix. In this test, the patient's cervix is scraped with a cytology brush to obtain tissue cells. The specimen is then spread on a glass slide or placed in a vial of transport fluid. It is taken to the laboratory, where it is examined by a pathologist.

The specimen is collected in the physician's office, where the patient is asked to undress from the waist down. She may be given a gown to wear or a drape to place over her lower body. The patient lies on the examination table with her knees bent and her feet supported in stirrups. In order to visualize the cervix, the physician gently inserts a speculum to open the vagina. The examination only takes a few minutes and causes little or no physical discomfort.

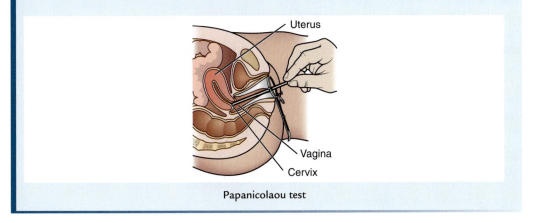

Papanicolaou test

Prognosis

The survival rate for patients with preinvasive cancer is almost 100%. For patients with invasive cervical cancer, the survival rate is approximately 91%. About 35% of patients with invasive cervical cancer experience recurrence.

Uterine Cancer
  ICD-9-CM: 179 (primary)   [ICD-10: C54.0–C54.9]
Uterine cancer is called an *adenocarcinoma* since it begins in the endometrial cells of the uterus, usually in the glandular tissue.

Flashpoint
The survival rate for women with cervical cancer is quite high.

Incidence

Uterine cancer is the most common malignancy of the female reproductive system. Over 40,000 American women are diagnosed with it each year, and nearly 7,500 die. Uterine cancer typically affects postmenopausal women between ages 50 and 60. The incidence is higher in Caucasian women than those in other ethnic groups, but the death rate is higher in African American women.

Etiology

The cause of uterine cancer is not fully understood; however, some risk factors have been identified. They include advanced age, obesity, Caucasian race, history of colon or rectal cancer, and history of endometrial hyperplasia. Other risk factors are estrogen related, such as the use of hormone replacement therapy—especially when estrogen is used alone—or the drug tamoxifen (which is used to treat breast cancer), early onset of menstruation, late menopause, and having had no children.

Signs and Symptoms

Signs and symptoms of uterine cancer include bleeding in the postmenopausal patient; yellow, watery discharge with a foul odor; and cramping or pressure in the abdomen or pelvis.

Diagnosis

Results of a uterine biopsy will show cellular changes consistent with cancer. If the biopsy is inconclusive, the physician will perform dilation and curettage, a procedure in which cells are scraped from the uterine lining, to obtain an adequate sample to determine malignancy.

Treatment

Flashpoint

Treatment for uterine cancer usually includes a total hysterectomy.

Treatment for uterine cancer is most commonly a total hysterectomy, to prevent recurrence of cancer in any of the reproductive organs. The physician may prescribe radiation therapy before surgery, if the tumor is poorly defined. The physician may also prescribe chemotherapy after surgery to prevent the growth of cancer in adjacent organs. Administration of progesterone before surgery reduces uterine bleeding during the procedure.

Prognosis

The 1-year survival rate for patients with uterine cancer is 92%. The 5-year survival rate varies from 65% to 70%, based on the timeliness of diagnosis.

Ovarian Cancer
ICD-9-CM: 183.0 (primary)   [ICD-10: C56]

Ovarian cancer is the development of malignancy of the ovaries.

Incidence

Approximately 21,000 American women are diagnosed with ovarian cancer each year, and more than 15,000 die from it. It accounts for 4% of all cancers among women.

Etiology

Many patients who develop ovarian cancer have the BRCA1 or BRCA2 gene, suggesting that they have a hereditary predisposition to ovarian cancer.

Ovarian tumors arise from three different types of ovarian cells:

- *Epithelial tumors* involve malignant changes to the surface cells of the ovary.
- *Germ cell tumors* involve abnormal changes to the cells that produce the ova.
- *Stromal tumors* involve changes to cells of connective tissues that hold the ovary together and produce estrogen and progesterone.

Signs and Symptoms

Early-stage symptoms of ovarian cancer include mild abdominal pain, abdominal bloating, diarrhea or constipation, indigestion, gas, upset stomach, fatigue, and abnormal menstrual or vaginal bleeding.

Diagnosis

Flashpoint

Ovarian cancer is usually not detected in the early stages.

Because symptoms are vague, many patients with ovarian cancer are not diagnosed in the early stages. Most cases are diagnosed when the disease has already progressed and symptoms include ascites (a buildup of fluid in the abdominal cavity), shortness of breath, persistent dry cough, nausea, vomiting, abdominal tumors, and weight loss.

Treatment

Treatment of ovarian cancer depends on the stage and grade of the tumor. It includes surgical removal of the reproductive structures and affected nearby tissues, along with radiation and chemotherapy (see Box 17-11).

Prognosis

Because most ovarian cancers progress to a late stage before diagnosis, only 25% of patients survive for 5 years.

Cancer of the Lymphatic/Immune Systems

The most common cancers affecting the immune and lymphatic systems are Hodgkin disease and non-Hodgkin lymphoma.

Hodgkin Disease

ICD-9-CM: 201.90   [ICD-O-3: M9650/3]   [ICD-10: C81]

Hodgkin disease, also known as *lymphoma*, is a malignancy of the lymph system. It initially affects lymph nodes but eventually spreads throughout the lymphatic system, involving the spleen, liver, and bone marrow.

Incidence

Nearly 8,000 new cases of Hodgkin disease are diagnosed each year in the United States. Most commonly affected are young adults between the ages of 15 and 40 and those over age 55.

Etiology

The cause of Hodgkin disease is not fully understood. However, the Epstein-Barr virus has been found in approximately 50% of those with the disease. Therefore, a link between the two is suspected. Another risk factor is a weakened immune system caused by chemotherapy, radiation, infection with HIV, or immunosuppressive therapy related to organ transplantation. A family history of Hodgkin disease is also a risk factor.

Signs and Symptoms

In the early stages of Hodgkin disease, patients may be asymptomatic except for a painless lump in the axilla (armpit) or neck. Other signs and symptoms are similar to those of influenza and include fever, anorexia, weight loss, fatigue, itching, and night sweats. Eventually, tumors develop.

Flashpoint

A link between the Epstein-Barr virus and Hodgkin disease is suspected.

Box 17-11 Wellness Promotion

TAKING CARE DURING RADIATION AND CHEMOTHERAPY

Radiation and chemotherapy are used to kill cancer cells. Unfortunately, most of these treatments also kill healthy cells of the body. This accounts for many of the typical side effects, such as nausea, vomiting, diarrhea, hair loss, fatigue, stomatitis (inflammation of the tissues of the mouth), tissue necrosis, and weakening of the immune system. To ease these symptoms and prevent complications, health-care providers should advise patients undergoing radiation and chemotherapy to:

- eat cool, soft, bland foods to reduce nausea and prevent vomiting
- eat iron-rich foods or take a multivitamin and mineral combination to replace red blood cells lost during treatment
- consider using acupuncture to treat nausea and stimulate appetite
- use a soft toothbrush to avoid irritation and infection of the gums
- use an electric razor to avoid injury to and infection of the skin
- pace activities and rest frequently; ask friends or family to help with daily chores and driving to the hospital or clinic for treatments
- report symptoms of infection, such as fever, cough, sore throat, and dysuria
- report sudden, severe headaches

Diagnosis

Diagnosis of Hodgkin disease is confirmed upon finding the giant Reed-Sternberg cells in biopsied lymph-node tissue. Staging is done to determine how advanced the disease is and to determine the best course of treatment. Stage I indicates early disease involving a single lymph structure. Stage IV is widespread disease. Chest, abdomen, and pelvic CT scans may be done to determine the extent of disease.

Treatment

Treatment for Hodgkin disease includes chemotherapy alone or in combination with radiation therapy. Bone-marrow transplantation may also be performed.

Prognosis

Approximately 1,300 Americans die from this disease each year—a 60% drop in mortality since the 1970s. Prognosis depends on the stage of metastasis at the time of diagnosis. Early disease is confined to one or a few nodes, while advanced disease spreads to both sides of the diaphragm or throughout the body. Those with early disease have a 5-year survival rate as high as 90%.

Non-Hodgkin Lymphoma
ICD-9-CM: 202.8   [ICD-O-3: M9591/3]   [ICD-10: C82.0–C82.9]

Non-Hodgkin lymphoma is a group of more than 30 types of malignancies of B or T lymphocytes, which are specialized kinds of white blood cells.

Incidence

Non-Hodgkin malignancies affect approximately 65,000 Americans each year, men more frequently than women. Approximately 19,000 people die each year from the diseases.

Etiology

Flashpoint

Prior immunosuppressive therapy significantly increases the risk of developing non-Hodgkin lymphoma.

The cause of non-Hodgkin lymphoma is unclear. However, those who have received previous treatment with immunosuppressive therapies have a risk 100 times greater than those who have not. Other risk factors include AIDS, infections with Epstein-Barr virus or *Helicobacter pylori*, and exposure to some chemicals used to kill weeds and insects.

Signs and Symptoms

Early symptoms of non-Hodgkin lymphoma are similar to those of Hodgkin disease and include painless enlargement of the lymph nodes. Other possible signs and symptoms include fever, night sweats, fatigue, abdominal pain or swelling, and weight loss.

Diagnosis

Diagnosis of non-Hodgkin lymphoma is determined by identifying malignant cells via lymph-node biopsy and bone-marrow examination. CT scans and MRI are performed to help determine the extent of the cancer's spread.

Treatment

Treatment of non-Hodgkin lymphoma includes radiation therapy, chemotherapy, and bone-marrow transplantation.

Prognosis

The prognosis for patients with non-Hodgkin lymphoma depends on the specific type of lymphoma involved and the timeliness of diagnosis and treatment. Some types spread slowly and respond well to treatment, while others spread quickly, respond poorly to treatment, and are rapidly fatal.

Cancer of the Cardiovascular System

The most common malignancy affecting the cardiovascular system is leukemia.

Leukemia
ICD-9-CM: 204.0–205.1   [ICD-O-3: M9800/   [ICD-10: C91.0–C95.9]
**   3–M9940/3]   (code by type, for all codes)**

Leukemia is a malignancy of the blood and blood-forming tissues, including the bone marrow, spleen, and lymph nodes. There are a number of different types of leukemia, both acute and chronic forms. The chronic forms have a relatively slow course that averages 4 years, while the acute forms are fatal within months or even weeks.

Incidence

In the United States, approximately 29,000 adults and 2,000 children are diagnosed with some form of leukemia each year. Acute lymphocytic leukemia is the most common type affecting children. The other three types—acute myelogenous leukemia, chronic lymphocytic leukemia, and chronic myelogenous leukemia—may occasionally affect children but develop mostly in older adults.

Etiology

In all types of leukemia, abnormally rapid proliferation of one type of white blood cell results in reduced production of other types of white blood cells, red blood cells, and platelets. The underlying cause is not always fully understood. Suspected triggers or contributors include viruses, the use of tobacco, chemical exposure, some drugs, previous radiation treatment, other types of cancer, and genetic factors.

Flashpoint

All types of leukemia affect the white blood cells.

Signs and Symptoms

Signs and symptoms of leukemia include fatigue, fever, frequent infections, pallor, *petechiae* (tiny purple-red hemorrhagic spots under the skin), and easy bruising or bleeding. Individuals may also experience hepatomegaly, splenomegaly, enlarged axillary or cervical lymph nodes, tenderness over bony areas, headache, weight loss, and bone and joint pain.

Diagnosis

Diagnosis is based on signs and symptoms, physical-examination findings, and examination of the blood and bone marrow. Complete blood count with differential may reveal anemia as well as an abnormal count of the different types of white blood cells, red blood cells, and platelets. A lumbar puncture may be done to obtain spinal fluid for examination.

Treatment

Treatment of leukemia varies with the specific type and usually involves chemotherapy, bone-marrow transplantation, or both.

Prognosis

The prognosis for individuals suffering from leukemia depends on the specific type of leukemia, the timeliness of diagnosis and treatment, and other factors, such as whether a suitable bone-marrow donor is identified. Survival rates vary dramatically, from 20% to 75%, depending on the type of leukemia and other factors.

Cancer of the Respiratory System

Cancers affecting the respiratory system are common. They include nasopharyngeal carcinoma, laryngeal cancer, and lung cancer.

Nasopharyngeal Carcinoma
ICD-9-CM: 230.0   [ICD-10: C11.0–C11.9]

Nasopharyngeal carcinoma (NPC) is cancer that that develops in the nasopharyngeal area, behind the nose. NPC arises from the epithelial cells that help make up the lining of the nasopharynx and oropharynx.

Incidence

Approximately 2,000 cases of NPC are diagnosed in the United States each year, with a disproportionate percentage in Alaska. It is more common in northern Africa, Southeast Asia, and southern China. It is estimated that 50% to 80% of NPC cases occur in teens and young adults, men twice as often as women.

Flashpoint

Most cases of NPC occur in teens and young adults.

Etiology

The exact cause of NPC is not fully understood. However, there is evidence of a connection with Epstein-Barr virus and some dietary practices. In some individuals, Epstein-Barr virus is thought to infect epithelial cells and affect their DNA, prompting them to begin growing abnormally. As these mutated cells continue to proliferate, they metastasize to other parts of the body. Other risk factors include a family history of NPC and a diet high in salt-cured food and nitrates.

Signs and Symptoms

Symptoms of NPC can often be attributed to other causes; therefore, it is rarely identified early. The most common first complaint is of a lump, caused by lymph-node enlargement, in the neck. Other signs and symptoms may include nasal stuffiness, nosebleeds, headache, neck or facial pain, visual disturbances, and difficulty opening the mouth. Patients may also experience unilateral ear symptoms, such as tinnitus (ringing in the ears), a feeling of ear fullness or hearing loss, and otitis media (middle ear infection).

Diagnosis

Once NPC is suspected, a thorough physical examination is performed; referral may be made to an ear, nose, and throat specialist for endoscopic examination of the nasopharynx. Physical examination is followed by a variety of other tests. Neurological evaluation is recommended to determine whether any of the cranial nerves are involved. Radiological studies to detect evidence of spreading cancer may include CT and MRI of the head and neck, and bone scans. X-ray or CT scan of the lungs may also be performed. Blood may be tested for evidence of Epstein-Barr virus. Cells may be obtained via fine needle aspiration for microscopic study. Biopsy of the lymph nodes may be performed to confirm diagnosis and stage the cancer.

Flashpoint

Lymph-node biopsy is usually the best way to confirm diagnosis and stage the cancer.

Treatment

Treatment for NPC is individualized for each patient and is based upon staging of the cancer, the patient's personal preferences, and anticipated side effects. Treatment includes chemotherapy, radiation therapy, or a combination of both. Surgery is rarely effective with this type of cancer.

Prognosis

Prognosis for NPC depends upon how far the cancer has spread at the time of diagnosis. Unfortunately, this type of cancer is often not detected until after metastasis has occurred. Side effects and complications of treatment must also be considered. Because radiation therapy is aimed at structures in the head and neck, possible side effects include hearing loss, dry mouth, dysphagia, hypothyroidism, and hypopituitarism. Radiation therapy may also lead to infertility in males.

Laryngeal Cancer
ICD-9-CM: 161.9   [ICD-10: C32.0–C32.9]

Laryngeal cancer is the growth of malignant cancer cells in the larynx.

Incidence

More than 93,000 individuals are currently diagnosed with laryngeal cancer in the United States. It is four to five times more common in men than in women and is more common in those over the age of 65.

Etiology

The main risk factors for laryngeal cancer are tobacco use (smoking and chewing) and heavy alcohol drinking. A combination of the two greatly increases the risk. Other contributors are thought to include infection with human papillomavirus; a weakened immune system; environmental exposure to wood dust, paint fumes, asbestos, and other chemicals; and a diet poor in vitamins A and B and retinoids.

Flashpoint

The main risk factors for laryngeal cancer are tobacco use and heavy drinking.

Signs and Symptoms

Common signs and symptoms of laryngeal cancer include persistent pharyngitis, chronic cough, dysphagia, persistent ear pain, dyspnea, weight loss, prolonged hoarseness, and a lump in the neck.

Diagnosis

Diagnosis is based upon presenting symptoms and careful physical examination of the mouth and throat, and it is confirmed via tissue biopsy. Studies to determine the extent of the cancer may include a CT scan, MRI, chest x-ray, positron emission tomography (PET) scan, and barium swallow (series of x-rays after the patient swallows a liquid with barium).

Treatment

Common treatment options include surgery, radiation, chemotherapy, or a combination of all three. Vocal-cord stripping is a surgical procedure used for very early cancers that involves removal of the top layers of the vocal cords. Cordectomy involves removal of part or all of the vocal cords and may be used to treat limited cancers of the glottis. Laser surgery is useful for treating some early forms of cancer. Partial laryngectomy is done to remove small cancers of the larynx while sparing part of the larynx, in the hope of saving the patient's ability to speak. A total laryngectomy (see Fig. 17-10) involves removal of the entire larynx and creation of a tracheostomy (artificial opening into the trachea). Total or partial pharyngectomy involves the removal of all or part of the pharynx and usually the larynx as well. Radiation therapy is often the main form of treatment for small cancers that can be destroyed without surgery, or for those who are poor surgical candidates.

Prognosis

The prognosis for laryngeal cancer depends upon the timeliness of diagnosis and treatment as well as the individual's age and underlying health status. In general, the 5-year survival rate is approximately 65% to 70%.

Lung Cancer
ICD-9-CM: 162.9   [ICD-10: C34.0–C34.9]

Lung cancer causes 90% of all cancer-related deaths in the United States. There are two general types of lung cancer. Small cell lung cancer accounts for 20% of all lung cancer and develops almost exclusively in smokers. Non–small cell lung cancer comprises the other 80% of lung cancer and can often be surgically removed, if identified early.

Types of non–small cell lung cancer include squamous cell carcinoma, which is most common in men; adenocarcinoma, which is most common in women and nonsmokers; and large cell carcinoma.

Incidence

Approximately 215,000 Americans are diagnosed with lung cancer each year. Over 160,000 die from it annually. African Americans have a higher risk, develop cancer at an earlier age, and are less likely to survive; this is thought to be related to poorer access to health care rather than to genetics.

Etiology

There are many forms of cancer, and the cause in each case is still not fully understood. However, it is well established that the single largest contributor to the development of lung cancer is cigarette smoke (active and secondhand), which is known to contain over 3,500 chemicals, many of them carcinogens as well as toxic metals and radioactive compounds. Other contributors to lung cancer include asbestos, air pollution, and radon, which is an odorless gas released from the breakdown of uranium in water and soil. As tissue cells are damaged by these substances, they change and in some cases, become cancerous.

> **Flashpoint**
> A laryngectomy is the removal of the voice box.

> **Flashpoint**
> Non–small cell lung cancer is the most common type and may be surgically removed if diagnosed early.

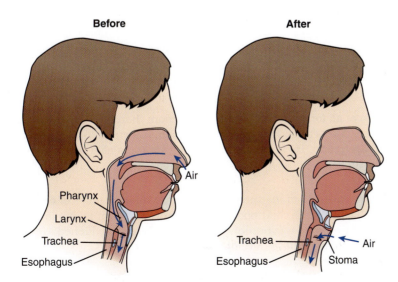

FIGURE 17-10 Before and after total laryngectomy with a tracheostomy

Signs and Symptoms

Individuals with lung cancer are often asymptomatic until the disease is far advanced. The most common first symptom is an unexplained cough or a chronic "smoker's cough" that worsens or changes in character. Other signs and symptoms include hemoptysis, dyspnea, chest pain, new onset of wheezing, prolonged hoarseness, fatigue, anorexia, weight loss, bone pain, headache, and repetitive episodes of bronchitis or pneumonia.

> **Flashpoint**
>
> The most common symptom in patients with lung cancer is an unexplained chronic cough.

Diagnosis

Screening for lung cancer is controversial and is not currently recommended by the American Cancer Society. Chest x-rays and CT scans will reveal abnormal lesions or masses. However, the definitive way to diagnose any form of cancer is through examination of a biopsied tissue specimen. Such specimens may be obtained through a sputum specimen, bronchoscopy, mediastinoscopy, transthoracic needle biopsy, thoracentesis, or video thoracoscopy. Tests used to determine staging include MRI and PET scans.

Treatment

Treatment for patients with lung cancer depends upon the type and stage of the cancer and on the patient's underlying health status and personal preferences. Surgery may be done if the cancer remains localized. Surgical procedures (see Fig. 17-11) include wedge resection (removal of only the affected part of the lung), lobectomy (removal of an entire lobe of a lung), and pneumonectomy (removal of an entire lung). In addition, sample lymph nodes will also be removed and studied to identify whether the cancer has spread into the lymphatic system. Small cell lung cancer does not respond as well to surgery as do other types. Regardless of the type of cancer, most patients undergo chemotherapy or radiation.

> **Flashpoint**
>
> Pneumonectomy is the surgical removal of an entire lung.

Prognosis

The prognosis for individuals with lung cancer is generally poor but varies somewhat, depending upon the type of cancer and the earliness of its detection. Small cell cancer grows and spreads rapidly, with a very poor prognosis; patients have a very low 5-year survival rate. All forms of lung cancer that respond well to initial treatment often reappear months or years later, and they are less responsive to treatment at that time. The 5-year survival rate for patients of all types of lung cancer combined is only 15%.

Cancer of the Gastrointestinal System

Cancer may develop anywhere along the gastrointestinal system, although most malignancies occur in the mouth (oral cancer), esophagus (esophageal cancer), stomach (gastric cancer) and colon (colorectal cancer), as well as the pancreas (pancreatic cancer) and liver (liver cancer). Because of the high incidence of gastrointestinal cancers, all patients should be encouraged to adopt lifestyle practices that reduce their general risk (see Box 17-12).

Oral Cancer

ICD-9-CM: 145.9 (mouth, unspecified)   **[ICD-10: C00.0–C06.9 (code by site)]**

Oral cancer includes cancerous changes to the tissue of any oral structures, including the lips, tongue, gums, inner cheek, and mouth floor.

Incidence

Oral cancer makes up 8% of all forms of malignancy, with more than 23,000 new cases diagnosed each year and more than 5,000 deaths. It is twice as common in men as in women, and it is most prevalent in the over-40 age group. However, an elevated incidence is also seen among young men who use chewing tobacco.

Etiology

Risk factors for oral cancer include the use of chewing tobacco (80% of cases) or alcohol, poor oral hygiene, jagged teeth, and poorly fitting dentures. Oral leukoplakia is a known precursor in some cases; it is a condition marked by white or reddened areas in which precancerous tissue changes have developed.

> **Flashpoint**
>
> Most cases of oral cancer are associated with the use of chewing tobacco. Therefore, oral cancer is nearly always preventable.

Signs and Symptoms

The most common symptom of oral cancer is the development of white, patchy lesions or mouth ulcers that fail to heal. Such lesions are usually not tender until late in the

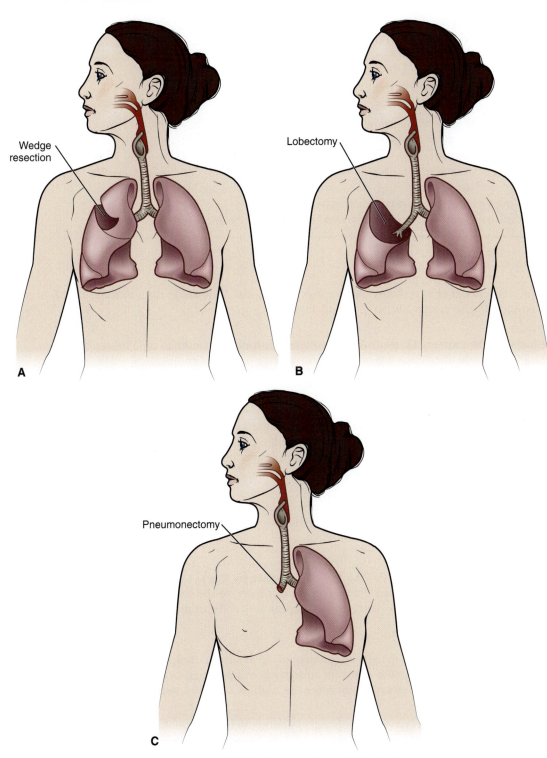

FIGURE 17-11 Surgeries for lung cancer: (A) Wedge resection; (B) Lobectomy; (C) Pneumonectomy

> ## Box 17-12 Wellness Promotion
>
> ### REDUCING RISK OF GASTROINTESTINAL CANCER
> Follow these general measures to reduce your risk of developing gastrointestinal cancers:
>
> - Have regular oral and dental hygiene checkups.
> - Minimize your alcohol intake.
> - Avoid tobacco products.
> - Prevent or treat gastroesophageal reflux disease.
> - Eat a diet that is high in fiber, rich in fruits and vegetables, and low in fat.
> - Follow measures to avoid contracting hepatitis B.
> - Follow measures to protect and strengthen your immune system.

disease process. Other symptoms include dysphagia, bleeding, difficulty chewing, numb areas, referred pain to the ear or jaw, and weight loss.

Diagnosis
Diagnosis of oral cancer is based upon physical-examination findings and tissue biopsy. Staging is possible after data are collected through a variety of radiological tests, including contrast-enhanced CT scan, MRI, or PET scan. These tests may also identify invasion of bone and cartilage.

Treatment
Treatment depends upon whether the cancer is localized or has spread. Surgery is commonly done to remove cancerous tissue and may include lymph-node dissection. Radiation therapy and chemotherapy are often used to destroy remaining cancer cells. In some cases, a form of heat therapy called hyperthermia treatment is used.

Prognosis
Oral cancers tend to spread quickly and invade bone, liver, and lung tissues. As a result, the 5-year survival rate is only 50%. However, survival depends upon the stage of the cancer at the time of diagnosis and treatment.

Esophageal Cancer
ICD-9-CM: 150.9   [ICD-10: C15.0–C15.9 (code by site)]
Esophageal cancer develops when tissue cells in the lining of the lower esophagus develop cancerous changes. Such cancer is nearly always squamous cell carcinoma but may occasionally be adenocarcinoma.

Incidence
Nearly 17,000 Americans are diagnosed with esophageal cancer each year, and over 14,000 die. The vast majority are male. Rates of squamous cell esophageal cancer are highest in Iran, Asia, and Africa; adenocarcinoma rates are highest in Caucasians.

Flashpoint

The majority of patients with esophageal cancer are men.

Etiology
Risk factors for both types of esophageal cancer include alcohol and tobacco use, obesity, swallowing caustic substances, poor nutrition, gastroesophageal reflux disease, and underlying esophageal disorders, such as stricture or achalasia.

Signs and Symptoms
Early symptoms of esophageal cancer include dysphagia, weight loss, substernal chest pain, a sensation of pressure or burning, hiccups, and hoarseness of the voice.

Diagnosis
Diagnosis of esophageal cancer is based upon presenting symptoms, x-rays, a barium swallow, and tissue biopsy via upper endoscopy. CT scan helps confirm the location of the tumor. CT and endoscopic ultrasound may help identify whether cancer has spread into nearby tissues.

Treatment

Esophageal cancer is usually treated with surgery and chemotherapy or radiation, depending on the stage of the cancer and the patient's general heath. Surgical procedures include esophagectomy (removal of the esophagus) and esophagogastrectomy (removal of the lower esophagus and upper stomach). Photodynamic therapy may be done to relieve pain or obstruction in the esophagus. In this form of treatment, a laser is aimed at the esophagus after the patient is injected with a light-sensitive drug that becomes concentrated in the cancer cells.

Prognosis

The prognosis for patients with esophageal cancer depends upon how early diagnosis occurs. Tracheoesophageal fistulas may form, in which the cancer erodes a hole between the trachea and the esophagus. There is a 30% rate of metastasis to the liver, bone, or lungs, at which point the prognosis becomes less favorable.

Gastric Cancer
ICD-9-CM: 151.9   [ICD-10: C16.0–C16.9]

Gastric cancer occurs when tissue cells in the stomach wall develop cancerous changes.

Incidence

More than 21,000 Americans are diagnosed with gastric cancer each year, and nearly 11,000 die from the disease. Populations with the highest rates of gastric cancer include Japanese and African American men over the age of 50.

Etiology

Risk factors for the development of gastric cancer include Barrett esophagus (precancerous cellular changes), infection with *H. pylori* bacteria early in life, and genetic and dietary factors. High-risk diets include those that are high in complex carbohydrates but low in fresh fruits, vegetables, and fiber.

Signs and Symptoms

People with early-stage gastric cancer are often asymptomatic. As the cancer advances, symptoms include weight loss, abdominal pain, nausea, vomiting, fatigue, dysphagia, feelings of fullness, **melena** (tarry black stool caused by the presence of digested blood), anorexia, and abdominal mass.

Diagnosis

Diagnosis is based upon presenting symptoms, medical history, double-contrast barium study, and gastroscopy. A CT scan may be done to detect metastasis and staging.

> **Flashpoint**
> People often have no symptoms until gastric cancer is advanced.

Treatment

Treatment of gastric cancer depends on the stage of the disease. It usually includes partial or total gastrectomy (surgical removal of part or all of the stomach) along with radiation or chemotherapy (see Fig. 17-12).

Prognosis

Metastasis has already occurred in half of all patients initially diagnosed with gastric cancer. Recurrence after remission is common, with an overall 5-year survival rate of only 20%.

Colorectal Cancer
ICD-9-CM: 154   [ICD-O-3: M8140/3   [ICD-10: C18.0–C20.9
(95% of cases)]   (code by site)]

Colorectal cancer is one of the most common types of cancer. It affects the large intestine and rectal area (see Fig. 17-13).

Incidence

Colorectal cancer is the second leading cause of cancer-related deaths in the United States, with nearly 150,000 new cases diagnosed each year. Nearly 50,000 individuals die from the disease annually. More than 90% of cases occur in the over-50 age group.

> **Flashpoint**
> Colorectal cancer is one of the most common causes of cancer-related deaths in the United States.

Etiology

Risk factors for colorectal cancer include a history of inflammatory bowel disease and family history of colorectal cancer. Lifestyle factors may include sedentary lifestyle; low-fiber, high-fat diet; obesity; and alcohol and tobacco use.

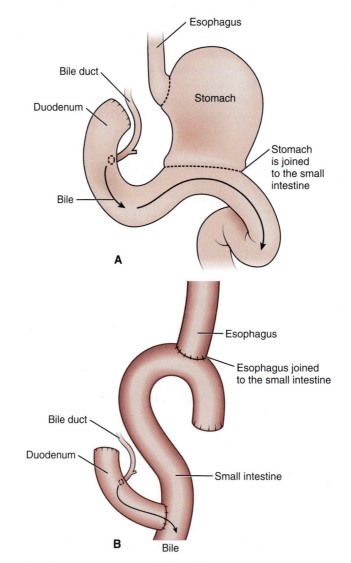

FIGURE 17-12 Surgeries for gastric cancer: (A) Partial gastrectomy; (B) Total gastrectomy

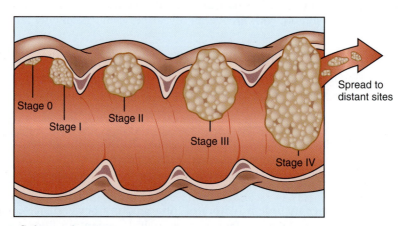

FIGURE 17-13 Colorectal cancer

Signs and Symptoms

Patients are often asymptomatic in the early stage of colorectal cancer. When symptoms occur, they include a change in bowel-elimination pattern, blood in the stools, abdominal pain, pallor, anemia, and intestinal obstruction.

Diagnosis

Screening for colon cancer includes fecal occult blood test and lower endoscopy. If findings are suspicious, a tissue biopsy is obtained. Barium enema may also be done.

Treatment

Treatment for colorectal cancer depends on the location and stage of the cancer and includes surgery, chemotherapy, or radiation therapy. Newer forms of treatment also include medications that help to shrink cancerous tumors or to inhibit blood flow to tumors.

Prognosis

Among patients whose colorectal cancer is detected early, the survival rate is 90%. However, in 61% of cases, metastasis has occurred by the time of diagnosis.

Liver Cancer

ICD-9-CM: 155.0   [ICD-O-3: M8170/3]   [ICD-10: C22.0–C22.9 (code by site)]

Primary liver cancer is cancer that originates in the liver.

Incidence

Liver cancer is the number one cause of cancer death in Africa and Asia, and it is the fifth-most common cancer worldwide. Primary liver cancer is uncommon in the United States but is becoming more common due to hepatitis C. Approximately 21,000 Americans are diagnosed with primary liver cancer each year, and more than 18,000 die from the disease. It is more common in men than women. Secondary liver cancer—that is, cancer that has spread to the liver from another site—is very common. Incidence is higher in men than in women.

Etiology

The cause of liver cancer is not always clear. However, some contributing factors have been identified, including chronic hepatitis B or C infection, cirrhosis, and exposure to toxins. Other potential risk factors are nonalcoholic fatty liver disease, obesity, alcohol abuse, and some inherited liver disorders.

Flashpoint

Chronic hepatitis B or C increases the risk of developing liver cancer.

Signs and Symptoms

Patients with liver cancer are often symptom free in the early stages. When signs and symptoms develop, they include abdominal pain, hepatomegaly (enlargement of the liver), weight loss, poor appetite, ascites, splenomegaly (enlargement of the spleen), nausea and vomiting, fatigue, weakness, and jaundice (a condition of increased bilirubin in the blood, which results in yellow staining of the skin and mucous membranes).

Diagnosis

Diagnosis of liver cancer is made through liver function tests, which reveal elevated alpha-fetoprotein (over 500 grams per liter). Other diagnostics include ultrasound, CT, and MRI. Biopsy may be done but is considered risky.

Treatment

Treatment of liver cancer often includes surgery to remove the tumor. Occasionally, liver transplantation may be considered. Several other treatment options exist. Cryosurgery is the application of liquid nitrogen to freeze cancerous tissue. Radiofrequency ablation involves the use of electric current to heat and destroy cancerous tissue. Alcohol injection involves the injection of pure alcohol directly into the tumor. During chemoembolization, agents are injected into the liver to interfere with the blood supply. Targeted drug therapy and traditional radiation therapy may also be used.

Prognosis

The prognosis for patients with liver cancer depends upon whether the condition is primary liver cancer or secondary cancer that has metastasized from another location, as well as on the patient's age and underlying health status. Metastasis to the bones, lungs, brain, peritoneum, and adrenal glands is common, and the mortality rate is high.

Pancreatic Cancer
ICD-9-CM: 157.9 (unspecified)   [ICD-10: C25.0–C25.9 (code by site)]

Pancreatic cancer is a condition in which pancreatic cells become malignant and proceed to grow and multiply.

Incidence
Pancreatic cancer is the fourth-most common cause of cancer-related death in the United States. Approximately 38,000 Americans are diagnosed with it each year, men slightly more than women. Approximately 34,000 Americans die from it each year.

Etiology
Risk factors include family history of pancreatic cancer, a diet high in fat and meats, cigarette smoking, history of chronic pancreatitis, and diabetes.

Signs and Symptoms
Patients may be asymptomatic until pancreatic cancer has spread. Symptoms include abdominal pain, nausea, vomiting, weight loss, anorexia, jaundice, steatorrhea (presence of fat in the stool), hepatomegaly, weakness, fatigue, and diarrhea.

Diagnosis
Because patients are frequently asymptomatic in the early stages, pancreatic cancer often goes undetected until it is advanced. Occasionally, pancreatic masses are detected when the patient undergoes radiological procedures for other purposes. Diagnosis is based upon history, physical examination, abdominal ultrasound, CT, endoscopic retrograde cholangiopancreatography, and MRI. A biopsy is required for definitive diagnosis.

Treatment
Surgery is generally useful only when pancreatic cancer is detected early or when performed for palliative purposes. Radiation and chemotherapy are frequently used.

Prognosis
The prognosis for patients with pancreatic cancer is very poor. Those who elect to undergo a high-risk surgery known as the Whipple procedure have a 5-year survival rate of only 10% to 25%. The Whipple procedure is a complex operation in which the proximal duodenum, head of the pancreas, common bile duct, and gallbladder are removed (see Fig. 17-14). For those who do not have this surgery, the survival rate is just over 3%.

> **Flashpoint**
> The prognosis for pancreatic cancer is very poor.

Cancer of the Endocrine System

Most cancers of the endocrine system are extremely rare. They can affect any structures within the system, including the thyroid, parathyroid, adrenal and pituitary glands, hypothalamus, and portions of the pancreas. The most common form of endocrine system cancer is thyroid cancer.

Thyroid Cancer
ICD-9-CM: 193   [ICD-10: C73]

Thyroid cancer is cancer that develops in tissue of the thyroid gland. There are four types of thyroid cancer; papillary thyroid cancer is the most common, comprising approximately 80% of all cases.

Incidence
Approximately 37,000 individuals are newly diagnosed with thyroid cancer each year in the United States, women three to four times more often than men. Approximately 1,600 people die each year from this disease. The most common type of thyroid cancer, papillary thyroid cancer, most often affects people between the ages of 30 and 50.

> **Flashpoint**
> Women are much more likely to develop thyroid cancer than men.

Etiology
The cause of thyroid cancer is uncertain. However, certain risk factors have been identified: high-level radiation exposure, especially to the head and neck; history of thyroid enlargement (goiter); and a family history of medullary thyroid cancer.

Signs and Symptoms
Individuals with early thyroid cancer may be asymptomatic. As the disease progresses, they may notice a firm, nontender lump in the front of the neck, changes in the voice, dysphagia, discomfort in the throat or neck, and enlarged lymph nodes in the neck.

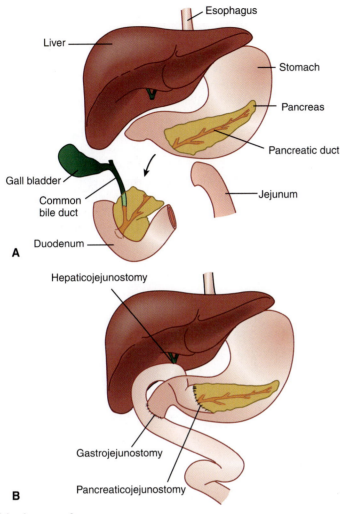

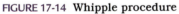

FIGURE 17-14 **Whipple procedure**

Diagnosis

Diagnosis of thyroid cancer may be suspected based upon the patient's signs and symptoms, but most people with these symptoms do not have thyroid cancer. Therefore, diagnostic testing is necessary to rule out or confirm the diagnosis. Blood may be drawn to check hormones such as thyroid-stimulating hormone and calcitonin. Ultrasound or other imaging studies may be done to evaluate thyroid nodules. A thyroid scan may be done to identify "cold" nodules that are suspected of malignancy (see Box 17-13). Needle biopsy is commonly done to collect cells for microscopic examination, in order to confirm the diagnosis. Less commonly, surgical biopsy may be done to remove a nodule for examination.

Treatment

The treatment plan for each patient is individualized and depends upon the specific type of cancer, the stage of the cancer, and the individual's underlying health status, age, and personal preferences. Options include surgical removal of part or all of the thyroid, often including removal of nearby lymph nodes. Radioactive iodine treatment in the form of a liquid or capsule is also usually used. Less commonly, standard external beam radiation therapy and chemotherapy may be used. After any treatment that removes or destroys the thyroid, the patient will begin lifelong supplementation of thyroid hormones.

Prognosis

The prognosis for individuals with thyroid cancer is usually very good. However, it is possible that the cancer can recur, even when thyroidectomy is done. Should this happen, the patient will need to undergo treatment a second time.

Flashpoint
Treatment may involve surgical removal of the thyroid.

Box 17-13 Diagnostic Spotlight

THYROID SCAN

A thyroid scan uses a radioactive substance as a tracer detectable by a special camera. The camera measures how much tracer is absorbed by thyroid tissue. The scan is done in the nuclear-medicine section of a radiology department, by a trained technologist. The patient must lie still and supine, with the head tipped backward and neck extended. There may be a brief warm, flushed sensation and mild nausea when the substance is administered. The test takes only about 10 minutes and is repeated 24 hours later. The patient is cautioned to be sure to flush the toilet and wash hands thoroughly after urinating over the next 24 hours, as the tracer is eliminated in the urine.

An abnormal scan may reveal a thyroid gland that is abnormally large, or small or "cold" nodules (areas of hypoactivity) and "hot" nodules (areas of hyperactivity). Cold nodules may indicate thyroid cancer. A whole-body thyroid scan may also be done to identify whether the cancer has spread to other areas of the body.

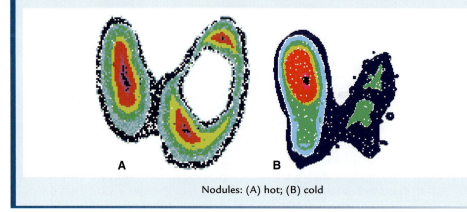

Nodules: (A) hot; (B) cold

Cancer of the Musculoskeletal System

Cancers affecting the musculoskeletal system are uncommon. Examples include osteosarcoma (bone cancer) and two forms of cancer affecting muscle tissue, rhabdomyosarcoma and leiomyosarcoma.

Osteosarcoma

ICD-9-CM: 170.0–170.9   **[ICD-O-3: M9180/3]**   **[ICD-10: C40.0–C41.9**
(code by site)   **(code by site)]**

Osteosarcoma, also called *osteogenic sarcoma*, is the most common type of bone cancer. It is a deadly form of cancer that originates in the rapidly growing parts of long bones in children and adolescents (see Fig. 17-15). It most commonly affects the ends of the femur, tibia, and upper humerus, although it can affect any bone.

Incidence

An estimated 400 to 900 individuals are diagnosed with osteosarcoma each year in the United States. It can affect people of all ages but most commonly affects children and teenagers between the ages of 10 and 19, a time when the body experiences rapid growth.

Flashpoint

Osteosarcoma most commonly strikes children and teenagers.

Etiology

The cause of osteosarcoma is not certain. In some cases there may be a genetic link. Risk factors for this form of cancer include tall stature, previous radiation treatment, osteochondroma (benign bone tumors), and prior bone disease, such as Paget disease.

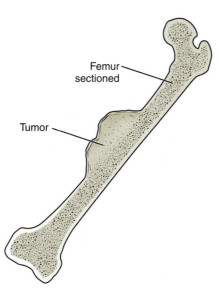

Femur sectioned

Tumor

FIGURE 17-15 **Osteosarcoma**

Signs and Symptoms

The most common symptom of osteosarcoma is tenderness or pain that worsens with use and at night. Other signs and symptoms may include pathologic fractures and limited range of motion. A palpable mass may be present, with increased prominence of blood vessels over the area.

Diagnosis

As with most forms of cancer, definitive diagnosis is determined though evaluation of biopsied tissue. Incisional or core needle biopsies are most commonly done. Other tests may include standard x-rays, MRI, CT scan, and bone scan. These tests can identify the primary bone tumor and detect spreading to surrounding areas. Chest CT may also be done to identify whether the cancer has spread to the lungs.

Treatment

A team approach to treating osteosarcoma is most effective, especially when the patient is a child. Treatment includes chemotherapy to shrink the tumor, followed by surgery to remove the tumor and any nearby malignant tissue. Whenever possible, the limb is spared (limb-salvage surgery), although amputation is sometimes required.

Prognosis

The prognosis for individuals with osteosarcoma has improved substantially in the past 40 years. At one time, amputation was the only treatment option and survival beyond 2 years was extremely low. Currently, the 5-year survival rate for patients with nonmetastatic osteosarcoma is over 70%. For those with metastasis at the time of diagnosis, the outlook is less favorable: The 5-year survival rate is around 30%. The mortality rate is highest among those in whom the cancer has spread to the lungs by the time of diagnosis.

Flashpoint

An attempt is made to save the limb, but amputation is sometimes necessary.

Rhabdomyosarcoma and Leiomyosarcoma

ICD-9-CM: 171	[ICD-O-3: M8900/3 (rhabdomyosarcoma), M8890/3 (leiomyosarcoma)]	[ICD-10: C49.0–C49.9 (code by site)]

The two cancers most likely to affect muscle tissue are rhabdomyosarcoma and leiomyosarcoma, although they are both rare. Rhabdomyosarcomas are cancerous tumors of skeletal muscle that most often grow in the arms or legs, although they can arise in other areas. Leiomyosarcomas are cancerous tumors of smooth muscle. Therefore, they can develop anywhere there is smooth muscle, such as the abdomen, blood vessels, and uterus.

Incidence

Malignancies of muscle tissue are uncommon. Rhabdomyosarcoma is the most common soft-tissue sarcoma in children, usually affecting areas in the head or neck.

Etiology

The cause of either type of muscle malignancy is unclear. Genetics and environmental factors, such as high-dose radiation or exposure to herbicides, may play a role. Whatever the cause, something damages the DNA and uncontrolled proliferation of cancerous cells occurs.

Signs and Symptoms

> **Flashpoint**
> Patients with rhabdomyosarcoma may complain of a lump in the muscle.

Patients with rhabdomyosarcoma may complain of a lump that has been present for several weeks or months. It may be painless, but may also cause discomfort if it compresses other structures, such as nerves. Signs and symptoms of leiomyosarcoma vary with the location and type of muscle involved.

Diagnosis

Diagnosis involves examination of the muscle tumor with MRI and core needle biopsy. Chest CT may be done to assess for lung involvement.

Treatment

Treatment usually involves surgical removal of the primary tumor and any adjacent malignant tissue, followed by chemotherapy or radiation therapy. In some cases an affected limb may require amputation.

Prognosis

The prognosis for patients with muscle malignancy is variable and depends upon the type of cancer, the timeliness of diagnosis and treatment, and the occurrence of metastasis.

Cancer of the Eyes

Cancers of the eyes are uncommon but may be devastating to those who develop them. There are numerous types of eye cancer; the most common form in adults is intraocular melanoma, and the most common form in children is retinoblastoma.

Intraocular Melanoma

> **Flashpoint**
> Intraocular melanoma is the most common form of primary eye cancer in adults.

ICD-9-CM: 190.9   [ICD-O-3: M8720/3]   [ICD-10: C69.0–C69.9 (code by site)]

Most cancers of the eye are cancers that have spread from elsewhere in the body, usually the breasts or lungs. The most common form of ***primary eye cancer*** (cancer that originates within the eyes) in adults is intraocular melanoma (see Fig. 17-16). Because it often develops within the uvea of the eye, it is also sometimes called *uveal melanoma*; however, it can develop in other parts of the eye, especially the iris.

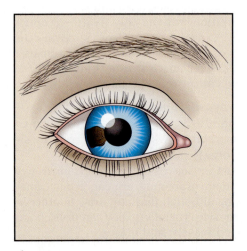

FIGURE 17-16 **Intraocular melanoma**

Incidence

Although intraocular melanoma is the most common form of primary eye cancer in adults, it is still uncommon. It comprises the bulk of the 2,400 new cases of eye cancer diagnosed each year in the United States. More than 200 Americans die from it each year. Primary eye cancer can strike individuals of all ages, but it is most common in those over age 50. Incidence is higher in Caucasians than other racial groups, especially in those with blue eyes.

Etiology

The exact cause of intraocular melanoma is not understood. Risk factors are similar to those for melanoma of the skin and include personal or family history of melanoma, advancing age, fair complexion, freckles, red or blond hair, blue or green eyes, and exposure to sunlight or some chemicals.

Signs and Symptoms

Individuals with intraocular melanoma are usually symptom free until the cancer becomes advanced. When signs and symptoms develop, they include blurred vision, loss of visual field, seeing floaters (cobwebs, strings, or specks in the visual field), the appearance of a dark spot on the iris, change in pupil shape, change in eyeball movement or position, and bulging of the eye. Pain is felt only rarely.

Diagnosis

The diagnosis of intraocular melanoma may be suspected by an ophthalmologist who notes enlargement of the blood vessels upon examination. Further diagnostic tests may be done to confirm the diagnosis. These include ultrasound and fluorescein angiography. MRI scan may be used to examine the eye tumor and detect spreading outside of the eye. Chest x-ray and CT scan may also be done to identify whether the cancer has spread to other parts of the body. Biopsy is rarely done in the case of eye cancer, because the delicate structures of the eye make it challenging to complete without causing damage to the eye or spreading cancerous cells outside of the eye.

Treatment

Treatment of intraocular melanoma includes a variety of therapies or surgeries. External beam radiation therapy is aimed by an external machine toward the cancer within the eye. Internal radiation therapy involves the placement of tiny seeds (disks), wires, or catheters directly into or near the cancerous tissue. This allows very precise radiation treatment of the cancerous cells. Photocoagulation is a procedure in which laser light is used to destroy vessels that supply blood flow to the tumor. Thermotherapy involves the use of heat to destroy cancerous cells; it may comprise variations of ultrasound and laser, microwave, and infrared radiation.

Surgical techniques vary depending upon the size and location of tumor. Iridectomy removes part of the iris and is useful for small melanomas affecting the iris. Iridotrabeculectomy removes part of the iris and a small portion of the outer eyeball. Iridocyclectomy removes part of the iris and ciliary body. Resection removes cancer of the ciliary body or choroid. Enucleation removes the entire eyeball.

Prognosis

The prognosis for patients with intraocular melanoma depends upon the exact location of the cancer, the type of melanoma cells, the size of the tumor, and whether the cancer is confined to the eye or has spread to other structures. Cancers of the iris are generally spotted earlier than those in other locations. They also grow more slowly than others and rarely spread. Therefore, the prognosis is usually quite good in these cases.

Retinoblastoma

ICD-9-CM: 190.5   [ICD-O-3: M9510/3]   [ICD-10: C69.2]

Retinoblastoma, though rare, is the most common form of eye cancer in children. It develops from immature cells within the retina (light-sensitive layer). It is usually unilateral (affecting one eye), but in 25% of cases it is bilateral (affecting both eyes).

Incidence

Approximately 300 American infants and children under age 5 are diagnosed with retinoblastoma each year. It affects approximately 5,000 individuals of all races worldwide, boys and girls equally. Approximately 40% of individuals have a type of retinoblastoma that can be passed on to their children. This hereditary form of the disorder is usually bilateral.

Flashpoint
Retinoblastoma is the most common form of eye cancer in children.

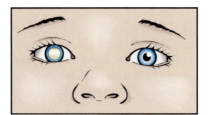

FIGURE 17-17 Leukocoria caused by retinoblastoma

Etiology

Most cases of retinoblastoma are caused by a mutation of the RB1 gene on chromosome 13. It is a tumor suppressor gene, which means that its job is to slow cell division, repair DNA errors, and trigger normal cell death. Mutations in this gene prevent the suppressor cells from effectively doing their work. As a result, some cells within the retina proliferate in an uncontrolled fashion, creating a cancerous tumor.

Signs and Symptoms

The most common sign of retinoblastoma is **leukocoria** (white pupil) that is especially obvious in dim lighting or in a photograph taken with a flash (see Fig. 17-17). This is also sometimes called *cat's eye reflex*. Other signs and symptoms include strabismus (crossed or misaligned eyes), redness, irritation, pain, an abnormally dilated pupil, differently colored eyes, and poor vision or blindness in the affected eye.

> **Flashpoint**
>
> The most common sign of retinoblastoma is a white pupil seen in dim light or in a photograph.

Diagnosis

To diagnose retinoblastoma and differentiate it from other disorders, the physician performs a careful examination of the eye under anesthesia, along with digital photography, ultrasound, and CT and MRI scans. This means of diagnosis is 95% accurate. Biopsy is rarely done, because it can result in the spread of the cancer to other areas outside of the eye.

Treatment

The treatment plan is individualized for each patient. It may include external beam radiation, temporary insertion of radioactive plaques (radioactive disks), eye-sparing radiotherapy, laser therapy, cryotherapy, chemotherapy, and enucleation.

Prognosis

The prognosis for patients with retinoblastoma depends upon how early the cancer is diagnosed and treated and whether it is unilateral or bilateral. In most cases, retinoblastoma can be successfully treated when caught early. Sadly, nearly 90% of children affected by this disease worldwide do not survive; most of these are in developing countries, where access to health care is extremely limited. Potential complications of the disease and its treatment include visual deficits and metastasis to other structures.

Student Resources

American Cancer Society: http://www.cancer.org
Breastcancer.org: http://www.breastcancer.org
CancerCare: http://www.cancercare.org
Eye Cancer Network: http://www.eyecancer.com
Healthcommunities.com Oncology Channel: http://www.oncologychannel.com
Kidney Cancer Association: http://www.kidneycancer.org
The Leukemia and Lymphoma Society: http://www.leukemia-lymphoma.org
Lungcancer.org: http://www.lungcancer.org
National Brain Tumor Society: http://www.braintumor.org
National Cancer Institute: http://www.cancer.gov

Ovarian Cancer National Alliance: http://www.ovariancancer.org
Prostate Cancer Foundation: http://www.prostatecancerfoundation.org
Skin Cancer Foundation: http://www.skincancer.org

Chapter Activities

Learning Style Study Strategies

Try any or all of the following strategies as you study the content of this chapter:

Visual learners: Create acronyms, which are abbreviations using the first letters or word parts in names or phrases you need to remember. Examples of acronyms from this chapter are CAUTION and ABCDE. Now create some of your own.

Kinesthetic, auditory, and verbal learners: Write out definitions of pathological terms or abbreviations. Read them several times aloud as you do so.

Practice Exercises

Answers to practice exercises can be found in Appendix D.

Case Studies

CASE STUDY 1

Arcelia is a medical assistant who just recently transferred from the internal medicine department to the dermatology department. She realizes that she needs to increase her knowledge about skin conditions and is therefore studying various forms of skin cancer. She has identified the three most common forms as basal cell carcinoma, squamous cell carcinoma, and malignant melanoma. Now she needs to find answers to the following questions.

1. Which of these types of skin cancer is Arcelia most likely to see among the patients that come to her department?

2. Which type of skin cancer is the most aggressive and the deadliest?

3. Which form of skin cancer often arises from a brown or black mole?

4. What country has the highest rate of malignant melanoma?

5. What are the risk factors that contribute to the development of malignant melanoma?

6. What are the warning signs of malignant melanoma, and what is an easy way Arcelia can teach her patients to remember them?

CASE STUDY 2

Nathaniel Blakemore is a 25-year-old man visiting his health-care provider with questions about testicular cancer. He states that a good friend of his recently died of testicular cancer and it "really freaked [him] out." He decided to examine his own testicles and thinks he might have noted a small lump on one of them. After performing an examination, the physician assures Nathaniel that his testicle is normal. However, he realizes that this is a good opportunity to teach this patient about testicular cancer and asks him what questions he has about it. What answers might the health-care provider give to this patient?

1. What causes this kind of cancer?

2. How would I know if I did have it?

3. If you thought someone had testicular cancer, how would you find out for sure?

4. Do people always die from this type of cancer, like my friend did?

5. Well, I feel kind of dumb for coming here today. I guess I was just being paranoid. So how can I tell if I'm feeling something that is abnormal or not?

CASE STUDY 3

Isaiah Cohen is a 65-year-old patient at the gastroenterology clinic. He was recently diagnosed with colorectal cancer after surgery for a bowel obstruction. He now has several questions for his health-care provider. What answers might his health-care provider give him?

1. My wife says this type of cancer is very common. Is this true?

2. Why did I get this? My wife says it's because I am overweight and drink too much.

3. I felt fine until I had that bowel obstruction. If I had bowel cancer, shouldn't I have belly pain?

4. Well, shouldn't I have seen blood in my bowel movements?

5. Is there a better way to diagnose this problem than just waiting to see if you get an obstruction?

6. So what is the usual prognosis?

Multiple Choice

1. All of the following terms are matched with the correct definition **except:**

    a. Palliative surgery: surgery done to ease pain and improve quality of life

    b. Staging surgery: surgery done to identify the extent of cancer

    c. Reconstructive surgery: surgery done to restore the body as close as possible to its original appearance and function

    d. Supportive surgery: surgery done to remove cancerous tissue and cure the patient

2. All of the following terms are matched with the correct definition **except:**

   a. Lymphoma: cancer arising from lymphatic cells

   b. Carcinoma: cancer arising from epithelial tissue

   c. Myeloma: cancer that originates within the eyes

   d. Melanoma: cancer arising from pigmented skin cells

3. Which of the following is a known risk factor for breast cancer?

   a. Late onset of menses

   b. Presence of the BRCA1 or BRCA2 gene

   c. Low body weight

   d. Having many children

4. All of the following are closely related **except:**

   a. Oral cancer: young men who chew tobacco

   b. Gastric cancer: Japanese and African American men over the age of 50

   c. Wilms tumor: postmenopausal Caucasian women

   d. Liver cancer: chronic hepatitis B or C

5. Which statement is LEAST appropriate as patient education for a patient undergoing chemotherapy?

   a. Avoid iron-rich foods, because they can cause constipation.

   b. Eat cool, soft, bland foods to reduce nausea and vomiting.

   c. Report sudden, severe headaches.

   d. Use a soft toothbrush to avoid irritation and infection of the gums.

Short Answer

1. **What are the common general warning signs of cancer?**

2. **List the treatment options for breast cancer, include the various surgical options.**

3. **What general measures can be followed to reduce the risk of gastrointestinal cancer?**

18 MENTAL HEALTH DISORDERS

Learning Outcomes

Upon completion of this chapter, the student will be able to:

- Define and spell key terms related to mental health disorders
- Identify characteristics of common mental health disorders, including:
  - description
  - incidence
  - etiology
  - signs and symptoms
  - diagnosis
  - treatment
  - prognosis

KEY TERMS	
affect	emotional reaction or mood
agoraphobia	condition of overwhelming symptoms of anxiety upon leaving home, especially about being trapped in crowded public areas, where a rapid escape might be difficult
antisocial personality disorder	disorder that features manipulation of others without regard for their feelings or for right and wrong
avoidant personality disorder	disorder that features feelings of inadequacy, social inhibition, and hypersensitivity to criticism
bargaining	irrational attempt to negotiate for unlikely or impossible changes
borderline personality disorder	disorder that features a "black or white" view; unstable self-image, relationships, and moods; and unpredictable and impulsive behavior
cataplexy	sudden, brief loss of muscle control triggered by strong emotion, excitement, surprise, or anger, during which the person remains fully conscious
cognition	thinking process that includes language use, calculation, perception, memory, awareness, reasoning, judgment, learning, intellect, social skills, and imagination
compulsions	behaviors performed repeatedly, in a ritualistic manner, in order to relieve the fear or anxiety caused by obsessive thoughts
delusion	false, unfounded belief
denial	refusal to accept the reality of a situation
dependent personality disorder	disorder that features a chronic, excessive psychological dependence on others
exposure therapy	therapy that involves exposing the patient repeatedly to the situation or object that triggers anxiety

KEY TERMS—cont'd

grandiosity	inflated sense of self-importance
hallucination	false sensory perception
histrionic personality disorder	disorder that features chronic attention-seeking and emotionalism, dramatic behavior, exaggeration, and angry outbursts
impulse control disorder	failure to resist performing socially unacceptable or even harmful behaviors
mental health	state that allows individuals to function effectively in all dimensions of life
mental illness	state of having one or more psychological disorders that affect mood or behavior and create mental or emotional pain, disability, or distress
motor tic	sudden, spasmodic, involuntary muscular contraction, usually involving the face, mouth, eyes, head, neck, or shoulders
narcissistic personality disorder	disorder that features a pattern of superiority and grandiosity combined with oversensitivity to criticism and a tendency to become easily enraged or depressed
obsessions	persistent, recurring, and distressing thoughts, images, feelings, or impulses that are unwanted and intrusive
obsessive-compulsive personality disorder	disorder that features rigid conformity to rules and moral codes combined with inflexibility and an excessive need for order; differs from obsessive-compulsive disorder in that it does not include an unwanted pattern of obsessions and compulsions
paranoid personality disorder	disorder that features unwarranted suspicion and mistrust
phobia	any persistent, intense anxiety about and irrational fear of an object, activity, or situation
physical dependence	condition of physical tolerance and, with sudden discontinuation of the substance, display of a withdrawal syndrome
psychological dependence	emotional and behavioral symptoms of craving, compulsive drug-seeking, hoarding, and use of substances purely for emotional and mental euphoria
schizoid personality disorder	disorder that features shyness, oversensitivity, withdrawal, eccentricity, daydreaming, and an inability to express normal anger or joy
schizotypal personality disorder	disorder that features odd behavior and thinking similar to that of people with schizophrenia; social and emotional detachment; magical thinking; and possible paranoid thoughts
social anxiety disorder	persistent irrational fear of, and need to avoid, social-performance situations in which the individual might be exposed to potentially embarrassing or humiliating scrutiny by others; also called *social phobia*
specific phobia	intense fear and anxiety related to a specific object or situation
substance abuse	persistent maladaptive pattern of substance use over a 12-month period, in which an individual continues substance use in spite of significant adverse consequences
substance dependence	continued substance abuse, compulsive use behaviors, development of tolerance, and withdrawal symptoms with discontinuation
vocal tic	involuntary sound such as clearing the throat, grunting, or uttering words

Abbreviations

Table 18-1 lists some of the most common abbreviations related to mental illness.

Mental Health and Mental Illness

Mental health is a state that allows individuals to function effectively in all dimensions of life, to be productive at work and home, and to develop and maintain fulfilling relationships. It also provides them with the ability to respond and adapt to expected and unexpected changes and to cope effectively with adversity. People who are mentally healthy have a high level of self-esteem, are self-confident, and are able to acknowledge their strengths and positive qualities. At the same time, they are willing to acknowledge their flaws and seek to improve areas of weakness.

Flashpoint

People who are mentally healthy are adaptable and flexible.

Mental illness is the state of having one or more psychological disorders that affect mood or behavior and create mental or emotional pain, disability, or distress. The condition creates dysfunction in one or more dimensions of life, impedes the development or maintenance of fulfilling relationships, and leads to increased risk of pain, disability, and death.

Most individuals fluctuate somewhat along a continuum or range of health and illness (see Fig. 18-1). At one end is a state of extreme mental health; at the other end is a state of extreme mental illness. Fortunately, most people spend the majority of their lives nearer to the healthy end. However, fluctuations do occur as individuals experience life changes and respond to life events. What causes some individuals to develop mental illness while others do not is often unclear. Mental health is thought to be influenced by many factors, including genetics, biological functioning, and the environment. Mental health is generally supported by being raised by biologically healthy parents who teach and model effective coping strategies and provide a loving, nurturing environment. General risk factors for mental illness include a family history of mental illness, substance abuse within the family, and conditions of child abuse and neglect. Yet individuals from dysfunctional homes often achieve a good state of mental health and go on to lead healthy productive lives; and conversely, individuals sometimes come from healthy homes with good parents, yet struggle with various forms of mental illness.

TABLE 18-1			
ABBREVIATIONS			
Abbreviation	**Meaning**	**Abbreviation**	**Meaning**
ADD	attention deficit disorder	OCD	obsessive-compulsive disorder
ADHD	attention deficit-hyperactivity disorder	ODD	oppositional defiant disorder
ECT	electroconvulsive therapy	PTSD	post-traumatic stress disorder
GAD	generalized anxiety disorder	SAD	seasonal affective disorder; social anxiety disorder
MDD	major depressive disorder	SSRI	selective serotonin reuptake inhibitor
MMPI	Minnesota Multiphasic Personality Inventory	TS	Tourette syndrome

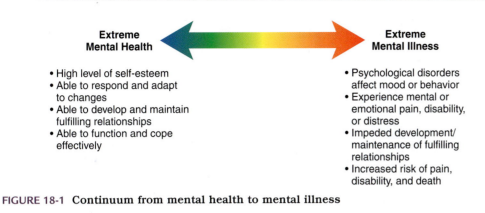

FIGURE 18-1 Continuum from mental health to mental illness

The American Psychiatric Association's *Diagnostic and Statistical Manual of Mental Disorders*, fourth edition text revision (DSM-IV-TR), is the most common reference used by mental health professionals in the clinical setting. (A new edition, the DSM-V, is due out in 2012.) This reference provides guidelines for diagnosing mental disorders and provides a standardized diagnostic code similar to the ICD-9-CM coding system. It categorizes mental illnesses by axes that pertain to different characteristics:

Axis I: Clinical disorders, including major disorders of mood and thought as well as developmental and learning disorders; often referred to as the main diagnosis (schizophrenia, depression, etc.)

Axis II: Developmental disorders (mental disability, autism, etc.) and personality disorders (antisocial, paranoid, borderline, etc.)

Axis III: Medical or physical conditions that may or may not contribute to the psychological condition (brain injury, etc.)

Axis IV: Stressors, such as psychosocial and environmental influences, that contribute to the psychological condition (unemployment, divorce, death of a loved one, etc.)

Axis V: Global assessment of functioning; includes an evaluation of the patient's highest level of function at present and within the previous year

> **Flashpoint**
> The DSM-IV-TR is the reference most widely used by mental health professionals.

Emotional Response to Illness

Physical health affects emotional and mental health. Individuals with healthy coping skills may respond to physical injury and illness reasonably well; those who lack such skills may not. Many people respond to permanent health loss in a manner similar to how they respond to other significant losses in their lives. The typical stages of grief and loss, as identified by researcher Elisabeth Kübler-Ross, are denial, anger, bargaining, depression, resolution, and acceptance (see Fig. 18-2). A grief reaction along these lines is normal and, to a certain extent, even healthy.

The stages of grief are fluid, meaning that patients may fluctuate between them and even exhibit signs of multiple stages at once. However, over time patients should progress to the point of acceptance.

Patients experiencing the initial stage of **denial** refuse to accept the reality of the situation that the injury or illness has caused in their lives. They may appear withdrawn and refuse to discuss health issues.

As patients begin to progress though stages of grief, they may feel and express anger, which is rage that masks the pain and grief, hiding what they feel. Initially it manifests in the form of emotional outbursts and statements of blame directed at others.

Bargaining is an irrational attempt to negotiate for unlikely or impossible changes. As patients display signs of the bargaining stage, they may offer to make behavior changes in exchange for a promise of better health.

> **Flashpoint**
> Physical health impacts mental health and vice versa.

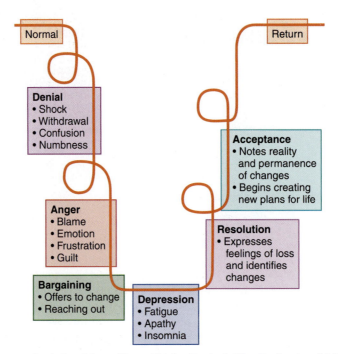

FIGURE 18-2 **Stages of grief and loss** (From Eagle, S, et al. *The Professional Medical Assistant: An Integrative Teamwork-Based Approach.* 2009. Philadelphia: F.A. Davis Company, with permission.)

Many patients will enter a period of depression as they face the inevitability of their health loss. During this time, they may exhibit typical depressive symptoms, such as fatigue, apathy, loss of interest in usual activities, and insomnia. As patients enter the resolution phase of the grieving process, they express emotions more freely and begin to identify changes caused by the health loss.

Acceptance is the stage in which patients acknowledge the reality and permanence of changes and begin to actively move forward in their lives.

Working through the stages of grief and loss requires time and physical and emotional resources that patients may or may not possess. In some cases, dysfunctional grieving can trigger or worsen mental illness; for example, some patients may enter into severe depression, requiring referral to a psychologist or psychiatrist for therapy.

Mental Health Disorders

A comprehensive discussion of mental health disorders is beyond the scope of this book. However, an attempt has been made to provide an overview of disorders that are likely to be seen in the medical office.

Intellectual Disability

ICD-9-CM: 317 (mild), 318.0 (moderate), 318.1 (severe), 318.2 (profound), 319 (severity unspecified)

[ICD-10: F70.0–F70.9 (mild), F71.0–F71.9 (moderate), F72.0–F72.9 (severe), F73.0–F73.9 (profound), F79 (severity unspecified)]

Intellectual disability, also called *developmental disability, mental challenge,* and *developmental delay,* is a condition marked by below average **cognition** (thinking process that includes language use, calculation, perception, memory, awareness, reasoning, judgment, learning, intellect, social skills, and imagination). It also includes deficits in adaptive and functional ability. These deficits are all apparent before age 18. Numerous other terms have been used in the past to describe this condition, but they have taken on negative meanings over the years and are no longer considered acceptable terms. A recent one, *mental retardation*, is falling out of favor because the term *retarded* is frequently used in an insulting manner.

Incidence

Intellectual disability is estimated to affect up to three million Americans.

Etiology

A specific cause of intellectual disability can only be identified about 25% of the time and can be an infection such as encephalitis, meningitis, congenital rubella, cytomegalovirus, or toxoplasmosis. A number of genetic and chromosomal syndromes, such as Down syndrome and Klinefelter syndrome, can also cause intellectual disability. Other causes are too numerous to list but include phenylketonuria, congenital hypothyroidism, Reye syndrome, severe malnutrition, intrauterine exposure to toxins such as alcohol or amphetamines, lead or mercury poisoning, and trauma before, during, or after birth.

Signs and Symptoms

Signs and symptoms of intellectual disability depend upon the severity of the disability. Most individuals are able to learn new information and skills but do so at a rate that is slower than that of individuals of average intelligence. Intellectual disability may appear as a delay or deficit in an infant's learning and ability to perform expected developmental tasks, such as sitting up, crawling, walking, and talking. Older individuals demonstrate memory deficit, lack of curiosity, difficulty learning, and difficulty following social norms (unwritten rules governing behavior in social settings). These individuals also struggle to perform their own activities of daily living, such as eating, dressing, toileting, and bathing. Those with intellectual disability often have other additional disabilities, such as seizure disorders, cerebral palsy, attention deficit-hyperactivity disorder (ADHD), and sensory deficits such as vision or hearing impairments. Signs and symptoms in those with mild intellectual disability may not be obvious until the child begins school. Even then, the condition may be confused with behavioral disorders or learning disabilities. The condition will be more obvious in those with moderate disability. Their need for ongoing assistance will require them to live with parents or in a structured setting on an ongoing basis. Those with severe conditions will require intensive care and support for their entire lives.

Diagnosis

Diagnosis of intellectual disability may be necessary for the individual to qualify for education-based services, home and community services, and Social Security Administration benefits. Intellectual disability may be suspected when the family and caregivers notice the child's developmental skills lagging behind those of other children of similar age. An official diagnosis, according to the DSM-IV-TR, is based upon three criteria. First, the limitation must be apparent before the individual reaches the age of 18. Second, the results of a measured intelligence (IQ) test must fall below 70. Third, an adaptive-behavior rating scale must indicate significant limitations in two or more areas of function (see Box 18-1).

Treatment

There is no cure for intellectual disability. However, many forms of treatment are available to support individuals in developing and living to their fullest potential. After a careful and thorough diagnosis, an individualized treatment plan is created. It may include special education services, home or community-based care and therapies, and Social Security Administration benefits.

Prognosis

The prognosis for individuals with intellectual disability depends upon the severity of the condition and the availability of supportive care and resources. With appropriate education and guidance, individuals with mild conditions can learn to live independently, seek and maintain gainful employment, and develop meaningful relationships. Those with moderate impairment require more structured living arrangements and some degree of supervision and assistance; however, in many cases they too can maintain certain

Flashpoint

The term *mental retardation* is falling out of favor.

Flashpoint

The IQ test has been used for many years to evaluate intelligence.

Flashpoint

People with intellectual disability can be helped to live satisfying lives to their fullest potential.

Box 18-1 Diagnostic Spotlight

ADAPTIVE-BEHAVIOR ASSESSMENT
An adaptive-behavior assessment measures the individual's abilities in three areas. *Activities of daily living* include abilities in self-care activities, such as toileting, feeding, dressing, work, using the telephone, managing a schedule, handling money, safety issues, health care, and transportation. *Communication skills* include the ability to understand what others are saying and the ability to respond. *Social skills* include interactions with family, peers, and adults, as well as following rules and laws, problem-solving in the social arena, and avoiding being victimized by others who would take advantage of the individual.

types of limited employment and can lead productive, satisfying lives. Those with severe conditions require continual supervision by caregivers who provide for their care and safety.

Learning Disorder

ICD-9-CM: 315.2   [ICD-10: F81.0–F81.9 (code by type)]
A learning disorder is a condition that affects the manner in which a person's brain receives, processes, analyzes, comprehends, and utilizes certain types of information. Specifically affected are the ability to understand and use written or spoken language and certain types of calculations. As a result, the individual may have greater difficulty with some types of learning than do people without learning disorders. There are numerous types of learning disorders, and many individuals are affected by more than one (see Table 18-2). Learning disorders are not caused by low intelligence; in fact, most individuals with learning disorders have normal or above normal IQs (see Box 18-2).

Flashpoint
There are many types of learning disorders.

TABLE 18-2	
LEARNING DISORDERS	
Disorder	**Description**
reading disability	difficulty processing language (speaking, reading, spelling, handwriting) and recognizing and comprehending words the individual already knows; often called *dyslexia*
dyscalculia	difficulty comprehending math concepts, solving math problems, using money, and understanding time
dysgraphia	difficulty forming letters, spelling, writing, and organizing ideas
information-processing disorder	difficulty using information gained through the senses (sight, sound, smell, touch, taste)
language-related learning disability	difficulty with age-appropriate communication, including reading, writing, spelling, speaking, and listening
dyspraxia	difficulty with manual dexterity, hand-eye coordination, and balance
auditory processing disorder	difficulty discriminating differences in sounds, leading to problems with reading and language comprehension
visual processing disorder	difficulty interpreting visual data, leading to problems with math and reading maps

Box 18-2 Diagnostic Spotlight

INTELLIGENCE TESTING

Intelligence testing, usually called *intelligence quotient (IQ) testing*, involves one or more standardized tests that measure intellectual ability based on a number of factors. These include language, vocabulary, numeric reasoning, motor speed, memory, and analytical ability. Most IQ tests measure a variety of factors, including knowledge of facts, reasoning, short-term memory, common sense, and visual-spatial abilities. Different tests must be used for children under age 16 than for adults. While IQ tests are known to provide accurate information predicting academic performance, they are not effective in measuring creativity or interpersonal skills. It is also important to note that factors other than intellectual ability can influence outcomes; some are cultural bias, language differences, depression, and anxiety. In general, scores are designated as follows:

Below 19: profound mental disability
20–34: severe mental disability
35–49: moderate mental disability
50–69: mild mental disability
70–79: borderline intelligence
80–95: low average intelligence
96–105: average intelligence
106–120: high average intelligence
121–129: superior intelligence
130 and higher: genius

Incidence

Learning disorders occur in very young children but are generally not noticed until children enter the school system. It is estimated that four million American children struggle with some type of learning disability.

Etiology

The brain is extremely complex, as is the manner in which it takes in, processes, and stores information. The information itself is also complex and varied. It may be presented as visual images, sounds, words, symbols, and so on. As the brain notes this complex array of data, it must sort, interpret, and determine their significance. Many of these different functions occur in different parts of the brain. Because people with learning disorders are thought to have differences in certain areas of the brain, the manner in which they process information is altered.

The exact cause of learning disorders is not fully understood. Some theories involve genetics, because learning disorders tend to be common in families. Others include physiological and environmental influences such as low birth weight, hypoxia (lack of oxygen), prematurity, birth injury, toxic exposure, and poor nutrition.

Signs and Symptoms

Learning disorders are actually considered variations within the normal range of human development. They are only considered disabilities if they significantly impede the individual's ability to perform and succeed in certain activities. Signs and symptoms of learning disorders are often subtle and may go undetected for years or even for a lifetime. Individuals with learning disorders typically evidence delays and struggle within certain areas, while other aspects of development and performance are normal. People with verbal learning disorders typically struggle with written or spoken language. Among the most common verbal learning disorders are variations of dyslexia. Individuals with dyslexia struggle to correctly recognize and process letters and to match letters with correct sounds. Consequently, they struggle with tasks that require reading, writing, spelling, or other language skills.

Individuals with nonverbal learning disorders struggle with processing visual images. For example, they may confuse symbols such as addition and division signs. Consequently, these

Flashpoint

Some people may have more than one type of learning disorder.

individuals struggle with tasks involving mathematics. For some the first real sign of a learning disorder is when they recognize a discrepancy between the large amounts of time spent studying for exams and the low scores they earn. Unfortunately, the signs and symptoms first noted are often misinterpreted by teachers or parents as low motivation, low self-esteem, depression, or acting out.

Diagnosis

To be accurately diagnosed for a learning disorder, the individual should first undergo vision and hearing testing to rule out sensory deficits that might be the real cause of their struggles. Next, they should be evaluated by a psychologist or learning specialist who is qualified to diagnose learning disorders. Early diagnosis and treatment are critical in reducing the negative impact of the disorder and increasing the child's success in school.

Flashpoint

Concerned parents can request that their child be evaluated by the school psychologist.

Treatment

There are many types of learning disorders. Therefore, treatment is variable and is designed according to the needs of the individual. Help may be given by education specialists, psychologists, or speech and language therapists. In some cases, students benefit from learning specific study skills, organizational strategies, and note-taking techniques, or from working with a tutor on specific subjects. If attention deficit is a contributing factor, medication may help the child focus and stay on task.

Prognosis

The prognosis for individuals with learning disorders is very good if diagnosis and appropriate interventions are timely. While some individuals dislike feeling "labeled" with a diagnosis, many feel a sense of relief in finally having an understanding of what has been impeding their efforts. They are also happy to know that help is available. As they begin to experience greater success in their activities, self-confidence and self-esteem improve.

Stuttering

ICD-9-CM: 307.0   [ICD-10 F98.5]

Stuttering, sometimes called *disfluency* or *stammering,* is a communication disorder in which speech is disrupted by the repetition of syllables, word fragments, prolongations, or hesitations. The condition may be mild or severe. *Acquired stuttering* is the sudden appearance of stuttering in a person over age 10 with no previous history of a speech disorder.

Incidence

A number of children experience some degree of stuttering during their early years, but in most cases the symptoms resolve within several weeks or months. Fewer than 5% experience a more significant and longer-lasting problem. However, the condition usually resolves by late childhood. An estimated three million American adults stutter; males are affected four times more often than women.

Flashpoint

Most cases of stuttering resolve on their own without treatment.

Etiology

The exact cause of stuttering is not well understood. It is suspected that individuals who stutter may process speech and language information in different parts of the brain. Genetics is considered a possible factor, since the problem appears to run in families. Acquired stuttering may occur after a stroke, after administration of certain drugs, or as a reaction to unusually stressful circumstances.

Signs and Symptoms

Individuals who stutter produce speech that is disrupted by the repetition of words, syllables, word fragments, prolongations, or hesitations. At times the speech may become totally blocked, with no sound produced. In addition, patients may exhibit physical tension evidenced by rapid blinking, trembling of the lips and jaw, and other unusual facial movements. The symptoms may be exaggerated during times of stress and may be worsened by some medications, diseases, and conditions.

Diagnosis

Stuttering is easily noted by listening to the individual speak. However, a certified speech and language pathologist must evaluate the individual to provide an accurate diagnosis of the type and severity of the condition. Evaluation includes observation, interview, and a variety of tests. Factors that may indicate a more severe stuttering condition include duration of 6 months or more, family history of stuttering, significant fear and anxiety for the patient or family, and the presence of other speech or language problems.

Treatment

Treatment of stuttering is aimed at helping patients speak and communicate more smoothly and effectively, to be able to participate more fully in desired activities. Patients are taught to monitor the pace at which they speak, to pronounce words in a slower, more relaxed manner, and to control their breathing. Other therapies include relaxation techniques, hypnosis, and delayed auditory feedback (a technique that enables speakers to hear their own voices a fraction of a second later, similar to an echo). In some cases, medications such as neuroleptics may also provide some benefit.

Prognosis

The prognosis for most individuals with stuttering is very good, since the condition usually resolves spontaneously by adulthood. Those with chronic stuttering may experience impairment in personal and professional communication, and as a result may feel hesitant to participate in certain activities. However, early diagnosis and therapy can improve fluency and increase self-confidence and self-esteem.

Oppositional Defiant Disorder

ICD-9-CM: 313.81   [ICD-10: F91.3]

Oppositional defiant disorder (ODD) is a condition in which a child demonstrates a pattern of extreme uncooperative, defiant, and hostile behaviors toward parents and other figures of authority. The behavior impairs functioning within school, social, and family settings.

Incidence

Estimates of the incidence of ODD vary, but the true figure is most likely around 6% to 10%. The disorder usually affects boys and generally begins before the age of 8.

Etiology

The cause of ODD is not fully understood. Genetics may play a role, since it has been noted that children with ODD often have other family members with the same or a related disorder. Biological contributors may include brain injuries and defects that impact the balance of neurotransmitters. Other forms of mental illness and environmental factors also play a role; for example, children whose family members struggle with substance abuse are more likely to exhibit ODD.

Flashpoint
ODD usually affects boys.

Signs and Symptoms

Individuals with ODD exhibit a pattern of behaviors that include some or all of the following:

- temper tantrums
- angry outbursts
- resentful attitude
- arguing, especially with adults
- resisting or questioning the rules
- refusing to cooperate
- deliberately annoying others
- blaming others for the individual's own mistakes
- becoming annoyed or irritated easily
- acting spitefully, vindictively, and revengefully
- using obscenities

Individuals with ODD have a low tolerance for frustration and suffer from low self-esteem. They frequently struggle with other problems, such as ADHD, learning disorders, mood disorders, anxiety disorders, and conduct disorder (marked by repetitive, persistent, aggressive, destructive, and disruptive behaviors that violate the rights of others).

Diagnosis

The diagnostic process may include a medical history and testing to rule out other disorders. The child is then referred to a child psychologist or psychiatrist for further evaluation. Data are gathered from parents, teachers, and others who have observed the child's behaviors, and further through conversation, testing, and observation of the child. A child is diagnosed with ODD when behavior includes four or more of the listed criteria; the behaviors interfere with functioning at home, at school, or in the community; the behaviors are not caused by another disorder; and the pattern of behavior is of 6 months' duration or greater.

Treatment

Treatment depends upon the severity of symptoms and the child's age and ability to participate in therapies. Psychotherapy may help the child with anger-management skills. Cognitive behavioral therapy may help the child gain insight into the behaviors and make adjustments to them. Parents may benefit from training programs aimed at positively influencing the child's behavior (see Box 18-3). Other therapies assist children in developing problem-solving and social skills. Family therapy may help all members of the family interact more effectively with the child, communicate better with one another, and better cope with their own feelings. Medication may be useful in controlling some symptoms and treating related conditions.

Flashpoint

Parents of children with ODD need education and support to provide effective parenting.

Prognosis

Children with ODD may experience rejection by peers and others because of their inappropriate and aggressive behaviors. They are at high risk of later developing conduct disorder, especially if they go untreated. Individuals with conduct disorder can then go on to develop antisocial personality disorder. However, early diagnosis and treatment significantly reduce these risks and increase the likelihood that individuals will go on to experience productive lives and rewarding relationships.

Tourette Syndrome

ICD-9-CM: 307.23   [ICD-10: F95.2]

Tourette syndrome (TS) is a neurological disorder marked by motor and vocal tics. A ***motor tic*** is a sudden, spasmodic, involuntary muscular contraction, usually involving the face, mouth, eyes, head, neck, or shoulders. A ***vocal tic*** is an involuntary sound such as clearing the throat, grunting, or uttering words. Tics can develop in anyone but are most common in children ages 7 to 10.

Box 18-3 Wellness Promotion

POSITIVE PARENTING TECHNIQUES

A mental health professional can help parents develop positive techniques to aid in managing the behaviors of children with ODD. Some examples are:

- Set reasonable limits with consequences you know you can and will enforce.
- Allow time for play and recreation.
- Talk with and *listen* to your child.
- Be accessible; be willing to interrupt your activities and give your child time.
- Give positive feedback and praise any time the child behaves in a cooperative manner.
- Support your child's interests.
- Support your child's efforts to be successful in school.
- Take time-outs if you notice conflict escalating and your temper rising.
- Encourage your child to also take time-outs for similar reasons.
- Model and encourage healthy habits (proper nutrition, exercise, avoidance of alcohol, tobacco, and illegal drugs, etc.)
- Do not verbally compare your child to siblings.
- Frequently voice genuine love, acceptance, and appreciation of your child.
- Choose your battles; don't make everything a power struggle.
- Set a good example by using effective coping strategies to manage your own stress.

Tics that last more than a year are called chronic tics and may be related to Tourette syndrome.

Incidence

An estimated 100,000 to 200,000 individuals in the United States have TS, but the numbers may be much higher, since many mild cases go undiagnosed. TS occurs in all racial and ethnic groups and is much more common in males than females. It usually is first noted during childhood, between 7 and 10 years old.

Etiology

The cause of TS is not fully understood. Genetics may play a role, since it often appears in multiple family members—although they may each have different symptoms. It also may be related to abnormal activity of neurotransmitter chemicals, such as dopamine.

Signs and Symptoms

Signs and symptoms of TS vary among individuals, but most cases are mild. Individuals with TS display multiple motor tics and one or more vocal tics, though they may not all occur at the same time. Motor tics include blinking, jerking or twisting the head, grimacing, twitching the nose, shrugging the shoulders, and swinging the arms. More complex motor tics may include grasping or touching others or objects, twirling, kicking, making obscene gestures, stamping, and hitting or biting oneself. Vocal tics include grunting, clicking the tongue, clearing the throat, yelping, barking, sniffing, shouting or uttering words or phrases, and in a small percentage of cases, uttering obscenities. These behaviors occur multiple times throughout the day. Symptoms may disappear for days or even weeks only to return again. While individuals can sometimes suppress their symptoms briefly for a matter of minutes or even hours, the symptoms eventually burst forth in a more severe fashion. Tics may noticeably increase when the individual experiences greater stress and may decrease with relaxation or focus on a task. Individuals with TS sometimes also have learning disorders, attention deficit disorder (ADD) or ADHD, depression, anxiety disorders, oppositional defiant disorder, sleep disorders, or any of the following:

impulse control disorder: failure to resist performing socially unacceptable or even harmful behaviors

obsessions: persistent, recurring, and distressing thoughts, images, feelings, or impulses that are unwanted and intrusive

compulsions: behaviors performed repeatedly, in a ritualistic manner, in order to relieve the fear or anxiety caused by obsessive thoughts

Diagnosis

TS is diagnosed through observation of symptoms. There is no particular test for TS, although testing may be done to rule out other disorders.

Treatment

Individuals with very minor symptoms may require no treatment. Others may benefit from medications to help control symptoms. While no one medication works equally well for everyone, the most commonly used class of medications for suppressing symptoms is the neuroleptics. Another class occasionally used is the alpha-adrenergic agonists. Side effects can be problematic with both classes of drugs, though; therefore, patients are counseled to work closely with healthcare providers and use the lowest effective dose. Other therapies may be helpful as well. Psychotherapy and other forms of counseling help patients and families cope with the disorder. Therapies such as biofeedback and relaxation strategies may help reduce stress. This does not cure the disorder but can reduce the frequency of symptoms and improve coping.

Prognosis

TS is a chronic disorder with no known cure. Children and teens may find themselves rejected by their peers, who find their behaviors bizarre and puzzling and respond with prejudice or even ridicule. Parents who are ignorant about the disorder may exclude the child from activities or threaten other forms of punishment. Early diagnosis and intervention can minimize these problems. Furthermore, most people experience marked improvement in their late teens or early 20s, and get better as they mature. Therefore, most people are able to lead productive, fulfilling lives.

Flashpoint
People with Tourette syndrome have motor or vocal tics.

Flashpoint
Individuals with minor symptoms may not need treatment.

Substance Abuse Disorders

ICD-9-CM: 303.90 (alcohol), 305.90 (other mixed or unspecified drug abuse)   [ICD-10: F10.0–F10.9 (alcohol), F11.0–F11.9 (opioids), F13.0–F13.9 (sedatives), F14.0–F14.9 (cocaine)—code by presenting symptoms]

Substance disorders include a variety of conditions involving dysfunctional use of legal and illegal substances. Intoxication is reversible physical and psychological symptoms specific to the ingested substance, caused by an episode of overuse. **Substance abuse** is defined as a persistent, maladaptive pattern of substance use over a 12-month period, in which an individual continues substance use in spite of significant adverse consequences. Addiction refers to a compulsive and maladaptive dependence on a substance of abuse. However, the term has come to be overused, misused, and misunderstood. More accurate terms are **physical dependence** and **psychological dependence.** Physical dependence is a condition of physical tolerance, which is the need for greatly increased dosages to achieve the same effect, or experience of a significantly reduced effect with the same dose. It also includes the display of a withdrawal syndrome if the substance is suddenly discontinued. Psychological dependence involves emotional and behavioral symptoms of craving, compulsive drug-seeking, hoarding, and using substances purely for emotional and mental euphoria (commonly referred to as getting high).

The general term *substance dependence* is defined as continued substance abuse, compulsive use behaviors, development of tolerance, and withdrawal symptoms with discontinuation. Craving may or may not be a factor, depending upon the substance. Abused substances are many, and the list seems to grow continually. It includes alcohol, prescription medications, opiates, marijuana, cocaine, hallucinogens, ecstasy, inhalants, amphetamines, and phencyclidine (PCP). Nicotine is often also included on the list, while caffeine generally is not.

Incidence

Statistics related to substance abuse in the United States are numerous and overwhelming. A general estimate of the total costs related to all forms of abuse, including tobacco and alcohol, exceeds $500 billion each year. Substance abuse accounts for more than 40 million annual accidents and injuries. It contributes to numerous diseases and is a known contributor to serious social problems, such as violent crime, unemployment, domestic violence, child abuse, and homelessness.

Etiology

Substance abuse disorders are thought to be caused by a combination of biological and environmental factors. Substance abuse is sometimes called a brain disease because many abused substances lead to changes in the structure and functioning of the brain. These changes become a part of the pathology that contributes to ongoing substance use and abuse. Some substances of abuse, such as marijuana and heroin, act on the brain by imitating neurotransmitter chemicals or by stimulating the reward and pleasure part of the brain. Others, such as the stimulants methamphetamine and cocaine, cause the release of large amounts of neurotransmitters. Most substances of abuse stimulate the reward and pleasure part of the brain with increased amounts of dopamine, which produces feelings of euphoria or feeling high; this is often the experience that users try to reproduce with repeated dosing. However, the brain quickly adapts by producing less dopamine or decreasing its response to it. Thus it becomes more difficult for the individual to achieve the same effect without increasing dosage. Some people are more prone to becoming psychologically dependent or physically dependent on drugs than are other people. Exactly why this happens is not clear, although genetic and environmental factors are thought to play a role. Risk factors include family history of substance abuse, history of physical or sexual abuse, and young age when abuse behaviors first begin.

Signs and Symptoms

Signs and symptoms of substance abuse and dependence include evidence of impairment, increasing tolerance, increasing amounts of time spent seeking and using the substance, and continued use despite adverse consequences. These consequences may include damaged personal relationships, missed days of work, job loss, traffic citations related to impaired driving, vehicle accidents, and substance-related illness or injury.

Flashpoint

Substance abuse is a huge problem that costs the United States over half a trillion dollars each year!

Flashpoint

Key signs of substance abuse are impairment in the ability to function and continued use in spite of adverse consequences.

Diagnosis

The criteria for a diagnosis of substance abuse include repeated or persistent use of the substance over a 12-month period with an associated failure to meet major role obligations, and use in spite of serious negative consequences. It is important that other underlying disorders, such as untreated depression or chronic pain, be considered. In such cases, patients may be attempting to self-medicate to alleviate their discomfort, rather than seeking to achieve physical or psychological euphoria.

Treatment

Treatment for substance abuse usually includes a combination approach. Therapies include detoxification, sometimes with hospitalization, psychotherapy, behavior therapy, and involvement in 12-step programs (see Box 18-4). Treatment approaches must be tailored to each patient's patterns of drug abuse and individual needs. Coexisting medical and psychiatric illnesses must also be addressed.

Prognosis

The prognosis for patients with substance abuse disorders is variable and depends upon the patient's motivation to recover and access to health care, the type of substance involved, and the duration of the substance use. In many cases patients can achieve recovery and return to an excellent quality of life. Relapses are common, but with appropriate intervention and treatment, most people can again return to recovery. Many individuals find that they can prevent relapse by maintaining some type of ongoing treatment or involvement in a support system, such as those provided by 12-step programs.

Flashpoint

Twelve-step programs provide support and education for people in recovery.

Mood Disorders

A mood disorder is any mental disorder that has a disturbance of mood as the predominant feature. Mood disorders described in this text are major depressive disorder and bipolar disorder.

Major Depressive Disorder

ICD-9-CM: 296.2 (single episode, fifth digit codes for severity), 296.3 (recurrent episodes, fifth digit codes for severity)   **[ICD-10: F32.0–F32.9 (single episode, code by severity), F33.0–F33.9 (recurrent episodes, code by severity)]**

Major depressive disorder (MDD) is sometimes called *unipolar depression*, *clinical depression*, or just *depression*. It is defined as a condition in which a person experiences five or more depressive symptoms for 2 weeks or longer. It is experienced as persistent feelings of sadness and hopelessness that significantly impair the person's ability to function in all aspects of life.

Box 18-4 Wellness Promotion

TWELVE-STEP PROGRAMS

Twelve-step programs are designed to aid people in recovery from addiction to substances or compulsion to perform certain behaviors. Originally developed by Alcoholics Anonymous in 1939, the successful strategy has since been modified and used by more than 200 different groups, according to their needs. Examples include Narcotics Anonymous, Overeaters Anonymous, and Gamblers Anonymous. Each 12-step group conducts regular open or closed (members-only) meetings for the purpose of providing group support to members working toward recovery. All 12-step programs share the following principles:

- Admitting that one cannot control the addiction or compulsion
- Recognizing that strength can be received from a greater power
- Working with a sponsor to examine and make amends for past mistakes
- Creating a new life lived according to a new code of behavior
- Extending help to other people who struggle with the same addiction or compulsion

Incidence

MDD is a significant disorder: It affects approximately 15 million Americans at any given time and is the leading cause of disability in the United States. Furthermore, it is believed to affect approximately 55 million Americans at some point during their lives. It is most often diagnosed in young adults but affects people of all ages, women more often than men.

Etiology

The cause of MDD is not fully understood. Psychological, biological, and environmental factors are thought to play significant roles. Initial episodes of depression may be triggered by a painful life event, such as a divorce or the death of a loved one. Postpartum depression may trigger MDD, with onset within 4 weeks of giving birth; seasonal affective disorder may be triggered in the fall, when natural light is decreased.

In some cases people evidence maladaptive responses to significant life events, such as a divorce, the death of loved ones, or job loss. They may interpret the cause and meaning of such events in negative terms and experience feelings of guilt, worthlessness, or inferiority. Other individuals feel victimized by life events and feel powerless to influence the course of their lives. In some cases, environmental events largely beyond the individual's control do occur; these might include natural disasters, some forms of major illness or injury, or oppression related to race, gender, or sexual orientation. This can cause the person to feel overwhelmed and emotionally bankrupt.

Biological causes of MDD include deficiencies in neurotransmitters in the brain, differences in brain structure, and genetics. Regardless of the triggering cause, major depression is a very real psychological and biological disorder that deserves real treatment.

Signs and Symptoms

The key feature of major depression is a pervasively sad, gloomy, or hopeless mood that the person feels unable to overcome. Numerous other symptoms may include sleep difficulties (sleeping too much or too little), decreased libido (sex drive), physical aches and pains, fatigue, irritability, low tolerance for frustration, faulty memory, feelings of worthlessness, difficulty concentrating and making decisions, and possible thoughts about suicide. Appetite may be increased, leading to obesity, or decreased, leading to unhealthy weight loss. There is a general lack of interest in activities the person once found enjoyable. Responsibilities related to work, home, or child care may feel overwhelming and burdensome. In severe cases the patient may experience psychotic symptoms, including ***delusions*** (false, unfounded beliefs) and ***hallucinations*** (false sensory perceptions). Depression often manifests in children or adolescents as irritability.

Flashpoint

The main symptom of MDD is a pervasive and overwhelming feeling of hopelessness.

Diagnosis

A diagnosis of depression may be suspected when patients, or concerned friends or relatives, complain of some of the described signs and symptoms. For a diagnosis of MDD, the patient must evidence at least five of the listed symptoms, which must persist for most of the day, nearly every day, for at least 2 consecutive weeks. The episode must be accompanied by clinically significant distress or impairment in social or occupational functioning or in other important areas of functioning. The disorder must not be due to bereavement, drugs, alcohol, or the direct effects of a disease, such as hypothyroidism. A screening tool such as the Beck Depression Inventory may be used to clarify the patient's symptoms and risk factors (see Box 18-5). Diagnosis is often complicated by the fact that patients may suffer from other coexisting mental health disorders.

Box 18-5 Diagnostic Spotlight

BECK DEPRESSION INVENTORY

The Beck Depression Inventory (BDI and BDI-II) is a commonly used tool for assessing the severity of depression. It is a 21-question multiple-choice questionnaire used for patients 13 years and older. The first 13 questions assess psychological symptoms, such as mood, feelings of guilt, and suicidal ideas, while the remaining questions assess physical symptoms, such as insomnia, fatigue, and loss of libido. All questions are related to symptoms of major depression. A seven-item shorter version is also available and often used in primary care settings.

Treatment

Treatment of major depression involves psychotherapy, medication, and sometimes electroconvulsive therapy. A variety of antidepressant medications are available. Most commonly used are selective serotonin reuptake inhibitors (SSRIs) and serotonin and norepinephrine reuptake inhibitors. Antidepressant medications are sometimes combined with antipsychotics or other classifications of drugs to achieve the most therapeutic response. Education for patients and family members is critically important in ensuring successful treatment (see Box 18-6).

Psychotherapy helps patients gain a clearer perspective on their disorder, manage symptoms, change negative thinking, and improve interpersonal relationships. For some patients, psychotherapy alone is all that is needed. For others, it is combined with medication for an optimal response. Light therapy, sometimes called *phototherapy*, is also useful for individuals who suffer from depression and seasonal affective disorder. In this form of therapy the person sits near a light box or device for a few minutes each day. The device produces bright light that imitates natural outdoor light (see Fig. 18-3). This exposure is thought to affect circadian rhythms (the 24-hour human biological clock) and causes the body to suppress the release of melatonin (a hormone that induces sleep-wake cycles).

Electroconvulsive therapy may be necessary for patients with severe symptoms who do not respond to psychotherapy and medication (see Box 18-7). General lifestyle changes can also help boost mood and well-being for any patients suffering from depression. Recommendations include eating a healthy diet, getting regular exercise, avoiding tobacco and alcohol, getting enough sleep, and seeking positive, supportive relationships. Some individuals find the use of complementary

---

Box 18-6 Wellness Promotion

TAKING ANTIDEPRESSANTS

General information related to medication therapy for patients with depression includes the following:

- The patient may experience increased energy and ability to make decisions before mood improves; consequently, risk of suicidal thoughts and actions is greatest at this point.
- About half of all patients experience troublesome side effects of antidepressant medication. There are many possible solutions, but the patient must communicate closely with the health-care provider to find the best one.
- Many medication side effects diminish with time.
- Most antidepressant medications require several weeks before the patient experiences maximal effect.
- Patients should never suddenly discontinue medications without consulting with their health-care provider.

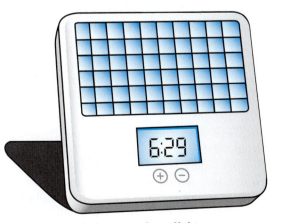

FIGURE 18-3 Light-therapy devices mimic natural sunlight

Box 18-7 Wellness Promotion

ELECTROCONVULSIVE THERAPY

Electroconvulsive therapy was discontinued at one time in favor of psychiatric medications; however, it has made a comeback in recent years. In its new form it is a modified, more comfortable, and more effective form of therapy than in the past. During treatment, a carefully calculated amount of electrical current is delivered to the brain of the sedated patient. The treatment is safe and has been found to achieve an effect that is as good as or better than that of many antidepressant medications. This form of therapy has been found to improve the mood and level of functioning of patients suffering from severe depression who have been unresponsive to other therapies. It is especially useful for patients in danger of harming themselves or others because of the severity of their depression.

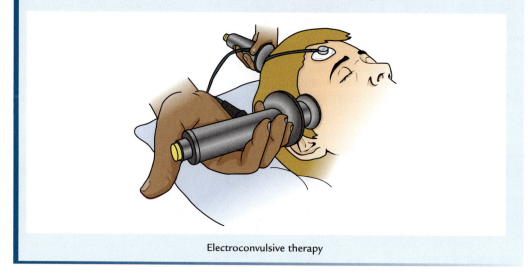

Electroconvulsive therapy

therapies beneficial. Herbal supplements sometimes used include Saint John's wort and ginkgo biloba. However, these can interact with other medications, including some antidepressants; it is therefore very important that patients inform their health-care providers of any supplements they are taking. Other complementary therapies include acupuncture, meditation, yoga, aromatherapy, music therapy, pet therapy, massage, and humor. While such measures are unlikely to cure severe depression, they have been found to decrease anxiety and stress, relieve or decrease pain, promote relaxation, increase endorphins, and promote general feelings of well-being.

Prognosis

Major depression can be devastating when left untreated, because symptoms tend to worsen over time. It is the most common contributor to suicide; 15% of patients with major depression die by suicide. In addition, depressed patients tend to engage in other self-destructive behaviors, such as tobacco use and abuse of drugs and alcohol. The good news, however, is that depression is highly treatable. Within 1 year of therapy, approximately 60% of patients achieve recovery or significant improvement, and up to 90% are able to return to an effective level of functioning in their personal and professional lives. Recurrence is common. Therefore, patients should be counseled about the need for ongoing maintenance therapy.

Flashpoint

Depression is a very treatable disorder.

Bipolar Disorder

Flashpoint

People with bipolar disorder fluctuate dramatically between euphoric and depressive states.

ICD-9-CM: 296.4 (manic, fifth digit codes for severity), 296.5 (depressed, fifth digit codes for severity), 296.6 (mixed, fifth digit codes for severity)

[ICD-10: F31.0–F31.9 (code by symptoms)]

Bipolar disorder, also called *manic-depressive disorder*, is a mental health disorder in which the individual's **affect** (emotional reaction or mood) shifts dramatically between highs and lows to such a severe extent that the normal ability to function at work or school or in relationships is impaired.

Incidence
An estimated six million Americans suffer from bipolar disorder.

Etiology
The cause of bipolar disorder is not clear; however, it tends to run in families. Emotional or physical trauma may serve as a trigger for those who are predisposed to this disorder.

Signs and Symptoms
Symptoms typically develop during the late teens or early adult years and vary depending upon whether the individual is experiencing a manic or a depressive state. During a manic state the individual typically demonstrates increased levels of energy. This can manifest as euphoria (extreme good mood), restlessness, little need for sleep, rapid speech, racing thoughts, extreme irritability, increased sex drive, aggressive behavior, drug or alcohol abuse, and poor judgment. During a depressive state the individual typically demonstrates decreased energy, feelings of sadness and hopelessness, and loss of interest in activities that are normally enjoyed, including sex. The individual may exhibit difficulty making decisions, remembering, and concentrating. Other symptoms include changes in appetite and in sleep pattern, sleeping either too much or too little. Suicidal thoughts or suicidal attempts may occur. Between manic and depressive states, the individual may experience relatively normal mood and behavior.

Diagnosis
Diagnosis is based upon family history and personal history, including a description of moods and behaviors. A manic state is identified if extreme mood elevation accompanies three or more other symptoms daily for a week or more. A depressive state is identified if a depressive mood accompanies five or more symptoms on a daily basis for 2 weeks or more.

Treatment
Treatment of bipolar disorder is aimed at stabilizing mood and behavior. This is usually done through a combination of medication and therapy. Mood-stabilization medications include lithium carbonate, anticonvulsants, calcium channel blockers, and beta-adrenergics. Antidepressants and other types of medication may also be used in some instances. Various forms of psychosocial therapy have been found helpful in providing support and guidance and in increasing the individual's mood stability, resulting in fewer crisis episodes. Education should focus on the importance of consistency in medication use, even when the person is feeling well and maintaining contact with health-care providers.

Prognosis
Bipolar disorder is considered a long-term disorder. However, most of those affected can achieve stabilization of mood and behavior, resulting in a high quality of life, through effective management.

Anxiety Disorders

Most people experience anxiety at times in their lives. A certain degree of anxiety is considered normal for many situations, such as awaiting the results of important medical tests or undergoing a job interview. However, most people recognize such anxiety as situational and experience relief when the situation passes. Furthermore, although the anxiety they felt may have been mildly distressing, they have sufficient coping skills to manage their feelings and to continue functioning within the given set of circumstances.

Some individuals, however, experience episodes of anxiety that are extreme and difficult or impossible to manage. Others experience a degree of chronic anxiety that is excessive. In either case, excessive anxiety interferes with functioning for approximately 18% of American adults. Common types of anxiety disorders include generalized anxiety disorder, panic disorder, phobic disorder, obsessive-compulsive disorder, and post-traumatic stress disorder.

Generalized Anxiety Disorder
ICD-9-CM: 300.02   [ICD-10: F41.1]
Generalized anxiety disorder (GAD) is a chronic condition in which individuals experience pathological anxiety—that is, anxiety that is excessive and is not triggered by any specific situation. GAD develops gradually, usually beginning between childhood and middle age. As it worsens it begins to interfere with normal daily functioning.

Flashpoint
People with GAD suffer from a chronic, excessive level of anxiety.

Incidence

GAD affects more than six million Americans, women slightly more often than men.

Etiology

The cause of GAD is not fully understood but is likely a complex combination of biological, environmental, and genetic factors. It has been noted that relatives of patients with GAD have a 20% higher likelihood than normal of having the disorder. Low or irregular levels of neurotransmitters, such as serotonin, norepinephrine, and gamma-aminobutyric acid, affect the individual's mood and sense of well-being. Environmental factors such as school, work, relationships, and quality and quantity of sleep all affect physical, mental, and emotional well-being. The condition may be worsened by problems with health or finances. Other risk factors include childhood trauma or adversity, serious illness, and personality disorders.

Signs and Symptoms

The primary symptom of GAD is chronic, excessive worry about everyday things, especially things beyond the individual's control. Other signs and symptoms include an inability to relax, difficulty falling or staying asleep, feeling on edge, irritability, restlessness, and difficulty concentrating. Physical symptoms are many and include headaches, fatigue, depression, nausea, diarrhea, sweating, muscle aches and tension, difficulty swallowing, and feeling short of breath or light-headed.

Diagnosis

To diagnose GAD, a mental health professional performs a thorough psychological evaluation. A physical examination may also be done to rule out other disorders. The patient may be asked to complete one or more questionnaires. The specific diagnostic criteria for GAD are:

- excessive anxiety and worry most days of the week for 6 months or more, about numerous issues
- inability to control feelings of anxiety
- worry focused on subjects not related to another identified condition, such as substance abuse, obsessive-compulsive disorder, or panic attacks

Additionally, at least three of the following symptoms must be experienced for 6 months or more:

- restlessness
- fatigue
- difficulty concentrating
- irritability
- muscle tension
- sleep disturbance

Treatment

There is no cure for GAD. However, patients generally respond well to combination therapy, including psychotherapy and medications such as antidepressants, anxiolytics, beta blockers, and benzodiazepines. Psychotherapy helps the patient to develop coping strategies for managing anxiety and to replace irrational, negative thoughts with healthy, positive ones. Techniques include meditation, biofeedback, and desensitization.

Prognosis

Flashpoint

People with GAD are prone to developing panic disorder and depression.

GAD is a chronic disorder that can worsen during times of extreme stress. Individuals with GAD are more prone than others to developing panic disorder and depression. They may also develop alcohol or substance abuse problems if they use these substances to self-medicate.

Panic Disorder
ICD-9-CM: 300.01   [ICD-10: F41.0]

Panic disorder is a condition in which the individual experiences recurring *panic attacks*, which are episodes of overwhelming anxiety, fear, and discomfort that strike suddenly and without warning. The intensity of the emotion felt is extreme and disproportional to the triggering event. Episodes usually only last a few minutes but can recur at any time. Individuals with panic disorder often have other mental or physical disorders, such as substance abuse disorder, depression, other anxiety disorders, irritable bowel syndrome, or asthma.

Incidence

Approximately four million Americans suffer from panic disorder. It is two to three times more common in women than in men and usually begins during adolescence or young adulthood. It affects members of different ethnic and economic groups equally.

Etiology

The cause of panic disorder is not fully understood. In some cases the patient is able to identify a stressful or traumatic event that precedes the first attack, such as the loss of a significant other. However, this is often not the case. Genetics may play a role, since panic disorder tends to run in families. After having one or two panic attacks, the individual becomes extremely anxious about the possibility of having more, and consequently fear of the panic attacks themselves becomes the overriding fear. Anticipatory anxiety can then cause the individual to become reclusive and avoid public places for fear of having an attack in an airplane, bus, shopping mall, or other such places.

Signs and Symptoms

The classic symptom of panic disorder is a recurring pattern of panic attacks. These are episodes of intense anxiety accompanied by at least four of the following symptoms: palpitations; racing heartbeat; sweating, trembling, or shaking; shortness of breath or sensation of smothering; choking sensation; chest pain or discomfort; nausea or abdominal distress; dizziness or light-headedness; feeling of detachment; feeling of losing control or going crazy; fear of dying; numbness or tingling; and chills or hot flushes. The onset of a panic attack is sudden; the attack builds to a peak within 10 minutes or less. It may include a sense of imminent danger or an urge to escape. Panic attacks become a part of a larger panic disorder if they occur repeatedly. The symptoms caused by a panic attack are physically real—patients may feel a sense of doom and fear that they are having a heart attack.

Diagnosis

Many of the symptoms of panic disorder imitate those of other disorders, such as heart disease or thyroid problems. This can make it difficult to make the diagnosis. Patients often make numerous visits to the emergency department or to their physicians, over a lengthy period of time, before an accurate diagnosis is made.

Flashpoint

The physical symptoms of a panic attack are very real and frightening to the patient.

Treatment

People with panic disorder frequently lack insight regarding the true nature of the problem and are embarrassed to seek care. This often delays treatment. A common form of treatment is cognitive behavioral therapy. It involves learning about the disorder, creating a treatment plan, monitoring the attacks and triggers, learning breathing and relaxation techniques, learning to reinterpret the physical symptoms in a realistic, less threatening manner, and desensitizing the self to triggers. Medications that are often helpful include antidepressants, benzodiazepines, and occasionally beta blockers. Many people also find participation in support groups to be very helpful. Friends and family members can help by first understanding that the symptoms the patient feels are very real. Then they can provide calm reassurance until the episode passes (see Box 18-8).

Box 18-8 Wellness Promotion

CALMING THE PATIENT WHO IS HAVING A PANIC ATTACK

Care providers, family members, and friends of patients with a panic disorder can help them deal with panic attacks by following these guidelines:

- Provide for safety.
- Provide a calm, quiet environment.
- Speak slowly, in short, simple sentences, using a clear, calm voice.
- Give one instruction at a time and avoid long explanations.
- Demonstrate deep, slow breathing.
- Avoid touching, pushing, or hurrying the patient unless absolutely necessary for safety reasons.
- Gently remind the patient that the attack will pass within a few minutes.

Prognosis

The prognosis for individuals with panic disorder is very good if diagnosis and treatment occur. Most people experience significant improvement within 2 to 5 months. Untreated panic disorder can lead to the development of other disorders. For example, if a person with panic disorder happens to have a panic attack while riding in a car or shopping at a grocery store, that place or activity may then become associated with the panic attack, and the person may become extremely fearful of going there again. This can lead to the development of a phobia (any persistent, intense anxiety about and irrational fear of an object, activity, or situation). In some cases the individual may even develop agoraphobia, which is a condition of overwhelming symptoms of anxiety upon leaving home, especially about being trapped in crowded public areas, where a rapid escape might be difficult. As the disorder increasingly impairs the person's ability to function, depression may develop. In addition, substance abuse sometimes develops as patients begin to self-medicate.

Flashpoint

Untreated panic disorder can evolve into phobias and even agoraphobia.

Phobic Disorder

ICD-9-CM: 300.20   [ICD-10: F40.0–F40.9 (code by type)]

A *phobia* is any persistent, intense anxiety about and irrational fear of an object, activity, or situation. The experience is so uncomfortable that affected people may go to great lengths to avoid the object or situation, even though they are often aware that their reaction is irrational. Phobic disorder is a condition in which the phobia has become a chronic and significant influence in the individual's life. There are three types of phobias: social anxiety disorder, agoraphobia, and specific phobias.

Social anxiety disorder, formerly called *social phobia,* is a persistent irrational fear of, and the need to avoid, social-performance situations in which the individual might be exposed to potentially embarrassing or humiliating scrutiny by others. Even the anticipation of a phobia-producing situation, such as speaking or eating in public, socializing, or using a public toilet, may cause anxiety or terror. Needless to say, this type of phobia can significantly interfere with many social and professional aspects of life.

Agoraphobia is a condition of overwhelming symptoms of anxiety upon leaving home, especially about being trapped in crowded public areas, where a rapid escape might be difficult. More than 75% of patients with agoraphobia also have panic disorder.

Specific phobias involve intense fear and anxiety related to a specific object or situation. There are numerous types. Some include fear of animals, such as spiders, snakes, mice, or dogs; others involve environmental situations, such as heights or storms. Some people fear specific situations, such as enclosed spaces (elevators, closets, public transportation, etc.). Some involve bodily issues, such as fear of injury, injections, or blood. For some people specific phobias are a minor inconvenience, while for others they can pose a significant hardship.

Incidence

Specific phobias affect an estimated 12 to 17 million Americans, women two to three times more often than men. Onset is usually early in life, during childhood or teenage years; the disorder may improve or even completely resolve during the adult years. Specific phobias are the most common type of phobia, but they often have less impact on the patient's life than other types do.

Flashpoint

Specific phobias of things like heights, snakes, or enclosed spaces are very common.

Agoraphobia affects an estimated 6 to 7 million Americans, women twice as often as men. It usually develops during the late teens or 20s.

Social anxiety disorder affects approximately 13 million Americans, women slightly more often than men—although men are more likely to develop avoidant personality disorder, which is the most severe form of social anxiety. This type of phobia has an early onset, usually during childhood or the teenage years.

Etiology

Numerous theories have been offered to explain phobias. While perhaps none fully explain them, they all offer useful information and insight into human behavior. Some theories suggest that phobias are symptoms of the patient's deep inner conflicts. Genetic influences have also been suggested as having some bearing on phobias, based upon the results of some studies of families and twins. The most popular theories suggest that phobias develop as a result of conditioned responses learned through the patient's past experiences. This is often the case with many specific phobias. For example, consider the small child who is bitten or knocked down by a large dog while playing at the park one day. When this occurs, the child is frightened and has a physical reaction that triggers the fight-or-flight response. The child's body doses itself with epinephrine, the heart begins to race, the blood pressure increases, the palms become sweaty, and the child feels shaky. The next time the child sees a large dog, even if it poses no physical threat, the same physiological responses may well occur. The child's body is sending a message of danger. Feeling these physical symptoms reinforces the child's fear of large dogs, and a phobia is born.

Social anxiety disorder may have a similar origin, although many people with social phobias are shy and timid by nature. This greatly increases the likelihood that they will feel fearful of performing in social situations. Their fear and anxiety then increase the odds that they too will experience many of the physical symptoms associated with the fight-or-flight response. Consequently, they may become flustered and perform poorly, leading to feelings of embarrassment and humiliation. These feelings then further reinforce their fear and anxiety related to any future public situations.

Agoraphobia often develops after patients suffer panic attacks in public areas. Their fear of suffering another panic attack in a crowded, public area leads them to avoid such situations. For others, the agoraphobia may begin more gradually, because of the person's general feelings of discomfort in crowded public areas. These individuals slowly change their behaviors and activities to avoid such settings. Panic attacks may or may not occur as a part of their disorder.

Signs and Symptoms

The key feature of phobias is the behavior of patients to avoid the feared object or situation. For some people this is barely noticeable, but other individuals may go to great lengths to rearrange their life and activities. In the most extreme cases, individuals with severe agoraphobia may become completely housebound for many years. A person with phobic disorder who is confronted with the feared object or situation will very likely experience a panic attack.

Diagnosis

Patients with suspected phobic disorder should first undergo physical examination to rule out physiological reasons for their symptoms. In this regard a variety of tests may be done, depending upon the patient's complaints. These may include thyroid function, electrolytes, kidney function, and a variety of cardiac tests. Once physiological conditions have been ruled out, a thorough mental health evaluation is done. Unless the patient has a coexisting psychiatric disorder, the findings will be completely normal except with regard to the fears of and response to the object or situation that triggers the phobic response. In most cases the patient is able to acknowledge the irrational nature of the fear and anxiety, yet still feels them intensely.

> **Flashpoint**
>
> Agoraphobia can cause people to become completely housebound.

Treatment

Treatment for patients with phobic disorder varies somewhat depending upon the individual patient's disorder and personal health factors. In general, treatment falls into three categories. Psychotherapy may help patients learn to recognize and modify their thinking and behavior. Medications such as antidepressants (usually SSRIs) and anxiolytics help alleviate anxiety and reduce the symptoms of panic response. Beta blockers may be useful in reducing some of the symptoms associated with anxiety, but they do not treat the anxiety itself. **Exposure therapy** is considered the most effective form of therapy. It involves exposing the patient repeatedly to the situation or object that triggers anxiety. It is most effective when combined with relaxation and deep-breathing techniques. Over time, the patient becomes desensitized to the object or situation that triggers the phobic response. Other general recommendations may include reducing or eliminating stimulants, such as caffeinated beverages, from the diet.

Prognosis

The prognosis for patients with phobic disorder depends upon the type and severity of the disorder, as well as the patient's coping strategies, motivation for treatment and recovery, support system, and degree of compliance with treatment recommendations. Without treatment, phobias will continue to affect the individual to varying degrees. The person may develop self-imposed restrictions on activity and consequently on relationships. With treatment, most patients' symptoms improve significantly, as does the quality of their lives.

> **Flashpoint**
>
> Exposure therapy is the most effective form of treatment for phobias.

Obsessive-Compulsive Disorder
ICD-9-CM: 300.3   [ICD-10: F42.0–F42.9 (code by type)]

Obsessive-compulsive disorder (OCD) is a condition marked by obsessive thoughts and compulsive behaviors. Obsessions are persistent, recurring, and distressing thoughts, images, feelings, or impulses that are unwanted and intrusive. The person is usually aware that the thoughts are not logical but feels as if they are beyond control. Compulsions are behaviors performed repeatedly, in a ritualistic manner, in order to relieve the fear or anxiety caused by obsessive thoughts.

Incidence

Approximately 7.5 million Americans suffer from OCD at some point in their lives. It occurs in individuals of all ages, although it generally develops before age 40, often during childhood. It affects men and women equally, and people of all races. Nearly half of those with Tourette syndrome also have OCD.

Etiology

The cause of OCD is not completely understood. Genetics is thought to play a role, since the disorder runs in families. There is some indication that areas of the brain that control judgment and planning are involved. Furthermore, inadequate levels of serotonin, a neurotransmitter, seem to be a factor, since medications that increase the concentration of serotonin improve symptoms. In some cases, streptococcal infection has been linked with the onset of OCD in children. Individuals who are already predisposed toward developing OCD may have the disorder triggered or worsened by environmental conditions, such as abuse, illness, the death of a loved one, or relationship problems.

Signs and Symptoms

People with OCD typically manifest a variety of obsessive thoughts and compulsive behaviors. Examples of common obsessions include fear of contamination with germs or dirt; fear of making mistakes; imagining having harmed others or the self; fear of losing control; intrusive sexual urges or thoughts; thoughts that are deemed to be sinful, evil, or forbidden; and fear of behaving in a socially unacceptable manner. Anxiety produced by these thoughts leads to compulsions, which are ritualistic behaviors. Examples of common compulsions include repeating specific words, phrases, or prayers; repeatedly checking locks and doors; touching specific items; and refusing to touch certain items, like doorknobs, or to shake hands. Others include counting, cleaning, bathing, hand washing, creating order and symmetry in one's surroundings, eating foods in a specific order, performing a task a specific number of times, and hoarding items with no apparent value. Performing these rituals temporarily resolves the person's anxiety, but it then builds again and the pattern continues.

Diagnosis

Diagnosis of OCD is based upon observation or upon a description of the individual's obsessive thoughts and compulsive behaviors, including the approximate amount of time spent on them each day. A diagnosis is established if distress is present, the acts are time consuming, or the illness significantly interferes with the individual's normal routine, occupation, or social activities. Many individuals go undiagnosed because they are too embarrassed to seek help or lack insight into the problem. Others lack access to health-care resources.

Treatment

Treatment of patients with OCD is based upon a combination of medications and cognitive behavioral therapy. Medication usually includes antidepressants or SSRIs. Cognitive behavioral therapy assists patients in confronting their fears and managing anxiety without the performance of ritual behaviors.

Prognosis

The prognosis for individuals with OCD is generally good but depends upon the timeliness of diagnosis and treatment. While the disorder is rarely curable, most people can experience a significant reduction in symptoms and can lead normal or near-normal, satisfying lives.

Post-Traumatic Stress Disorder
ICD-9-CM: 308.3 (brief, acute), 309.81 (prolonged)   [ICD-10: F43.1]

Post-traumatic stress disorder (PTSD) is a condition that develops after exposure to an event in which the individual felt terrified or significantly threatened. It has been known by many names in the past, especially in relation to military combat. American Civil War veterans suffered from *soldier's heart*, World War II veterans experienced *gross stress reaction*, and Vietnam War veterans suffered from *post-Vietnam syndrome*, *battle fatigue*, and *shell shock*.

Incidence

PTSD affects approximately five million Americans at some point in their lives. The incidence is as high as 30% among war veterans and victims of sexual assault.

Etiology

PTSD can be caused by any event that the individual perceives as life-threatening. Examples include being a victim of physical or sexual assault, abuse, or kidnapping; witnessing a murder; being exposed to or witnessing a natural or man-made disaster; and being involved in military combat. Risk factors for developing PTSD include mental health or emotional disorders, increased duration of exposure to the event, lack of social or emotional support, and membership of a vulnerable group (the frail elderly, children, women, the disabled, etc.).

When the individual feels threatened, the body's fight-or-flight response is triggered. This normally self-protective mechanism causes changes within the body that ordinarily enable the person to flee from danger or fight to survive. As this occurs, stress hormones are released in the body, which causes changes such as increased heart rate and increased blood pressure. Some people recognize this as an "adrenaline rush." PTSD episodes are a faulty resurfacing of the fight-or-flight response and the emotional feelings associated with the original trauma at later, unexpected times. This occurs when subsequent events remind the person, consciously or unconsciously, of the original event.

> **Flashpoint**
> The incidence of PTSD rises during times of military conflict.

Signs and Symptoms

Patients with PTSD suffer from persistent memories and thoughts of the event, yet they may feel a sense of emotional numbness and lose interest in activities they once enjoyed. Signs and symptoms of PTSD generally fall into three categories:

- **resurfacing**, in the form of distressing memories, nightmares, persistent thoughts, and flashbacks in which the person relives the trauma, including physical and emotional responses to it; triggers can be sights, sounds, or smells
- **avoidance**, which is blocking some or all memories associated with the event, avoiding events or places that act as reminders of the experience, becoming emotionally numb and losing interest in activities, and experiencing strong feelings of guilt or depression
- **hypervigilance**, as evidenced by feeling chronically tense and angry, startling easily, having insomnia, struggling to focus or concentrate, and experiencing emotional, angry outbursts

Individuals who develop chronic PTSD experience a more severe and ongoing form of the disorder. They may become more detached, experience persistent feelings of guilt or despair, and have suicidal thoughts.

Diagnosis

Diagnosis of PTSD can be challenging, because patients often lack insight into the cause of their symptoms and may complain instead of physical bodily symptoms or manifest symptoms of depression, substance abuse disorder, or other disorders. Diagnosis of PTSD is based upon evidence that the patient has a minimum of one symptom of resurfacing, three symptoms of avoidance, and two symptoms of hypervigilance for 1 month or longer and that these symptoms are causing significant distress or impairment in the ability to function.

The acute phase occurs within 3 months of the initial trauma. Chronic PTSD may be diagnosed if symptoms continue for 3 months or more. Delayed PTSD may be diagnosed if symptoms develop 6 months or later after the initial trauma. Evaluation and diagnosis must be done by a qualified mental health professional familiar with PTSD. Appropriate structured-interview tools, such as the PTSD scale, should be administered by the clinician. Physical and psychiatric evaluation should also be done to rule out other disorders.

> **Flashpoint**
> People often do not realize that their symptoms are related to PTSD.

Treatment

Treatment for patients with PTSD is somewhat variable, since patients have varying symptoms and needs. A combination of medication and psychotherapy is usually most effective. In psychotherapy, patients are educated about the disorder to help them gain insight and to dispel feelings of guilt or shame. They are encouraged to discuss their feelings and are given practical strategies for reducing symptoms, managing anger and anxiety, and improving communication. Therapies aimed at resolving sleep problems have a twofold effect. First, they help to alleviate some of the distressing PTSD symptoms; second, they aid the patient in getting refreshing sleep and being rested enough to cope with daily stressors. Both results can significantly reduce anxiety and increase the patient's ability to cope. Family therapy can help significant others and children of the patient. Antidepressants and select antihypertensive medications have been found most useful in reducing feelings of anxiety, depression, panic, impulsivity, aggression, and suicidal ideation. Other medications may be helpful for some patients, depending upon their symptoms. These include mood stabilizers and antipsychotics.

Prognosis

The prognosis for patients with PTSD is generally good if they receive timely, professional diagnosis and treatment. However, the severity and manifestations of the disorder vary, as do individual patient responses to treatment. Left untreated, the disorder can have a devastating impact on the individual and on family members.

Conversion Disorder

ICD-9-CM: 300.11   [ICD-10: F44.0–F44.9 (code by type)]

Conversion disorder, once called *hysteria* or *hysterical neurosis*, is a condition in which patients manifest psychological stress in the form of physical neurological symptoms.

Incidence

Conversion disorder can affect individuals of all ages but is most common among older children, teens, and young adults. Women are affected more often than are men.

Etiology

Symptoms of conversion disorder usually develop after the person experiences some type of emotional trauma. The cause is not fully understood, but there is some speculation that a part of the brain that controls neuromuscular and sensory functions may be involved. Risk factors include other coexisting physical or mental disorders, a history of physical or sexual abuse, economic struggles, and a family member who has had conversion disorder. Although diagnostic tests reveal no cause for the symptoms, it is important that health-care providers understand that the symptoms are very real and not within the patient's conscious control.

Flashpoint

Conversion disorder causes physical neurological symptoms that are very real to the patient.

Signs and Symptoms

Signs and symptoms of conversion disorder include paralysis, blindness, numbness, impaired balance or coordination, seizures, hallucinations, urinary retention, and loss of the ability to speak, hear, or swallow. Symptoms begin suddenly, shortly after the person experiences some type of emotional trauma. The patient may also seem to lack the degree of concern over their physical symptoms that would normally be expected.

Diagnosis

The diagnosis of conversion disorder can be reached only after physical causes have been ruled out. Therefore, a variety of neurological diagnostic tests may be done, depending upon the patient's presenting signs and symptoms. Diagnosis requires at least one symptom beyond the patient's control that involves sensory or neuromuscular function. Furthermore, the symptoms must not be related to pain or sexual dysfunction, must arise after a stressful event, must not be explicable by another medical or psychiatric condition or any medication, and must cause the patient significant impairment or distress.

Treatment

The main therapy for patients with conversion disorder is psychotherapy. The patient is also taught stress-management strategies to help resolve the current condition and prevent a recurrence. Hypnosis may be used in this regard. Physical therapy is provided as needed, depending upon the body part and specific symptoms involved. Anxiety and depressive disorders are treated, as appropriate.

Prognosis

The prognosis for patients with conversion disorder is generally very good. Some cases resolve without any intervention. Episodes usually last less than 2 weeks. However, as many as 25% of patients experience recurrences or even develop chronic conditions. Therefore, professional intervention is recommended.

Hypochondriasis

ICD-9-CM: 300.7 [ICD-10: F45.2]

Hypochondriasis, sometimes called *health phobia*, is a condition in which people feel an abnormal degree of concern about their health, with a false belief that they are suffering from some disease despite medical reassurances to the contrary. Furthermore, they often interpret minor physical problems as symptoms of serious illness. In spite of sometimes acknowledging that their fears are exaggerated or baseless, they continue to feel anxious about their health.

Incidence

Hypochondriasis of varying degrees is thought to affect between nine and 20 million Americans. However, many cases are likely not full-blown hypochondriasis but may instead involve some degree of preoccupation with illness. The disorder affects individuals of all ages but often begins during the early adult years. It affects men and women equally.

Etiology

The exact cause of hypochondriasis is not fully understood. Risk factors include history of physical or sexual abuse, a parent or other significant figure who is excessively concerned about illness, an immediate relative with OCD, and history of serious illness as a child. People with the tendency toward hypochondriasis may also be influenced by the Internet, television, and movies, where certain illnesses are commonly portrayed or discussed, often inaccurately. Other influences may be major outbreaks or predictions of outbreaks, as well as the illness or death of friends or relatives; patients with hypochondriasis may begin to believe they are experiencing symptoms of the same diseases. Some of the very real symptoms that hypochondriacs experience are thought to be caused by a decreased level of serotonin or an elevated level of norepinephrine. It is also theorized that hypochondriacs are more tuned in to the physical sensations within their bodies. Whereas other people generally ignore or shrug off unexplained sensations, hypochondriacs are more likely to interpret them as signifying illness or disease.

Signs and Symptoms

The key symptom of hypochondriasis is obsession with and exaggerated fears about illness. This may manifest as frequently describing symptoms verbally, frequently researching feared diseases, and visiting one physician after another with various complaints. When the patient's fears about one potential disorder resolve, renewed fears arise about a different one. Complaints are frequently of a minor and common nature, such as a mild cough, general aches and pains, and fatigue, or about normal physical variations, such as mild light-headedness upon standing. Patients may also demonstrate signs and symptoms associated with depression or an anxiety disorder. This can amplify the situation, since these disorders present their own array of symptoms that may then be interpreted by patients as an indication of their feared illness.

> **Flashpoint**
>
> People with hypochondriasis seem to be suggestible and may become convinced they are having symptoms of a disorder they learn about on TV.

Diagnosis

It may take some time for patients to be diagnosed with hypochondriasis. Legitimate physical explanations for their signs and symptoms must first be investigated and ruled out. The diagnosis likely first occurs to physicians when patterns of patient behavior become apparent and examinations fail to find actual illnesses. At this point, screening tests may be administered to identify hypochondriasis, anxiety, or depression. Depending upon the results and the patient's willingness, a referral may be made to a psychotherapist. The criteria for diagnosis are:

- behavior pattern lasting 6 months or more
- patient's concerns not related solely to physical appearance
- absence of delusional beliefs

- physical causes all ruled out
- preoccupation with illness and disease
- patient's obsession with illness not completely explicable by another mental health disorder
- a significant degree of distress and interference in the patient's life

Treatment

Treatment for hypochondriasis includes a combination of therapies. Psychotherapy, if patients are willing to participate, helps them to modify their thinking and behavior and to cope more effectively with stress. Medication is used as needed to treat mood or anxiety disorders. SSRI medications are especially useful in helping hypochondriacs decrease the severity of obsession and worry.

Flashpoint

SSRIs may help decrease obsession and worry.

Prognosis

Untreated, hypochondriasis is usually a chronic disorder; only a small percentage of patients fully recover. Complications include patients' undergoing unnecessary tests and treatments when they don't have a real illness and their not being taken seriously when they do. The behavior of obsessing over suspected physical ailments also grows tiresome to others and can have a detrimental effect on personal and professional relationships. Taking frequent sick days becomes a detriment to employment and a hardship on the patient's employer and coworkers.

Munchausen Syndrome and Munchausen Syndrome by Proxy

ICD-9-CM: 301.51   [ICD-10: F68.1]

Munchausen syndrome is a bizarre, severe mental health disorder in which the patient feigns illness, or may even create self-induced illness or injury, out of an abnormal need to be injured or ill. Munchausen syndrome by proxy is a disorder in which a parent, usually the biological mother, repeatedly brings a child to the health-care provider, describing a variety of signs and symptoms that are either untrue or intentionally induced. The parent generally acts extremely attentive and protective of the child, yet the child's symptoms usually mysteriously disappear when the parent is absent and return when the parent is present. This disorder is actually a dangerous form of child abuse, with a mortality rate as high as 50%.

Flashpoint

Munchausen syndrome by proxy is a dangerous form of child abuse, with a 50% mortality rate.

Incidence

The exact incidence of Munchausen syndrome is unknown, although it is thought to be uncommon both globally and in the United States. Most patients are male, although females may also have the disorder, and exhibit a strong pattern of forming a personal attachment with a particular physician or physician group. It can occur in individuals of all ages but is most common among young or middle-aged adults.

Etiology

Munchausen syndrome is a puzzling disorder without a clearly identifiable cause. Efforts to gather statistical data and to gain an understanding of the disorder have been complicated by the fact that patients excel in concealing the true cause or nature of their symptoms, sometimes conceal their true identities, and are extremely resistant to psychiatric evaluation. Patients seem not to be motivated by secondary gain, as with many other disorders, but rather seek the illness, hospitalization, and invasive procedures as a primary goal. The disorder also differs from hypochondria in that hypochondriacs truly believe they are ill whereas patients with Munchausen syndrome *desire* to be. Risk factors for the disorder that have been identified thus far include childhood abuse or neglect, history of frequent illness, a relative with a serious illness, loss of a loved one, low self-esteem, working in health care, and personality disorders.

Signs and Symptoms

The typical patient with Munchausen syndrome travels from one health-care provider or hospital to another with a variable list of symptoms or injuries. In some cases the complaints are fabricated; in other instances the illness or injury is real but has been self-induced. Patients are eager for, and sometimes insist upon, risky and unnecessary tests and procedures. When test results are negative, patients may suddenly develop new or additional symptoms. They often describe dramatic but vague medical problems that develop or worsen for no identifiable reason; make frequent requests for medications, including pain relievers; have a history of multiple hospital admissions; are hesitant to let health-care providers talk with family members or friends; and display an extensive command of medical terminology and diseases. They embellish or even totally fabricate a history of illnesses.

Patients with Munchausen syndrome create self-inflicted illness in a variety of creative ways, such as injecting themselves with toxic or contaminated substances (including feces) and taking unnecessary medications, such as anticoagulants to cause bleeding or diabetic medications to alter blood glucose levels. They frequently relapse after improvement by intentionally doing things that hinder their own recovery. Examples include reopening healing wounds and contaminating wounds with bacteria-laden substances. Furthermore, they may manipulate the results of laboratory tests by tampering with medical instruments or contaminating laboratory specimens— for example, heating a thermometer to falsely indicate a fever or placing blood or feces into a urine specimen. Their symptoms may change dramatically and without reasonable explanation once treatment has started. There is sometimes evidence that the patient has lied about a variety of information.

Diagnosis

Diagnosis of Munchausen syndrome is extremely challenging because of the elaborate efforts by the patient to be deceptive. Actual physical disorders must be ruled out or treated as appropriate. When the disorder is suspected, a psychiatric evaluation is necessary. However, patients are generally very resistant to this and may respond angrily by "firing" their physician and leaving to seek out another physician at another facility, to repeat the pattern there. Whenever possible, a psychiatrist performs an evaluation. To make the diagnosis, certain criteria must be met, including evidence that the patient is either faking or self-inducing the disorder and that the patient is motivated to be viewed as ill but is not motivated by financial or legal gain.

Treatment

While patients with Munchausen syndrome are eager to undergo treatment for physical ailments, they are extremely resistant to admit to or accept treatment for their psychiatric disorder. A gentle approach that helps the patient avoid embarrassment is most effective. Psychotherapy is aimed at behavior modification to reduce the use or misuse of medical care. When possible, family members are included in therapy aimed at eliminating any rewarding of the illness behaviors. Medication may be useful in treating related disorders, such as anxiety or depression. However, this must be carefully monitored, since the patient may misuse prescribed medications. In some cases hospitalization in a psychiatric facility may be necessary.

Prognosis

The prognosis for patients with Munchausen syndrome is poor because of an incomplete understanding of the disorder, their own resistance to treatment, and a lack of highly effective treatment methods. The disorder is usually chronic. Patients who go untreated or respond poorly to treatment interventions may create real illness or injury in their ongoing efforts to seek attention. Consequently, they may indeed suffer from a variety of very real, potentially life-threatening complications of their self-induced conditions or of the associated procedures and treatments. Individuals with this disorder also frequently have substance abuse disorders, financial problems, and significant problems in their personal relationships and professional lives.

> **Flashpoint**
>
> Patients with Munchausen syndrome are very eager to undergo medical treatment, yet are very resistant to psychiatric treatment.

Sleep Disorders

Disrupted sleep is a common problem suffered by most people at one time or another. Fortunately, for most people it is of limited incidence and duration and usually resolves on its own. However, a large number of people suffer from chronic sleep disruptions, which then have a significant impact on their quality of life. Common sleep disorders include insomnia, narcolepsy, and sleep apnea.

Insomnia

ICD-9-CM: 780.52   [ICD-10: G47.0]

Insomnia is a condition marked by insufficient quantity or quality of sleep. Primary insomnia refers to sleep problems unrelated to any other health conditions. Secondary insomnia is defined as sleep problems caused by another health condition, such as arthritis or cancer. Acute insomnia is short-term, lasting from 1 night to several weeks. Chronic insomnia is defined as insomnia that occurs three or more times per week, for a month or longer.

Flashpoint

Mild, temporary insomnia is common and usually requires no treatment.

Incidence

It is estimated that over one-third of adults experience insomnia at some point in their lives and up to 15% struggle with chronic insomnia. Insomnia is twice as common in women as in men.

Etiology

The cause of primary insomnia is not clear. Causes of secondary acute insomnia are numerous and include alcohol or substance use, travel across time zones, acute stress, acute illness, environmental stimuli (light, noise, etc.), some medications, caffeine, nicotine, and work at night or on a rotating shift. There are many causes of chronic insomnia; some are chronic anxiety or stress, chronic health issues, sleep apnea, depression, and chronic pain. Risk factors for insomnia include advanced age and female gender.

Signs and Symptoms

People troubled by insomnia often report difficulty falling or staying asleep, feeling unrefreshed in the morning, daytime fatigue, difficulty concentrating, irritability, depression, tension headaches, and an increased rate of accidents or errors on the job.

Flashpoint

Sleep studies are extremely helpful in diagnosing the specific cause of insomnia and identifying the most effective treatment plan.

Diagnosis

Diagnosis of insomnia is based upon a physical examination, medical history, and sleep history. The patient may be asked to complete a questionnaire and keep a sleep diary. Some patients are referred to a sleep center for a sleep study (see Box 18-9). Blood tests are generally not needed, although thyroid levels might be checked in select cases.

Box 18-9 Diagnostic Spotlight

SLEEP STUDY

Sleep studies include a variety of tests performed while the patient spends the night in a sleep laboratory located in a hospital or in a sleep clinic. During the tests a variety of body activities are measured, including respiration, heart rate, body movements, brain waves, and eye movements. Analysis of the results identifies whether the patient is experiencing normal, uninterrupted sleep cycles. The patient reports to the laboratory in the evening. After the patient has had time to prepare for bed and get comfortable, technicians place sensors on the patient's head, face, chest, and legs, and a clip-type sensor on a finger. These are not painful; they are connected to a computer for data collection with wires long enough to allow the patient to move about freely during sleep. Although most patients do not sleep as well as they normally do at home, this does not affect the quality of information obtained. Sleep studies help diagnose a variety of sleep disorders, including insomnia, narcolepsy, parasomnias, sleep apnea, and sleep-related seizure disorders.

A *polysomnogram* records brain activity, eye movement, heart rate and rhythm, general body movement, and muscle tension. Indicators of effective breathing are also measured. These include air flow through the mouth and nose, snoring, episodes of breathing cessation, chest and abdominal movement, and levels of oxygen and carbon dioxide in the blood.

A *multiple wake test* measures whether the person is able to remain awake during normal waking times.

A *multiple sleep latency test* measures how long it takes the patient to fall asleep.

Box 18-9 Diagnostic Spotlight—cont'd

Actigraphy measures movement during sleeping and awake times. It helps to assess times during the day that the patient unintentionally falls asleep.

Sleep study

Treatment

Acute insomnia often requires no treatment, since it is short lived. Mild cases of insomnia, whether acute or chronic, will generally respond to the adoption of good sleep habits (see Box 18-10). More severe cases of chronic insomnia may need more intensive treatment. A good health evaluation will help to identify whether any health problems are interfering with sleep. A therapist can help patients develop behaviors that promote sleep, such as biofeedback, progressive relaxation, meditation, and breathing exercises. These techniques can relieve or reduce anxiety and muscle tension, calm the mind, and create a more restful state. Other techniques include using the bed and bedroom only for sleep and sex, creating mild sleep deprivation by restricting and then slowly increasing the number of sleep hours allowed, and light therapy.

Some people find over-the-counter sleep aids helpful. However, caution must be used: Many of these medications contain antihistamines that may be contraindicated for people with some conditions and may interact with some other medications. Prescription sleep medications are most effective and safest when used only for a few days, or at most a few weeks. They may be appropriate for insomnia related to temporary situations in a person's life. However, prolonged use creates a high risk of dependency, and the medication tends to become less effective over time. Another complication is rebound insomnia, which occurs when the medication is discontinued. Depending upon the length of time the person has taken the medication, rebound insomnia may be severe. Melatonin may help some people improve sleep when jet lag or shift work interferes with normal sleep cycles. Patients who struggle with depression and insomnia may find that both problems improve with the use of certain antidepressant medications.

Prognosis

The prognosis for most people with insomnia is very good if appropriate measures are taken. However, sleep deprivation can leave people feeling irritable, fatigued, depressed, and unable to focus. This can have a negative impact on relationships as well as performance in school or at work. Sleep deprivation also contributes to illness and obesity and increases the risk of accidents.

Box 18-10 Wellness Promotion

GETTING A GOOD NIGHT'S SLEEP
A good night's sleep provides rest for the body and mind and restores energy. Strategies that improve quantity and quality of sleep include:

- going to bed and getting up at the same times each day (the human body likes a regular schedule)
- avoiding stimulants such as caffeine or tobacco in the evening
- eating a light, low-fat snack in the evening if hungry but avoiding large, high-fat meals
- exercising during the day, not before bedtime
- using meditation or relaxation exercises to relax the body and mind
- creating a calm, quiet, dark, soothing environment in which to sleep
- creating a bedtime routine or ritual, such as reading, taking a warm bath, or stretching
- avoiding performing activities in the bedroom that are not related to sleep (working, watching TV, eating, etc.)
- not napping during the day
- masking environmental noise by wearing earplugs or creating white noise with a fan or sound machine
- getting out of bed for a while if you are awake for more than 30 minutes
- getting up, writing yourself a note, and putting it where you are sure to see it in the morning (if you are worried about forgetting to do something)
- making a prioritized list of items that you must complete the next day, items that can be delegated, and items that can be postponed
- giving yourself permission to simply rest rather than sleep; as you focus on simply relaxing and resting your body and mind, there is a very good chance that you will "accidentally" fall asleep without even realizing it

Narcolepsy
ICD-9-CM: 347.00 (fourth and fifth digits code for involvement of cataplexy and other conditions)   **[ICD-10: G47.4]**

Narcolepsy is a chronic disorder, related to unregulated sleep-wake cycles, marked by recurrent, uncontrollable episodes of falling asleep without warning during the daytime.

Incidence

Narcolepsy is estimated to affect approximately 150,000 Americans, although it is considered an underdiagnosed condition, so the rate may actually be higher. Symptoms usually develop between ages 10 and 30, although they can occur at any time. The condition is more common in men than in women and affects members of all ethnic and racial groups.

Etiology

Most adults sleep 7 to 8 hours at night and experience four to six sleep cycles in a given night. A sleep cycle normally lasts around 100 minutes and is made up of a phase called non–rapid eye movement sleep followed by rapid eye movement (REM) sleep, when dreaming usually occurs. Patients with narcolepsy experience too little non–rapid eye movement sleep at night and consequently fall directly into REM sleep at unpredictable times during the day. When this occurs, they may experience vivid dreams.

The cause of narcolepsy is not fully understood, but it is probably due to multiple factors. In a small percentage of cases, genetics is thought to play a role, since the disorder sometimes clusters in families. Specific human leukocyte antigens have been identified in most of these individuals. It has also been noted that patients with this disorder have lower levels of orexins, also called hypocretin, in their brains; these are substances that affect sleep-wake cycles and consciousness level. This diminished supply may be due to factors such as infection, hormones, stress, trauma,

Flashpoint

Narcolepsy causes uncontrollable episodes of falling asleep during the daytime.

or immune system problems. Levels of hypocretin are especially low in those who experience *cataplexy,* a sudden, brief loss of muscle control triggered by strong emotion, excitement, surprise, or anger, during which the person remains fully conscious. Episodes may last from a few seconds to several minutes, causing problems such as slurring of speech, drooping of the head, and leg weakness. Cataplexy occurs in about 70% of people with narcolepsy. Furthermore, it is thought that the areas of the brain responsible for regulating REM sleep may be different in narcolepsy patients.

Signs and Symptoms

Signs and symptoms of narcolepsy tend to be most severe in individuals who develop the disorder during their childhood years. The most prominent symptom is extreme daytime sleepiness, regardless of the amount of sleep obtained at night. Other symptoms include exhaustion, feelings of mental dullness, difficulty concentrating, faulty memory, and depression. Other symptoms may include cataplexy and, less commonly, sleep paralysis and hallucinations. Sleep paralysis is a temporary inability to speak or move while the person is falling asleep or waking up. This can last a few seconds or several minutes. Episodes of sleep paralysis may be recalled by the individual. Sleep paralysis can also affect individuals who do not have narcolepsy. Hallucinations are delusional episodes that are usually quite vivid and may seem real; consequently, they are sometimes frightening for the patient. Hallucinations may be primarily visual or may involve other senses.

Narcoleptic sleep attacks can occur at any time and can last from a few seconds to half an hour. They can be very disruptive and even dangerous, particularly if they occur when the person is in the midst of important work or operating a vehicle or other machinery.

Nighttime sleep for people with narcolepsy is often restless and disrupted by frequent awakenings. Patients may display episodes of automatic behavior at night while sleeping or during the daytime during a sleep attack. This may involve acting out their dreams by yelling and flailing their arms and legs about. It may also involve talking and continuing to perform routine tasks while sleeping. However, the quality of their task performance is usually impaired and they have no memory of the episode. Consequently, they may forget where they placed things or may suffer accidents or injury. Up to 40% of individuals with narcolepsy experience automatic behavior to varying degrees.

Flashpoint

Sleep attacks can last a few seconds or half an hour.

Diagnosis

Diagnosis of narcolepsy can be challenging, since many of the signs and symptoms may also be indicative of other disorders. Furthermore, most laypeople and even most health-care providers are unfamiliar with the disorder. Consequently, many people are not properly diagnosed for 10 years or more after the initial onset of symptoms. In addition to a thorough medical history, sleep history, and physical examination, the patient may undergo a sleep study and keep a sleep diary. Actigraphy and results of the sleep study identify whether the person is experiencing normal sleep cycles and may help to rule out other disorders. The multiple sleep latency test measures the patient's tendency to fall asleep during the day and helps to identify whether inappropriate episodes of REM sleep occur during the day. In this test, the patient takes several short naps throughout the day.

Treatment

Narcolepsy is a chronic disorder for which there is no cure. However, the most troublesome symptoms can usually be managed with stimulant medication and antidepressants. Certain behavioral changes can also help with symptom control. These include establishing a regular routine of meals and exercise, going to bed and getting up at the same time each day, and avoiding caffeine, nicotine, and alcohol. Some patients also take routinely scheduled naps at the time of day they usually feel sleepiest.

Prognosis

Narcolepsy is a chronic disorder. However, with appropriate diagnosis and treatment, most people can manage their symptoms effectively. Untreated narcolepsy can result in accident or injury. It also can have a detrimental effect on the patient's personal and professional relationships. Narcolepsy may contribute to behavioral disorders, such as ADHD; therefore, it should be considered and, if present, treated first. Medications used to treat narcolepsy can have significant side effects, and physical dependence and tolerance can occur with long-term use. Patients should therefore work closely with their health-care providers in creating the

Flashpoint

There is no cure for narcolepsy, but there are helpful forms of treatment.

medical regimen that is best for them. Furthermore, they should make changes in scheduling or dosing of medication only in consultation with their health-care provider.

Sleep Apnea
ICD-9-CM: 780.57 (unspecified)   [ICD-10: G47.3]

Sleep apnea, sometimes called *sleep-disordered breathing*, is a common condition in which individuals stop breathing, possibly hundreds of times, during sleep. It is classified as obstructive, the most common form; central, a less common form; or complex, a mix of the two. See Chapter 11 for a detailed description of sleep apnea.

Personality Disorders

A personality disorder is a chronic psychiatric condition in which the person demonstrates a rigid and maladaptive pattern of relating to and perceiving the world. The pattern is chronic and affects all areas of social, professional, and personal behavior. It affects the individual's perception, thinking, and manner of communicating and behaving. Patterns generally begin during adolescence or early adulthood and may affect cognition, affect, interpersonal function, or impulse control. Personality disorders have been grouped into clusters A, B, and C.

Flashpoint

There are many types of personality disorders.

Cluster A
ICD-9-CM: 301.0 (paranoid), 301.20 (schizoid), 301.22 (schizotypal)   [ICD-10: F60.0 (paranoid), F60.1 (schizoid), F21 (schizotypal)]

Patients with cluster A personality disorders are generally distrustful, emotionally detached, and isolated, and they may be considered eccentric. The group includes paranoid, schizoid, and schizotypal personality disorders.

The key features of ***paranoid personality disorder*** include unwarranted suspicion and mistrust, suspecting others of hidden, harmful motives; hypersensitivity to criticism; a tendency to hold grudges and be easily offended; reluctance to confide in others; and coldness and distance toward others. These individuals frequently threaten or take legal action against other people yet fail to recognize their own roles in conflicts.

The key features of ***schizoid personality disorder*** include shyness, oversensitivity, withdrawal, reluctance to develop interpersonal or competitive relationships, eccentricity, and daydreaming. These individuals prefer solitary activities, are unable to express anger or joy in situations that normally evoke such feelings, are emotionally and socially distant, and may be viewed by others as cold or aloof.

The key features of ***schizotypal personality disorder*** include odd behavior and thinking similar to that of people with schizophrenia, yet most individuals do not develop schizophrenia. They display social and emotional detachment, magical thinking (believing their thoughts or actions can control people or things), and possible paranoid thoughts.

Cluster B
ICD-9-CM: 301.7 (antisocial), 301.83 (borderline), 301.81 (narcissistic), 301.50 (histrionic)   [ICD-10: F60.2 (antisocial), F60.3 (borderline), F60.8 (narcissistic), F60.4 (histrionic)]

Individuals with cluster B personality disorders share a high sense of entitlement and have a general disregard for, and lack of empathy toward, others. They also display attention-seeking behaviors, are highly excitable and unpredictable, and develop intense and unstable relationships. This group includes antisocial, borderline, narcissistic, and histrionic personality disorders.

The key feature of ***antisocial personality disorder,*** formerly called *sociopathic personality* and *psychopathic personality*, is manipulation of others without any regard for their feelings or for right and wrong. Signs of antisocial personality disorder include a variety of behaviors, some obviously destructive or negative, such as fire-setting, cruelty to animals, theft, aggression toward others, intimidation of others, commission of crimes, abuse of drugs and alcohol, and abuse or neglect of children. Other behaviors are more subtle, but just as destructive, such as lying and manipulating others for selfish gain, usually in a completely charming manner. Because of their complete disregard for others, these individuals may jeopardize the safety of themselves or others yet feel no guilt or remorse for their actions. Instead, they rationalize their behavior or blame others. They are usually unable to anticipate the potentially negative consequences of their actions and tend to be impulsive and irresponsible. They are easily frustrated and prone to irritation and anger. Symptoms tend to worsen and peak when patients are in their 20s and then decrease over time.

The key features of ***borderline personality disorder*** include a "black or white" view and unstable self-image, relationships, and moods. These individuals demonstrate impulsive behaviors that are sometimes manifested as promiscuity and substance abuse. They may also have episodes of psychotic thinking, hallucinations, and paranoia, and they are prone to irritability and angry outbursts. They may feel sad, empty, and fearful. They develop intense and dramatic relationships; their fear of abandonment is usually expressed as intense anger. Self-mutilation and suicidal behavior may occur. Patients with borderline personality disorder are usually female.

Key features of ***narcissistic personality disorder*** include a pattern of superiority and ***grandiosity*** (inflated sense of self-importance) and preoccupation with fantasies of unlimited success, power, brilliance, or beauty; yet these individuals are overly sensitive to failure and criticism. They are easily enraged or depressed, thrive on admiration and attention from others, and often believe that other people envy them. They have a high sense of entitlement and lack empathy toward others, which is demonstrated by their willingness to exploit others for their own gain. Furthermore, they believe their problems are unique and can only be understood by a few special people. People with this personality disorder are often viewed by others as arrogant, self-centered, and offensive, although they may be high achievers.

Key features of ***histrionic personality disorder*** include chronic attention-seeking and emotionalism and a tendency to be overly dramatic and prone to exaggeration. Individuals may also be prone to angry outbursts or tantrums. Their exaggerated emotions and behaviors often appear childish and contrived. They tend to become bored with routine activities and crave novelty and excitement. Their behavior in interpersonal relationships is shallow, vain, demanding, and dependent. Their desire to be protected and cared for may be acted out as sexually provocative behavior. They also display a tendency toward hypochondriacal behavior or exaggeration of physical problems to get attention.

Cluster C

ICD-9-CM: 301.6 (dependent), 301.82 (avoidant), 301.4 (obsessive-compulsive) **[ICD-10: F60.7 (dependent), F60.0 (avoidant), F60.5 (obsessive-compulsive)]**

Those with cluster C personality disorders share a desire to avoid social situations; a tendency to be fearful, anxious, and submissive; and a preoccupation with order, rules, and details. This group includes dependent, avoidant, and obsessive-compulsive personality disorders.

The key feature of ***dependent personality disorder*** is a chronic, excessive psychological dependence on others. These individuals may surrender responsibilities and control to others and may sacrifice their needs to the needs of others. They lack self-confidence and tend to feel insecure.

The key features of ***avoidant personality disorder*** include feelings of inadequacy, social inhibition, and hypersensitivity to criticism. These tendencies become most prominent in relationship situations at school and work. Patients desire affection, security, certainty, and acceptance, and they may fantasize about an idealized relationship, yet they avoid intimate relationships for fear of rejection.

The key features of ***obsessive-compulsive personality disorder*** include rigid conformity to rules and moral codes and an excessive need for order. Individuals with this disorder tend to be methodical perfectionists who lack flexibility and adaptability. They have a strong need for control, yet may struggle with decision-making. They are generally high achievers and are dependable but may struggle with task completion. They have difficulty enjoying their successes because of anxiety. They are usually uncomfortable with feelings and consequently are not comfortable in relationships. This disorder differs from OCD in that it does not include an unwanted pattern of obsessions and compulsions.

Incidence

The general incidence of personality disorders in the United States is estimated at 3 to 4.5 million people. The exact incidence varies with the disorder, as does the ratio of males to females

Flashpoint

People with antisocial disorder manipulate others for selfish gain without guilt or remorse.

Flashpoint

People with histrionic personality disorder are dramatic attention-seekers who tend to be shallow, vain, demanding, and dependent.

affected. In general, more men have antisocial and obsessive-compulsive personality disorders and more women have borderline, dependent, and histrionic disorders.

Etiology

The cause of personality disorders is not well understood, and causes vary somewhat by disorder. In most cases, genetic, biological, and environmental factors are all thought to play a role. Risk factors that increase the likelihood of an individual's developing a personality disorder include history of child abuse, emotional neglect, and one or both parents who are antisocial or involved in abuse of alcohol or other substances.

Diagnosis

Individuals with personality disorders rarely seek help on their own, because they are usually unaware that their thoughts or behaviors are inappropriate. However, they may seek help related to problems in their lives caused by their disorder, or they may be referred to professional help by concerned family or friends. In some cases professional intervention may also be suggested by social services or even ordered by a court in a legal proceeding.

Flashpoint

People with personality disorders rarely seek help, because they believe their behavior is appropriate.

A personality disorder may be suspected when an individual persists in patterns of thinking and behavior despite negative results. For an accurate diagnosis, they must be willing to undergo thorough psychiatric evaluation by a qualified mental health professional, such as a psychologist or psychiatrist. Information is gathered about family history, personal history, behavior patterns, thought processes, and coping mechanisms. A variety of psychological-evaluation tools may be used. Specific criteria for diagnosing individual personality disorders vary and are determined by the DSM-IV-TR.

Treatment

Treatment of personality disorders is tailored to the individual and the diagnosis. Because patients are often in denial that a problem exists, confronting them with the negative results of their behaviors is sometimes helpful. Psychotherapy sometimes helps patients recognize their problematic behaviors and attitudes. Family and group therapy provides opportunities for individuals to modify socially undesirable behaviors. Other therapies may include anger management, reduction of environmental stress, medication, and hospitalization. A team approach is generally used and may involve the physician, psychiatrist, psychotherapist, pharmacist, and family members. However, some patients—such as those with antisocial personality disorder—are resistant to therapy because they rarely believe they need it. Treatment of other coexisting psychiatric disorders is more complicated in people with antisocial personality disorder, and vice versa.

Flashpoint

Individuals with antisocial personality disorder are the most resistant to treatment.

Prognosis

Personality disorders are chronic conditions that are resistant to treatment, some more than others. Left untreated, people with these disorders may develop a worsening of their disorders or worsening of coexisting mental health disorders. Potential complications of personality disorders that are untreated or unresponsive to treatment vary widely; some are deviant sexual behavior, legal problems, relationship problems, substance abuse, professional problems, violence toward others, and suicidal behavior. Some disorders may improve as the individual ages. Patients usually require a minimum of a year of therapy to experience benefit, and many require several years of ongoing therapy.

Attention Deficit Disorder and Attention Deficit-Hyperactivity Disorder

ICD-9-CM: 314.00 (childhood attention deficit disorder), 314.01 (childhood attention deficit-hyperactivity disorder)

[ICD-10: F90.0 (attention deficit disorder), F90.1 (attention deficit-hyperactivity disorder)]

Attention deficit disorder (ADD) and attention deficit-hyperactivity disorder (ADHD) are behavioral disorders. In ADD, a patient displays an inability to focus attention for more than short periods of time and has trouble prioritizing and completing tasks. In ADHD, the patient has trouble focusing and finishing tasks and, in addition, has trouble sitting still for long and prefers to be moving around.

Incidence

ADHD affects as many as 30 million Americans, males 5 to 10 times more often than females.

Etiology

There is growing evidence that ADD and ADHD may be caused, at least in part, by genetic factors. Other contributors may include differences in brain structure and neurotransmitters, medical conditions, learning disabilities, and some mental health conditions.

Signs and Symptoms

Signs and symptoms of both disorders include difficulty getting organized, prioritizing, and staying on task; impulsivity and distractibility; losing things; failure to complete tasks; making careless mistakes; failure to pay attention; and struggles with schoolwork. In addition, the patient with ADHD is fidgety, struggles to stay seated, feels restless, may talk excessively, blurts out comments or answers, interrupts others, and has difficulty waiting in lines or taking turns.

Diagnosis

Diagnosis of ADD or ADHD involves a patient interview by a pediatrician or psychologist. A minimum of six of the characteristic symptomatic behaviors must be noted for each diagnosis, to a degree that is considered abnormal.

Treatment

While there is no known cure, stimulant medication and counseling can help the child focus. Parents can be educated about behavioral approaches that may be more effective with their children. It is also important that parents communicate with the child's teachers, so that the teachers can better understand the child's behavior and address the child's learning needs (see Box 18-11). The physician may recommend restricting food additives if they are found to contribute to the child's hyperactivity.

Prognosis

The prognosis for patients with ADD and ADHD is generally very good, with timely diagnosis and treatment. Most people are able to achieve a reduction in their symptoms with therapy and to lead productive and satisfying lives. Furthermore, symptoms of both disorders often subside or disappear completely with age.

Flashpoint

ADD and ADHD are much more common in males than in females.

Flashpoint

Understanding ADD and ADHD helps parents and teachers help the child.

Flashpoint

Symptoms of ADD and ADHD tend to lessen with age.

Autism

ICD-9-CM: 299.0   [ICD-10: F84.0]

Autism, often called a spectrum disorder, is a complex developmental disability that affects people differently. It affects communication with others and is accompanied by repetitive, characteristic behaviors. Autism spectrum disorder is also known as *pervasive developmental disorder*.

Incidence

Autism affects approximately 1.5 million Americans, males four times more often than females. The annual cost of providing care for patients with autism in the United States is nearly $90 billion.

Etiology

The cause of autism is not fully understood. Current theories suggest that abnormalities in brain structure or function may play a role. Other factors under investigation include genetics, viral infections, environmental toxins (such as mercury), and other medical problems.

Signs and Symptoms

Symptoms of autism are variable and can include any of the following:

- failure to make eye contact
- repetitive behaviors, such as rocking
- delayed language development

Box 18-11 Wellness Promotion

HELPING THE CHILD WITH ADD/ADHD LEARN

Succeeding in school can be a real challenge for children with ADD and ADHD, but it is important that they experience success. Here are some tips for teachers and parents to help children do well in school.

Tips for Teachers

- Don't expect these children to sit still for long periods. Trying to do so will only make their symptoms worse.
- Don't scold or punish these children for mildly inappropriate behavior that is a manifestation of the disorder.
- Provide accommodations for the child as recommended by the psychologist.
- Offer praise and rewards for good behavior.
- Establish a signal that allows you to cue the child that current behavior is inappropriate, in a way that is not demeaning or embarrassing.
- Modify the classroom to minimize distractions for the child, such as seating the child facing away from the door and windows or placing the child in front of your desk.
- Provide instructions one at a time and be prepared to repeat them.
- Provide instructions verbally and in writing.
- Tackle the most difficult or complex material early in the day.
- Use multisensory teaching methods (auditory, visual, tactile, etc.).
- Designate a quiet area for studying or taking tests.
- Break work up into short segments.
- Plan frequent breaks with physical activities.
- Allow the child to expend physical energy in some type of quiet activity when sitting is required (squeezing a small foam ball, etc.).
- Limit the number of timed tests.
- Be flexible and creative in finding alternative ways for the child to test or demonstrate knowledge (oral discussion, dramatic presentations, filling in blanks, drawing diagrams, etc.).
- Allow the student to do work on the computer.
- Be flexible on due dates.
- Show the child techniques for organizing work (binders with dividers, color-coding, etc.).
- Communicate directly with parents frequently (when child is struggling or doing well) by telephone or e-mail.

Tips for Parents

- Educate yourself about your child's disorder.
- Communicate frequently with the teacher and be sure to go to conferences.
- Check with your child every day about homework or notes from the teacher.
- Provide an uncluttered area for your child to do homework.
- Designate a regular homework time but allow frequent breaks.
- Do not expect perfection; reward your child for good behavior.
- Help your child develop organizational skills. Ideas might include a designated place for the child's backpack and a large calendar for the wall that the child can write on.
- Consult with the school psychologist if you are concerned that your child's needs are not being met.

- poor cognitive functioning
- extreme agitation with changes in routine
- preference for solitary play activities
- indifference or lack of attachment to people

Flashpoint
Symptoms of autism vary widely.

Diagnosis

Autism is usually not diagnosed until age 3 or later. Diagnosis of autism is based on behaviors defined in the DSM-IV-TR. To meet the criteria, the patient must exhibit at least two symptoms of impaired social interaction, at least one symptom of impaired communication, and at least one symptom of repetitive behavior.

Treatment

There is no cure for autism and no one single form of treatment that suits all patients. Early intervention by a referral to specialists will initiate a variety of therapies that can increase the child's speech development and interactions with others. Special-education programs, along with behavior and occupational therapies, help children learn self-care and social and job skills. Some children benefit from anticonvulsant, antidepressant, stimulant, or antipsychotic medications, depending upon their symptoms.

Prognosis

The prognosis for patients with autism depends upon the type and severity of the disorder and the timeliness of diagnosis and treatment. Those with high-functioning autism do well with proper support and care and may go on to lead semi-independent lives. Others will require more care and structure on a permanent basis.

Alzheimer Dementia

ICD-9-CM: 331.0   [ICD-10: F00.0–F00.9 (code by onset and type)]

Alzheimer dementia is the most common form of dementia, a neurological disorder characterized by chronic, progressive, irreversible decline in mental function. It is marked by deficits in reasoning and judgment. It progressively impairs a person's ability to participate in occupational and social activities. For more details about Alzheimer dementia, see Chapter 6.

Schizophrenia

ICD-9-CM: 295.90   [ICD-10: F20.0–F20.9 (code by type)]

Schizophrenia is a group of chronic thought disorders that result in varying degrees of impaired function. There are several subtypes of schizophrenia: paranoid, catatonic, disorganized, and residual.

Flashpoint
There are several different types of schizophrenia.

Incidence

Schizophrenia affects approximately three million Americans, men and women equally. It affects members of all ethnic groups. Onset typically occurs in the late teens to early 30s.

Etiology

The cause of schizophrenia is not fully understood. However, genetics is thought to play a role.

Signs and Symptoms

Symptoms of schizophrenia usually impair the individual's ability to function at work, at school, or in relationships. These include hallucinations in which the individual feels, sees, smells, or hears things that are not there, and delusions, which are false beliefs in things that are untrue. An example is the belief that messages are being sent specifically to them through the television ("thought insertion") or that others are able to read their thoughts ("thought broadcasting"). Other symptoms include disorganized speech, movement disorders, difficulty expressing emotion, and deficits in speaking, memory, attention, or organization.

Paranoid schizophrenia is marked by delusions of persecution, grandiosity, jealousy, and hallucinations with persecutory or grandiose content. Those with paranoid schizophrenia believe that others are plotting against them, and they may accuse others of spying on them or trying to poison them.

Catatonic schizophrenia is marked by motor features such as immobility or stupor; excessive, purposeless motor activity; and peculiar voluntary movements, such as posturing (moving body parts in a peculiar manner or holding a specific body position). Other features include extreme negativism or mutism (inability or unwillingness to speak), echolalia (involuntary repetition of words spoken by others), and echopraxia (meaningless imitation of motions made by others).

Disorganized schizophrenia is marked by disorganized thought processes and impairment in the ability to perform common daily activities. Emotions may appear unstable or inappropriate to the situation.

Residual schizophrenia is marked by continuing evidence of flat affect, impoverished or disorganized speech, and eccentric or odd behavior. There may still be evidence of delusions, hallucinations, or disorganized speech, but it has lessened in intensity.

Diagnosis

Diagnosis is based upon personal history, including a description of moods, thoughts, and behaviors. Psychological tests may also be used. The Thematic Apperception Test is used to evaluate aspects of the patient's personality that have been repressed. In this test, patients are shown a series of ambiguous pictures and asked to tell a story about them. The story must include prior events, a description of what is happening in the picture, what the characters (if any) are thinking and feeling, and an ending. The test is evaluated through analysis of the pattern of reactions, attitudes, and needs revealed by the patient. Another test commonly used is the Minnesota Multiphasic Personality Inventory (MMPI—see Box 18-12).

Flashpoint

The MMPI is one of the most commonly used mental evaluation tools.

Treatment

There is no cure for schizophrenia. Antipsychotic medications are used to alleviate many of the symptoms; newer antipsychotics are used first, because they have a lower risk of side effects than the older ones. Many side effects will go away with continued use.

Patients should be informed that it can take several weeks for full therapeutic benefits to be realized. They must also be cautioned to not discontinue medications without checking with their physician, since this can cause a sudden increase in symptoms. After individuals are stabilized on antipsychotic medications, they will benefit from psychosocial therapy, which helps them with communication, self-care, and work and personal relationships. Those in psychosocial therapy also demonstrate greater consistency in compliance with medication regimens and experience fewer relapses.

Flashpoint

Patients should be told that medication may take several weeks for full benefit to be felt.

Prognosis

Schizophrenia is considered a long-term disorder. However, many of those affected can achieve a good quality of life with consistent medication and therapy. Approximately

---

Box 18-12 Diagnostic Spotlight

MMPI

The Minnesota Multiphasic Personality Inventory (MMPI) is one of the most common tools used by mental health professionals to assess patients age 18 or over for mental illness. The current version is composed of 567 true-or-false questions and usually takes patients 1 to 2 hours to complete. Questions are designed to help assess hypochondriasis, depression, hysteria, psychopathy (measures social deviation, resistance to authority, and amorality), masculinity or femininity, paranoia, obsessive-compulsive disorder, schizophrenia, hypomania (measures elevated mood, accelerated speech and motor activity, irritability, etc.), and social introversion (measures social withdrawal). The test is given and analyzed by a psychologist or psychiatrist and used along with other assessment tools to aid in diagnosis. The MMPI also has built-in features that help to detect whether patients falsified responses, marked answers inconsistently, or simply answered questions randomly. These features increase the reliability and validity of testing results.

80% suffer frequent relapses that may require hospitalization, intensive treatment, or crisis management.

Eating Disorders

Eating disorders are serious, potentially life-threatening disorders that have physical and psychological components. The two most common are anorexia nervosa and bulimia nervosa.

Anorexia Nervosa
ICD-9-CM: 307.1   [ICD-10: F50.0]

Anorexia nervosa is a physical and psychiatric disorder. It involves a combination of an intense fear of weight gain and severe self-imposed restriction of food intake.

Incidence
Anorexia nervosa affects 1.5 to 3 million Americans, most commonly highly intelligent high achievers, 90% of them female.

Etiology
The cause of anorexia nervosa is not well understood. Contributors include genetic, neurobiological, nutritional, and psychological factors. Childhood sexual abuse is a common contributor. Social and cultural norms reinforce anorexic behaviors by placing excessive emphasis on being thin.

Signs and Symptoms
Characteristics of anorexia nervosa include self-imposed starvation, a distorted body image (see Fig. 18-4), obsession with food, and the compulsion to be thin. Malnutrition and weight loss may be mild or severe. Menstrual periods may cease as body fat drops below normal. Other physical symptoms associated with poor nutrition may include slowed growth, anemia, hypothermia, thinning hair, dizziness, and dry, pale skin. Psychological and emotional symptoms may include perfectionism, memory difficulties, obsessive or compulsive tendencies, low self-esteem, depression, and moodiness.

Diagnosis
Patients must be evaluated by a clinical psychologist or psychiatrist in addition to their primary care provider. Diagnosis is based upon a variety of criteria, such as history and behaviors. These include eating patterns, distorted body image, refusal to maintain normal weight, intense fear of gaining weight, and weight loss to less than 15% below ideal. Blood and urine tests are done to identify electrolyte and nutritional imbalances. Cardiac tests,

> *Flashpoint*
> Anorexia nervosa includes self-imposed starvation, obsession with food, compulsion to be thin, and a distorted body image.

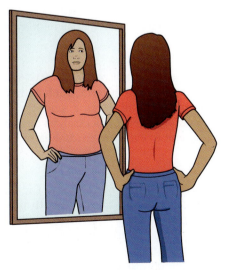

FIGURE 18-4 Distorted body image causes people with anorexia nervosa to see themselves as too fat.

such as an electrocardiogram, may be done to evaluate cardiac rhythm, since severe weight loss can affect heart function.

Treatment

A team approach is vital to effective management of anorexia nervosa. Members of the team may include physicians, nurses, medical assistants, psychiatric and mental health professionals, and nutritionists. Goals are to restore normal body weight and healthy eating behaviors and to aid the patient in regaining a normal body image. Underlying psychological issues must be addressed to prevent recurrence or worsening of symptoms. In severe cases, patients may be hospitalized for replacement of fluids, electrolytes, and nutrition. Vitamin supplements containing zinc have been shown to help with weight gain and improvement of neurological functioning.

Prognosis

Prognosis is variable and depends upon the adequacy and timeliness of treatment interventions as well as the individual's acceptance of psychological therapy. Complications include heart failure, osteoporosis, and loss of muscle mass and strength. Anorexia nervosa has one of the highest reported mortality rates of psychiatric disorders, at 5% to 6%.

Flashpoint

The mortality rate for anorexia nervosa is one of the highest of all psychiatric illness.

Bulimia Nervosa
ICD-9-CM: 307.51   [ICD-10: F50.2]

Bulimia nervosa, often just called *bulimia*, is a psychiatric disorder marked by preoccupation with weight, size, and shape, and feelings of shame and guilt. Classic behavior includes binge eating followed by purging (some means to rid the body of calories).

Incidence

Bulimia most commonly affects women (80% of cases) and affects 1% to 2% of all young women in the United States.

Etiology

The cause of bulimia is not well understood, although it is believed to be complex and to include genetic, neurobiological, nutritional, psychological, social, and environmental factors. Childhood sexual abuse is a common contributor. There are usually issues of depression, conflict, anger, denial, low self-esteem, and perfectionism. Binge-and-purge episodes are often triggered by emotional distress. Social and cultural norms reinforce such behaviors by placing excessive emphasis on being thin.

Signs and Symptoms

The key characteristic of bulimia is an identified pattern of binge eating large quantities of food followed by purging through self-induced vomiting, laxative abuse, diuretic abuse, use of enemas, and periods of fasting or extreme exercise. Esophagitis, sore throat, or sore mouth may develop, and teeth may begin to erode from stomach acids. Eyes may display small broken vessels from the stress of self-induced vomiting. Weight may be normal but fluctuate often. Sores, calluses, or scars may be present on the hands or knuckles, from self-induced vomiting. Irregular heartbeat may develop from electrolyte abnormalities. Other physical signs may include abnormal bowel function, fatigue, and dehydration.

Diagnosis

Patients must be evaluated by a clinical psychologist or psychiatrist in addition to their primary care provider. Diagnosis is based upon a variety of criteria, such as history and behaviors. Diagnostic criteria include a pattern of binging and purging more than twice a week for at least 3 months. Blood tests are done to detect low levels of electrolytes and protein. Cardiac tests, such as an electrocardiogram, may be done to evaluate cardiac rhythm, since abnormal electrolytes can impact heart function.

Treatment

A team approach is vital to effective management. Members of the team may include physicians, nurses, medical assistants, psychiatric and mental health professionals, and nutritionists. Goals are to restore healthy eating behaviors, to control the urge to purge, and to aid the patient in regaining a normal body image. Underlying psychological issues must be addressed to prevent recurrence or worsening of symptoms. Medications may include antidepressants. Nutritional counseling and referral to a support group may also be helpful.

Prognosis

Prognosis is variable and depends upon the adequacy and timeliness of treatment interventions as well as the individual's acceptance of psychological therapy. Complications include heart failure and life-threatening hemorrhage caused by the rupture of esophageal vessels, the esophageal wall, or even the stomach.

> **Flashpoint**
>
> A deadly complication of bulimia is massive hemorrhage caused by damage to the esophagus or stomach.

 STOP HERE.
Select the flashcards for this chapter and run through them at least three times before moving on to the next chapter.

Student Resources

1on1health.com Depression page: http://www.depression.com
Alzheimer's Association: http://www.alz.org
American Association on Intellectual and Developmental Disabilities: http://www.aamr.org
Children and Adults with Attention Deficit/Hyperactivity Disorder: http://www.chadd.org
International OCD Foundation: http://www.ocfoundation.org
Learning Disabilities Association of America: http://www.ldanatl.org
National Association of Anorexia Nervosa and Associated Disorders: http://www.anad.org
National Eating Disorder Information Centre (Canada): http://www.nedic.ca
National Eating Disorders Association: http://www.nationaleatingdisorders.org
National Institute of Mental Health: http://www.nimh.nih.gov
National Stuttering Association: http://www.westutter.org
SleepEducation.com: http://www.sleepeducation.com
Tourette Syndrome Association: http://www.tsa-usa.org

Chapter Activities

Learning Style Study Strategies

Try any or all of the following strategies as you study the content of this chapter:

Visual learners: Being a student is stressful, so try these visualization exercises to help you reduce stress and do your best.

1. The night before and the morning of written exams, class presentations, or performance of clinical skills, spend at least 10 minutes in a meditative exercise with your eyes closed. Breathe slowly in and out and picture yourself going through the steps you will take to take the exam, present the project, or perform the skill. As you do so, picture yourself as calm, focused, confident, efficient, and successful.

2. Regularly perform a long-term variation of the previous exercise. The more you clarify your long-term career goals, the easier this will be. Spend a few minutes each day with your eyes closed in a meditative state. You may wish to play calm, soothing music to help you relax. As you breathe slowly in and out, relax all parts of your body. Once you are relaxed, picture yourself in the role you plan to achieve. You can begin with sessions in which you see yourself receiving your college diploma and then earning your license or other professional credentials. Successive sessions might include visualizing yourself in successful job interviews, during your first day on the new job, and

earning promotions. Ultimately, picture yourself employed, happy, and working productively in the role you desire to achieve.

Kinesthetic learners: Write terms, definitions, or key concepts in the air using your hands and fingers.

Auditory learners: Select music that evokes feelings of peacefulness and well-being and play it when you notice yourself feeling tense and stressed about school. This might be a great way to begin and end a study session.

Verbal learners: Recite key data or definitions that you need to remember in overly dramatic and expressive ways. You may feel silly (and wish to do this alone), but this will enhance your ability to recall the data later.

Practice Exercises

Answers to practice exercises can be found in Appendix D.

Case Studies

CASE STUDY 1

Mr. and Mrs. Villanueva are visiting Valley Clinic with their 8-year-old son, Marco. Based on some comments from Marco's teacher and some of their own observations, they are wondering whether Marco might have ADD. They have some questions for their health-care provider.

1. What is the difference between ADD and ADHD? How would we know which one he might have?

2. It sounds like Marco may have ADHD rather than ADD. Did we do something wrong to cause him to get this?

3. Marco does seem to wiggle and move around a lot, he can't seem to get his room cleaned up like his sister, and he is always losing things. Is this is part of the ADHD? What other symptoms should we look for?

4. Is there anything that we can do to help Marco to do better in school?

CASE STUDY 2

Holly is a certified medical assistant. She has worked in a pediatrician's office 4 days per week for the past 2 years. Because of this, her friends and family sometimes come to her for medical advice. Today, Holly is enjoying a day off and is working in her front yard. Her neighbor, Mrs. Lawson, stops by to chat and begins asking Holly what she knows about people who have problems with stuttering. Mrs. Lawson has noticed that her grandson Josh, age 5, has been stuttering in the past week or two, and she is a bit concerned. How should Holly answer her questions?

1. Is this something that we should be worried about?

2. What causes stuttering?

3. What kind of treatment should Josh get?

Practice Exercises **671**

CASE STUDY 3

Thomas Sinclair is a 28-year-old patient who has been to the medical clinic a number of times since establishing care there just six months ago. He usually complains of multiple vague symptoms and seems eager to undergo medical testing and take medications. In some cases, he has actually insisted upon it. The clinic has been unable to obtain complete medical records for him since he keeps forgetting to provide them with the necessary information to do so. However, according to him, he has been hospitalized "more than a dozen times" in the past few years. He states that he works as a maintenance worker for a local industry yet displays an extensive knowledge of human anatomy and medical vocabulary. When asked, he simply states that "medicine has always interested me, and I like to look things up." Currently, he is being treated for an infected laceration on his arm. Although it seemed to be healing well after the initial injury, he has returned for follow-up care several times, once with the sutures torn out and now with obvious signs of infection. As the medical assistant involved in this patient's care, answer the following questions.

1. Based on your limited information and your observation of Mr. Sinclair's behaviors, you suspect he may have which mental health disorder?

2. Describe why it is usually difficult to confirm a diagnosis of this disorder.

3. How might the physician go about confirming the diagnosis of this disorder?

4. Describe how this disorder is treated.

Multiple Choice

1. All of the following terms are matched with the correct information **except:**

   a. Histrionic personality disorder: attention-seeking, emotionalism, tendency to be overly dramatic and prone to exaggeration and tantrums

   b. Avoidant personality disorder: chronic, excessive psychological dependence on others

   c. Antisocial personality disorder: manipulation, disregard for others and for right and wrong

   d. Schizoid personality disorder: shyness, oversensitivity, withdrawal, eccentricity, daydreaming, and an inability to express normal anger or joy

2. All of the following terms are matched with the correct information **except:**

   a. Grandiosity: inflated sense of self-importance

   b. Cataplexy: sudden, brief loss of muscle control triggered by strong emotion, excitement, surprise, or anger, during which the person remains fully conscious

   c. Compulsions: ritualistic behaviors performed to relieve fear or anxiety caused by obsessive thoughts

   d. Hallucination: false, unfounded belief

3. Which of the following statements is correct?

   a. According to an IQ test, "average" intelligence is 106–130.

   b. The most commonly used reference tool for the diagnosis of mental health disorders is the Physicians' Desk Reference (PDR).

   c. Dysgraphia is a type of learning disorder.

   d. Shouting obscenities is a common sign of Tourette disorder.

4. Which of the following statements is correct?

   a. Compulsions are persistent, recurring, and distressing thoughts, images, feelings, or impulses that are unwanted and intrusive.

   b. Electroconvulsive therapy is an outdated and barbaric form of treatment that is no longer legal.

   c. Delirium is an acute, reversible state of agitated confusion marked by disorientation, hallucinations, or delusions.

   d. Cluster B personality disorders include the dependent, avoidant, and obsessive-compulsive personality disorders.

5. When providing education to a patient taking antidepressant medication, all of the following information is appropriate **except:**

   a. Your mood and energy level should both improve within 7 to 10 days.

   b. Many side effects of medication diminish with time.

   c. You should never suddenly stop taking your medication without talking with your doctor.

   d. About half of all patients have some troublesome side effects. There are many possible solutions, so please communicate closely with your doctor to find the best one.

Short Answer

1. **Describe some techniques the average person can use to develop good sleep habits.**

2. **Describe the key feature of antisocial personality disorder and list common signs.**

3. **Compare anorexia nervosa and bulimia nervosa with regard to the following criteria:**

   - population most commonly affected
   - social norm conformed to
   - amount of food eaten
   - body weight
   - physical signs and symptoms
   - shared deadly complications

19 BIOTERRORISM

Learning Outcomes

Upon completion of this chapter, the student will be able to:

- Define and spell key terms related to bioterrorism
- Identify category A biological pathogens and their characteristics, including:
  - description
  - incidence
- etiology
- signs and symptoms
- diagnosis
- treatment
- prognosis
- potential use as a biological weapon

KEY TERMS	
aerosol	suspension of tiny droplets or particles in a gas or floating form
antitoxin	antibody produced in response to and capable of neutralizing a specific biological toxin
bioterrorism	form of terrorism in which biological agents, such as viruses and bacteria, are used as weapons to kill, injure, threaten, intimidate, or coerce; also called *biowarfare*
category A agents	biological agents meeting specific criteria that identify them as having a high risk of use as biological weapons
disseminate	to spread, scatter, or disperse
mycotoxin	poison produced by a fungus
terrorism	violent act or threat with the intention of intimidating or coercing the government or civilian population to behave in a particular manner

Abbreviations

Table 19-1 lists some of the most common abbreviations related to bioterrorism.

History of Bioterrorism

Terrorism is a violent act or threat with the intention of intimidating or coercing the government or civilian population to behave in a particular manner. The goal of terrorists is usually to promote their social, political, or religious agenda. **Bioterrorism,** sometimes called *biowarfare,*

TABLE 19-1
ABBREVIATIONS

Abbreviation	Meaning	Abbreviation	Meaning
BSL	biosafety level	VHF	viral hemorrhagic fever
CDC	Centers for Disease Control and Prevention	WHO	World Health Organization
HPS	hantavirus pulmonary syndrome		

is a form of terrorism in which biological agents, such as viruses or bacteria, are used as weapons in an effort to kill, injure, threaten, intimidate, or coerce these same populations.

Bioterrorism is not new. Examples have been recorded as far back as 600 BC:

- 600 BC—Assyrians poisoned their enemies' wells with ergot that contained **mycotoxins** (poisons produced by fungi).
- 184 BC—Hannibal's army launched earthen pots filled with poisonous snakes onto their enemies' ships.
- 1346 (and later)—Plague-infected corpses were launched by military troops over the walls of enemy cities.
- 1767—British soldiers gave smallpox-infested blankets to Indians as "gifts" to intentionally cause an epidemic.
- 1930s—Japan used biological weapons against China, killing tens of thousands.
- 1940s and 1950s—The United States developed sites in Maryland, Mississippi, Utah, and Arkansas to make and study biological weapons.
- 1960s—The Vietcong placed feces-contaminated spears in pits to trap and kill their enemies.
- 1979—An explosion in a military compound in the USSR resulted in the accidental release of anthrax spores, killing approximately 1,000 people.
- 1984—Members of the Rajneeshee group in Oregon contaminated salad bars in The Dalles in an effort to influence the outcome of an election, making more than 750 people ill and hospitalizing 40.
- 2001—Twenty-one people in the United States developed anthrax after exposure by mail; several of them died.

Flashpoint

Bioterrorism is a form of terrorism with biological agents, such as bacteria or viruses.

Biological Agents

Biological agents in the hands of terrorists could be **disseminated** (spread, scattered, or dispersed) via water, food or air. Those that meet the criteria that identify them as having a high risk of use as biological weapons have been classified as **category A agents.** They include agents that cause anthrax, botulism, plague, smallpox, tularemia, and viral hemorrhagic fever. Other organisms are placed in categories B and C because their potential for threat, though real, is lower than that of the category A agents. Criteria for classification in category A are:

- potential for dissemination as an **aerosol** (suspension of tiny droplets or particles in a gas or floating form)
- potential for mass casualties
- initially benign presentation of victims
- need for a sophisticated medical and governmental response

Flashpoint

Agents most likely to be weaponized have been classified as category A agents.

- potential for widespread panic
- potential to cause diseases that can be transmitted from person to person

Anthrax

| ICD-9-CM: 022 (unspecified), 022.1 (pulmonary), 022.0 (cutaneous), 022.2 (gastrointestinal), 022.3 (anthrax septicemia) | [ICD-10: A22.1 (pulmonary), A22.0 (cutaneous), A22.2 (gastrointestinal), A22.7 (anthrax septicemia)] |

Anthrax is a serious disease caused by the bacterium *Bacillus anthracis.* It can manifest in three different forms, depending upon the type of exposure: cutaneous (skin), gastrointestinal (digestive system), and inhalation (lungs). The cutaneous form of anthrax has long been known as a threat to cattle and sheep. Anthrax in humans has been very rare; however, the cases after September 11, 2001, increased fears of the use of anthrax as a biological weapon.

Incidence

The first documented case of cutaneous anthrax in the United States occurred in 1992. Inhalation anthrax is very rare, but 21 cases occurred in 2001 when mail that had been intentionally contaminated with the bacterium was delivered to members of the national news media and the U.S. Senate. Five of those people died. Gastrointestinal anthrax is caused by the ingestion of contaminated meat; there have not been any cases of this form of the disease in the United States.

Flashpoint

Five people in the United States died when anthrax was used as a biological weapon in 2001.

Etiology

The cause of anthrax varies somewhat by type. Cutaneous anthrax is contracted through contact with infected animals or animal tissue or other direct contact with the bacterium. This most often occurs during slaughter or the handling of infected hides, meat, or other animal products. It is not contagious from person to person but can be contracted by touching infected animals or animal products, such as hides and wool. Anthrax can also be contracted through inhaling spores or eating raw or undercooked meat from animals infected with anthrax.

Signs and Symptoms

Signs and symptoms of anthrax vary with the form of infection. Cutaneous anthrax manifests as an itchy bump that progresses to a vesicle and then to a painless ulcer with an escharotic (blackened) center (see Fig. 19-1). Gastrointestinal anthrax causes symptoms associated with acute gastrointestinal inflammation, including nausea, anorexia, bloody diarrhea, fever, and severe stomach pain.

Inhalation anthrax initially produces symptoms typical of the common cold, including mild fever, sore throat, nonproductive cough, malaise, fatigue, and muscle aches. This is followed by progressive dyspnea, cyanosis, and the development of enlarged, tender lymph nodes. In severe cases, death occurs from septic shock.

Diagnosis

In addition to physical examination, diagnostic testing is done to identify *B. anthracis* from the blood, respiratory secretions, or skin lesions, or to identify specific antibodies in the blood of infected individuals (see Box 19-1). Which specimen is needed depends upon which type of anthrax is suspected. Blood samples and secretions from vesicles are tested for those suspected of having cutaneous anthrax. Blood and cerebrospinal fluid are tested for those suspected of having inhalation anthrax. Blood samples are tested for those suspected of having gastrointestinal anthrax. Other tests include chest x-ray and a study of secretions obtained from nasal swabs.

Treatment

All forms of anthrax are treated with antibiotics. Anyone with known exposure to anthrax bacteria may also be treated with prophylactic (preventive) antibiotics. Production of anthrax vaccine has recently been resumed due to its potential use as a weapon, and vaccination is currently available to some members of the armed forces, laboratory workers, and those who need to work in contaminated areas. Research continues to try to develop a vaccine that causes fewer side effects.

Flashpoint

Anthrax can be treated with antibiotics.

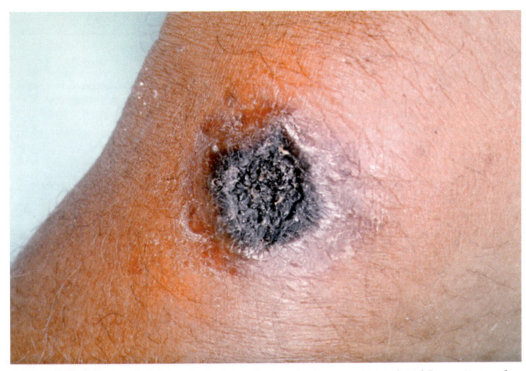

FIGURE 19-1 Anthrax ulcer (Courtesy of the Centers for Disease Control and Prevention and James H. Steele.)

Box 19-1 Diagnostic Spotlight

ANTHRAX TESTING
A new test recently approved by the Food and Drug Administration is available for detecting anthrax. The Anthrax Quick ELISA test, produced by Immunetics, detects antibodies produced by *B. anthracis*. The test can be completed in less than 1 hour, which is much shorter than previously available tests. It will also be much more widely available than previous tests, which were performed only in facilities operated by the CDC or the U.S. Army.

Prognosis

The survival rate for patients with anthrax depends upon the type of tissue infected and the earliness of treatment. Untreated cutaneous anthrax has a mortality rate of 20%, but early intervention is generally curative. Gastrointestinal anthrax has a mortality rate between 25% and 50% (depending on if or when treatment is initiated), while the mortality rate of inhalation anthrax is approximately 50%.

Potential Use as a Biological Weapon

A number of nations and terrorist groups have devoted energy and resources to the research and development of anthrax as a biological weapon. It is difficult to know the extent of this threat, since such efforts require sophisticated biotechnical capabilities and resources. The anthrax spores used would need to be incredibly small to be able to enter the smallest airways of the lungs. Furthermore, they would need to be treated with chemicals that eliminate static electricity in order to disperse readily. An individual would need to inhale between 8,000 and 50,000 spores to become ill. These factors make anthrax a difficult disease to use effectively as a bioweapon. Members of the Aum Shinrikyo group in Japan realized this when they attempted, unsuccessfully, on several occasions to infect large numbers of people.

Flashpoint
Inhalation anthrax is the deadliest form.

Botulism

ICD-9-CM: 040.41 (infant), 040.42 (wound),   [**ICD-10:** A05.2]
040.4 (other, specified), 005.1 (foodborne)

Botulism is a rare disease caused by toxins released by *Clostridium botulinum*, a bacterium usually found in the soil. It grows best in conditions with low oxygen and forms spores that can remain dormant until conditions become conducive to growth. Three types of botulism are foodborne, wound, and gastrointestinal (GI) botulism, sometimes called *infant botulism* because it most commonly occurs in infants.

Incidence

On average, 110 cases of botulism are reported in the United States each year. Approximately 25% of these are foodborne, 72% are gastrointestinal, and the other 3% are wound botulism. While this last group is quite small, it has been increasing in recent years due to the use of black-tar heroin.

Etiology

Foodborne botulism is contracted by eating food contaminated with botulism toxins. GI botulism is contracted by ingesting botulinum spores in honey or other foods. Wound botulism occurs when wounds become infected with *C. botulinim*.

Signs and Symptoms

Symptoms of foodborne botulism manifest 6 hours to 10 days after individuals eat contaminated food. The classic triad of symptoms is symmetric descending paralysis, absence of fever, and intact sensory ability. Related symptoms include visual impairment, drooping eyelids, dysphasia (difficulty speaking), dysphagia, dry mouth, muscle weakness, and fatigue. Infants with botulism are lethargic and have poor muscle tone and a weak cry. They also tend to be constipated and eat poorly.

Diagnosis

Initially, the diagnosis of botulism may not be clear. Other neuromuscular disorders may need to be ruled out, including Guillain-Barré syndrome, stroke, and myasthenia gravis. Tests that help with this process include nerve conduction velocity tests, Tensilon test (for myasthenia gravis), brain scan, and a study of cerebrospinal fluid. Diagnosis is most easily confirmed by identifying the botulinum toxins in the patient's stool or blood.

Treatment

There is no cure for botulism. However, administration of **antitoxin** may reduce symptoms if it occurs early enough. An antitoxin is an antibody produced in response to and capable of neutralizing a specific biological toxin. The antitoxin blocks the action of the toxin in the body. For those with GI botulism, the intestinal tract may be emptied by the induction of vomiting and the use of enemas to remove contaminated food. Many cases of GI botulism could be prevented by following proper food-preservation techniques (see Box 19-2). Those with cutaneous botulism may undergo surgical wound débridement to remove toxin-producing bacteria. If muscles important to breathing are affected, respiratory support is provided. This may include placing the person on a ventilator for an extended period of time. Other care includes physical therapy and other forms of rehabilitation.

Prognosis

Any type of botulism can be fatal: Paralysis of muscles that are essential for breathing can result in death unless life-support measures are initiated. The good news is that the mortality rate for botulism has dropped from 50% to just 8% over the past 50 years. Those who survive may experience prolonged shortness of breath and fatigue for a number of months. Most of those who contract botulism eventually recover after weeks or months of care and rehabilitation.

Potential Use as a Biological Weapon

Botulinum toxin is considered a threat as a biological weapon because it is extremely lethal, and it is easy to produce, transport, and use. It would be most effectively used in aerosolized form. Fortunately, however, it is a difficult agent to successfully disseminate due to its instability when exposed to oxygen, heat, or humidity.

Box 19-2 Wellness Promotion

SAFE FOOD PRESERVATION

Improperly canned food can lead to the growth of *C. botulinum*. These bacteria thrive in environments that are moist, low in acid, and anaerobic (with little or no oxygen). People who preserve their own food must be sure to follow specific guidelines to ensure that botulinum spores are destroyed and their food is safe:

- Examine jars carefully and do not use any with cracks or nicks in the rim.
- Use only new lids.
- Examine rings and use only those in excellent condition.
- Prepare food according to manufacturer recommendations.
- Do not overfill containers.
- Follow instructions carefully for processing times and temperatures.
- Never tamper with a processed jar to try to hurry it or force it to seal.
- Immediately use or discard the contents of any jars that do not seal; do not save for later use.
- Do not process foods in a water bath if guidelines recommend a pressure cooker.
- Contact an extension office of the Department of Agriculture for guidance if you are unsure about food-preservation techniques (http://www.usda.gov).

Attempts to use botulinum toxin as a bioweapon have already occurred. During the 1930s, Unit 731—a covert unit of the Imperial Japanese Army assigned to biological research and development—experimented with botulinum toxin by feeding it to war prisoners in Manchuria, who died as a result. More recently, the toxin was disseminated in downtown Tokyo and at U.S. military bases in Japan by the Aum Shinrikyo group on at least three occasions in the early 1990s. Fortunately, their efforts failed, because of inefficient aerosol-generating equipment, ineffective microbiological technique, or internal sabotage.

Plague

ICD-9-CM: 020.0 (bubonic), 020.2 (septicemic), 020.3 (primary pneumonic), 020.9 (pneumonic, unspecified)	[ICD-10: A20.0 (bubonic), A20.7 (septicemic), A20.2 (primary pneumonic), A20.9 (pneumonic, unspecified)]

The term *plague* refers to any widespread contagious disease with a high mortality rate. However, it is most commonly used to refer to the disease caused by a bacterium sometimes found in rodents and their fleas, called *Yersinia pestis*.

Incidence

According to the World Health Organization, there are an estimated 1,000 to 3,000 cases of plague each year, with 10 to 15 occurring in the United States. Most are bubonic plague. Cases of pneumonic (respiratory) plague are uncommon, but incidence might increase if the plague were weaponized in aerosol form.

Flashpoint
A plague is any widespread contagious disease with a high mortality rate.

Etiology

Bubonic plague is contracted from the bite of infected fleas or from exposure through broken skin. It is not spread from person to person. Pneumonic plague, by contrast, which develops as a result of *Y. pestis* infection in the lungs, is very contagious. It is spread by coughing or sneezing. This is why it might be viewed as an attractive weapon by terrorists.

Signs and Symptoms

Signs and symptoms of plague develop 1 to 6 days after infection. The form they take varies depending upon which form of the disease the individual has. Those with bubonic plague develop tender, swollen lymph glands, called buboes. They also develop severe malaise, muscle aches, high fever with chills, restlessness, confusion, headache, nausea, and vomiting. In addition to these symptoms, those with pneumonic plague develop hemoptysis (coughing bloody sputum), bruising, weakness, septicemia, and shock. Without early and aggressive treatment, death results from respiratory and circulatory failure.

Flashpoint

Pneumonic plague is a deadlier version of the disease because it affects the lungs.

Diagnosis

Diagnosis is based upon physical examination and testing of blood and sputum samples. Lymph nodes may be aspirated for fluid specimens as well.

Treatment

Treatment with antibiotics should be started within 24 hours. Those with known exposures should begin treatment within 7 days.

Prognosis

Bubonic plague has a mortality rate of up to 15% if treated early, but 40% to 60% if left untreated. If septicemia develops, the mortality rate jumps to 100% in untreated cases. The pneumonic form has a 100% mortality rate if not treated within the first 24 hours.

Flashpoint

Pneumonic plague has a 100% mortality rate!

Potential Use as a Biological Weapon

If used as a biological weapon, *Y. pestis* would most likely be aerosolized. This would result in pneumonic plague, which is highly contagious and has a very high mortality rate. The organism can live for up to an hour in the air but fortunately is readily destroyed by sunlight and drying.

Smallpox

ICD-9-CM: 050.9 (smallpox, unspecified)   [ICD-10: B03]

Smallpox is a serious, contagious disease caused by the variola virus. Though it historically existed in human populations for thousands of years, it has been virtually eliminated in recent years, except for what is used in laboratory research. Because of this, routine smallpox vaccinations were stopped over 30 years ago. However, since the events of September 11, 2001, there has been concern that it might be used as an agent of bioterrorism. The U.S. government has thus been developing a plan of response in the event of an outbreak.

The term *pox* is from a Latin word that means "spotted," and refers to the rash of raised bumps that develops on those who are infected with smallpox (see Fig. 19-2). There are several categories of smallpox, including four types of variola major, which are the most severe, and variola minor, which is less common and less severe.

Incidence

Historically this disease affected individuals of all ages and all racial groups. There have been no documented naturally occurring cases of smallpox in the United States since 1949. There were cases documented in Somalia as late as 1977. However, the increasing frequency of terrorist activities around the globe in recent years has given rise to concerns about the potential use of smallpox as a biological weapon by terrorists.

Etiology

Smallpox is quite contagious and is spread through respiratory secretions and secretions from lesions. It may also be spread indirectly through contact with contaminated objects, such as clothing or blankets. The only known natural hosts of smallpox are human beings; it is not transmitted by animals or insects. Those who are infected become contagious with the onset of fever but are most infectious during the rash phase and remain so until the last of the scabs falls off.

Flashpoint

Smallpox is spread through respiratory secretions and secretions from lesions.

Signs and Symptoms

Those exposed to smallpox usually feel fine during the incubation period, which varies between 7 and 17 days. They are not contagious during this time. This is followed by a fairly sudden onset of acute flu-like symptoms that last 2 to 4 days. Symptoms include fever as high as 104°F, chills, headache, backache, body aches, severe malaise, sore throat,

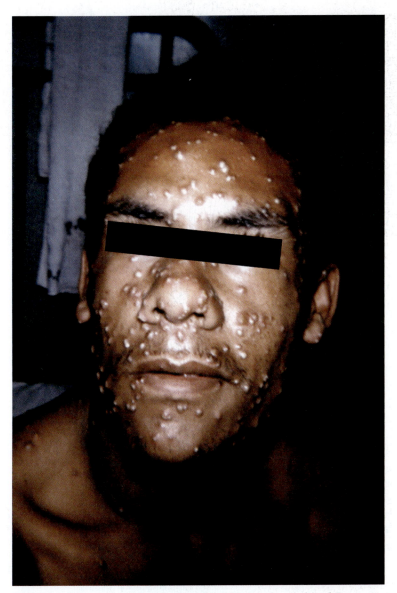

FIGURE 19-2 Smallpox (Courtesy of the Centers for Disease Control and Prevention and Dr. Noble.)

and cough. Individuals may also experience abdominal pain, nausea, and vomiting. With the onset of acute symptoms, a macular rash develops in the mouth and then spreads quickly to the rest of the body. It progresses through papular (bumps), vesicular (clear blisters), and pustular (pus-filled blisters) stages. The pustules subsequently rupture and form scabs that leave disfiguring scars. The acute symptomatic stage typically lasts 14 to 21 days.

Diagnosis

Diagnosis of smallpox is based upon a history of known exposure, physical examination, and culture of fluid from the lesions. A key way to distinguish smallpox from chickenpox is that smallpox lesions spread over the body very quickly (within 24 hours) and are all in the same stage at the same time. Furthermore, the lesions are most prevalent on the face, hands, and legs. The lesions of chickenpox, by contrast, appear over a much longer period of time (14 days), are in multiple stages of development at the same time, and are most prevalent on the face and trunk (see Fig. 19-3).

Flashpoint

Smallpox and chickenpox appear similar, but their onset and distribution are very different.

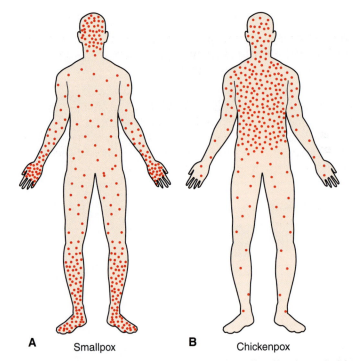

FIGURE 19-3 Distribution of smallpox lesions compared to distribution of chickenpox lesions

Treatment

There is no cure for smallpox once an individual is infected. Therefore, treatment is supportive and is aimed at providing comfort through fluids, nutrition, and medications to reduce fever and relieve pain. Measures are taken to prevent secondary bacterial infection and to minimize risk of spreading the disease to others. Vaccination for smallpox has been provided to limited populations, such as military personnel and medical-response teams, but it has not been made available to the general public.

Prognosis

Based upon past statistics, the mortality rate for smallpox ranges between 20% and 40%. Those who survive are left with disfiguring scars.

Potential Use as a Biological Weapon

As a category A agent, the variola virus is believed to pose a potential threat to the public and has the potential for large-scale dissemination. The deliberate release of variola virus as an aerosol might cause the highly fatal form of respiratory infection and would also cause widespread panic. The good news is that it is actually considered a fragile virus, which would die or dissipate within 24 hours.

Tularemia

ICD-9-CM:021.1 (enteric), 021.2 (pulmonary), 021.9 (unspecified) **[ICD-10: A21.3 (enteric), A21.2 (pulmonary), A21.9 (unspecified)]**

Tularemia is a serious illness caused by the bacterium *Francisella tularensis*, found in animals such as rabbits and rodents.

Incidence

Between the years 1990 and 2000, there were 1,368 cases of tularemia in the United States reported to the Centers for Disease Control and Prevention (CDC). More than half of the cases occurred in the four states of Arkansas, South Dakota, Oklahoma, and Missouri.

Etiology

Tularemia is acquired in several ways: eating or drinking contaminated water or food, being bitten by an infected insect, touching infected animal carcasses, and breathing in the bacteria. It is not contagious from person to person.

Signs and Symptoms

Incubation usually lasts from 3 days to 2 weeks, followed by the onset of symptoms. These include the sudden onset of fever with chills, headache, joint and muscle aches, diarrhea, weakness, and dry cough. Pneumonia may develop, with chest pain, dyspnea, and hemoptysis. Other symptoms depend on the type of exposure and include ulcers of the skin or mouth; tender, swollen lymph nodes; sore throat; and painful, puffy eyes.

Diagnosis

Tularemia should be suspected when patients in areas where it is known to develop present with the described signs and symptoms. It is confirmed by identifying the bacterium in a culture of blood or other fluid specimen.

Treatment

Patients with tularemia respond well when antibiotic therapy is initiated quickly. Currently there is no vaccine.

Prognosis

Tularemia has a 30% mortality rate when left untreated. However, those who receive timely treatment usually recover.

Potential Use as a Biological Weapon

If *F. tularensis* were used as a biological weapon, it would likely be aerosolized. Inhalation of the organism causes severe, life-threatening respiratory illness and systemic infection without rapid, aggressive treatment. Because the bacteria exist readily in nature, they could be isolated and developed in sizable quantities in the laboratory. However, the manufacture of an efficient and effective aerosol weapon would take significant sophistication.

> **Flashpoint**
> Tularemia is not spread between people; however, it can be spread many other ways.

Viral Hemorrhagic Fevers

ICD-9-CM: 065.9 (arthropod-borne hemorrhagic fever, unspecified), 065.8 (specified arthropod-borne hemorrhagic fever)   **[ICD-10: A96.0–A98.9 (code by virus)]**

Viral hemorrhagic fevers (VHFs) are a group of illnesses caused by four families of viruses: arenaviruses, filoviruses, bunyaviruses, and flaviviruses. They normally live in animal hosts, such as rodents, or insects, such as ticks and mosquitoes. The viruses are dependent on their hosts for their survival. Because of this, most of the viruses are distributed in areas of the world in which their hosts naturally reside. Therefore, the risk of contracting each virus is usually limited to individuals who live in the associated geographic region. However, when hosts live in widely distributed areas—such as hosts for the agents of hantavirus pulmonary syndrome, which live throughout North and South America—the virus is more widespread.

Furthermore, it is possible for individuals to become infected by a host that has been moved from its natural environment. For example, animals that have been exported to other countries for use as pets or in laboratory research can infect people in their new environment. An example is the outbreak of Marburg virus disease in parts of Germany and Yugoslavia, when monkeys infected with the Marburg virus were imported and used in laboratories. On the other hand, human beings sometimes travel to areas where the virus naturally occurs, become infected, and then return home or travel elsewhere. If the virus is one that is transmitted from person to person, the risk of spread is high. Because people are traveling more than ever before, such risk is on the rise. Examples of viruses that are transmitted between people and cause hemorrhagic fever are Lassa virus, Marburg virus, the Ebola viruses, Dengue fever, and Crimean-Congo hemorrhagic fever virus.

VHFs are called "hemorrhagic" because bleeding is a common characteristic of these illnesses, but the bleeding is usually not life-threatening. Rather, it is the involvement and deterioration of multiple body systems that becomes potentially fatal.

> **Flashpoint**
> VHFs include a large group of viral illnesses that cause fever and hemorrhagic symptoms.

Incidence

Incidence of viral hemorrhagic fevers is quite variable depending upon the type. Most are more common in Africa. Some are on the rise there as well as in some other countries. Crude estimates for Lassa virus number as high as 300,000 per year, with as many as 5,000 deaths per year. In the past 40 years, there have just been 450 confirmed cases of Marburg and over 2,300 confirmed cases of Ebola. Crimean-Congo fever is common to many countries in Africa, Europe, and Asia. In the past 10 years, outbreaks also have been recorded in Kosovo, Albania, Iran, and Pakistan. It has a mortality rate of 30%. Dengue fever has the highest estimated incidence of any VHF at 50 to 100 million people infected yearly in more than 110 countries.

Etiology

VHFs are initially contracted when human beings come in contact with the urine, saliva, feces, or other excretions of infected reservoir hosts, such as rodents, or when human beings are bitten by vectors, such as mosquitoes. In some cases the illness is spread to animals, such as livestock, by vectors; human beings then contract the illness when they handle or slaughter the livestock. Because some viruses are spread from person to person, secondary transmission then occurs through contact with body fluids of infected individuals.

Flashpoint
VHFs are highly contagious.

Signs and Symptoms

The signs and symptoms of VHFs vary with the specific virus involved. In general, the early manifestations are deceptively flu-like and include fever, malaise, muscle and joint aches, fatigue, dizziness, sore throat, conjunctivitis, rash, and chest or abdominal pain. As the illness progresses, bleeding begins from the mouth, eyes, and ears, and under the skin (see Fig. 19-4). Internal bleeding can also occur, although massive hemorrhage is uncommon. Rather, death occurs more commonly due to multisystem failure and shock.

Diagnosis

Diagnosis of VHFs is based in part upon physical-examination findings, signs and symptoms, and information about the individual's travel history during the preceding 3 to 4 weeks. Information about the individual's recent exposure to other ill people is also important. The presence of sore throat, conjunctivitis, skin rash, and eventual hemorrhage and shock support the diagnosis of VHFs. Testing includes blood smears, to rule out malaria, as well as blood cultures and a complete blood count. The diagnosis is confirmed by identifying the virus or the presence of antibodies in the blood. However, antibodies may not be present in the infected patient's blood until the second week of illness. Some types of virus can also be recovered from the individual's throat or urine—or, postmortem, from the liver. Such testing should only be done in CDC facilities at biosafety level 4 (see Box 19-3) or in the CDC mobile laboratory, which is available upon

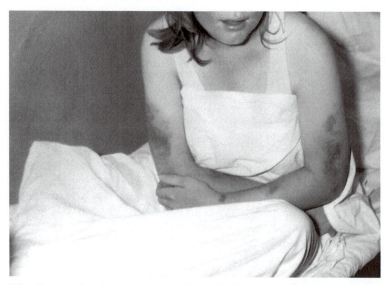

FIGURE 19-4 Bleeding under the skin caused by VHF (Courtesy of the Centers for Disease Control and Prevention and Dr. B.E. Henderson.)

Box 19-3 Diagnostic Spotlight

CDC BIOSAFETY LEVEL 4 LABORATORIES

Biosafety levels (BSLs) are specified by the CDC; they refer to the precautions needed to isolate biological agents (pathogens) within a facility. Minimal precautions are designated as level 1 (BSL-1), and strictest precautions are level 4 (BSL-4). Highly dangerous microorganisms, such as airborne pathogens that cause a fatal disease with no available vaccine or therapy, are studied in BSL-4 laboratories. Examples of pathogens studied in this type of lab are the Marburg virus, the Ebola viruses, and other hemorrhagic fever viruses. BSL-4 labs are designed with a number of safety features:

- High-level security allows only specially designated, carefully trained people to enter.
- Scientists wear fully protective hazmat suits, with head gear and an air supply delivered through overhead lines that plug into the suits.
- Flood hoods create negative pressure by pulling air into the experimental area; this keeps pathogens from spreading into the general laboratory area.
- Individual rooms are sealed with multiple airlocks, and special procedures are followed for decontamination when scientists enter and exit rooms (multiple showers, a vacuum room, an ultraviolet room, etc.).

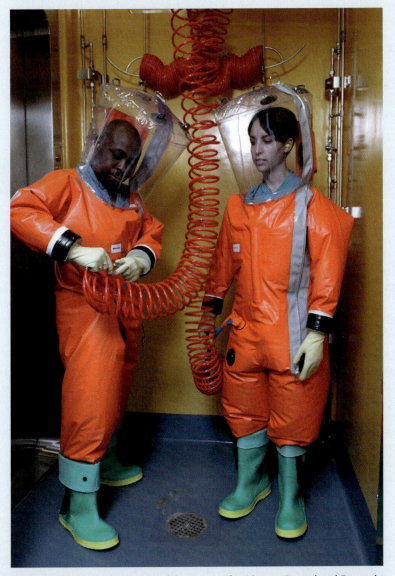

CDC biosafety level 4 laboratory (Courtesy of the Centers for Disease Control and Prevention and Dr. Scott Smith.)

request. This enables appropriate testing to be done by trained individuals who understand the precautions necessary to prevent the spread of the disease.

Treatment

If VHFs seem a likely diagnosis, the patient should be immediately isolated. Immediate notification must also be sent to local and state health departments and the CDC. The aim of management is twofold. First, the patient is provided with supportive care. Second, care must be taken to protect health-care staff and prevent the spread of the disease. There is no cure for VHFs. With a few viruses, antiviral drugs may be helpful; for example, ribavirin has been helpful in treating some people ill with Lassa fever.

Prognosis

The mortality rate varies with the individual virus and the aggressiveness of care. The mortality rates for the Ebola viruses vary between 53% and 88%. The mortality rate for Crimean-Congo hemorrhagic fever varies between 15% and 40%. Other types, such as Lassa fever, have had mortality rates as low as 1%.

Potential Use as a Biological Weapon

According to the CDC, hemorrhagic fever viruses have been weaponized in the past. The Soviet Union and Russia produced sizable amounts of Ebola, Lassa, and Marburg virus and New World arenaviruses until 1992. The United States developed yellow fever virus and Rift Valley virus as biological weapons before the termination of its biological weapons program in 1969. It has been reported that North Korea may have weaponized the yellow fever virus.

There is some debate among experts about whether VHFs currently pose a high risk as potential biological weapons. Most agree that there is some risk, given the early flu-like presentation of some types and the facts that some may be transmitted from person to person and that most health-care providers are unfamiliar with these diseases. In light of these factors, there is some concern that accurate diagnosis and clear identification of the threat may be delayed. In addition, though ribavirin therapy may be useful in some cases, there are currently few vaccines available for VHFs.

Preparation and Response

Developing an organized plan for the prevention of, and response to, bioterrorism is challenging, given the variety of organisms involved and the unpredictability of terrorist groups. Furthermore, with only two exceptions (Argentine hemorrhagic fever and yellow fever), there are no vaccines available to provide protection against VHFs. Agencies such as the CDC, the Department of Homeland Security, and the American Red Cross are working to provide information and resources in this endeavor. The CDC, in partnership with a number of other health organizations, has developed a national program for bioterrorism preparedness and response that includes a range of resources. A few measures that have been taken or are currently underway are:

- creation of a response plan
- identification and training of response teams to work at local and state levels
- ensuring the availability of resources to provide accurate testing and appropriate treatment
- collection and storage of antibiotics
- creation of a national database to facilitate the identification and tracking of cases
- coordination of nationwide sharing of information
- creation of educational programs and resources for the media, the general public, and health-care professionals

Anthrax

Researchers are working on developing a type of protective antigen they hope will inhibit the release of lethal toxins and possibly provide protection against future exposures to anthrax.

Botulism

The CDC maintains a surveillance system for botulism cases based upon reports from health-care providers. Two antitoxins are available and are being stored in a variety of locations across the nation. An investigational botulism vaccine has been used for military and high-risk laboratory personnel in the recent past. While this vaccine is no longer in production, another one is currently under development. In addition, efforts are planned to develop a means of rapidly detecting and diagnosing botulism by the year 2013.

Viral Hemorrhagic Fevers

The CDC and the World Health Organization (WHO) have collaborated to develop hospital-based guidelines to help improve the recognition of VHF cases and to prevent further transmission. National and state public-health officials in the United States have sizeable quantities of the drugs needed in case of a bioterrorism event involving VHFs and report that these drugs can be quickly made available anywhere in the country. Furthermore, ongoing efforts are aimed at:

- identification of strategies to contain and treat VHFs
- production of vaccines
- development of a more rapid means of diagnosis
- study of disease transmission
- improved preventive measures

Student Resources

Center for Biosecurity of UPMC: http://www.upmc-biosecurity.org/index.html
Centers for Disease Control and Prevention Bioterrorism page: http://www.bt.cdc.gov/bioterrorism
United States Department of Homeland Security: http://www.dhs.gov

Chapter Activities

Learning Style Study Strategies

Try any or all of the following strategies as you study the content of this chapter:

Visual and kinesthetic learners: Collect photos and illustrations of pathological conditions from journals, Internet image search engines, and other sources. Visit the CDC website for information about pathogens most likely to be used as biological weapons. Create a poster or collage with the images and information you find. Be sure to write the name of each disorder and a *brief* description next to each image. Tape the poster somewhere that you will see it frequently and review the information on it at least once each day.

Auditory and verbal learners: Verbally describe photos or illustrations in this book to a real or imaginary friend who cannot see them. Be especially detailed in your description of any skin lesions caused by the various diseases. Use language that allows your friend to accurately picture the images without ever having seen them. Explain to your friend the differences between the typical manifestations of the diseases as they might naturally occur and how they might present if they were used as biological weapons.

Practice Exercises

Answers to practice exercises can be found in Appendix D.

Case Studies

CASE STUDY 1

During a conversation with friends, someone comments, "Bioterrorism is a terrible invention of the 21st century."

1. Describe how you might approach your friend to correct and educate her on this matter without offending her.

2. List at least eight examples of bioterrorism that occurred throughout history (before the 21st century).

CASE STUDY 2

You have recently returned from a workshop about bioterrorism and are telling a coworker about it. As you tell her about category A biological agents, you explain to her why they have been identified as having the potential for use as weapons. What are the six characteristics you will list?

CASE STUDY 3

Angel is a CMA at a local medical clinic. She is learning about biological microorganisms that could potentially be used as biological weapons and is currently researching smallpox. In doing so she must answer the following questions:

1. Why were smallpox vaccinations discontinued over 30 years ago?

2. Where does the term pox come from, and what does it mean?

3. How is smallpox spread?

4. What is the progression of smallpox lesions, and how do they differ from chickenpox lesions?

Multiple Choice

1. Which of the following disorders is **not** matched with the correct information or definition?

    a. Anthrax: the cutaneous form manifests as an itchy bump that progresses to a vesicle and then a painless ulcer with an escharotic (blackened) center

    b. Viral hemorrhagic fevers: a group of illnesses caused by arenaviruses, filoviruses, bunyaviruses and flaviviruses

    c. Plague: the disease caused by a bacterium sometimes found in rodents and their fleas, called *Yersinia pestis*

    d. Botulism: the classic symptoms include nausea, anorexia, bloody diarrhea, fever, and severe stomach pain

2. Which of the following statements is true regarding anthrax?

    a. Vaccination is currently available to some members of the armed forces, laboratory workers, and those who need to work in contaminated areas.

    b. It is contagious from person to person.

    c. There is no cure, and patients are treated symptomatically.

    d. It manifests in one form only, which affects the skin.

3. Which of the following groups is known for making a number of attempts in recent years to disseminate several different category A biological organisms?

    a. The Branch Davidians

    b. The followers of Jim Jones

    c. The Aum Shinrikyo group

    d. The Unification Church

4. Which of the following statements is true regarding botulism?

    a. Most cases are foodborne.

    b. The causative organism is usually found in the soil.

    c. Wound botulism in on the rise because of the use of cocaine.

    d. A vaccine is available.

5. Which of the following statements is true regarding viral hemorrhagic fevers?

    a. The causative organism normally lives in the soil.

    b. Death is usually due to massive hemorrhage.

    c. Early symptoms are similar to those of influenza.

    d. They have never been weaponized before.

Short Answer

1. **The CDC has developed a national program for bioterrorism preparedness and response. List five measures that have been taken or are currently underway.**

2. **What measures are being taken to minimize the risk that botulism will be used as a biological weapon?**

3. **How would weaponized *Francisella tularensis* behave? What factors make its weaponization more and less likely?**

Learning Outcomes

Upon completion of this chapter, the student will be able to:

- Define and spell key terms related to pain
- Differentiate between objective and subjective data
- Briefly describe the gate control theory of pain
- Describe the effects of age, physical factors, emotional factors, psychosocial factors, and cultural factors on the experience of pain
- List 10 common myths about pain, and explain the truth about each one
- Discuss the ethical duty that health-care providers have to treat their patients' pain
- List the classifications of drugs commonly used to treat pain, and include an example of one drug in each class
- Describe ethical and unethical uses of placebos
- Describe eight nonpharmacological means of treating various forms of pain
- Discuss the impact that locus of control and self-efficacy have on a patient's ability to provide self-care

KEY TERMS	
acute pain	pain lasting 6 months or less that has an identifiable cause and resolves when healing occurs
adjuvant	medication that hastens or increases the action of other agents
biofeedback	type of therapy that teaches patients to control their autonomic (involuntary) nervous system
chronic pain	pain lasting 6 months or longer that has a cause that is often unclear
endorphins	opiatelike substances produced in the body
enkephalins	opiatelike substances produced in the body
gate control theory	generally accepted theory that suggests that the experience of pain depends upon the results of competition between neurotransmitters and neuromodulators
malignant pain	cancer pain
neuropathic pain	nerve pain
nociception	transmission of impulses along peripheral nerves to the central nervous system, where the stimulus is perceived as pain
nonmalignant pain	noncancer pain
nonopioid analgesic	pain-relieving medication that contains no opiates
NSAID	nonsteroidal anti-inflammatory drug; nonsteroid medication used to relieve pain and reduce inflammation
objective	observable, measurable, and analyzable

Continued

KEY TERMS—cont'd	
opioid analgesic	pain-relieving medication that contains opiates
physical dependence	condition of physical tolerance and, with sudden discontinuation of the substance, display of a withdrawal syndrome
placebo	inactive substance that has no inherent medicinal value
pseudoaddiction	behavior that is often mistaken for drug-seeking but is in reality relief-seeking due to poor pain relief
psychological dependence	emotional and behavioral symptoms of craving, compulsive drug-seeking, hoarding, and using substances purely for emotional and mental euphoria
subjective	knowable only by the person involved
synergistic effect	enhanced action when two or more agents work together
tolerance	phenomenon that develops over time, in which the body loses sensitivity to opioids and their pain-relieving effects
trigger point	tender, painful area that may cause pain elsewhere

Abbreviations

Table 20-1 lists some of the more common abbreviations related to pain.

Definitions of Pain

Pain has been defined by the International Association for the Study of Pain as an "unpleasant sensory and emotional experience associated with actual or potential tissue damage or described in terms of such damage." Other sources define pain as strong discomfort, the perception of an uncomfortable stimulus, or the sensation of hurting. Regardless of how one chooses to define pain, most would agree it is a distressing experience that negatively affects one's quality of life. In fact, complaints of pain are what prompt the majority of patients to seek medical care.

TABLE 20-1

ABBREVIATIONS

Abbreviation	Meaning	Abbreviation	Meaning
EDR	electrodermal response	PENS	percutaneous electrical nerve stimulation
IASP	International Association for the Study of Pain	SNRI	serotonin and norepinephrine reuptake inhibitor
MS*	morphine sulfate	TENS	Transcutaneous electrical nerve stimulation

*Currently included on the "Dangerous Abbreviations" list from The National Coordinating Counsil for Medication Error Reporting and Prevention because of potential for confusion with abbreviations for other substances, such as magnesium sulfate. It is now recommended that *morphine sulfate* be spelled out.

When evaluating patients, health-care providers look for ***objective*** findings to aid them in identifying the diagnoses. These are observable, measurable, and analyzable findings. Such data are usually obtained through physical examination and diagnostic testing. One of the most challenging aspects of treating pain is that the experience is completely ***subjective.*** This means that it is knowable only by the person involved; it cannot be seen or measured. Consequently, when the cause of pain (an injury or illness) is not readily apparent, patients often feel frustrated as they attempt to describe it and try to convince others of its presence or severity. The subjectivity of pain is what led nurse researchers Margo McCaffery and Alexandra Beebe to define pain as "whatever the experiencing person says it is, existing whenever the experiencing person says it does." This definition emphasizes the subjective nature of pain and also emphasizes health-care providers' ethical obligation to believe their patients.

While there are many types of pain, most have been grouped into one of two categories: acute and chronic. These designations are somewhat arbitrary, and some forms of pain may have characteristics of both.

> **Flashpoint**
>
> **O**bjective findings are **o**bserved, and **s**ubjective information is what the patient **s**ays.

Acute Pain

Acute pain has been defined as pain of 6 months' duration or less that has an identifiable cause, occurs soon after injury to body tissues, and resolves when healing occurs. Severity of pain is generally in proportion to the type and extent of tissue damage. Acute pain is often accompanied by objective physical changes such as diaphoresis (profuse sweating) and increased respiratory rate, pulse, and blood pressure. Pain behaviors may be present as well; these might include frowning, muscle tension, tearfulness, guarding of the painful body part, and moaning.

Acute pain is considered protective because it warns of an injury or physical threat, such as inflammation or infection. This usually prompts the person to respond with self-care measures. The onset of acute pain may be sudden or slow, and the intensity may vary from mild to severe. Acute pain is better understood than chronic pain and is more easily treated.

Chronic Pain

Chronic pain was initially defined as pain lasting 6 months or longer that has a cause that is often unclear. A more recent definition describes it as pain that lasts longer than the typical time associated with healing of a particular type of injury or disease process. Chronic pain may be continuous or intermittent. In either case, it is present much of the time over an extended period of time.

Compared with acute pain, chronic pain is less well understood. Unlike acute pain, it seems to serve no useful purpose. It is often present when a cause is unclear and long after an initial injury seems to have healed. Some view chronic pain as a disease itself, rather than a symptom, given its harmful physical and emotional effects. It is sometimes divided into the two groups of ***malignant pain*** (cancer pain) and ***nonmalignant pain*** (noncancer pain). Examples of nonmalignant chronic pain include the pain associated with rheumatoid arthritis and peripheral neuropathy (nerve pain). Malignant pain is pain caused by any form of cancer (lung cancer, pancreatic cancer, bone cancer, etc.).

The objective physical changes seen in acute pain are rarely present with chronic pain except during acute exacerbations, in which the pain temporarily escalates. Instead, it is more common to see signs and symptoms of depression. However, health-care providers should be cautious about assuming that depression is the patient's only problem. Certainly there is a common connection between the two, but it is usually the chronic pain that leads to depression, rather than the reverse (see Fig. 20-1). Depression, in turn, then leads to difficulty in effectively coping with the pain.

> **Flashpoint**
>
> Chronic pain is less well understood than acute pain.

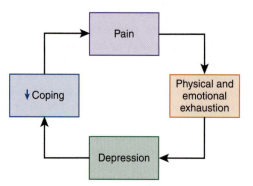

FIGURE 20-1 The cycle of chronic pain and depression

Physiology of Pain

There is much about pain that is not yet fully understood. Theories about the transmission of pain generally include discussions of **nociception** and **gate control theory.** Nociception is the transmission of impulses along peripheral nerves to the central nervous system, where the stimulus is perceived as pain. Gate control theory is a generally accepted theory that suggests that the experience of pain depends upon the results of competition between neurotransmitters and neuromodulators. It explains how pain is perceived, how pain signals are transmitted, and why some pain-relieving measures are effective.

Pain is usually triggered by some type of tissue damage. This damage stimulates the release of chemicals that cause inflammation and its related signs (redness, swelling, and tenderness). Messages are immediately sent to nociceptors, which are free nerve endings that serve as receptors for painful stimuli. There are two types of nerve fibers that conduct pain messages. A fibers are myelinated (covered by an insulating sheath). They send messages of sharp, distinct pain that help the brain identify the source and intensity of the pain. The slower C fibers send messages that are more persistent and burning but less specific about the location of the pain. Pain messages travel rapidly to the spinal cord and then move up to the brain. When they reach the cerebral cortex in the brain, the pain is interpreted and processed. The body then releases chemicals such as **endorphins** and **enkephalins** (opiatelike substances produced by the body), serotonin (a mood elevator), norepinephrine (adrenaline), and other substances that reduce the transmission of pain impulses and help to produce an analgesic (pain-relieving) effect.

Flashpoint

The body produces chemicals that help relieve pain.

Gate control theory involves neurotransmitters, such as acetylcholine, that transmit pain signals and neuromodulators, such as endorphins, that block pain signals. When neurotransmitters dominate, pain signals make their way to the brain. When neuromodulators dominate, the pain is blocked. It is also thought that large-diameter nerves carry sensory data that is not pain, such as cold, heat, and touch, while small-diameter nerves carry pain messages. In some forms of treatment, such as the use of transcutaneous electrical nerve stimulation (TENS) units, the goal is to overwhelm nerves with sensory data unrelated to pain in order to block pain messages and prevent them from reaching the brain.

Interpretation of Pain

A person's perception and expression of pain are influenced by age and by physical factors such as energy level and neurological impairment. They are also influenced by emotional factors, such as fear; psychosocial factors, such as coping ability; and cultural factors, such as family values and religious beliefs.

Age

Age has little impact on an individual's ability to feel pain, but it may affect the expression of pain. For example, the very young are likely to respond to pain with crying and physical movement, while some teens and adults may refrain from such a response, believing that it is a sign of weakness. The elderly are more prone to forms of chronic pain yet will often refrain from complaining, out of a desire to avoid being labeled as bothersome. Others deny pain out of fear that it may be signaling a worsening of their condition.

Flashpoint

Elderly patients are often afraid to complain about pain.

Physical Factors

Physical energy level affects the individual's perception of pain and ability to cope with it. Fatigue caused by insufficient sleep, by stress, or by physical activity increases pain perception and diminishes coping ability. Sleep, as well as rest from emotional distress, helps to restore energy and coping ability. This diminishes the perception of pain and increases tolerance of it.

Impaired neurological functioning may interfere with the individual's perception of pain. For example, a person who has ingested alcohol or medications that depress the central nervous system will likely have a decreased sensitivity to pain. Diseases that cause nerve damage may also decrease pain perception. For example, diabetics who have developed peripheral neuropathy have decreased sensitivity in their hands and feet. While this might seem like a useful thing, it actually puts them at risk for injury, since they may not notice small injuries right away. This compounds the risk of further injury and the onset of infection.

Emotional Factors

Experience with severe or unremitting pain increases the fear of its return and actually serves to increase pain perception. Thus, pain and the emotions of fear and anxiety it causes can become something of a vicious cycle. Pain actually activates parts of the brain that control emotions; it often triggers feelings of anxiety in response to the physical discomfort and feelings of helplessness. Health-care providers must remember this and respond to both.

Flashpoint

Experience with severe pain can increase the fear of its return.

Psychosocial Factors

Effective coping skills learned through past events in an individual's life can help the individual respond to and manage injury, pain, and fear. People with dysfunctional coping strategies often respond poorly. For example, individuals who respond to pain by using prayer, deep breathing, or meditation techniques are more relaxed and feel less fearful. This helps reduce their perception of pain. Those who respond with emotional displays of anger and anxiety by crying, moaning, or shouting deplete their energy more quickly and increase their muscle tension and perception of pain.

Cultural Factors

Cultural factors have little impact on the physical experience of pain; however, they may affect how people interpret it, how they respond to it, and how they choose to express it. Members of some cultures believe that loud, emotional responses are appropriate, while members of others may believe that expressions of pain indicate weakness. Individuals from these two types of cultures may experience similar levels of pain yet present very differently. Members of some cultures view pain as punishment for sin or for mistakes that have been made, while members of others view it as an opportunity to purify themselves or demonstrate faithfulness.

Common Myths About Pain

Sadly, myths about pain have persisted for many years and continue to contribute to the under-treatment of pain by health-care professionals. Some relate to confusion about pain behaviors and the use of opioid medications for the treatment of pain; others relate to biases about gender or age.

Myth: Health-care providers can determine whether or not the client's pain is real.

The pain experience is completely subjective. Health-care providers have no way to see, feel, or measure a patient's pain. Objective physical changes may or may not be apparent, but their absence should never be considered proof of the absence of pain. It is important to remember that physical indicators associated with acute pain are rarely seen in those suffering from chronic pain. It is also important to remember that people express pain differently based upon a variety of personal, social, and cultural factors. Finally, health-care providers should remember to treat their patients in the same manner that they themselves would wish to be treated—which means that they choose to believe them, or at least to give them the benefit of the doubt, and then respond in a compassionate manner.

Myth: The very young and the very old have a decreased perception of pain.

There is little evidence that age affects pain perception. Individuals in these two groups often have a compromised ability to communicate what they are feeling, which may lead others to mistakenly assume that they feel less pain. Health-care professionals must be very careful never to make such assumptions and should always err on the side of providing more, rather than fewer, comfort measures.

Myth: Men or women perceive pain more (or less) than those of the opposite gender.
Myth: Men or women have a greater (or lesser) tolerance for pain than those of the opposite gender.

Such topics always generate a lively discussion, with opinions going both ways. However, there is no evidence to support the belief that men or women experience more or less pain or have a higher or lower tolerance for it. Such beliefs generally arise from assumptions based upon differences that may be seen in the expression of pain. However, it is important to remember that pain is subjective and may be expressed in a wide variety of ways by men and women of different cultures.

Myth: Individuals who take opioid analgesics run a high risk of becoming addicted.

According to the American Pain Society, misunderstandings about addiction and unfair labeling of patients as addicts have resulted in unjustified withholding of opioid medications. Studies show that the risk of addiction from the treatment of acute pain with opioid medication is nearly zero (less than 1%). Evidence shows that individuals who take opioid analgesics for pain stop taking the medication when the pain ends.

The use of opioid medications by those with chronic pain has not been well studied, so the risk of addiction is not clearly known. However, there is reason to believe that opioid use by patients with chronic pain who are properly evaluated and well managed increases their productivity and overall quality of life without producing the feared ramifications.

Myth: People with chronic pain should never be treated with opiates.

Given the long-standing concerns that health-care providers have had about the potential for abuse of medication among those with chronic pain, it is important to point out the difference between *physical dependence, tolerance,* and *psychological dependence.* Both physical dependence and tolerance occur naturally in those who take opioid medication on a regular basis for an extended period of time. Tolerance is a phenomenon that develops over time, in which the body loses sensitivity to opioids and their pain-relieving effects. As a result, there may be the need for an increased dosage to achieve the same results. Physical dependence is said to have occurred if the individual experiences a withdrawal syndrome when the medication is suddenly discontinued. Neither of these phenomena reflects immoral, unethical, or illegal behavior or intent on the part of the individual. Nor do they indicate anything about the individual's moral character. They simply describe a physiological response to the continued presence of the opioid medication. Psychological dependence occurs when the individual desires the substance for psychological effects such as feelings of euphoria and general well-being.

Health-care providers should refrain from using the terms *addict* and *addiction* in reference to their patients, because of the negative implications associated with such terms. Addiction has been commonly described in a variety of negative ways: compulsive, maladaptive, disabling, relapsing, chronic disease, drug-seeking, and dependence. The results of addiction are also usually described in terms of adverse or negative psychological, physical, economic, social, health, and legal consequences. Therefore, more accurate and less judgmental terms should be used, such as *physical dependence* and *psychological dependence.*

Drug abuse is a real problem, and health-care providers are sure to encounter some patients who may be drug-seeking. However, they must be very careful about labeling patients as drug seekers, since such labels can easily promote bias against patients and negatively affect the quality of the care provided. Furthermore, it is important to note that health-care providers are making assumptions which may or may not be true. The behaviors of patients who are drug-seeking might be very similar to those of patients who are relief-seeking due to poor pain relief. This is called ***pseudoaddiction.*** These people seem preoccupied with obtaining opioids because of the poor pain relief they have experienced. Once their pain is well managed, the drug-seeking behavior in such individuals will generally disappear.

In an effort to respond to misconceptions about the risk of addiction when treating patients with chronic pain, the World Health Organization has issued a recommended approach to pain management:

Step 1: Use of NSAIDs and adjuvant medication
Step 2: Use of weak opioids and adjuvants
Step 3: Use of strong opioids and adjuvants

These steps are to be taken in the order listed until the patient has achieved satisfactory relief and management of pain. In the case of patients with cancer pain, the recommended order is reversed: Strong opioids should be used initially, if needed, to get the patient's pain under control, followed by a reduction to the point that adequate pain management is maintained.

Myth: The risks of adverse effects of opioid medications outweigh the benefits.

Common adverse effects of opioid medications are respiratory depression, sedation, and gastrointestinal problems, including nausea, vomiting, and constipation. Health-care providers often recite the risks of these adverse effects as reason to discontinue or withhold opioids. Certainly these adverse effects are a potential problem for any patient taking opioids; but they can usually be minimized or managed, and they are not an acceptable reason to withhold treatment. The risk of sedation and respiratory depression is greatest when opioid medication is first given to an individual who has little or no experience with them. Therefore, dosage strength and frequency should be conservative until the patient's response has been determined. Medication can then be increased as necessary, as indicated by the physician, to achieve the best result. Over time, people actually develop a tolerance for these side effects and will experience less of a problem with either sedation or respiratory depression.

It is also worth noting that unrelieved pain is exhausting. When individuals finally achieve pain relief, they may be able to relax and sleep for the first time in a long while. This is not the same thing as being oversedated; the two can be easily distinguished by noting whether the person's respiratory rate is depressed and whether the person is easily awakened.

Gastrointestinal side effects tend to be more ongoing but in most cases can be minimized or managed through a variety of strategies. Nausea is lessened by taking medication with food and by the administration of antiemetic (antinausea) medication. Constipation may be prevented or managed by dietary modification (increase of fluid and fiber) and the use of medications such as stool softeners and laxatives. Lastly, it is worth noting that people respond differently to different medications; a certain amount of trial and error may be necessary to find the best medication for any given individual.

Flashpoint

Health-care providers should refrain from using the terms *addict* and *addiction.*

Flashpoint

Relief-seeking is too often confused with drug-seeking.

Myth: People with a history of chemical dependency should never be treated with opioid medication.

There is no question that patients with a history of chemical dependency present unique challenges. However, to accept this statement as an ironclad rule does a grave disservice to this patient population. Health-care providers should treat each patient individually, taking all factors into consideration. A careful medical history should be gathered, along with information about the individual's history of substance abuse. Whenever possible, it is generally considered preferable to avoid prescribing opioid medication if adequate pain control can be achieved by other means. However, there are times when this is not possible, and it is never acceptable to withhold opioid medication as a viable treatment option for those suffering severe, unrelieved pain. The American Pain Society states that those with known addiction have been shown to benefit from the judicious use of opioids to manage postoperative pain, cancer pain, and even forms of recurrent pain.

Flashpoint

Pain medication should never be withheld from any patient in severe pain.

When health-care providers do prescribe opioid medication for such individuals, their tendency is to keep doses low, out of fear of worsening the patient's dependency. However, these patients often require more than the typical dose of opioids to achieve adequate pain relief, because of tolerance. In addition, they typically are more sensitive to pain than the average person, because their bodies have stopped producing endorphins. When the decision is made to prescribe opioids for such patients, it should be done thoughtfully, and such patients should be monitored carefully by their primary health-care provider.

Myth: People with chronic pain can learn to develop a greater tolerance for it.

The phrase "just learn to live with it" has been recited all too often to patients who endure chronic pain. Such statements send the message that health-care providers no longer care and are abandoning all efforts to help. They also imply that patients should somehow be able to turn down their sensitivity to pain and feel it less. The first message is sad indeed; the second is totally absurd. Both are unacceptable.

Patients with chronic pain sometimes accept the reality of continued pain, but this is not the same thing as developing a tolerance for it. Their suffering continues and is actually worsened by their feelings of abandonment and isolation.

Myth: Those who complain of chronic pain are really just depressed.

Living with chronic pain takes a severe toll. It is physically, emotionally, psychologically, and spiritually exhausting. Add to this feelings of abandonment and isolation, and the result may be feelings of helplessness and hopelessness. Is it any wonder, then, that such individuals are prone to depression?

Flashpoint

Unrelieved chronic pain can lead to depression.

Depression is indeed a problem among those who suffer from chronic pain. However, it is unfair to assume that depression caused the pain when in fact the reverse is more likely true. In any case, one certainly compounds the other. Unrelieved pain contributes to feelings of depression, and depression certainly impairs the individual's ability to cope effectively with pain. Furthermore, depression seems to actually increase sensitivity to pain. Caring and compassionate health-care providers should address both issues without implying judgment.

Ethics of Pain Control

In recent years the medical community has acknowledged that its response to patients in pain has been woefully inadequate. This has been due in part to an inadequate understanding of pain, inadequate strategies for managing pain, and exaggerated fears about the abuse of medication and about side effects. In an effort to address the problem, some health-care organizations have developed standards and guidelines for the evaluation and management of pain. Pain has been labeled as the fifth vital sign as a reminder that it should be evaluated as frequently as temperature and blood pressure. The Joint Commission has developed the following standards:

Flashpoint

Extensive research shows that most patients' pain has been grossly undertreated for years.

- All patients have the right to have their pain assessed and managed.
- Staff are to be competent in the assessment and management of pain.

- Patients and family members are to be educated about effective pain management.
- Symptom management is to be addressed during discharge planning.
- All care (described above) is to be documented.

The American Academy of Pediatrics' policy statement indicates, among other things, that appropriate tools and techniques should be used for the assessment of pain, and that pain medication should be effectively used for children to ensure compassionate and competent management of pain.

Evaluation of Pain

Effectively treating pain begins with effectively evaluating the patient and the patient's complaints of pain. According to the American Pain Society, the evaluation should begin with a medical history, including a history of the patient's pain, the impact it has had on the patient, and the patient's ability to function on a daily basis. Although pain cannot be objectively measured, the pain scale has emerged as a useful evaluation tool. The scale is used by the patient to rate pain on a scale from zero to 10 (see Box 20-1). This gives the examiner a somewhat accurate indicator of the patient's pain and helps to establish baseline information. As

Box 20-1 Diagnostic Spotlight

PAIN SCALES
The pain experience is totally subjective and does not lend itself to observation or measurement by a second person. Therefore, the pain scale has been identified as a valid tool for assessing pain. The keys to accuracy are identifying a pain scale the patient can relate to and making sure that the patient, rather than the health-care provider, is the person assigning the number rating.

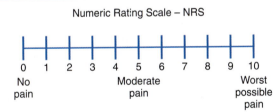

The numeric scale works well for people who are able to assign a number to their pain.

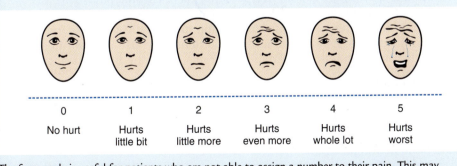

The faces scale is useful for patients who are not able to assign a number to their pain. This may include children or patients who do not speak English.

various interventions are initiated, the scale continues to be a useful indicator of the patient's response. A physical examination should be completed, including a review of any prior diagnostic tests, all treatments and interventions tried, medication history, and evaluation of any other underlying diseases or disorders. Once this information has been gathered, the healthcare provider develops a management plan in collaboration with the patient.

Management of Pain

There are many types of pain and they do not respond equally well to all types of interventions. Therefore, a pain-management plan must be individualized for each person. A variety of strategies might be employed, including medications, surgery, physical therapy, and nontraditional interventions, such as chiropractic and acupuncture. In some cases the patient may be referred to a specialist in pain medicine.

Medications Commonly Used to Treat Pain

There are three groups of medications commonly used to treat and manage pain (see Table 20-2). The first two are *nonopioid analgesics* and *opioid analgesics.* Nonopioid analgesics are pain-relieving medications that contain no opiates; opioid analgesics are pain-relieving medications that contain opiates. The nonopioids include medication that relieves pain and reduces fever by mechanisms that are not fully understood. This group includes *NSAIDs,* which act to reduce the level of inflammatory chemicals released at the site of injury. This action makes NSAIDs an especially good choice for treating painful musculoskeletal and inflammatory problems, such as sprains, strains, and arthritis. NSAIDs also have fever-reducing properties.

Opioid analgesics, formerly called *narcotics*, are a class of potent pain medications that are all opiate derivatives. An example is morphine. Medications in this class have been designated as controlled substances because of their potential for abuse. Therefore, they can only be obtained with a prescription. Combination products are very popular, due to their lower potential for abuse and their *synergistic effect* (enhanced action when two or more agents work together). These medications include an opioid medication and a nonopioid medication (see Table 20-3). This combination helps patients achieve better pain relief while using a lower dose of the opioid medication than if they had used it alone.

The third group of medications is sometimes called *adjuvants* (medications that hasten or increase the action of other agents). These are not analgesics per se, but they have the ability to enhance the effect of analgesics or in some cases, to relieve or reduce certain types of pain on their own. Included in this group are skeletal-muscle relaxants and some types of antidepressants and anticonvulsants. Skeletal-muscle relaxants promote the relaxation of skeletal muscle through their effect on the central nervous system. They have been found useful in treating patients with acute musculoskeletal pain, especially low back pain.

Some types of antidepressants aid in relieving some forms of chronic pain. They are thought to do this by increasing the level of certain neurotransmitters, which then act to block pain signals. They are sometimes helpful in treating *neuropathic pain* (nerve pain) caused by diabetes and shingles. A variety of other conditions may also respond to antidepressants, including fibromyalgia, chronic fatigue syndrome, migraine headaches, arthritis, and back or pelvic pain.

Anticonvulsant medication sometimes helps to relieve certain forms of chronic pain by affecting the action of sodium and calcium on nerve cells. This causes the nerve cells to send fewer pain signals. Anticonvulsants have been found useful in treating some types of cancer pain, trigeminal neuralgia, diabetic neuropathy, migraine headaches, and postherpetic neuralgia.

Corticosteroid medication sometimes helps to relieve acute pain because of its potent anti-inflammatory effect. When inflammation and swelling are reduced, so are the pain they contribute to.

Flashpoint

The most commonly used medications for pain are opioid analgesics and nonopioid analgesics, which include NSAIDs.

Flashpoint

Muscle relaxants are not pain relievers, but they can help relieve painful muscle spasms.

TABLE 20-2

MEDICATIONS USED TO TREAT PAIN

Generic name	Trade name	Common uses
Miscellaneous analgesics		
acetaminophen	Tylenol	most types of mild to moderate pain
NSAIDs		
aspirin	Empirin, Ecotrin	most types of mild to moderate pain; inflammatory conditions
ibuprofen	Motrin, Advil	
naproxen	Aleve, Naprosyn	
ketorolac	Toradol, Acular	
Opiate analgesics		
morphine	Roxanol, MS Contin	moderate to severe postoperative pain, cancer pain, and some types of chronic pain
hydromorphone	Dilaudid	
oxycodone	Oxycontin	
fentanyl	Sublimaze, Duragesic	
methadone	Methadose	
tramadol	Ultram	
Antidepressants		
amitriptyline	Elavil	some types of chronic pain, such as nerve pain, arthritic pain, and cancer pain
paroxetine	Paxil	
fluoxetine	Prozac	
Anticonvulsants		
carbamazepine	Tegretol	trigeminal neuralgia and other types of nerve pain
gabapentin	Neurontin	
valproic acid	Valproate	
phenytoin	Dilantin	
Corticosteroids		
prednisone	Deltasone	exacerbations of inflammatory conditions, such as rheumatoid arthritis
methylprednisolone	Solu-Medrol	

Placebos

A *placebo* is an inactive substance that has no inherent medicinal value. Yet in some cases, individuals who take placebos report a therapeutic response. Because of this, it was sometimes practiced in the past to give placebos instead of opioids to patients who complained frequently of pain. If patients reported pain relief, it was concluded that they had been lying

TABLE 20-3

COMMON COMBINATION PRODUCTS USED TO TREAT PAIN

Trade name	First ingredient (nonopioid analgesic)	Second ingredient (opioid analgesic)
Percocet 5/500	acetaminophen, 500 mg	oxycodone, 5 mg
Tylenol With Codeine #3	acetaminophen, 300 mg	codeine, 30 mg
Vicodin	acetaminophen, 500 mg	hydrocodone, 5 mg

about their pain or that their pain was "all in their heads." In either case, the patients' integrity and honesty were questioned.

As research has led to a greater understanding of the human body, it has come to be acknowledged that the psychological expectation of a response sometimes causes the body to produce that response. In this case, the body sometimes produces endorphins and other pain-relieving chemicals when the brain believes that pain medication has been administered. Therefore, if patients who are given placebos report pain relief, it is entirely possible that their pain and their pain relief are both real. Research shows a response rate as high as 50% among patients who receive placebos; yet the other 50% experience no pain relief at all.

This understanding has led the American Pain Society to issue a statement that the use of placebos is unethical and is to be avoided. If patients are deceptively given a placebo, they may be left wondering why the medication did not work and why they are still in pain. Furthermore, when they learn of the deception, the trust relationship between them and their health-care providers is destroyed. Sadly, they tend to mistrust health-care providers thereafter.

Flashpoint

The use of placebos is unethical except within the context of research studies.

Patients deserve to be treated with respect, dignity, and honesty. They also are legally and ethically entitled to make informed decisions. This isn't possible when critical information is kept from them. For these reasons, it is now recognized that the use of placebos is completely unethical and unacceptable. The exception is when placebos are used within the context of research studies, where patients are informed at the outset that they may be given a placebo instead of the research drug.

Nonpharmacological Interventions

When possible, nonpharmacological strategies should be used to manage pain. In some cases this prevents the need for medication. In other cases it allows for lower doses of medication. Many nonpharmacological treatment methods exist. Common ones include surgery, biofeedback, physical therapy, massage, chiropractic, acupuncture, various forms of meditation, and distraction.

Flashpoint

There are many types of nonpharmacological options for treating pain.

Surgery

Surgical procedures can, in some cases, be performed to relieve or reduce pain. There are many possibilities; the choice depends upon the specific condition being treated. Two examples are diskectomy and laminectomy to relieve back pain. Diskectomy involves the removal of the herniated portion of a disk that is compressing the spinal cord or a spinal nerve. Laminectomy involves the removal of a part of a vertebra to reduce pressure on the spinal cord or nerve roots. In either case, pain relief often occurs as pressure on the spinal cord or spinal nerves is relieved.

Biofeedback

Biofeedback is a type of therapy that teaches patients to control their autonomic (involuntary) nervous system. This involves the use of a variety of technologies that provide feedback about physiological functions. These include electromyography, which provides feedback about muscle tension; skin sensors, which provide feedback about skin temperature; electroencephalography, which provides feedback about brain-wave activity; and electrodermal response, which provides feedback about the activity of the sweat glands. Feedback is given by way of sounds through headphones or blinking lights when changes occur in pulse, blood pressure, brain waves, or muscle contractions. This helps patients to develop an increased awareness of their bodies, thereby gaining greater control over them. The patient then attempts to reproduce the conditions that caused the desired changes. Once the technique is learned, patients are able to reproduce the results without the need for technology. Through this process they learn how to exercise voluntary control over bodily functions that were previously involuntary or unconscious. Because some types of pain respond to improved circulation and muscle relaxation, mastery of this skill helps some patients to relieve or reduce their own pain. Patients usually master the skill after 10 or 12 sessions and are able to use it when pain relief is needed. Biofeedback has been found useful with a number of other conditions as well, including anxiety, hypertension, urinary and fecal incontinence, constipation, migraine and tension headaches, irritable bowel syndrome, and attention deficit-hyperactivity disorder and attention deficit disorder.

Physical Therapy

Physical therapists are experts in providing a variety of treatment modalities, including stretching, exercise, massage, application of heat and cold, and low-impact aerobic conditioning. They also provide treatment through iontophoresis and with devices like TENS units. Iontophoresis provides the transdermal (through the skin) delivery of a substance, usually medication, using positive and negative electrical charges. It is a noninvasive, painless procedure that generally takes 20 to 30 minutes. TENS units are used to deliver small electrical pulses to specified parts of the body with electrodes placed on the skin (see Fig. 20-2). TENS units do not work for everyone, but they seem to relieve or reduce the perception of pain in some people for some types of painful conditions. They produce a painless tingling sensation in the area of application that is thought to interfere with pain messages. They are also thought to increase the body's production of endorphins.

Some physical therapists are also trained in the use of manual physical-therapy techniques that help relax tense muscles and increase flexibility. This generally includes soft-tissue work such as massage and manipulation. These therapies improve circulation, break up scar tissue, ease pain, and realign joints.

Some physical therapists are trained in hydrotherapy, which is ideal for some patients (see Fig. 20-3). Such therapy typically occurs in specially designed therapy pools. In the water, patients are able to participate in weight-bearing exercises that they could not tolerate on dry land. Water creates buoyancy and supports a large percentage of the patient's body weight. This allows greater participation in therapy without causing damage or excessive discomfort. It also

Flashpoint
Biofeedback has been shown to help relieve tension and migraine headaches.

Flashpoint
Physical therapists are able to provide many different types of therapy.

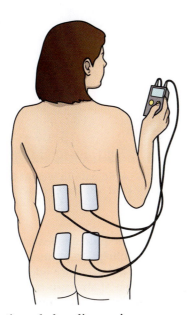

FIGURE 20-2 **TENS units sometimes help relieve pain**

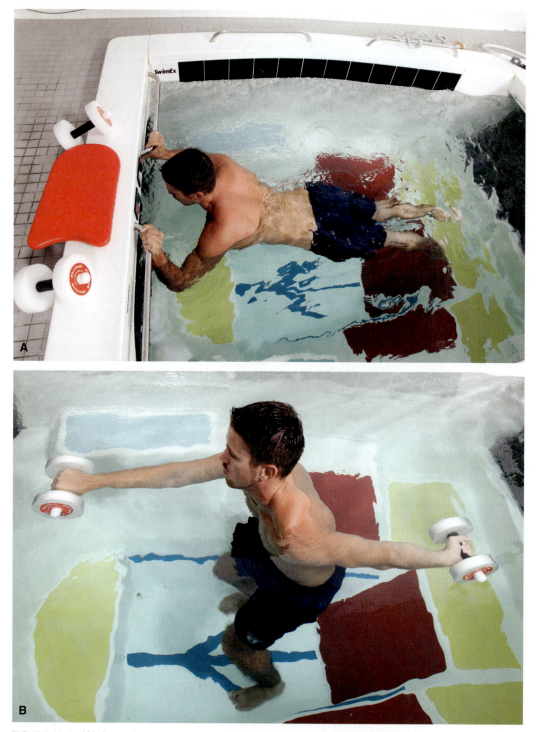

FIGURE 20-3 (A) Aquatherapy allows patients to participate in weight-bearing exercises and other maneuvers they could not tolerate on dry land. (B) Water provides resistance against body movement.

removes the fear of falling, thereby decreasing the patient's fear and anxiety. The water is kept warmer than in a typical swimming pool, which helps to promote relaxation and flexibility. Hydrostatic pressure exerted by the water also helps reduce edema. Water provides resistance against body movement, which adds a dimension of strength training that is not possible on dry land. Finally, most patients find therapy in the water to be much more enjoyable than dry-land therapy. This enjoyment promotes consistency in attendance and enthusiastic participation.

Massage

Massage is useful in relieving or reducing some forms of pain. Many types of massage exist; specific techniques can be adapted to the patient's specific problem and the body parts involved. Rhythmic application of pressure, kneading, and friction produces muscle relaxation, promotes circulation, and stimulates increased production of endorphins and enkephalins. Therapists may focus on specific **trigger points** (tender, painful areas that may cause pain elsewhere), which is known to promote pain relief. Patients also receive the less quantifiable but very real therapeutic benefits created by direct, warm, nurturing human contact.

Chiropractic

The term chiropractic comes from Greek words that mean *done by hand*. It is a form of therapy that involves manipulation of the spine and joints to relieve or reduce pain and stiffness. The profession, founded in the late 1800s, focuses on realigning joints and vertebrae so that nerves, joints, and muscles work more properly. The goal of chiropractic adjustments is to correct any distortions so that nervous system function is optimal. *Straight* chiropractors focus strictly on spinal adjustments, while *mixer* chiropractors combine adjustments with other therapies, such as massage, application of heat and cold, nutrition, and exercise. All forms of pain are treated with chiropractic, including back pain, neck pain, joint pain, and headaches.

Acupuncture

Acupuncture is one of the oldest known forms of therapy; it has been practiced for at least 5,000 years. According to traditional Chinese medicine, there are over 2,000 acupuncture points on the body that connect 20 meridians or channels. It is believed that pain and disease occur when these channels become blocked. The insertion of very fine needles at specific acupuncture points along these channels is thought to restore energy flow (see Fig. 20-4).

A more modern view, according to Western medicine, is that acupuncture therapy releases endorphins, the body's natural painkillers, and may stimulate the immune system and increase production of certain neurotransmitters. The needles are sometimes twirled, and in a Westernized

> **Flashpoint**
> Massage promotes relaxation and circulation and increases production of endorphins.

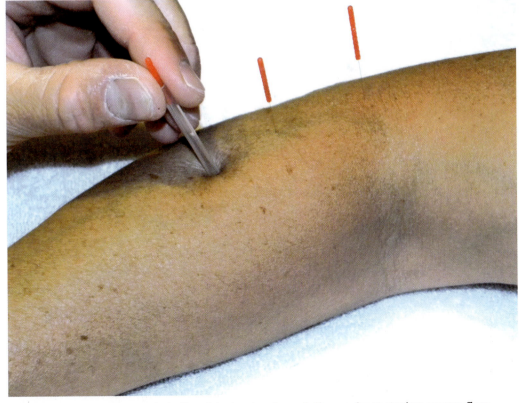

FIGURE 20-4 **Acupuncture is believed to treat pain and disease by restoring energy flow**

version known as percutaneous electrical nerve stimulation, are connected to a very weak electrical current. Each treatment involves a small number of needles and lasts for up to an hour. Patients typically report no pain but occasionally describe a very minor pricking sensation when some needles are inserted. Once needles have been placed, there is no discomfort; many patients find themselves quite relaxed and even doze off during the session. Acupuncture has been found useful in treating many forms of pain, including headaches, neck pain, dental pain, and postoperative pain.

Meditation and Relaxation

Many kinds of relaxation and meditative techniques are useful in reducing pain, relieving anxiety, easing depression, and promoting healing. Many forms exist; all work by inducing a deep state of relaxation. Some of the most common techniques are slow, rhythmic breathing; progressive relaxation of muscle groups; calming of the mind; and imagery or visualization. When using imagery, the person usually imagines an environment that is safe, pleasant, and relaxing. Visualization of a healing blue, pink, or white light on a part of or all of the body may also be used. These techniques promote physical and emotional relaxation and promote the production of endorphins and enkephalins. They are most effective when practiced regularly. Conditions that respond to meditation include insomnia, backache, anxiety, headache, and hypertension.

Flashpoint

Meditation promotes relaxation and the production of endorphins.

Distraction

Many activities can be useful in reducing pain perception through distraction. Some of the possibilities are reading, watching television or movies, playing games, listening to music, and visiting with others. Such activities are effective because they help to take the individual's attention away from the pain and focus it elsewhere. Furthermore, some activities, such as laughing, have been shown to actually increase production of endorphins and enkephalins. Therefore, especially useful activities are watching funny movies, telling jokes, reading humorous books, and any other activity the patient finds humorous.

It is important for health-care providers to note that distraction activities are most useful during the daytime when patients are awake. When patients are trying to relax and calm their minds for sleep, their pain can seem greater and more difficult to ignore. For this reason, many patients can do well taking little or no pain medication during the day but may need it at night to be able to sleep.

A word of caution to health-care providers is appropriate here. They have often been guilty of assuming that a patient's pain can't be that bad because they observe the patient reading, laughing, visiting with friends, or participating in other distraction activities. In fact, the patient may have severe pain but be actively following the advice of health-care providers who have urged the use of distraction as a strategy for managing pain. Yet when the patient does so, the very same providers make accusations that the complaints of pain were exaggerated because the patient now looks like it doesn't hurt. These health-care providers apparently require proof in the form of moaning, crying, or other objective behaviors. This puts patients in a no-win situation: If they act like they are hurting, they may be accused of being overly dramatic and manipulative; on the other hand, if they do not, then their reports of pain are doubted. Such attitudes on the part of health-care providers are actually partly responsible for the exaggerated pain behaviors of some patients, who have learned that they must demonstrate "proof" of their pain in order to be believed. This backfires when such behaviors lead them to be labeled as manipulative and histrionic (theatrical, artificial, and melodramatic). To prevent such situations, health-care providers must remember what they have learned about the subjectivity of pain and make the decision to believe their patients—or at least to give them the benefit of the doubt.

The Partnership Between Patient and Health-Care Provider

The relationship between patient and health-care provider is important in creating successful outcomes for everyone. With this in mind, health-care providers must strive to establish trust and rapport. This takes time and depends upon treating patients with courtesy, respect, and consideration. It is also helpful if health-care providers understand the concepts of locus of control and self-efficacy.

Locus of Control

Locus of control is a concept that relates to the degree of control (or lack of control) that people believe they have over events in their lives. People who believe that everything that happens to them is controlled by fate, chance, luck, God, or any other external source are said to have an external locus of control.

On the other hand, people who believe that they are in control of the events in their lives and that their destinies are largely up to them are said to have an internal locus of control. Of course, many people believe in a combination of the two. In general, it has been found that people whose locus of control is more internal than external are more goal oriented and get higher-paying jobs. They are more likely to put in the study and work necessary to get ahead and earn promotions, because they believe their efforts will pay off. People who believe their fate is up to chance or some external power are less likely to see the value of such efforts. Consequently, their behaviors are more passive.

Understanding the concept of locus of control helps health-care providers better understand their patients. Patients with an internal locus of control are more likely to take charge of their health and demonstrate the willingness to invest time and effort into self-care activities, since they believe they can alter their own destiny. On the other hand, those with an external locus of control tend to be more fatalistic and less likely to adopt lifestyle changes or alter their self-care practices. It is also important to note that those with an external locus of conrol tend to feel more helpless and may at times feel victimized by God, fate, luck, or even their health-care provider.

Providing care for patients with pain, especially those in chronic pain, can be a rewarding experience. It can also be a challenging and frustrating one. A useful strategy is to enlist the patient as a partner and encourage the patient to take responsibility for managing pain. This is may be difficult to accomplish with patients whose locus of control is external. Influencing lifelong beliefs and habits is not easy. The development of locus of control happens over a lifetime but is most influenced during the early formative years, by family, culture, religion, and life experiences. Efforts to influence patients are best aimed at educating them about their illness and treatment plan and performing activities that help to foster their feelings of self-efficacy.

Flashpoint

Patients with an internal locus of control are more likely to make healthy behavior changes.

Self-Efficacy

Self-efficacy is an individual's beliefs about and confidence in that individual's capability of making changes. A number of factors affect a patient's feelings of self-efficacy, including locus of control, self-esteem, and past experience with success or failure. Helping increase a patient's self-efficacy is the key to helping the patient make changes. There are a number of things health-care providers can do to help boost the patient's feelings of self-efficacy (see Box 20-2).

Box 20-2 Wellness Promotion

INCREASING SELF-EFFICACY
The following strategies can help increase a patient's feelings of self-efficacy:

- Identify and address the patient's beliefs and concerns regarding health issues and needed changes.
- Help patients understand the *whys*. Most people feel more enthusiastic about making changes once they understand how they will benefit.
- Start with small, realistic, achievable steps.
- Invite the patient to identify individual learning goals.
- Work new behaviors into the existing routine; this makes change feel less drastic and more possible.
- Ask the patient for a commitment to take specific steps.
- Connect the patient to a support person or support group.

Continued

Box 20-2 Wellness Promotion—cont'd

- Consult with physicians about appropriate referrals for professional consultation. Examples include registered dietitians, diabetes educators, physical therapists, and psychologists.
- Identify a plan for follow-up and let the patient know that you will be monitoring progress.
- Express concern and care. A persuasive statement from a health-care professional can be influential.
- Express confidence in the patient's ability to succeed.

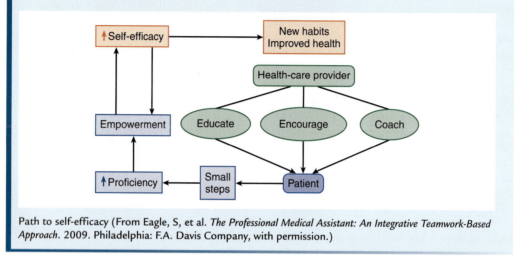

Path to self-efficacy (From Eagle, S, et al. *The Professional Medical Assistant: An Integrative Teamwork-Based Approach*. 2009. Philadelphia: F.A. Davis Company, with permission.)

Student Resources

American Chronic Pain Association: http://www.theacpa.org
American Pain Society: http://www.ampainsoc.org
Association for Applied Psychophysiology and Biofeedback: http://www.aapb.org
International Association for the Study of Pain: http://www.iasp-pain.org

Chapter Activities

Learning Style Study Strategies

Try any or all of the following strategies as you study the content of this chapter:

All learners: Study the two pain scales in this chapter, then draw them each from memory. Once you have completed the drawings, look at the scales again and correct any errors you may have made. Now teach your patient (real or imaginary) how to use the pain scale to rate pain. Do this twice, once as if your patient is an adult and once as if your patient is a 6-year-old child.

All learners: Assign each member of your study group to visit various medical or pain clinics and ask for any literature or brochures they may have regarding the pain-treatment strategies listed here. Read carefully through the brochures and take them to your next study-group session. Group members can take turns sharing what they learned and passing the literature around the group. Examples of information obtained may include the following:

- biofeedback
- physical therapy
- therapeutic massage
- chiropractic
- acupuncture
- meditation
- naturopathic care
- yoga

Practice Exercises

Answers to practice exercises can be found in Appendix D.

Case Studies

CASE STUDY 1

Marjorie McKenna is a 57-year-old woman with rheumatoid arthritis, a disease that has slowly caused destructive changes in her joints. Her hands and fingers are severely affected. This makes it difficult for her to perform daily self-care activities. The rheumatoid arthritis has caused her to have pain on a daily basis that has slowly worsened for the past 20 years.

1. Explain whether this patient's pain falls into the category of acute or chronic pain, and why.

2. What kind of subjective data would indicate that this patient has pain?

3. Is her pain malignant or nonmalignant?

4. What would be an appropriate response to a health-care provider who states that Ms. McKenna's pain is just caused by depression?

CASE STUDY 2

Rafael is a CMA who was recently hired to work in a clinic that specializes in providing care for patients with chronic pain. He is excited about the new challenges this job will present him but knows that he needs to learn more about pain management.

1. What factors should Rafael be aware of that can influence how patients perceive and express pain, and what should he know about each of those factors?

2. What should Rafael understand about the history of health-care professionals' response to their patients' suffering from pain?

3. What should Rafael understand about the Joint Commission's standards regarding pain management?

CASE STUDY 3

Rafael is at work one day in the Pain Clinic and is preparing for a new patient named Joyce O'Brien. Ms. O'Brien was injured at work 15 months ago and has been suffering from chronic back pain since then.

1. While getting acquainted with Ms. O'Brien, Rafael plans to gather information about her locus of control. How will this information be useful in her care?

2. Ms. O'Brien is interested in learning more about nonpharmacological means of controlling pain. Today she specifically wants to know about biofeedback and hydrotherapy. What can Rafael tell her about these therapies?

Multiple Choice

1. All of the following terms are matched with the correct definition **except:**

   a. Adjuvant: medication that hastens or increases the action of other agents

   b. Subjective: observable, measurable, and analyzable

   c. Enkephalins: opiatelike substances produced in the body

   d. Tolerance: phenomenon that develops over time, in which the body loses sensitivity to opioids and their pain-relieving effects

2. All of the following terms are matched with the correct definition **except:**

   a. Pseudoaddiction: behavior that is often mistaken for drug-seeking but is in reality relief-seeking due to poor pain relief

   b. Nociception: transmission of impulses along peripheral nerves to the central nervous system, where the stimulus is perceived as pain

   c. Endorphin: inactive substance that has no inherent medicinal value

   d. Subjective: knowable only by the person involved

3. Which of the following statements is true regarding pain?

   a. Pain is defined as patient behaviors such as muscle tension, frowning, and crying.

   b. Acute pain has been defined as pain that lasts 12 months or less.

   c. Acute pain serves no useful purpose.

   d. The cause of chronic pain is often unclear.

4. All of the following statements are true **except:**

   a. Gate control theory is a generally accepted theory that explains how pain is perceived, how pain signals are transmitted, and why some pain-relieving measures are effective.

   b. There are two types of nerve fibers that conduct pain messages.

   c. The body produces chemicals that reduce the transmission of pain impulses and help to produce an analgesic effect.

   d. TENS units work by delivering neurotransmitters to the central nervous system.

5. All of the following statements are true **except:**

   a. Iontophoresis delivers small electrical pulses to specified parts of the body with electrodes placed on the skin.

   b. Biofeedback can help patients reduce pain through control of the autonomic nervous system.

   c. Diskectomy and laminectomy may help relieve back pain.

   d. Physical therapists may be trained to use manual physical therapy to relax tense muscles and increase flexibility.

Short Answer

1. **Explain why it is unethical to give placebos to patients other than during a research study.**

2. **List at least three things a health-care provider can to do help increase a patient's level of self-efficacy.**

3. **List three myths about pain and tell the truth about each one.**

A

Abduction: Motion away from the midline of the body

Ablation: Destruction of electrical conduction pathways of the AV node

Abrasion: Area where skin or mucous membranes are scraped away

Abscess: Localized collection of pus

Absorption: Process by which nutrients move from the digestive tract into the bloodstream

Accommodation: Ability of the eye to see objects in the distance and then adjust to a close object

Acromegaly: Excessive growth of the bones and tissues of the face and extremities, caused by excessive levels of growth hormone

Acute glaucoma: Form of glaucoma in which a sudden blockage of outflow of the aqueous humor causes a rapid increase in intraocular pressure; also called *closed-angle glaucoma*

Acute pain: Pain lasting 6 months or less that has an identifiable cause and resolves when healing occurs

Adduction: Motion toward the midline of the body

Adhesive capsulitis: Loss of range of motion in the shoulder; also called *frozen shoulder*

Adjuvant: Medication that hastens or increases the action of other agents

Aerobe: Microorganism that needs oxygen to grow

Aerosol: Suspension of tiny droplets or particles in a gas or floating form

Afebrile: Without fever

Affect: Emotional reaction or mood

Agoraphobia: Condition of overwhelming symptoms of anxiety upon leaving home, especially about being trapped in crowded public areas, where a rapid escape might be difficult

Anaerobe: Microorganism that grows without oxygen

Angioplasty: Surgical repair of a vessel by placement of a stent or balloon inflation

Anomaly: Abnormality that develops in utero

Anorexia: Loss of appetite

Antibody: Substance produced by white blood cells in response to a specific antigen that then acts to destroy the disease-causing organism

Antigen: Marker that identifies a cell as being part of the body (self) or not part of the body (nonself)

Antisocial personality disorder: Disorder that features manipulation of others without regard for their feelings or for right and wrong

Antitoxin: Antibody produced in response to and capable of neutralizing a specific biological toxin

Anuria: Absence of urine production

Aphasia: Absence of speech

Apical pulse: Heartbeat heard over the apex of the heart, best for auscultating sounds from the mitral valve

Arrhythmia: Irregularity or loss of rhythm of the heartbeat; also called *dysrhythmia*

Arthrodesis: Surgical procedure to fuse a joint

Asbestosis: Form of pneumoconiosis caused by inhalation of asbestos fibers

Ascites: Abnormal fluid accumulation in the abdominal space between organs

Astigmatism: Abnormality of the eye in which the refraction of a ray of light is spread over a diffuse area rather than sharply focused on the retina

Asymptomatic: Free of symptoms

Ataxia: Lack of coordination

Atelectasis: Condition of collapse or airlessness in parts of the lung

Atrophy: Decrease in mass of a muscle or organ; also called *wasting*

Aura: Sensory warning prior to the onset of a migraine headache or a seizure

Autonomic dysreflexia: Serious nervous system response in those with spinal cord lesions to sensations that normally would be felt as painful; may progress to a stroke

Autosomal dominant disorder: Disorder that can be passed on when just one faulty gene is inherited from one parent

Autosomal recessive disorder: Disorder that can be passed on only when two faulty genes are inherited, one from each parent

Autosome: Any chromosome other than the sex chromosomes

Avoidant personality disorder: Disorder that features feelings of inadequacy, social inhibition, and hypersensitivity to criticism

B

Bacterium: One-celled organism; some bacteria are capable of producing disease

Bargaining: Irrational attempt to negotiate for unlikely or impossible changes

Benign: Noncancerous

Berylliosis: Form of pneumoconiosis caused by inhalation of or exposure to beryllium

Bilateral: Pertaining to both sides

Binge eating disorder: Eating pattern that includes consumption of large quantities of food over short periods of time at least twice a week for 6 months or more; also called *compulsive overeating*

Biofeedback: Type of therapy that teaches patients to control their autonomic (involuntary) nervous system

Biopsy: Removal of a tissue sample from the body for microscopic examination

Bioterrorism: Form of terrorism in which biological agents, such as viruses and bacteria, are used as weapons to kill, injure, threaten, intimidate, or coerce; also called *biowarfare*

Birth defect: Congenital anomaly

Blood pressure: Pressure created by pumping blood

Bolus: Rounded mass of chewed food that is ready for swallowing

Borderline personality disorder: Disorder that features a "black or white" view; unstable self-image, relationships, and moods; and unpredictable and impulsive behavior

Bradykinesia: Slow, hesitating pattern of movement

Bruit: Abnormal swooshing sound

Burnout: Syndrome of feeling physical, emotional, or mental exhaustion caused by ongoing intensive demands without sufficient physical or emotional rest

C

Carcinogen: Cancer-causing substance

Carcinoma: Cancer arising from epithelial tissue

Cardiac cycle: Contraction and relaxation of all chambers of the heart

Cardiac output: Volume of blood pumped by the heart each minute

Cardiomegaly: Enlargement of the heart

Cardioversion: Synchronized shock of electrical current delivered to the chest wall while the patient is under sedation and analgesia

Cataplexy: Sudden, brief loss of muscle control triggered by strong emotion, excitement, surprise, or anger, during which the person remains fully conscious

Category A agents: Biological agents meeting specific criteria that identify them as having a high risk of use as biological weapons

Central scotoma: Blind spot in the center of the visual field surrounded by an area of normal vision

Cholecystectomy: Surgical removal of the gallbladder

Cholinergic crisis: Episode of respiratory failure, paralysis, salivation, and sweating that can occur if a patient takes too much anticholinesterase medication

Chromosome: Linear strand of DNA that carries genetic information

Chronic glaucoma: Form of glaucoma in which the aqueous humor drains too slowly, leading to gradually increased intraocular pressure; also called *primary open-angle glaucoma*

Chronic hypoxia: Chronic lack of oxygen

Chronic pain: Pain lasting 6 months or longer that has a cause that is often unclear

Chyme: Liquid mixture of stomach acids and partially digested food in the stomach and intestines

Circumcision: Procedure in which part or all of the foreskin of the penis is removed

Circumduction: motion of a body part in a circle

Claudication: Sensation of tiredness, aching, cramping, pain, tightness, heaviness, or weakness in the leg (usually the calf) with exercise that is relieved with rest

Coal worker's pneumoconiosis: Form of pneumoconiosis caused by inhalation of coal dust; also called *anthracosis* or *black lung*

Cognition: Thinking that includes language use, calculation, perception, memory, awareness, reasoning, judgment, learning, intellect, social skills, and imagination

Comedones: Small skin lesions of acne that include whiteheads and blackheads

Communicable: Contagious, capable of being passed between individuals

Compulsions: Behaviors performed repeatedly, in a ritualistic manner, in order to relieve the fear or anxiety caused by obsessive thoughts

Conductive hearing loss: Partial or complete hearing loss caused by factors that interfere with sound transmission from the outer to the inner ear

Congenital: Present at birth

Congenital hypothyroidism: Congenital deficiency of thyroid hormones, characterized by arrested physical and mental development; formerly called *cretinism*

Contrecoup: Type of injury in which there is a rapid acceleration followed by deceleration, which throws the brain forward and backward within the skull

Crackles: Abnormal lung sound heard on auscultation that indicates fluid in the alveoli

Cryptorchidism: Undescended testicle(s)

Culture: Laboratory examination of growing microorganisms

Cyanosis: Bluish color due to lack of oxygen

D

Débridement: Removal of dead or damaged tissue

Decortication: Procedure done under general anesthesia in which scar tissue, pus, or other debris is removed from the pleurae and pleural space

Defecation: Elimination of feces from the bowel; also called *bowel movement*

Delirium: Acute, reversible state of agitated confusion marked by disorientation, hallucinations, or delusions

Delusion: False, unfounded belief

Denial: Refusal to accept the reality of a situation

Dependent personality disorder: Disorder that features a chronic, excessive psychological dependence on others

Depolarization: Electrical change in cardiac muscle cells that causes them to contract

Dermabrasion: Process in which outermost layer of skin is scraped away with a wire brush or burr impregnated with diamond particles

Dermatome: Area of skin associated with a pair of spinal nerves

Diabetic ketoacidosis: Condition of severe hyperglycemia

Diaphoresis: Profuse sweating

Diastolic pressure: Lower blood-pressure number, which measures the lowest pressure exerted against artery walls during ventricular relaxation

Digestion: Process by which food is broken down mechanically and chemically in the gastrointestinal tract and converted into absorbable forms

Disease: Any condition characterized by subjective complaints, a specific history, clinical signs, symptoms, and laboratory or radiographic findings

Disseminate: To spread, scatter, or disperse

Diuresis: Abnormal increase in urine production and excretion

DNA: Deoxyribonucleic acid; material inside cells that carries genetic instructions for the individual's development and survival

Dynamic equilibrium: Sense of balance when in motion

Dysentery: Group of disorders marked by intestinal inflammation and diarrhea

Dyspareunia: Pain with intercourse

Dysphagia: Pain or difficulty with swallowing

Dysphasia: Difficulty speaking

Dyspnea: Difficulty breathing

Dysuria: Pain, burning, or other discomfort during urination

E

Edema: Swelling

Empyema: Collection of fluid in the pleural space containing infectious matter, such as bacteria and white blood cells

Endorphins: Opiatelike substances produced in the body

Enkephalins: Opiatelike substances produced in the body

Equilibrium: Sense of balance

Ergonomics: Study of human ability relative to work demands

Erythema: Redness

Esotropia: Form of strabismus in which one or both eyes are turned inward

Etiology: Cause

Eversion: Motion that turns a body part outward

Exacerbation: Aggravation of symptoms or increase in severity

Excretion: Process of eliminating bulk waste (feces) from the anus

Exophthalmos: Protruding eyeballs

Exotropia: Form of strabismus in which one or both eyes are turned outward

Exposure therapy: Therapy that involves exposing the patient repeatedly to the situation or object that triggers anxiety

Extension: Motion that straightens a body part

Exudate: Substance that drains out

F

Fasting: Going without food or nutrition, usually for a specified period of time before laboratory tests or surgical procedures

Febrile: Having a fever

Flail chest: Injury in which three or more ribs are fractured in two or more places, creating a free-floating segment

Flatulence: Gassiness

Flexion: Motion that bends a body part

Fomite: Any object that adheres to and transmits infectious material (e.g., comb, countertop, drinking glass)

Frequency: Need to urinate frequently

Friction: Rubbing of skin against bedding, linens, a brace, a cast, etc.

Fungus: Organism such as yeast, mold, or mushroom; most are not pathogenic

G

Gait: Manner of walking

Gate control theory: Generally accepted theory that suggests that the experience of pain depends upon the results of competition between neurotransmitters and neuromodulators

Gene: Basic, self-replicating unit of heredity, made up of pieces of DNA

Genetic: Inherited

Genetic mutation: Permanent change in genetic structure within the sperm or egg cell that causes a change in the offspring that is different from the parents; or a permanent change in an individual's DNA triggered by exposure to an environmental factor

Gestation: Time from conception to birth

Gigantism: Form of hyperpituitarism that results in an abnormal increase in height and size

Gingivectomy: Excision of part of the gums

Glioma: Cancer arising from glial cells

Glucometer: Instrument used to measure glucose levels in the blood

Goiter: Enlarged thyroid gland

Goniometry: Process of measuring joint movements and angles

Grading: Standardized process of describing differentiation of cancer cells, from grade I to grade IV

Grandiosity: Inflated sense of self-importance

Graves disease: Autoimmune form of hyperthyroidism

Gustation: Sense of taste

H

Hallucination: False sensory perception

Hematopoiesis: Production and development of blood cells

Hematuria: Presence of blood in the urine

Hemiparalysis: One-sided paralysis

Hemiparesis: Altered sensation on one side of the body

Hemodialysis: Filtration of wastes and fluid from blood as it passes through selectively permeable membranes; also called *dialysis*

Hemoptysis: Spitting or coughing up blood from the respiratory tract

Hepatomegaly: Enlargement of the liver

Hirsutism: Male pattern of body-hair development

Histamine: Chemical which causes the dilation of blood vessels and other activities in the inflammatory response

Histrionic personality disorder: Disorder that features chronic attention-seeking and emotionalism, dramatic behavior, exaggeration, and angry outbursts

Homeostasis: Dynamic state of equilibrium in the body

Hypercapnea: Chronic retention of carbon dioxide, leading to symptoms of mental cloudiness and lethargy

Hyperextension: Extension of a body part beyond its normal limits

Hyperglycemia: High blood glucose

Hyperkeratosis: Thickening of the skin

Hyperplasia: Increased cell growth

Hypertropia: Form of strabismus in which one or both eyes are turned upward

Hypotropia: Form of strabismus in which one or both eyes are turned downward

Hypoxemia: Condition of low blood oxygen

I

Idiopathic: Having an unknown or uncertain cause

Impaction: Cavity that is tightly packed or overloaded

Impulse control disorder: Failure to resist performing socially unacceptable or even harmful behaviors

In situ: Confined to the original site

Incubation: Interval between exposure to infection and the appearance of the first symptoms

Infectious disease: Any disease transmitted directly or indirectly between individuals; also called *communicable disease*

Ingestion: Oral consumption

Interferon: Chemical produced by white blood cells in response to pathogen invasion that inhibits virus production within infected cells

Intussusception: Telescoping of the bowel into itself

Inversion: Motion that turns a body part inward

Ischemia: Temporary deficiency in blood supply

J

Jaundice: Condition of increased bilirubin in the blood that results in yellow staining of the skin and mucous membranes

K

Karyotype: Analysis based on a photomicrograph of the chromosomes of a single cell

Keratinized: Hardened

Kinins: Chemicals that increase blood flow and increase the permeability of small blood capillaries as a part of the inflammatory response

L

Laceration: Cut or tear in the flesh

Lactation: Production of breast milk

Laparotomy: Incision into the abdomen

Lavage: Irrigation or rinsing out of a body cavity

Legal blindness: Vision that is worse than 20/200 in the better eye with correction

Lesions: Skin wounds or sores

Leukemia: Cancer arising from blood-forming cells

Leukocytes: White blood cells that act against infection and tissue damage

Leukocoria: White pupil caused by retinoblastoma; also called *cat's eye reflex*

Lithotripsy: Procedure in which shock waves or sound waves crush stones in the kidneys or urinary tract

Lobectomy: Surgical removal of a lobe of the lung

Lower endoscopy: Visual examination of the lower digestive tract with a scope

Lymph: Clear, colorless, alkaline fluid found within lymph vessels; made up of water, protein, salts, urea, fats, and white blood cells

Lymphadenopathy: Enlarged, tender lymph nodes

Lymphocyte: White blood cell

Lymphoma: Cancer arising from lymphatic cells

Lysozyme: Enzyme present in tears, saliva, and other secretions which protects against pathogens

M

Malaise: Discomfort, weakness, fatigue

Malignant: Cancerous

Malignant pain: Cancer pain

Mastication: Chewing

Medical asepsis: Destruction of pathogenic organisms after they leave the body

Melanoma: Cancer arising from pigmented skin cells

Melena: Tarry black stool caused by the presence of digested blood

Menorrhagia: Excessive menstrual flow

Mental health: State that allows individuals to function effectively in all dimensions of life

Mental illness: State of having one or more psychological disorders that affect mood or behavior and create mental or emotional pain, disability, or distress

Metastasize: To spread to distant sites

Microorganism: Living organism too small to be seen by the naked eye

Micturition reflex: Urge to urinate

Mitral valve prolapse: Abnormal displacement of the mitral valve into the atrium each time it attempts to close

Motor tic: Sudden, spasmodic, involuntary muscular contraction, usually involving the face, mouth, eyes, head, neck, or shoulders

Myasthenic crisis: Potentially life-threatening episode of worsening of myasthenic symptoms

Mycotoxin: Poison produced by a fungus

Myeloma: Cancer arising from cells that comprise the blood-forming part of the bone marrow

Myringotomy: Procedure in which a tiny tube is placed in the tympanic membrane

Myxedema: Waxy, coarse changes in skin texture caused by a severe form of hypothyroidism

N

Narcissistic personality disorder: Disorder that features a pattern of superiority and grandiosity combined with oversensitivity to criticism and a tendency to become easily enraged or depressed

Necrosis: Tissue death

Negative feedback system: System in which an increase or decrease in a substance stimulates an opposite response

Neonatal: Newborn

Nephropathy: Diseased changes of the kidneys, with eventual kidney failure

Neuropathic pain: Nerve pain

Neuropathy: Motor and/or sensory nerve damage from long-standing diabetes

Neurotransmitter: Chemical released by an axon terminal (end of a neuron) to inhibit or excite a target cell

Nociception: Transmission of impulses along peripheral nerves to the central nervous system, where the stimulus is perceived as pain

Nocturia: Frequent need to urinate during the night

Nonmalignant pain: Noncancer pain

Nonopioid analgesic: Pain-relieving medication that contains no opiates

Normal flora: Organisms commonly found on and in the body that do not cause disease

Nosocomial: Acquired within the hospital

NSAID: Nonsteroidal anti-inflammatory drug; nonsteroid medication used to relieve pain and reduce inflammation

Nuchal rigidity: Pain and stiffness of the neck with a resulting reluctance to flex the head forward

Nystagmus: Involuntary back-and-forth or circular eye movement

O

Objective: Observable, measurable, and analyzable

Obsessions: Persistent, recurring, and distressing thoughts, images, feelings, or impulses that are unwanted and intrusive

Obsessive-compulsive personality disorder: Disorder that features rigid conformity to rules and moral codes combined with inflexibility and an excessive need for order; differs from obsessive-compulsive disorder in that it does not include unwanted pattern of obsessions and compulsions

Olfaction: Sense of smell

Oliguria: Deficient urine production

Ophthalmoscope: Handheld device used to examine the interior of the eye

Opioid analgesic: Pain-relieving medication that contains opiates

Opportunistic infections: Infections by pathogens that do not normally cause disease unless the immune system is impaired

Orchiectomy: Surgical removal of one or both testes

Orthopnea: Difficulty breathing that is eased by sitting rather than lying down

Otoscope: Handheld device used to view the outer ear canal and tympanic membrane

P

Palliative care: Treatment aimed at preventing or relieving pain and suffering associated with disease

Palliative surgery: Surgery done to ease pain and improve quality of life

Palpitation: Sensation of rapid or irregular beating of the heart

Panhypopituitarism: Condition of diminished secretion of all hormones secreted by the anterior pituitary gland

Paradoxical motion: Motion of a free-floating fractured rib segment in the opposite direction from the rest of the chest as the patient breathes

Paranoid personality disorder: Disorder that features unwarranted suspicion and mistrust

Parasite: Pathogen requiring another living organism in order to live

Paresthesia: Altered sensation, such as numbness, stinging, or burning, that results from injury to nerves

Paroxysmal-nocturnal dyspnea: Episodes of dyspnea at night that occur repeatedly and without warning

Pathogen: Disease-producing microorganism

Pathogenic: Disease-causing

Pathological fracture: Breaking of diseased, weakened bone from the stress of normal, everyday activities

Pathologist: One who is devoted to the study of human tissues, cells, and body fluids for evidence of disease

Perfusion: Circulation of blood, nutrients, and oxygen through tissues and organs

Pericardial effusion: Increased fluid collection between the heart and pericardium

Peristalsis: Rhythmic, wavelike muscular contractions of a tubular structure

Peritoneal dialysis: Filtration of fluid and wastes from the blood using the lining of the patient's peritoneal cavity as a dialyzing membrane

Petechiae: Tiny purple-red hemorrhagic spots under the skin

pH scale: Tool for measuring the acidity or alkalinity of a substance

Phagocytosis: Process in which specialized white blood cells engulf and destroy microorganisms, foreign antigens, and cell debris

Pharyngitis: Sore (inflamed) throat

Phimosis: Stenosis of the foreskin opening so that it cannot be pushed back over the glans penis

Phobia: any persistent, intense anxiety about and irrational fear of an object, activity, or situation

Phonophobia: Sensitivity to sound

Photophobia: Sensitivity to light

Physical dependence: Condition of physical tolerance and, with sudden discontinuation of the substance, display of a withdrawal syndrome

Pituitary dwarfism: Condition of reduced growth and development due to deficiency of growth hormone in childhood

Placebo: Inactive substance that has no inherent medicinal value

Pleural friction rub: Low-pitched scratching, creaking, grating sound made by the pleurae as they rub against one another

Pleurodesis: Procedure in which a sterile, irritating substance is infused into the pleural space, causing the pleural linings to develop scar tissue and fuse to one another

Pneumonectomy: Surgical removal of an entire lung

Polydipsia: Excessive thirst

Polyphagia: Excessive appetite

Polyuria: Excessive urination

Portal hypertension: Increased pressure in the vein entering the liver

Postphlebitic syndrome: Chronic condition, marked by edema and aching, that may develop after an episode of phlebitis

Prehypertension: Blood pressure in which the systolic pressure is between 120 and 140 or the diastolic pressure is between 80 and 90

Primary eye cancer: Cancer that originates within the eyes

Proctoscopy: Visual examination of the anus and rectum with a scope

Prodromal: Occuring between earliest symptoms and the appearance of a rash or fever

Pronation: Act of lying facedown or turning the hand so the palm faces downward

Prostaglandins: Hormones that stimulate receptors and produce localized vasodilation, vascular permeability, and platelet aggregation

Proteinuria: Presence of protein in the urine

Protozoan: Organism; most protozoans live in soil, and some are capable of producing disease

Pruritus: Itching

Pseudoaddiction: Behavior that is often mistaken for drug-seeking but is in reality relief-seeking due to poor pain relief

Psychological dependence: Emotional and behavioral symptoms of craving, compulsive drug-seeking, hoarding, and use of substances purely for emotional and mental euphoria

Pulmonary embolism: Obstruction by a blood clot of vessels in the lungs

Pulse points: Points on large arteries in the body that have a strong pulse and are easily palpated; also called pressure points

R

Range of motion: Normal range through which a joint moves

Rape: Forced vaginal, anal, or oral penetration

Reconstructive surgery: Surgery done to restore the body as close as possible to its original appearance and function

Reduction: Manual manipulation of a bone to return it to its normal position

Remission: Period of improvement or absence of disease activity

Renal colic: Severe, intermittent pain caused by spasm of the ureter

Retinopathy: Disease of the retina caused by poorly controlled diabetes

Rotation: Motion that turns a body part about its axis

Rhinophyma: Large, irregularly shaped, dark-red nose

S

Schizoid personality disorder: Disorder that features shyness, oversensitivity, withdrawal, eccentricity, daydreaming, and an inability to express normal anger or joy

Schizotypal personality disorder: Disorder that features odd behavior and thinking similar to that of people with schizophrenia; social and emotional detachment; magical thinking; and possible paranoid thoughts

Sciatica: Pain from compression of the sciatic nerve that radiates down the leg to the ankle

Self-care: Any activity which supports and nurtures one's physical, mental, spiritual, or emotional health and well-being

Sensorineural hearing loss: Partial or complete hearing loss caused by degeneration of or damage to the sound pathway from the hair cells of the inner ear to the auditory nerve and brain

Sepsis: systemic infection

Shearing: Sliding downward of deeper structures due to gravity while the skin remains in place

Silicosis: Form of pneumoconiosis caused by inhalation of silica (quartz) dust; also called *grinder's disease, progressive massive fibrosis,* and *potter's rot*

Social anxiety disorder: Persistent irrational fear of, and need to avoid, social-performance situations in which the individual might be exposed to potentially embarrassing or humiliating scrutiny by others; also called *social phobia*

Specific phobia: Intense fear and anxiety related to a specific object or situation

Spontaneous bleeding episodes: Episodes of bleeding with no identifiable cause that are sometimes seen in individuals with hemophilia

Staging: Identifying the extent of dissemination of the cancer, including tumor size and regional and distant metastasis

Staging surgery: Surgery done to identify the extent of cancer

Standard precautions: Guidelines for the handling of any blood or body fluids (except sweat) that might contain blood or infectious organisms

Stasis: Sluggish blood flow

Static equilibrium: Ability to maintain a steady position of the head and body in relation to gravity

Steatorrhea: Presence of fat in the stool

Strangulated hernia: Herniated tissue that has had the blood supply cut off, resulting in necrosis and possible septicemia

Stress incontinence: Leakage of urine with minor physical stress, such as coughing, sneezing, or laughing

Stridor: High-pitched breathing sound

Subjective: Knowable only by the person involved

Substance abuse: Persistent maladaptive pattern of substance use over a 12-month period, in which an individual continues substance use in spite of significant adverse consequences

Substance dependence: Continued substance abuse, compulsive use behaviors, development of tolerance, and withdrawal symptoms with discontinuation

Supination: Act of lying faceup or turning the hand so the palm faces upward

Supportive surgery: Surgery done to aid in the delivery of other therapies

Surgical asepsis: Destruction of pathogenic organisms before they enter the body

Sutures: Stitches used to hold tissue together

Symptomatic: Having symptoms, such as fever, sore throat, nausea, or vomiting

Syncope: Fainting

Synergistic effect: Enhanced action when two or more agents work together

Systolic pressure: Upper blood-pressure number, which measures the highest pressure exerted against artery walls during ventricular contraction

T

Tachycardia: Rapid heartbeat

Tachypnea: Rapid breathing

Telangiectasia: Appearance of dilated vessels on the skin of cheeks and nose

Terrorism: Violent act or threat with the intention of intimidating or coercing the government or civilian population to behave in a particular manner

Tet spells: Episodes in which an infant's arterial oxygen level drops, seen in infants with tetralogy of Fallot

Thyrotoxicosis: Severe episode of worsening symptoms of hyperthyroidism

Tinnitus: Ringing or other abnormal sounds in the ears

Tolerance: Phenomenon that develops over time, in which the body loses sensitivity to opiates and their pain-relieving effects

Trigger point: Tender, painful area that may cause pain elsewhere

U

Unilateral: Pertaining to one side

Uremia: Presence of increased nitrogenous waste products, especially urea, in the blood

Urge incontinence: Leakage of urine with the urge to void

Urgency: Need to urinate urgently

Urinalysis: Laboratory analysis of the urine

Upper endoscopy: Visual examination of the upper digestive tract with a scope

Uteropexy: Surgical fixation of the uterus

V

Vasopressin: Hormone that helps the body concentrate urine and conserve water

Vector: Carrier, usually an insect, that transmits a disease from an infected person to a noninfected person

Vertigo: Sensation of moving around in space and extreme dizziness

Virus: Pathogen which grows and reproduces after infecting a host cell

Vocal tic: Involuntary sound such as clearing the throat, grunting, or uttering words

Volvulus: Twisting of the bowel on itself resulting in obstruction

W

Wheezes: Musical sound caused by narrowed air passages

X

X chromosome: One of two chromosomes that determine gender in humans; determines female gender

X-linked recessive disorder: Disorder inherited by a man from his mother because the trait is attached to a gene error on the X chromosome

Y

Y chromosome: One of two chromosomes that determine gender in humans; determines male gender

ABBREVIATIONS

SYMBOLS

♀	female
♂	male

A

AAA	abdominal aortic aneurysm
Ab	antibody
ABG, ABGs	arterial blood gases
ac	before meals
ACTH	adrenocorticotropic hormone
ADD	attention deficit disorder
ADH	antidiuretic hormone
ADHD	attention deficit-hyperactivity disorder
ADL	activities of daily living
AFP	alpha-fetoprotein
Ag	antigen
AGA	appropriate for gestational age
AIDS	acquired immune deficiency syndrome
AK	above the knee
AKA	above-the-knee amputation
ALS	amyotrophic lateral sclerosis
ANA	antinuclear antibody
ANS	autonomic nervous system
APGAR	activity, pulse, grimace, appearance, respiration
ARDS	acute respiratory distress syndrome
ARF	acute renal failure
ARMD	age-related macular degeneration
AS	ankylosing spondylitis
ASD	atrial septal defect
ATN	acute tubular necrosis
AV	atrioventricular

B

BG	blood glucose; also called *blood sugar*
BK	below the knee

BKA	below-the-knee amputation
BM	bowel movement
BMD	Becker muscular dystrophy
BP	blood pressure
BPH	benign prostatic hypertrophy (hyperplasia)
BS	blood sugar; also called *blood glucose*
BSE	breast self-examination
BSL	biosafety level
BUN	blood urea nitrogen
Bx, bx	biopsy

C

C&S	culture and sensitivity
C1–C7	first cervical vertebra, second cervical vertebra, etc.
Ca	calcium
CA	cancer
CAD	coronary artery disease
CBC	complete blood count
CDC	Centers for Disease Control and Prevention
CF	cystic fibrosis
CFIDS	chronic fatigue and immune dysfunction syndrome
CFS	chronic fatigue syndrome
CIS	carcinoma in situ
CMC	chronic mucocutaneous candidiasis
CNS	central nervous system
CO_2	carbon dioxide
COPD	chronic obstructive pulmonary disease
CP	cerebral palsy
CPAP	continuous positive airway pressure
CPR	cardiopulmonary resuscitation
CRF	chronic renal failure
C-section	cesarean section
CSF	cerebrospinal fluid

CT	computed tomography
CTS	carpal tunnel syndrome
CVA	cerebrovascular accident
CVS	chorionic villus sampling
CWP	coal worker's pneumoconiosis

D

D&C	dilation and curettage
DD, DDx, ddx	differential diagnosis
DDH	developmental dislocation of the hip
decub	decubitus ulcer
derm	dermatology
DIC	disseminated intravascular coagulation
DKA	diabetic ketoacidosis
DM	diabetes mellitus
DMD	Duchenne muscular dystrophy
DNA	deoxyribonucleic acid
DRE	digital rectal examination
DTP	diphtheria-pertussis-tetanus (vaccine)
DTR	deep tendon reflex
DVT	deep vein thrombosis
Dx	diagnosis

E

EBV	Epstein-Barr virus
ECG	electrocardiography
ECT	electroconvulsive therapy
ED	erectile dysfunction
EDR	electrodermal response
EEG	electroencephalogram
EENT	eyes, ears, nose, and throat
EGD	esophagogastroduodenoscopy
EMG	electromyography
ENT	ears, nose, and throat
EOM	extraocular movement
ESR	erythrocyte sedimentation rate
ESRD	end-stage renal disease

F

FAS	fetal alcohol syndrome
FBG	fasting blood glucose; also called *fasting blood sugar*

FBS	fasting blood sugar; also called *fasting blood glucose*
FSH	follicle-stimulating hormone
FTT	failure to thrive
Fx	fracture

G

GAD	generalized anxiety disorder
GBS	Guillain-Barré syndrome
GC	gonorrhea
GFR	glomerular filtration rate
GH	growth hormone
GI	gastrointestinal
GVHD	graft-versus-host disease
GYN, gyn	gynecology

H

HAART	highly active antiretroviral therapy
HCG, hCG	human chorionic gonadotropin
HD	Huntington disease
HEENT	head, eyes, ears, nose, and throat
HPS	hantavirus pulmonary syndrome
HPV	human papillomavirus
HRT	hormone replacement therapy
HSV	herpes simplex virus

I

I&D	incision and drainage
IASP	International Association for the Study of Pain
IC	interstitial cystitis
ICP	intracranial pressure
ID	intradermal (injection)
IDDM	insulin-dependent diabetes mellitus; also called *type 1 diabetes*
IM	intramuscular
INR	international normalized ratio
IOP	intraocular pressure
ITP	idiopathic thrombocytopenic purpura
IUD	intrauterine device
IV	intravenous
IVF	in vitro fertilization
IVP	intravenous pyelography

J

JVD   jugular-vein distention

K

KUB   kidney, ureter, bladder

L

L1–L5   first lumbar vertebra, second lumbar vertebra, etc.

LA   left atrium

LASIK   laser-assisted in situ keratomileusis

LH   luteinizing hormone

LLE   left lower extremity

LMP   last menstrual period

LP   lumbar puncture

LUE   left upper extremity

LV   left ventricle

M

MDD   major depressive disorder

MI   myocardial infarction

MMPI   Minnesota Multiphasic Personality Inventory

MMR   measles-mumps-rubella (vaccine)

MMSE   Mini-Mental State Examination

MRSA   methicillin-resistant *Staphylococcus aureus*

MS   morphine sulfate; multiple sclerosis

N

N&V   nausea and vomiting

NCV   nerve conduction velocity

NG   nasogastric

NIDDM   non–insulin-dependent diabetes mellitus; also called *type 2 diabetes*

NPC   nasopharyngeal carcinoma; nonproductive cough

NPO, npo   nothing by mouth

NSR   normal sinus rhythm

NTD   neural tube defect

O

O$_2$ oxygen

OB   obstetrics

OC   oral contraceptives

OCD   obsessive-compulsive disorder

ODD   oppositional defiant disorder

OI   osteogenesis imperfecta

OM   otitis media

ORIF   open reduction and internal fixation

ortho   orthopedic; straight

OT   occupational therapy

OTC   over-the-counter

P

PAC   premature atrial contraction

PAD   peripheral artery disease

PAP, Pap   Papanicolaou smear, Papanicolaou test

pc   after meals

PCOS   polycystic ovary syndrome

PCP   *Pneumocystis carinii* pneumonia

PDA   patent ductus arteriosus

PE   pulmonary embolism

Peds   pediatrics

PENS   percutaneous electrical nerve stimulation

PERRLA   pupils are equal, round, reactive to light and accommodation

PFTs   pulmonary function tests

pH   potential of hydrogen

PID   pelvic inflammatory disease

PKD   polycystic kidney disease

PKU   phenylketonuria

PM   polymyositis

PMS   premenstrual syndrome

PND   paroxysmal-nocturnal dyspnea; postnasal drainage; postnasal drip

PNS   peripheral nervous system

PO, po   by mouth

PPD   purified protein derivative (TB test)

PR   per rectum

PSA   prostate-specific antigen

PT   physical therapy; prothrombin time

PTH   parathormone; also called *parathyroid hormone*

PTSD   post-traumatic stress disorder

PTT   partial thromboplastin time

PVC   premature ventricular contraction

PVD   peripheral vascular disease

R

RA	right atrium
RBC	red blood cell
RLE	right lower extremity
ROM	range of motion
RP	retrograde pyelogram
RSV	respiratory syncytial virus
RUE	right upper extremity
RV	right ventricle
Rx	prescription

S

S1–S5	first sacral vertebra, second sacral vertebra, etc.
SA	sinoatrial
SAD	seasonal affective disorder; social anxiety disorder
SCC	squamous cell carcinoma
SCI	spinal cord injury
SIDS	sudden infant death syndrome
SLE	systemic lupus erythematosus
SNRI	serotonin and norepinephrine reuptake inhibitor
SOB	short of breath
SS	Sjögren syndrome
SSRI	selective serotonin reuptake inhibitor
STI	sexually transmitted infection
Sub-Q	subcutaneous
supp	suppository
Sx	symptom

T

T&A	tonsillectomy and adenoidectomy
T1–T12	first thoracic vertebra, second thoracic vertebra, etc.
T_3	triiodothyronine
T_4	thyroxine

TAH	total abdominal hysterectomy
TAO	thromboangiitis obliterans
TB	tuberculosis
TENS	transcutaneous electrical nerve stimulation
THA	total hip arthroplasty; also called *total hip replacement*
THR	total hip replacement; also called *total hip arthroplasty*
TKA	total knee arthroplasty; also called *total knee replacement*
TKR	total knee replacement; also called *total knee arthroplasty*
TM	tympanic membrane
TMJ	temporomandibular joint
TNM	tumor, node, metastasis
Trich	trichomoniasis
TS	Tourette syndrome
TSE	testicular self-examination
TSH	thyroid-stimulating hormone
TSS	toxic shock syndrome
TUNA	transurethral needle ablation
TURP	transurethral resection of the prostate
Tx	treatment

U

UA	urinalysis
URI	upper respiratory infection
ung	ointment
UTI	urinary tract infection

V

VC	vital capacity
VHF	viral hemorrhagic fever
VSD	ventricular septal defect

W

WBC	white blood cell
WHO	World Health Organization

DRUGS AND DRUG CLASSIFICATIONS

There are thousands of prescription and OTC drugs on the market. New ones are added continually, and occasionally, old ones are pulled from the market. This table is not comprehensive. It simply reflects a list of most of the classifications of drugs mentioned in this text. Furthermore, many drugs have numerous trade names. This table lists only a few.

ADRENERGIC AGENTS

Other classifications	Generic name	Trade name	Common uses
	albuterol	Proventil	asthma, emphysema
	epinephrine	Adrenalin	asthma, COPD, anaphylaxis

ALPHA-ADRENERGIC BLOCKERS

Other classifications	Generic name	Trade name	Common uses
	phentolamine mesylate	Phentolamine	hypertensive episodes in patients with pheochromocytoma, prevention or treatment of dermal necrosis caused by norepinephrine, diagnosis of pheochromocytoma, blocking test

ALS AGENTS

Other classifications	Generic name	Trade name	Common uses
	riluzole	Rilutek	ALS

ANALGESICS

Other classifications	Generic name	Trade name	Common uses
antipyretics	acetaminophen	Tylenol	most types of mild to moderate pain, fever
antipyretics, NSAIDs, platelet inhibitors, salicylates	aspirin	Empirin, Bayer Aspirin	mild pain, inflammatory conditions, MI, ischemic stroke, TIA
antipyretics, cyclooxygenase-1 (COX-1) inhibitors, NSAIDs	ibuprofen indomethacin ketorolac naproxen	Motrin, Advil Indocin Toradol Aleve, Naprosyn	mild to moderate pain associated with inflammatory conditions, dysmenorrhea, fever
cyclooxygenase-2 (COX-2) inhibitors	celecoxib	Celebrex	mild to moderate pain associated with inflammatory conditions, dysmenorrhea
analgesics, topical	menthol	Blistex	pain caused by cold sores

Continued

725

ANALGESICS, OPIATE

Other classifications	Generic name	Trade name	Common uses
analgesics, opioid	codeine sulfate	Codeine	moderate to severe pain
	fentanyl	Sublimaze, Duragesic	
	hydrocodone	Vicodin	
	hydromorphone	Dilaudid	
	morphine	Roxanol, MS Contin	
	oxycodone	Oxycontin, Roxicodone	
	tramadol	Ultram	

ANALGESICS, COMBINATION PRODUCTS

Trade name	Opiate substance	Nonopiate substance	Common uses
Lortab	hydrocodone, 10 mg	acetaminophen, 500 mg	moderate to severe pain
Percocet 7.5/500	oxycodone, 7.5 mg	acetaminophen, 500 mg	moderate to severe pain
Percodan	oxycodone, 4.5 mg	aspirin, 325 mg	moderate to severe pain
Tylenol With Codeine #3	codeine, 30 mg	acetaminophen, 300 mg	moderate to severe pain
Vicodin	hydrocodone, 5 mg	acetaminophen, 500 mg	moderate to severe pain

ANDROGENS

Other classifications	Generic name	Trade name	Common uses
	fluoxymesterone	Androxy	male hypogonadism

ANESTHETICS

Other classifications	Generic name	Trade name	Common uses
anesthetics, topical	benzocaine 20%	Kanka	pain caused by canker sores
anesthetics, topical	viscous lidocaine 2%	Lidocaine	pain caused by mucositis

ANESTHETICS, GENERAL AND LOCAL

Other classifications	Generic name	Trade name	Common uses
anesthetics, general	propofol	Diprivan	general surgery, surgical procedures,
	thiopental	Pentothal	
anesthetics, local	lidocaine	Xylocaine	procedures such as suturing of a laceration or dentistry
	procaine	Novocain	

ANTACIDS

Other classifications	Generic name	Trade name	Common uses
calcium supplements	calcium carbonate	Tums, Caltrate	antacid, calcium supplement, hypertension in pregnancy, osteoporosis, hypocalcemia, hyperparathyroidism

ANTIACNE

Other classifications	Generic name	Trade name	Common uses
	isotretinoin	Accutane	severe cystic acne

ANTIANGINALS

Other classifications	Generic name	Trade name	Common uses
nitrates	nitroglycerin	Nitrostat, Nitro-Bid	angina
calcium channel blockers	diltiazem nifedipine	Cardizem Procardia	angina, hypertension

ANTIANXIETY

Other classifications	Generic name	Trade name	Common uses
	alprazolam	Xanax	anxiety
	lorazepam	Ativan	anxiety, insomnia

ANTIBIOTICS

Other classifications	Generic name	Trade name	Common uses
aminoglycosides	gentamicin streptomycin	Garamycin, Cidomycin, Septopal	bacterial infection
cephalosporins	cefaclor cefazolin cefixime cefotaxime cephalexin	Ceclor Ancef Suprax Claforan Keflex	bacterial infection
fluoroquinolones	ciprofloxacin levofloxacin	Cipro Levaquin	bacterial infection
penicillins	amoxicillin/ clavulanate ampicillin/ sulbactam dicloxacillin	Augmentin Unasyn Dyapen	bacterial infection
tetracyclines	doxycycline tetracycline	Oracea Sumycin	bacterial infection
sulfonamides	trimethoprim and sulfamethoxazole	Bactrim	bacterial and protozoal infection

ANTICHOLINERGICS

Other classifications	Generic name	Trade name	Common uses
	atropine	Atropine	treatment of bradycardia, given preoperatively to reduce oral secretions and prevent bradycardia
antispasmodics	dicyclomine	Bentyl	irritable bowel syndrome
antihistamines; sedative-hypnotics, miscellaneous	diphenhydramine	Benadryl	tremors and drooling caused by Parkinson disease

Continued

ANTICOAGULANTS

Other classifications	Generic name	Trade name	Common uses
	enoxaparin	Lovenox	prevention and treatment of thromboembolic disorders
	dalteparin	Fragmin	prevention and treatment of DVT
	fondaparinux	Arixtra	prevention and treatment of DVT
	heparin	Heparin	prevention and treatment of thromboembolic disorders and MI
	warfarin	Coumadin	prevention and treatment of thromboembolic disorders

ANTICONVULSANTS (ANTISEIZURE, ANTIEPILEPTICS)

Other classifications	Generic name	Trade name	Common uses
anticonvulsants, miscellaneous	carbamazepine	Tegretol	seizures, trigeminal neuralgia
barbiturates	phenobarbital	Luminal	seizures
benzodiazepines	diazepam	Valium	status epilepticus
benzodiazepines	lorazepam	Ativan	status epilepticus
antidysrhythmics, hydantoin	phenytoin	Dilantin	generalized tonic-clonic seizures, status epilepticus, migraines, trigeminal neuralgia, Bell palsy, ventricular dysrhythmias
	valproic acid	Depakote	seizures

ANTIDEPRESSANTS

Other classifications	Generic name	Trade name	Common uses
antidepressants, tricyclic	amitriptyline	Elavil	depression
selective serotonin reuptake inhibitors (SSRIs)	citalopram sertraline	Celexa Zoloft	depression
serotonin and norepinephrine reuptake inhibitors (SNRIs)	duloxetine	Cymbalta	depression

ANTIDIABETICS

Other classifications	Generic name	Trade name	Common uses
biguanide oral antidiabetics	metformin	Glucophage	Type 2 diabetes
first generation	chlorpropamide	Diabinese	Type 2 diabetes
second generation	glipizide glyburide	Glucotrol Micronase	Type 2 diabetes

ANTIDIABETICS—cont'd

Other classifications	Generic name	Trade name	Common uses
thiazolidinediones	rosiglitazone	Avandia	Type 2 diabetes
	insulin (lispro, regular, glargine, NPH human insulin)	Humalog, Humulin 70/30, Humulin N, Humulin R, and others	Type 1 diabetes

ANTIDIARRHEAL AGENTS

Other classifications	Generic name	Trade name	Common uses
local action	bismuth subsalicylate	Pepto-Bismol	diarrhea
systemic action	loperamide	Imodium	diarrhea
	diphenoxylate hydrochloride and atropine sulfate	Lomotil	diarrhea

ANTIDYSRHYTHMICS

Other classifications	Generic name	Trade name	Common uses
class Ia	quinidine	Quinaglute	atrial and ventricular arrhythmias
class Ib	lidocaine	Xylocaine	ventricular arrhythmias
class III	amiodarone	Cordarone	various arrhythmias
class IV; calcium channel blockers	verapamil diltiazem	Calan Cardizem	certain tachycardias
miscellaneous	digoxin	Lanoxin	atrial dysrhythmias

ANTIEMETICS

Other classifications	Generic name	Trade name	Common uses
anticholinergics used for motion sickness	dimenhydrinate diphenhydramine hydroxyzine	Dramamine Benadryl Vistaril	motion sickness
antipsychotics, dopamine antagonists, phenothiazines	prochlorperazine promethazine	Compazine Phenergan	nausea, psychosis
benzodiazepines	lorazepam	Ativan	nausea caused by chemotherapy
cannabinoids	dronabinol (THC)	Marinol	nausea and anorexia caused by chemotherapy
prokinetics, butyrophenones	metoclopramide	Reglan	nausea
serotonin antagonists	ondansetron	Zofran	nausea and vomiting caused by chemotherapy

Continued

ANTIFUNGALS

Other classifications	Generic name	Trade name	Common uses
imidazoles	clotrimazole	Lotrimin	fungal infections
	amphotericin B fluconazole ketoconazole metronidazole	Fungizone Diflucan Nizoral Flagyl	fungal infections

ANTIFLATULENTS

Other classifications	Generic name	Trade name	Common uses
	simethicone	Gas-X, Mylicon	disperses gas pockets in the GI tract

ANTIHISTAMINES

Other classifications	Generic name	Trade name	Common uses
	cetirizine	Zyrtec	seasonal allergies
	diphenhydramine	Benadryl	seasonal allergies, nausea, motion sickness, symptoms of Parkinson disease, nighttime cough
antianxiety, antiemetics, sedative-hypnotics	hydroxyzine	Vistaril, Atarax	anxiety, nausea, pruritus, sedation, potentiation of opioid analgesics
	loratadine	Claritin	seasonal allergies
phenothiazine derivatives	promethazine	Phenergan	motion sickness, allergy symptoms, nausea, sedation

ANTIHYPERTENSIVES

Other classifications	Generic name	Trade name	Common uses
angiotensin-converting enzyme inhibitors	enalapril lisinopril	Vasotec Zestril	hypertension, heart failure, post-MI
calcium channel blockers	diltiazem nifedipine	Cardizem Procardia	hypertension
alpha-adrenergic blockers	terazosin	Hytrin	hypertension, benign prostatic hyperplasia

ANTIHYPOGLYCEMIC AGENTS

Other classifications	Generic name	Trade name	Common uses
	glucagon	GlucaGen	hypoglycemia

ANTI-INFECTIVES, MISCELLANEOUS

Other classifications	Generic name	Trade name	Common uses
	metronidazole	Flagyl	bacterial, fungal, protozoal infections

ANTILIPIDEMICS

Other classifications	Generic name	Trade name	Common uses
HMG CoA-reductase inhibitors	atorvastatin rosuvastatin simvastatin	Lipitor Crestor Zocor	high cholesterol, high triglycerides
HMG CoA-reductase inhibitor combination products	atorvastatin and amlodipine simvastatin and ezetimibe	Caduet Vytorin	high cholesterol, high triglycerides
bile acid sequestrants	cholestyramine colestipol	Cholybar, Questran	high cholesterol, high triglycerides
antilipidemics, miscellaneous	gemfibrozil niacin	Gemcor, Lopid	high cholesterol, high triglycerides

ANTIPARASITICS

Other classifications	Generic name	Trade name	Common uses
	albendazole mebendazole ivermectin	Albenza Vermox Mectizan	parasitic infections

ANTIPARKINSONIANS

Other classifications	Generic name	Trade name	Common uses
	amantadine	Symmetrel	Parkinson disease
	carbidopa-levodopa levodopa selegiline	Sinemet, Parcopa, Atamet Eldepryl	Parkinson disease

ANTIPRURITICS

Other classifications	Generic name	Trade name	Common uses
antihistamines	diphenhydramine	Benadryl	itching related to allergic reaction
anesthetics, local	benzocaine	Lanocaine	itching or other skin pain or irritation

ANTIPSYCHOTICS

Other classifications	Generic name	Trade name	Common uses
phenothiazines, typical (first generation) antipsychotics	prochlorperazine	Compazine	psychiatric disorders such as psychosis, also nausea
atypical (second generation) antipsychotics	aripiprazole	Abilify	psychiatric disorders such as mania and schizophrenia
nonphenothiazines	haloperidol	Haldol	acute psychosis, schizophrenia, delirium
atypical (second generation) antipsychotics	olanzapine risperidone	Zyprexa Risperdal	bipolar disorder, schizophrenia

Continued

ANTISPASMODICS

Other classifications	Generic name	Trade name	Common uses
	atropine	Atropine	pylorospasm and spastic GI conditions
	dicyclomine	Bentyl	irritable bowel syndrome

ANTITUBERCULARS

Other classifications	Generic name	Trade name	Common uses
	isoniazid rifampin streptomycin	Laniazid, Nydrazid Rifadin	tuberculosis

ANTITUSSIVES

Other classifications	Generic name	Trade name	Common uses
	dextromethorphan	Robitussin CoughGels	disruptive cough

ANTIVIRALS

Other classifications	Generic name	Trade name	Common uses
	acyclovir	Zovirax, Zovir	Herpes viral infections (genital and oral herpes)
	ribavirin	Copegus, Rebetol, Ribasphere, Vilona, Virazole	RSV infection, hepatitis C

ANTIVIRALS/ANTIRETROVIRALS

Other classifications	Generic name	Trade name	Common uses
	acyclovir famciclovir	Zovirax Famvir	Herpes viral infections (oral and genital herpes)
	zidovudine	Retrovir	AIDS
	amantadine	Symmetrel	influenza
	docosanol	Abreva	cold sores

BARBITURATES

Other classifications	Generic name	Trade name	Common uses
	phenobarbital secobarbital	Luminal Seconal	preanesthetic sedation in pediatrics sedation

BENZODIAZEPINES

Other classifications	Generic name	Trade name	Common uses
	alprazolam	Xanax	anxiety
	diazepam	Valium	status epilepticus, preoperative sedation, anxiety

BENZODIAZEPINES—cont'd

Other classifications	Generic name	Trade name	Common uses
	lorazepam	Ativan	anxiety, status epilepticus, insomnia
	midazolam	Versed	preoperative anxiety, status epilepticus, insomnia, anesthesia induction, conscious sedation

BETA-ADRENERGIC BLOCKING AGENTS (BETA BLOCKERS)

Other classifications	Generic name	Trade name	Common uses
Selective beta-1 receptor blockers	atenolol metoprolol	Tenormin Lopressor	hypertension, angina hypertension, angina, heart failure, MI
Nonselective beta-1 and beta-2 receptor blockers	propranolol	Inderal	dysrhythmias, hypertension, angina, migraine

BRONCHODILATORS

Other classifications	Generic name	Trade name	Common uses
beta-adrenergic agonists	albuterol salmeterol	Proventil, Ventolin Serevent Diskus	relief and prevention of bronchospasm associated with asthma, emphysema, and other obstructive disorders
bronchodilators, anticholinergic	tiotropium bromide	Spiriva	treatment of reversible bronchospasm caused by COPD, bronchitis, and emphysema
	epinephrine	Adrenalin	bronchospasm associated with severe allergic responses

CALCIUM CHANNEL BLOCKERS

Other classifications	Generic name	Trade name	Common uses
	amlodipine diltiazem nifedipine verapamil	Norvasc Cardizem Procardia Covera-HS	hypertension

CARDIAC GLYCOSIDES

Other classifications	Generic name	Trade name	Common uses
	digoxin	Lanoxin	atrial fibrillation, heart failure

CHOLINERGICS

Other classifications	Generic name	Trade name	Common uses
	edrophonium pyridostigmine	Tensilon Mestinon	mayasthenia gravis diagnosis and treatment

Continued

CORTICOSTEROIDS

Other classifications	Generic name	Trade name	Common uses
glucocorticoids	dexamethasone methylprednisolone prednisone	Decadron Solu-Medrol Deltasone	autoimmune disorders, inflammatory disorders, and others
corticosteroids, intranasal	fluticasone	Flonase	seasonal allergies
corticosteroids, inhalant	fluticasone triamcinolone	Flovent Azmacort	reduction of airway inflammation, enhancement of effects of bronchodilators

DECONGESTANTS (NASAL)

Other classifications	Generic name	Trade name	Common uses
decongestants, topical	oxymetazoline	Afrin	nasal congestion
decongestants, systemic	pseudoephedrine	Sudafed	nasal congestion

DENTIFRICES

Other classifications	Generic name	Trade name	Common uses
	all dentrifices contain one or more abrasive agents, a foaming agent, and a flavoring material	Colgate, Crest	cleaning the teeth, preventing tooth decay and gingivitis

DIURETICS

Other classifications	Generic name	Trade name	Common uses
thiazides	chlorothiazide	Diuril	treatment of edema caused by heart failure, and various other disease states
diuretics, loop	bumetanide furosemide torsemide	Bumex Lasix Demadex	treatment of edema caused by heart failure, treatment of cirrhosis, renal disease, HTN, hypercalcemia
diuretics, potassium-sparing	spironolactone	Aldactone	treatment of edema and ascites that are not responding to other agents
osmotic	mannitol	Osmitrol	increased intracerebral pressure

ESTROGENS

Other classifications	Generic name	Trade name	Common uses
	conjugated estrogen estradiol	Premarin Estrace	treatment of symptoms of menopause

EXPECTORANTS

Other classifications	Generic name	Trade name	Common uses
	guaifenesin	Robitussin	thinning of mucus

FIBRINOLYTIC AGENTS

Other classifications	Generic name	Trade name	Common uses
	alteplase (rtPA)	Activase	destruction of blood clots

H_2 RECEPTOR ANTAGONISTS (H_2 BLOCKERS)

Other classifications	Generic name	Trade name	Common uses
	famotidine	Pepcid	treatment of gastric
	ranitidine	Zantac	ulcer and GERD

HEMORRHEOLOGIC AGENTS

Other classifications	Generic name	Trade name	Common uses
	pentoxifylline	Trental	intermittent claudication

IMMUNE GLOBULINS

Other classifications	Generic name	Trade name	Common uses
	respiratory syncytial virus immune globulin	RespiGam	RSV infection
	palivizumab	Synagis	prevention of serious lower respiratory tract infections

INSULINS

Other classifications	Generic name	Trade name	Common uses
rapid-acting insulin	lispro	Humalog	type 1 diabetes
short-acting insulin	regular	Humulin R	type 1 diabetes
intermediate-acting insulin	NPH	Humulin N	type 1 diabetes

KERATOLYTICS

Other classifications	Generic name	Trade name	Common uses
	salicylic acid, topical	Compound W, Dermarest Psoriasis Medicated Skin Treatment, Dr. Scholl's Callus Removers	acne, dandruff, corns, and warts

LAXATIVES

Other classifications	Generic name	Trade name	Common uses
laxatives, bulk	psyllium hydrophilic mucilloid	Metamucil	prevention or treatment of constipation
osmotics	lactulose	Cephulac	constipation, high blood ammonia related to liver disease

Continued

LAXATIVES—cont'd

Other classifications	Generic name	Trade name	Common uses
stimulants	bisacodyl senna	Dulcolax	constipation
stool softeners	docusate sodium	Colace	prevention or treatment of constipation

MOUTHWASHES

Other classifications	Generic name	Trade name	Common uses
mouthwashes, cosmetic	N/A (various ingredients)	Scope	freshening of breath and rinsing away of debris
mouthwashes, medicinal	N/A (various ingredients)	Listerine	reduction of plaque and gingivitis
mouthwashes, antibacterial	chlorhexidine	Peridex	treatment of oral mucositis

MUCOLYTIC AGENTS

Other classifications	Generic name	Trade name	Common uses
	acetylcysteine	Mucomyst	liquefaction of mucus

NEUROMUSCULAR BLOCKING AGENTS

Other classifications	Generic name	Trade name	Common uses
	pancuronium succinylcholine	Pavulon	emergency intubation

NSAIDS

Other classifications	Generic name	Trade name	Common uses
analgesics, antipyretics, platelet inhibitors, salicylates	aspirin	Empirin, Bayer Aspirin	mild pain, inflammatory conditions, MI, ischemic stroke, and TIA
analgesics, antipyretics, cyclooxygenase-1 (COX-1) inhibitors	ibuprofen indomethacin ketorolac naproxen	Motrin, Advil Indocin Toradol Aleve, Naprosyn	mild to moderate pain associated with inflammatory conditions, dysmenorrhea, fever
cyclooxygenase-2 (COX-2) inhibitors	celecoxib	Celebrex	mild to moderate pain associated with inflammatory conditions, dysmenorrhea
anti-inflammatories, topical	amlexanox paste 5%	Aphthasol	healing of canker sores

OXYGEN-RELEASING AGENTS

Other classifications	Generic name	Trade name	Common uses
	hydrogen peroxide	Colgate Peroxyl	treatment of canker sores, oral débridement and cleansing

PEDICULICIDE/SCABICIDE

Other classifications	Generic name	Trade name	Common uses
	lindane	Kwell	treatment of infestation with scabies, lice, or nits
	permethrin cream 5%, topical	Acticin, Elimite, Nix	treatment of infestation with lice, nits, ticks, or fleas

PLATELET INHIBITORS

Other classifications	Generic name	Trade name	Common uses
analgesics, anti-inflammatories, antipyretics	aspirin	Empirin, Bayer Aspirin	decreasing risk of MI and thrombotic stroke
	clopidogrel	Plavix	reduction of risk of MI and stroke

PROGESTINS

Other classifications	Generic name	Trade name	Common uses
	medroxyprogesterone	Provera	secondary amenorrhea, abnormal uterine bleeding

PROTON PUMP INHIBITORS

Other classifications	Generic name	Trade name	Common uses
	esomeprazole omeprazole pantoprazole	Nexium Prilosec Protonix	gastric reflux, ulcers

SALICYLATES

Other classifications	Generic name	Trade name	Common uses
analgesics, anti-inflammatories, antipyretics, platelet inhibitors	aspirin	Empirin, Bayer Aspirin	prevention of thrombus formation

SALIVA SUBSTITUTES

Other classifications	Generic name	Trade name	Common uses
mucopolysaccharides, parasympathetic alkaloids	pilocarpine	Mouth Kote, Orajel Dry Mouth, Moisturizing Spray	treatment of xerostomia (dry mouth)

SEDATIVE-HYPNOTICS, MISCELLANEOUS

Other classifications	Generic name	Trade name	Common uses
	eszopiclone zolpidem	Lunesta Ambien	insomnia

Continued

THROMBOLYTICS

Other classifications	Generic name	Trade name	Common uses
	alteplase (rtPA) streptokinase urokinase	Activase Streptase Kinlytic	destruction of thrombi (clots) associated with acute MI, PE, and DVT

THYROID HORMONES

Other classifications	Generic name	Trade name	Common uses
	levothyroxine	Synthroid	thyroid-hormone replacement

UTERINE RELAXANTS

Other classifications	Generic name	Trade name	Common uses
	magnesium sulfate		inhibition of preterm labor

UTERINE STIMULANTS

Other classifications	Generic name	Trade name	Common uses
	dinoprostone	Cervidil	starting and continuation of cervical ripening at term
	oxytocin	Pitocin	induction of labor, augmentation of contractions, control of postpartum bleeding

VASODILATORS

Other classifications	Generic name	Trade name	Common uses
	dipyridamole hydralazine	Persantine Apresoline	treatment of pulmonary hypertension

VITAMINS AND MINERALS

Other classifications	Generic name	Trade name	Common uses
fat-soluble vitamins	phytonadione (vitamin K) vitamin A vitamin C vitamin D		nutritional deficiencies
water-soluble vitamins	ascorbic acid (vitamin C) cyanocobalamin (vitamin B_{12}) pyridoxine (vitamin B_6) riboflavin (vitamin B_2) thiamine (vitamin B_1)		nutritional deficiencies
	copper		nutritional deficiencies
	zinc oxide		nutritional deficiencies
	iron		iron-deficiency anemia

ANSWERS TO PRACTICE EXERCISES

CHAPTER 1

True or False

1. True
2. False
3. False
4. True
5. True

Multiple Choice

1. b. Visual
2. b. Visual learners
3. a. They can recall information by seeing it in their mind's eye.
4. d. Rhymes
5. d. All of these
6. c. Their learning styles are probably a mix of visual and auditory.
7. c. Beware your tendency to get stuck in analysis paralysis.
8. b. They dislike following official procedures.
9. d. All of these
10. b. Emotional feelings affect whether some information is stored in long-term memory.

CHAPTER 2

Case Study 1

1. Use common sense measures to help break the chain of infection and prevent pathogen transmission. This includes information in Boxes 2-2 and 2-3 as well as wearing gloves, and—if the patient is coughing or sneezing—possibly wearing a mask and even eye protection.
2. Teaching the patient about appropriate precautions such as hand washing; avoiding touching her eyes, mouth, and nose; and avoiding sharing eating or drinking utensils with others.

Case Study 2

Remind her that she is professionally and ethically obligated to protect her patients and that her current practice puts them at a very high risk, since she could easily be transmitting microorganisms between patients. Furthermore, she is putting herself and everyone else in the office at risk as she touches doorknobs, charts, desks, and staff members. Assure her that your concern is for her as well as for everyone else. Remind her that she can use hand sanitizer if she is pressed for time, since it requires virtually no extra time—but that she must wash her hands with soap and water when they are visibly soiled and between every few uses of hand sanitizer.

Case Study 3

Use your imagination and remember that children are very visual and love to participate in hands-on activities. Some suggestions are:
- Have children draw or paint pictures of what they think germs might look like, and then show them magnified pictures of some real germs.
- Bring lotion or powder that glows under black lights, have the children apply it, then wash their hands, and then examine their hands under the special lights (with the room lights turned off). Any areas that glow represent germs they missed. For an even greater effect, wait a while after the children apply the lotion before they wash it off. See where else the glowing spots show up (faces, hair, books, etc.).
- Teach children about the chain of infection. Make it fun by letting them role-play with you; assign them roles to play, such as the germ, the means of entry, the means of exit, and so on.
- Teach children the importance of washing or sanitizing their hands frequently throughout the day, especially during cold and flu season, after using the toilet, after blowing their nose, and before eating.

- Have children create posters about how to stop the chain of infection and put them up around the room.
- Have children create their own brochure about infection control to take home and teach their families.

Multiple Choice

1. d. Idiopathic: having an unknown cause
2. a. Prodromal: interval between earliest symptoms and the appearance of a rash or fever
3. a. Antibody
4. d. Intermittent
5. b. Prostration stage

Short Answer

1. To help break the cycle in the chain of infection, health-care workers must team up in their efforts to keep the environment as clean as possible. Measures might include: cleaning countertops, windows, and other surfaces in the reception area; cleaning surfaces and equipment in the clinical areas between patients; keeping hand sanitizer and tissues in all areas; and teaching patients the importance of hand washing.

2. a. An acute infection usually has a quick onset and short duration, may or may not have a clear prodromal phase, and usually lasts 1 to 3 weeks.

   b. A chronic infection lasts a long time (years or a lifetime); the patient may be asymptomatic or symptoms may fluctuate.

   c. A latent infection has symptomatic periods (relapses) alternating with symptom-free periods (remissions). The infecting organism, usually a virus, never leaves the body but lies dormant between relapses.

3. Any three of the following:
   - Discontinuing medication early could cause a relapse and worsening of the illness.
   - Discontinuing medication early exposes the pathogens to the medication without fully destroying them. This brief but inadequate exposure is a major contributor to the rise in antibiotic-resistant organisms so prevalent today.
   - Taking more than the prescribed amount could put patients at risk of drug toxicity without increasing the healing benefit.
   - Taking less than the prescribed amount could lead to decreased effectiveness of the medication and provides no benefit to the patient.

CHAPTER 3

Case Study 1

She should flush her eye thoroughly at the eyewash station and then document the event by completing an incident report as soon as possible. Her employer will provide testing for HBV and HIV immediately to check her current status, and provide postexposure treatment if necessary. Counseling will also be provided if she desires. The employer is also required to follow up on the exposure incident.

The spill on the floor should be contained with paper towels and then covered with 10% bleach solution and left to stand for at least 20 minutes. When cleaning up the spill, a mechanical device must be used rather than the hands. All items should then be placed in a biohazard container and the bleach application repeated, waiting another 20 minutes. The incident must be documented in the incident report according to office policy.

Case Study 2

1. Fatigue, possible depression, loss of interest in or enthusiasm for the job, excessive need for sleep, loss of empathy for clients, and feelings of anger or frustration

2. Questions can vary but should address at least some of the following:
   - What do you do to nurture and renew yourself?
   - Do you feel guilty if you take time for yourself?
   - Is there a balance between work and other activities, like rest, play, and socializing?
   - What activities do you do to take care of your physical, emotional, and spiritual health?

3. Advice should include at least some of the following:
   - Consider seeing a therapist, or at least find a trusted friend you can talk to about how you are feeling.

- Make a commitment to doing something nice (nurturing) for yourself every day.
- Try to cut back on work hours if you can afford it.
- Find healthful activities to "escape" with, such as exercise, meditation, reading, etc.
- Resolve any conflicts or stressful issues in the workplace.
- Be sure to eat a balanced, healthful diet and take a multivitamin.
- Make a commitment to exercise at least three times each week.
- See your physician about any current health issues that may be draining your physical and emotional energy.
- Avoid unhealthful coping mechanisms, such as smoking, drinking, illegal drugs, etc.

Multiple Choice

1. c. Cilia
2. d. Enzymes
3. a. They are markers that identify cells as self or nonself.
4. b. It causes blood vessels to constrict to reduce blood loss.
5. c. Hand sanitizer

Short Answer

1. The hepatitis B vaccine is administered in a series of three injections; the shots are at 0 months, 1 month, and 6 months.
2. Examples of sharps include needles, scalpel blades, capillary tubes, and broken glass or slides. They must be disposed of in a puncture-resistant container.
3. Answers will vary.
4. Answers will vary.

CHAPTER 4

Case Study 1

1. High 5-day fever, lack of responsiveness to antibiotics, skin rash, swollen hands and feet, peeling skin around fingers and toes, eye redness without exudate, and swollen cervical lymph nodes
2. Diagnostic criteria for Kawasaki disease include a fever of at least 5 days accompanied by four or more of the principal symptoms

(high fever [102°F to 104°F] not responsive to antibiotics; red-purple palms and soles; swollen hands and feet; peeling skin around the fingers and toes; a diffuse red skin rash over the trunk and extremities; severe eye redness without exudate; red, cracked lips; reddened, swollen tongue; sore throat; and swollen cervical lymph nodes). Alternately, a patient meeting the temperature criterion who has fewer than four of the principal symptoms but also has coronary disease may be diagnosed.

3. Treatment includes high-dose intravenous gamma globulin and salicylate therapy in the form of high-dose aspirin.
4. Relapses may occur. If treatment is not initiated early, the child may develop vasculitis damage to the muscles, lining, and valves of the heart. Abnormal heart rhythm and even heart attack can occur. The mortality rate is 2%. Caution should also be taken when giving children aspirin, because of its association with Reye syndrome.

Case Study 2

1. Measles, mumps, rubella, pertussis, tetanus, diphtheria, chickenpox, and human papillomavirus
2. The reason the numbers of cases of these diseases has dropped so dramatically in the United States is that most of the population has been immunized. However, there are still individuals who are not immunized, and they can contract and spread these diseases. If she doesn't have her baby immunized, he will be one of them. Furthermore, he would be at risk for any of these diseases if he were exposed to someone who "imported" the disease from out of the country (immunizations are not widely available in all countries) or if he traveled abroad later in his life. The bottom line is that there is no way she can guarantee that he will not be exposed sometime in his life, so protecting him by having him immunized now is the safest thing to do.
3. Some of the following complications are uncommon, but all are possible:
   - Measles: croup, bronchitis, pneumonia, bronchiolitis, conjunctivitis, myocarditis, otitis media, encephalitis, and death
   - Mumps: meningitis, encephalitis, hearing loss, pancreatitis, and impaired fertility

- Tetanus: death
- Diphtheria: peripheral neuropathy, kidney damage, cardiomyopathy, and death
- Pertussis: secondary bacterial infection, pneumonia, encephalitis, pulmonary hypertension, and death
- Chickenpox: secondary bacterial skin infection and shingles
- HPV: cervical cancer and throat cancer (see Chapter 17)

Case Study 3

1. Injuries that are typical for the age of the child and match the explanation offered by the child or parent are probably not signs of abuse. Examples include bruised shins or a skinned knee on an active 8-year-old. On the other hand, any of the following should be cause for concern and would warrant further investigation by the physician: injuries that do not match the offered explanation; bruises in odd places in various stages of healing; bruises, welts, or red marks in the shape of handprints or long, narrow objects such as belts or sticks; human bite marks; burn marks in the shape of a cigarette or possibly from being dunked in hot water; rope burns; bald patches from hair being pulled out; greenstick fractures; retinal hemorrhages; skull fractures; and subdural hematoma.

2. Signs of emotional abuse include extremes in behavior, such as excessive cooperation or passivity, extreme aggression, depression, emotional detachment, or attempted suicide.

3. Signs of sexual abuse are subtle and include difficulty sitting or walking, hesitance to remove clothing for examination, sleep disturbance, bedwetting, inappropriate sexual knowledge for the child's age, bruising or injuries to the genitalia, and the presence of sexually transmitted disease.

4. Signs of neglect include inappropriate clothing for the weather, poor hygiene, malnutrition, lethargy, failure to seek health care, frequent school absenteeism, failure to thrive, and behavioral problems at school, including begging or stealing from classmates.

Multiple Choice

1. d. Bronchiolitis
2. a. Croup: severe viral respiratory illness that involves swelling and edema of the upper respiratory passages due to inflammation or spasms
3. a. Acetaminophen
4. b. A risk factor is exposure to cigarette smoke or high levels of air pollution.
5. d. Supine

Short Answer

1. Shaken-baby syndrome (SBS) occurs when a child, usually under 1 year of age, is shaken vigorously by a frustrated parent or caretaker in an effort to stop the child's crying. Almost 50% of infants who experience SBS die. Those that survive often experience irreversible brain damage that leads to blindness, seizures, and learning difficulties.

2. Munchausen by proxy syndrome is a form of child abuse in which a caretaker or parent, usually the mother, fabricates or deliberately causes illness in the child in order to receive the sympathy and attention of health-care providers. The child undergoes unnecessary testing and may be given medications, hospitalized, and even operated on to determine the cause of the illness. Health-care providers may not be suspicious because the parent appears to be very concerned, attentive, and cooperative.

3. Colic is described as crying in an infant less than 3 months of age that lasts more than 3 hours of the day and occurs at least 3 days per week (the "rule of three").

CHAPTER 5

Case Study 1

1. It sounds like he may have tinea pedis, although you are not qualified to diagnose him. If your friend is concerned about him, she should consider taking him to their family health-care provider. It is possible for her son to have caught ringworm from the stray cat, since ringworm is any fungal skin infection on the body. However, since his symptoms are localized to his feet, it is difficult to say if the cat is the source. He may have picked it up elsewhere, perhaps in the showers at school, from the local fitness club, or even from sharing someone else's shoes or socks.

2. Over-the-counter antifungal cream or powder can be effective for home treatment. Her son must continue to use it consistently for 2 weeks after all of his symptoms have resolved, or the infection may recur. If his symptoms don't begin to improve after several days, he should see a medical professional. He may need prescription-strength medication.

Case Study 2

1. Bedsores, more properly called decubitus ulcers, are areas of injury and tissue death caused by a variety of factors, especially unrelieved pressure that impedes circulation in the skin and underlying tissues.

2. Areas of the body most at risk of pressure ulcers are those where soft tissue becomes compressed between bony prominences and external forces. Consequently, decubitus ulcers are frequently found on the elbows, heels, sacrum, hips, and anywhere that may be subject to pressure.

3. Early signs of a decubitus ulcer include mild redness over a bony area and a dull ache that comes from remaining in the same position for too long, as well as itching or tenderness. The skin there may be warmer or cooler than surrounding skin and it may change color or consistency, becoming firmer or softer than normal.

4. • Inspect her skin, especially bony prominences like the heels, elbows, sacrum, and hips, at least once each day.
   • Turn or reposition her frequently—at least every 2 hours—using a written schedule if necessary.
   • Remind her to shift her weight and position, if she is able, every 15 minutes.
   • Place soft padding between bony body parts (such as her knees) to keep them from pressing on one another.
   • Provide heel protection, such as a soft pillow or cushion under her calf to keep her heels from pressing into the bed.
   • Keep her skin clean and dry, but moisturize if it becomes too dry and flaky.
   • Provide careful hygiene and skin protection if she is incontinent.
   • Provide cushioned or padded surfaces when she is sitting; consider special mattresses for her bed.
   • Use a turn sheet to turn and reposition her, to avoid friction and shearing trauma—consider getting and using a mechanical lifting device if necessary.
   • Provide good nutrition and hydration to promote optimal skin health.
   • Treat any areas of skin breakdown early and aggressively, and call her physician if you have concerns or notice an area that is getting worse in spite of your efforts.

Case Study 3

The development of calluses and corns is always related to pressure and friction, and it is nearly always preventable. Inserting friction-reducing material, such as a special insole, into shoes may help. Orthotics may also be helpful. Inspect your feet regularly for areas of redness or tenderness. Carefully select new shoes that are comfortable—do not sacrifice your feet for fashion! Stop wearing shoes that hurt your feet or toes. Avoid wearing heels more than 2 inches high (or avoid wearing heels at all). Avoid wearing pointy-toed shoes. Wear socks, but avoid those with seams that press against your toes. Avoid wearing shoes that are loose and rub against your skin.

Multiple Choice

1. c. Wheal: rounded, temporary elevation in the skin that is white in the center with a red-pink periphery; accompanied by itching
2. b. Warts
3. a. Melasma
4. d. Lyme disease
5. b. Callus

Short Answer

1. After an initial outbreak of varicella (chickenpox), the varicella-zoster virus incorporates itself into nerve cells and lies dormant until it is reactivated years later. When the virus reactivates, shingles is the result.

2. • Stage 1 ulcers exhibit temperature changes (warmer or cooler than surrounding skin), color changes—including redness in light-skinned people and blue or purple coloring in dark-skinned people—that do not blanch (become more pale) with briefly applied pressure or resolve after pressure is relieved,

discomfort (itching or tenderness), and change in consistency (firmer or softer).

- Stage 2 ulcers exhibit erosion of the epidermis or dermis without subcutaneous exposure; may appear as abrasions, blisters, or shallow wounds.
- Stage 3 ulcers exhibit erosion or necrosis of all layers of skin down to underlying fascia and appear as deep wounds which may or may not extend beneath the surrounding skin. For this reason they are often much larger than they appear (the "iceberg effect").
- Stage 4 ulcers exhibit erosion and tissue necrosis through all layers of skin and subcutaneous tissue, with damage to supporting structures such as muscle, tendons, and bones.

3. First-degree burns are caused by exposure to heat, or more commonly, the ultraviolet rays of the sun. They involve only the epidermis and are generally considered minor injuries. The skin is red, blanches with pressure, is moderately painful to the touch, and is dry with no blisters. Permanent tissue damage is rare and may consist of minor changes in skin color.

Second- and third-degree burns usually result from exposure to or direct contact with very hot objects, scalding liquids, flames, chemicals, or electricity. Second-degree burns involve the epidermis and part of the dermis. The skin appears red, edematous, and wet, shiny, or blistered, and is intensely painful. Third-degree burns destroy the epidermis, dermis, and subcutaneous layers of the skin. Fatty tissue, muscles, bones, and tendons may be involved as well, although some experts further classify such burns as fourth-degree burns. These burns may appear black and charred, brown, yellow, or even white. They are also dry and leathery. The patient feels no pain from third-degree burns because nerves are destroyed.

CHAPTER 6

Case Study 1

1. We don't really know, but we've identified a few things. For example, we know that the brain deteriorates and begins to lose the ability to function. Certain factors seem to increase the chances of developing Alzheimer dementia, including advanced age, genetics, some viruses,

previous brain injuries from head trauma or minor stroke, cardiovascular disease, deficiency of vitamins B_{12} and folate, brain infection, diabetes, and immunologic factors. The brain also develops tangled bundles of nerve cells and lacks certain chemicals important for nerve function.

2. Dementia is sometimes confused with depression. Here are some of the ways you can tell the difference: Depression may get better with therapy or medication; dementia gets continually worse. During the early stages of dementia, a person's short-term memory gets worse but the person can remember things from long ago. As time goes by, short-term memory gets really bad and the person struggles to remember things from long ago, eventually becoming unable to remember anything and perhaps even recognize his or her closest friends or family. A depressed person may have an unpredictable memory that works well sometimes and not so well at other times, but it doesn't progressively worsen like with dementia. The depressed person may have some difficulty focusing on things and may be apathetic; however, the person's judgment isn't too bad and he or she is still able to perform most tasks. On the other hand, the person with dementia displays judgment that becomes less predictable and less safe over time, as well as increasing difficulty communicating and performing routine, everyday tasks. Eventually the person with dementia needs someone else to take care of him or her all of the time.

3.
   - Keep doors and windows locked.
   - Install safety latches on cabinets and drawers that contain objects such as knives.
   - Lock up firearms or remove them from the home.
   - Install protective gates at the top and bottom of stairs.
   - Supervise the ingestion of all medications.
   - Keep car keys in a locked cupboard.
   - Place night-lights throughout the home, especially in the bedroom and bathroom.
   - Keep walkways clear.

4. Most communities have day services, respite care, support groups, and home health-care services. The nurse should give Mrs. O'Connor information for these resources in her area.

Case Study 2

1. Bell palsy is a disorder of the seventh cranial nerve that causes temporary weakness or paralysis of one side of the face.

2. Bell palsy is not contagious between people. It occurs when the seventh cranial nerve becomes inflamed, swollen, and compressed. The underlying cause is unknown, but a viral infection may serve as a triggering event.

3. Symptoms of Bell palsy vary somewhat. In most cases there is some degree of paralysis that causes drooping of the facial features on the affected side. Other symptoms may include twitching, weakness, drooling, eye dryness, impaired taste, excessive tearing, headache, ringing in the ears, and difficulty eating or drinking.

4. There is no cure for Bell palsy. You might be given corticosteroids to decrease inflammation and swelling of the involved nerve, or antiviral medication if a viral cause is suspected. Analgesics and warm, moist compresses may help relieve pain. If you have difficulty blinking or closing your eyes, you should protect them and keep them moist, by using artificial tears or an eye patch.

5. The prognosis is usually very good and most people recover completely, but it may take as long as 6 months. In some cases the symptoms may never fully resolve, and in a very small number of cases the paralysis may be permanent. Recurrences are rare.

Case Study 3

1. Indicators that these might be migraines include a report of an aura, throbbing pain on one or both sides of the head, nausea with or without vomiting, and sensitivity to bright light and sound. Headaches may last from 4 to 72 hours and are often described as more severe than other common headaches the individual may have. Frequency varies from once a week to once a year.

2. Tension headaches may be chronic or episodic, lasting for minutes or days. They are experienced as a dull, aching sensation that is usually bilateral. Pain may be centered in the forehead, base of the head, or neck. There may be a sensation of pressure or bandlike tightness encircling the head. The individual may notice a connection between situational stress and the headaches. Chronic forms may be present continuously or occur daily.

3. The cause of migraine headaches is not fully understood, although they tend to run in families, be worse early in life, and generally improve in later years. Current theories about causes include involvement of the trigeminal nerve, imbalances in such chemicals as serotonin, and vascular dilation and inflammation. Many risk factors and potential triggers have also been identified, including hormonal changes and such foods as red wine, beer, aged cheese, chocolate, aspartame, and monosodium glutamate. Other triggers include stress, bright lights, fumes, perfumes, smoke, exertion, fatigue, environmental changes, and some medications.

    Tension headaches are caused by muscle tightening, or tension, in the scalp, neck, jaw, or upper shoulders. This tension is generally related to situational, physical, or emotional stress, anxiety, or depression. Examples of physical stress include certain types of manual labor and prolonged work at a desk or computer. Emotional stress is anything that causes feelings such as anxiety, anger, or frustration. Contributors to tension headaches include poor posture, lack of sleep, alcohol use, and missed meals. Pain may be worsened with noise.

4. Some forms of treatment may be helpful for both types of headache, including the use of various types of analgesics and NSAIDs. However, migraine headaches do not always respond to these medications, so other forms of treatment may be necessary. Examples include triptans, which are a newer class of drugs that help to abort the migraine before it becomes severe. Other medications, such as antihypertensives, antidepressants, and antiseizure medications may help reduce the frequency and severity of migraines.

    Tension headaches generally respond better to over-the-counter analgesics than do migraines. They may also respond to measures such as relaxation, massage, biofeedback, and stress-management activities.

Multiple Choice

1. b. Aura: sensory warning prior to the onset of a migraine headache or a seizure

2. a. Altered sensation, such as numbness, stinging, or burning, that results from injury to nerves

3. d. Migraines can be cured with the use of medications called triptans.
4. c. It is definitively diagnosed with MRI.
5. d. Treatment may include the use of thrombolytic and anticoagulant medications.

Short Answer

1. Strokes have two general causes: ruptures and bleeding of a vessel in the brain and deficiency in blood supply. TIAs are commonly caused by tiny emboli; permanent brain damage does not occur because the emboli are quickly dissolved by the body's protective mechanisms.

   Signs and symptoms of stroke include vision loss or changes, dysphasia, dysphagia, severe headache, dizziness, confusion, altered consciousness, difficulty with gait and balance, and paresthesia and weakness on one side of the body. Many of these symptoms may become permanent deficits. Rehabilitation is needed to help the individual achieve optimal recovery. Signs and symptoms of TIA may be similar to strokes, but they are temporary.

2. Changes in movement include resting hand tremor, muscle rigidity, pill-rolling tremor of the hands, bradykinesia, shuffling gait, posture that is stooped with the neck bent forward, difficulty initiating movements, and difficulty swallowing.

3. Measures include avoiding the use of tobacco and illicit drugs, avoiding lead exposure, avoiding chronically high levels of stress, maintaining a healthy blood pressure, managing diabetes effectively, following all recommended measures to prevent heart disease, pursuing educational or mentally stimulating activities, exercising regularly, and participating in social activities.

CHAPTER 7

Case Study 1

1. Interstitial cystitis (IC)
2. Other symptoms might include feelings of pressure, aching, or severe pain in the low back area, pain in the urethra, vulva, or scrotum, and pain with intercourse. For many, pain is most severe during the early morning hours.
3. Cystoscopy and biopsy
4. Any two of the following:

- Pentosan (Elmiron) is thought to help the bladder resurface itself.
- Other medications that may relieve or reduce symptoms include analgesics, antihistamines, and antidepressants.
- Bladder distention may be done to increase bladder capacity; for some individuals it also reduces pain for a time.
- Instillation of medications such as dimethyl sulfoxide and heparin into the bladder is sometimes helpful.
- Patients with Hunner's ulcers may experience improvement with laser surgery.
- Some individuals respond to diet modification; recommendations are numerous, including eliminating or reducing intake of acidic or spicy foods such as tomatoes, citrus fruit, and chocolate as well as eliminating alcoholic and caffeinated beverages.

5. She should explain that IC is considered a chronic disorder with no known cure. For some people it is a minor annoyance; for others the impact on quality of life is significant. It can affect many aspects of life, including sleep, social life, and for some, sexual intimacy. As Ms. Bell learns more about the disorder and the treatments available, she can work with her health-care provider to create an effective management plan.

Case Study 2

1. Kidney stone
2. Radiological tests such as CT scan, ultrasound, IVP, MRI, or abdominal x-rays
3. Yes, he is a white male between the ages of 40 and 70. This is the group most commonly affected.
4. Conservative treatment of renal calculi includes opiate analgesics for pain; fluids; and smooth-muscle relaxants. The goal is to support him in passing the stone in his urine. If the stone is too large or the ureter is completely blocked, the physician may order surgery to remove the stone. Lithotripsy, another treatment option, involves the use of ultrasound to disintegrate the stone.
5. Hydronephrosis

Case Study 3

1. Diabetic nephropathy is a disease of the kidneys associated with diabetes. It results in

inflammation, degeneration, and sclerosis (scarlike tissue changes) of the kidneys. We aren't completely sure what causes it, but it is thought to develop as damage to the tiny structures within the kidneys is caused by inflammation and injury brought on by chronically high blood sugar levels. You also have several risk factors for this disease: high blood pressure, smoking, and Native American descent.

2. Most people have no symptoms in the early stages of diabetic nephropathy.

3. As the disease progresses, tests may indicate that you have severe proteinuria (protein in your urine), worsening high blood pressure, and high cholesterol and triglyceride levels. You may also begin to notice worsening anorexia (loss of appetite), weight loss, edema (swelling), fatigue, weakness, nausea, and insomnia.

4. Unfortunately there really is no cure. A treatment plan will be created just for you, most likely focusing on measures to lower and manage your blood pressure and achieve control of your blood glucose level. You may be given blood-pressure medication. Diet modifications may include a low-fat, low-salt, low-protein diet.

Multiple Choice

1. b. Anuria: need to urinate frequently
2. d. Uremia: temporary deficiency in blood supply
3. b. 1 to 2 liters
4. c. Common symptoms include frequency, urgency, and dysuria.
5. d. Definitive diagnosis usually requires a biopsy.

Short Answer

1. Prerenal acute renal failure is caused by inadequate blood flow to the kidneys. Specific causes, or triggering events, include hemorrhage, severe burns, shock, severe dehydration, liver failure, and renal vein thrombosis secondary to nephrotic syndrome.

2. Common symptoms of ARF include oliguria or anuria, generalized edema, altered mental status, tremors, anorexia, a metallic taste in the mouth, easy bruising or bleeding, flank pain, fatigue, hypertension, and seizures.

3. Diabetes and hypertension

CHAPTER 8

Case Study 1

1. HPV is transmitted sexually and is the most common STI in the United States today; more than half of all sexually active men and women become infected. Your boyfriend must have acquired it sometime in the past and has now given it to you.

2. Unfortunately, there is no complete cure for HPV—and because it is caused by a virus, antibiotics will not help. HPV can be destroyed with topical podophyllin or laser surgery but may return after treatment. Treatment should be administered weekly until all warts are removed. After treatment ends, you should schedule a follow-up examination to be seen in 3 months.

3. HPV may disappear without treatment; however, active infection may still be present, and transmission to a partner is possible. Therefore, even though his HPV went away, he very likely still has the virus in his body.

4. You should undergo testing for HIV and other STIs just to be safe. In addition, it is *very* important that you undergo regular Pap tests from here on, because HPV increases your risk of cervical cancer.

Case Study 2

1. Testicular torsion is a condition in which the testicles become twisted and the spermatic cord, blood vessels, nerves, and vas deferens become strangled. The cause of testicular torsion is often unclear. It may be related to vigorous physical activity or scrotal injury, though it frequently occurs during sleep.

2. Diagnosis is usually based upon the patient's presenting signs and symptoms and physical-examination findings. Color Doppler sonography may identify lack of circulation to the testicle, which is characteristic of torsion and is useful in ruling out epididymitis.

3. Treatment of testicular torsion includes an attempt at manual detorsion (untwisting) of the testicle. Surgical intervention may be necessary if this is not successful. Orchiectomy is necessary if necrosis has occurred. If the testicle can be saved, it is sutured to the wall of the scrotum to secure it.

Case Study 3

1. Dysmenorrhea

2. Causes of dysmenorrhea include endometriosis, uterine fibroids, and PID.

3. She can try taking analgesics but should ask her health-care provider which would be safest in the event of pregnancy. She can also try application of warm or cold compresses and should get plenty of rest and avoid caffeine and alcohol. She should be encouraged to eat a healthy diet and get moderate physical exercise, since these measures have also been shown to lessen symptoms of dysmenorrhea. Oral contraceptives would probably lessen her symptoms but would also prevent the pregnancy that she desires.

4. Lack of a pregnancy in just 3 months does not indicate infertility. However, her complaint of dysmenorrhea that worsened after she discontinued oral contraceptives indicates a possibility of endometriosis, which can impair fertility. To identify whether this is a factor, further testing will be needed.

Multiple Choice

1. a. Undescended testicle(s)

2. d. Phimosis

3. c. Phimosis is a common contributing factor.

4. d. Prognosis for mother and infant is usually excellent.

5. b. Patients are always female.

Short Answer

1. Fibrocystic breast disease is the presence of multiple nonmalignant lumps in the breast, consisting of fibrous tumors or fluid-filled cysts. Diagnosis is confirmed by a manual breast examination and mammography.

2. Herpes simplex √

   Chlamydia

   Genital warts (HPV) *

   Gonorrhea

   Syphilis □

   Trichomoniasis △

   Chancroid ○

3. *Sexual assault* is a broader term than *rape* (forced vaginal, anal, or oral penetration) and is therefore more useful for conveying the scope of the problem of sexual attack. Sexual assault is defined as any form of unwanted sexual contact forced upon an individual. The victim may or may not be known to the perpetrator and may even be a friend, date, or spouse. Victims may be subdued by chemical means through drugs or alcohol, physically restrained or overpowered, or coerced to cooperate though threats of harm. Forms of sexual contact vary and include, but are not limited to, forced vaginal, anal, or oral penetration, touching of the breasts or genitalia, masturbation, forced nudity, and photography or video recording.

CHAPTER 9

Case Study 1

1. She should tactfully remind her coworker that she cannot share any personal patient information with anyone not directly involved in that patient's care. However, she would be very happy to share what she knows about the disorder.

2. CMC is caused by *Candida* organisms, usually *Candida albicans*.

3. CMC causes large, circular skin lesions that manifest on the skin, nails, mucous membranes, or vagina. Infants generally develop recurrent diaper rash or oral thrush as their first symptoms. With older children, lesions often begin on the scalp or fingernails. In the later stages, some people may develop recurring respiratory infections. Other body systems may become involved as well; for example, endocrine system involvement manifests as hypoparathryoidism, hypocalcemia, and pernicious anemia. Individuals may also be more vulnerable to bacterial, viral, and other fungal infections.

4. CMC is treated with antifungal medication, immunosuppressive therapy, or a combination of the two. Systemic antifungals, oral antifungals, and transfer factor may also be helpful in some cases.

Case Study 2

1. The cause of CFS is not yet clearly known, although various theories have suggested endocrine, immune, and nervous system involvement. Environmental and genetic factors

may also be involved. Depression has been identified as a common coexisting disorder but not a cause.

2. The main symptom is pronounced fatigue, unrelieved by rest, that causes a significant reduction in the ability to perform activities of daily living. Physical exertion may be followed by extreme fatigue that lasts for 24 hours or more. Other symptoms vary greatly in type and severity and include insomnia, unrefreshing sleep, weakness, muscle aches, and difficulty with concentration and memory.

3. Sadly, there is no known cure. Treatment is aimed at relieving symptoms and improving function. Medications may provide symptom relief for pain, anxiety, gastrointestinal complaints, and insomnia. Lifestyle recommendations can help, such as stress-reduction strategies and dietary modification, including nutritional supplementation (under a physician's direction). Other measures are massage, meditation, and acupuncture. Moderate exercise and careful physical therapy may help maintain strength and health without causing undue fatigue.

Case Study 3

1. Transplant rejection occurs when a recipient's immune system identifies transplanted tissue as foreign and responds by attacking it. The incidence varies by transplant organ or tissue type. It occurs in 60% to 75% of first kidney transplants.

2. The most common signs and symptoms of kidney transplant rejection include hypertension, decreased urine output, fever, flu-like symptoms (body aches, fatigue, nausea, vomiting, chills, headache), increased pain over the transplant site, and fluid retention (indicated by swollen ankles, fingers, etc.).

3. Hyperacute rejection is usually prevented by careful crossmatching before surgery to identify antibodies. However, should rejection occur, the transplanted organ or tissue must be immediately removed to prevent a severe systemic inflammatory response.

   Acute organ rejection may be prevented by the use of immunosuppressive medications, but rejection can occur after months or even years. Acute rejection is treated with high doses of IV corticosteroids. In some cases,

plasma exchange may be done to remove antibodies that are attacking the transplanted tissue. Chronic rejection cannot be treated; re-transplantation is necessary.

Multiple Choice

1. b. Lymph nodes are distributed along lymphatic vessels, with higher concentrations in the neck, axillae, groin, and the mesentery of the abdomen.

2. d. Current life expectancy is 10 to 20 years from the time of diagnosis.

3. b. It is commonly triggered by depression.

4. a. Transplant rejection occurs in 25% of first kidney transplants.

5. c. The skin should be treated with sunlight or tanning beds.

Short Answer

1. Common signs and symptoms include gradual or sudden onset of muscle weakness in the trunk that progresses to affect muscles of the neck, shoulders, back, and hip, and possibly the hands and fingers. Affected individuals may experience muscle pain and difficulty with activities such as standing, climbing stairs, reaching overhead, and lifting objects. They may be at risk of falling. They may also notice dysphagia, fatigue, and thickening of the skin on their hands.

2. Corticosteroids and immunosuppressants

3. The mucous membranes of the eyes, mouth, and other areas of the body

4. Most commonly affected are postmenopausal women (nine times more often than men), although Sjögren syndrome can also strike younger individuals.

5. Epstein-Barr virus (EBV)

6. The exact cause of SLE is not fully understood, but it is an autoimmune disorder, meaning that the body produces antibodies that target "self" tissues, resulting in inflammation and degeneration. There is some thought that genetics, viruses, some drugs, female hormones, stress, and ultraviolet light (in the form of sunlight, fluorescent lights, and tanning beds) may play a role.

7. Lupus is marked by exacerbations and remissions. One of the most prominent features of both discoid lupus and SLE is the skin rash that may develop anywhere on the body but

is most obvious on the face and scalp. It is generally red and flat—but may have raised borders—and painless, and it doesn't itch. Other symptoms of SLE depend upon the body system affected. General whole-body symptoms include mild fever, fatigue, anorexia, and weight loss. Other symptoms include myalgia (muscle aches), arthralgia (aching joints), photosensitivity, splenomegaly, lymphadenopathy, and Raynaud phenomenon (a circulatory disorder of the fingers and toes). Arthritic changes develop in 90% of those with SLE and cause joint pain, stiffness, edema, and possible joint deformity.

8. Intrinsic factor

9. Signs and symptoms include fatigue, malaise, pallor, shortness of breath, and tachycardia. Gastrointestinal symptoms include diarrhea, nausea, constipation, abdominal pain, anorexia, and weight loss. The desire or ability to eat is also affected by common mouth problems, including sore, red tongue, burning tongue, and bleeding gums. The sense of smell may be impaired. Abnormal neuromuscular symptoms include paresthesia (abnormal sensation) of the hands and feet, muscle spasms, weakness, difficulty moving, and impaired reflexes. Other effects include fever, confusion, and memory deficits.

10. The mainstay of treatment is the administration of monthly vitamin B_{12} injections.

11. Ankylosing spondylitis (AS) is a type of inflammatory arthritis that causes degenerative changes in the spinal vertebrae and sacroiliac joints. It also causes inflammatory changes in connective tissues such as tendons and ligaments, and can affect joints of the hips, shoulders, knees, feet, and ribs. Tissues of the lungs, eyes, and heart valves may be affected as well.

    The signs and symptoms associated with AS include feelings of stiffness and difficulty moving, pain, chronic stooping, fatigue, difficulty breathing, anorexia, weight loss, and inflammation of the eyes and bowels.

CHAPTER 10

Case Study 1

1. Yes, because atrial fibrillation affects 5% to 10% of all individuals over the age of 70, which amounts to about 2.2 million Americans.

2. Depolarization of the atria is not triggered by signals from the sinoatrial node, as normally occurs; instead, rapid, irregular electrical activity occurs in muscle cells throughout the atria. As a result, the atria fail to contract in an organized fashion and instead fibrillate, or quiver in a disorganized and ineffective manner.

3. A Holter monitor is a portable device that records the patient's cardiac rhythm over a 24- or 48-hour period. This type of testing is useful for patients with an irregular heartbeat or other symptoms that may be intermittent.

    An event recorder is a small, portable monitor that the patient can wear around the neck like a pendant or place in a shirt pocket. The patient can activate it upon such symptoms as chest pain, dizziness, and palpitations. The data is then sent to the cardiology clinic via telephone for analysis. This type of device is most ideal for patients whose symptoms are intermittent and unpredictable and are therefore unlikely to manifest during an ECG test.

4. An antiarrhythmic such as digoxin (Lanoxin)

5. If medication is not successful, Mrs. Neibert may undergo cardioversion, which is a synchronized shock of electrical current delivered to the chest wall while she is under sedation and analgesia. If these measures are unsuccessful, she may undergo ablation of the atrioventricular node with subsequent placement of a pacemaker.

Case Study 2

1. Raynaud is a disorder that affects blood vessels in the fingers, toes, ears, and nose. Most people who develop primary Raynaud are young women.

2. We don't completely understand what causes it, but we know it is not contagious and cannot be passed from one person to another.

3. Symptoms are triggered by things like cold temperature. In response, blood vessels constrict, blood flow diminishes, and tissue doesn't get enough oxygen. The lack of blood flow causes the color change and the pain.

4. Here are some suggestions. You will need to try them all out and figure out a plan of care that works best for you.
   - Avoid directly touching cold objects.
   - Keep gloves or mittens next to the refrigerator and freezer and put them on before handling frozen or cold food.

- Always wear socks and shoes or warm house slippers.
- Dress warmly for cold environments, including overly air-conditioned areas.
- When possible, avoid medications or other substances that cause vasoconstriction, such as decongestants, oral contraceptives, caffeine, and nicotine.
- Keep hand warmers inside of coat pockets or even slip them inside gloves.
- Avoid using vibrating tools such as electric saws or sanders.
- Avoid excess stress.

Case Study 3

1. Deep vein thrombosis (DVT)

2. Common symptoms of DVT include a dull ache in the area of the clot, a feeling of heaviness, and localized edema, redness, and heat.

3. He is 62 years old, which puts him into the typical age group. The scenario does not tell us if he has other known risk factors for DVT.

4. DVT usually occurs secondary to vessel injury and blood stasis caused by poor circulation and immobility. Platelets begin to gather and fibrin formation occurs in areas of injury, creating a blood clot, and then inflammation ensues. Other contributing factors include clotting disorders, heart failure, estrogen use, malignancy, obesity, and pregnancy.

5. A D-dimer test may have been done, with a high result (greater than 300). Compression ultrasonography may have revealed failure of the vein to compress where the clot was located. Radiographic venography may also have been done.

6. Anticoagulants

7. Any two of heparin, enoxaparin, and warfarin

8. The physician may have told him to rest and refrain from vigorous exercise until the condition resolves and to elevate the limb and apply warm compresses.

9. A potential complication of DVT is embolization of the clot to the lungs, resulting in pulmonary embolism.

Multiple Choice

1. c. Claudication: abnormal fluid accumulation in the abdominal space between organs

2. d. Abnormal swooshing sound

3. a. Cardiac cycle

4. c. Agranulocytosis

5. b. Thromboangiitis obliterans

Short Answer

1. Similarities: Both conditions are very common. Both present with very similar signs and symptoms. Both have the same general risk factors, especially coronary artery disease. Diagnostic tests for both may include ECG and cardiac enzymes. When the patient is stable, both may require further diagnostic testing with cardiac catheterization. Both may be treated with nitrates and antihypertensive medication, or with angioplasty. Both should prompt patients to participate in lifestyle modification to reduce risk factors for future events.

    Differences: Angina does not kill heart muscle like MI does. A cardiac stress test would probably not be appropriate for the MI patient, unless done at a much later date, after full recovery. People die from MI but not from angina (although it is a warning that a future MI could occur).

2. Arteriosclerosis, commonly called *hardening of the arteries*, is the thickening and loss of elasticity and contractility of arterial walls. Atherosclerosis is a common form of arteriosclerosis marked by deposits of cholesterol, lipids, and calcium on the walls of arteries, which may restrict blood flow.

3.
- Stop or reduce the use of tobacco products.
- Limit alcohol intake to two drinks (1 ounce of alcohol each) or less per day.
- Participate in aerobic exercise several times per week.
- Maintain blood pressure within recommended ranges.
- For diabetics, maintain blood glucose level within the recommended range.
- Keep cholesterol, LDL, VLDL, HDL, and triglycerides within the recommended ranges.
- Schedule a screening examination to find out what your cholesterol levels are.
- Eat a diet low in cholesterol and saturated fat.
- Attain and maintain a healthy weight.

CHAPTER 11

Case Study 1

1. It is possible that Mr. Reeves has sleep apnea, a common condition in which individuals stop breathing, possibly hundreds of times, during sleep. He would need to discuss this with his physician to be sure.

2. Sleep apnea is diagnosed by history, physical examination, and sleep studies. During sleep studies he might stay overnight in a sleep lab. Tests might include continuous pulse oximetry, which is a test in which a small sensor is placed on his finger to detect abnormal drops in oxygen level during sleep. This test can also be done at home. During a sleep study he would likely have nocturnal polysomnography done. In this test, sensors would be applied to Mr. Reeves that detect heart, lung, and brain activity in addition to body movements, breathing patterns, and oxygen levels.

3. The information gathered in a sleep study identifies the number, frequency, and severity of apnea periods as well as the number of nighttime awakenings. Mr. Reeves might be surprised to find out just how many times he awakens during the night without knowing it.

4. Sleep apnea is pretty common, affecting an estimated 12 to 18 million Americans and about 10% of all middle-aged men. It does put individuals at risk of certain problems, including hypertension and cardiovascular disease, and increases risk of heart attack and stroke. It also contributes to obesity, memory impairment, impotence, headaches, irritability, depression, memory problems, daytime sleepiness, and impaired mental functioning. This can result in accidents, injury, and death on the job or on the road. The good news, however, is that the prognosis is very good if it is diagnosed and treated.

5. It depends upon the type of sleep apnea. In obstructive sleep apnea, air flow is blocked by upper-airway tissue but respiratory efforts continue. This results in a repetitive pattern of snoring, snorting, and gasping as the individual rouses from sleep just enough to finally take several effective breaths. As carbon dioxide is eliminated and the need for oxygen is satisfied, the person slips back into a deeper sleep. Then muscles in the throat relax and the airway becomes obstructed once again. Because this pattern repeats itself hundreds of times during the night, normal sleep patterns are disrupted, interfering with truly restful sleep. Individuals rarely feel rested in the morning and often struggle with daytime drowsiness. In addition, they may note morning headache, dry mouth, and sore throat. Signs and symptoms typical of sleep apnea include fatigue and daytime drowsiness, morning headache, dry mouth, and sore throat. The patient's spouse or significant other also notices snoring and observes the apnea periods.

6. Losing weight could certainly help: Obesity is a risk factor for sleep apnea. Others include age of at least 40, neck circumference greater than 44 centimeters (17.5 inches), narrowed airway, family history of sleep apnea, smoking, use of alcohol or sleeping medication, and being male. Some of these things cannot be changed, but some, like use of tobacco, alcohol, and sleeping aids, could be modified. Other things Mr. Reeves could try are sleeping on his side rather than his back and using a saline nasal spray before bed to help keep nasal passages open. He might also talk with his dentist about using an oral device or with his doctor about a CPAP breathing machine or even surgical options.

Case Study 2

1. A common sign of acute sinusitis is when a cold seems to improve and then worsens again. Pressure or pain is often felt in the face, including the cheeks and forehead, and between the eyes. Other symptoms may include nasal congestion, fever, malaise, and a cough and sore throat (due to postnasal drainage) that are worse in the mornings.

2. Diagnosis is usually based upon a description of symptoms and physical-examination findings. In some cases sinus films may be done, including standard x-rays, computed tomography (CT), or magnetic resonance imaging (MRI).

3. Antibiotics are prescribed for 10 to 14 days and should be taken until gone, even if symptoms begin to improve after a few days. Decongestants may also be prescribed. Other treatment includes rest, fluids, moist heat compresses, humidifiers, and hot showers (breathing in the steam).

4. A sinus infection, also called sinusitis, is caused when sinus cavities become blocked due to swelling or growth of polyps. As bacteria grow, an infection develops, which increases the inflammation. This all causes sinus pain. The sinuses are just above the teeth and share some of the same bones, so it's not surprising that sinusitis can make it feel like the teeth are hurting.

5. You might catch a cold or influenza virus from someone that could put you at risk of developing sinusitis, but the sinus infection itself is not transmitted between people.

Case Study 3

1. Approximately 20% of the U.S. population gets the flu each year, over 200,000 are hospitalized, and more than 35,000 die. Those at greatest risk are the very young, very old, and those with chronic health disorders and weakened immune systems.

2. There are a number of flu viruses, often categorized as types A, B, and C. Types A and B cause the flu that circulates almost every winter; occasionally, a stronger strain of these types causes a deadly pandemic or more serious local outbreak. Types A and B are constantly changing, with new strains appearing regularly, while type C is more stable. All three commonly spread from person to person in respiratory droplets and secretions through coughing, sneezing, and kissing. They may also be spread through contact with surfaces with viruses on them (doorknobs, etc.) followed by contact with the mouth or nose. A person may be infectious up to 1 day before symptoms develop and up to 5 days after.

3. The most common signs and symptoms of the flu include fever as high as 105°F, chills, sweats, anorexia, headache, muscle aches, nasal congestion or rhinitis, fatigue, sore throat, and dry cough. Occasionally, patients also complain of gastrointestinal symptoms such as nausea, vomiting, and diarrhea.

4. Treatment of the flu includes fluids, rest, and antipyretic and analgesic medication. Sore throat may be soothed by warm saltwater gargles and throat lozenges.

5. Children should not be given aspirin, because of the risk of Reye syndrome.

6. Vaccination is recommended for health-care providers and vulnerable individuals, such as the elderly, residents of long-term care facilities, those with cancer and lung disease, those with weakened immune systems, infants between 6 and 23 months old, and children on long-term aspirin therapy.

7. Possible complications of influenza are dehydration, bacterial pneumonia, bronchitis, and sinus or ear infections.

Multiple Choice

1. d. Pleural friction rub: motion of a free-floating fractured rib segment in the opposite direction from the rest of the chest as the patient breathes

2. b. Chronic retention of carbon dioxide, leading to symptoms of mental cloudiness and lethargy

3. a. A procedure done under general anesthesia in which scar tissue, pus, or other debris is removed from the pleurae and pleural space

4. d. Histoplasmosis

5. d. All of these

Short Answer

1. Oxygen (air) moves through the mouth or nose, through the nasopharynx or oropharynx, through the trachea, then through smaller and smaller bronchi and into the alveoli. From there, it crosses the thin walls of the alveoli and capillaries and enters the blood.

2. It is all related to blood pH. The urge to breathe is triggered by a lowered pH (caused by a rising CO_2 level). The act of inhalation brings fresh oxygen-rich air into the person's lungs so that the oxygen can be absorbed into the blood. By exhaling, or breathing out, the body eliminates excess CO_2, thus restoring a normal blood pH level. Therefore, when pH levels are low, breathing is faster and deeper (to blow off CO_2), and when pH levels are high, breathing is slower and shallower (to retain CO_2).

3. Apply direct pressure to the soft part of the nose for at least 10 minutes. To prevent nausea, the individual should lead forward and spit blood out rather than swallow it. More severe epistaxis may require treatment by a medical professional. Measures include cauterization by silver nitrate sticks, application of vasoconstricting decongestant nasal sprays, and nasal packing. A calcium alginate mesh called NasalCEASE may be placed to speed

coagulation. In rare cases endoscopic surgery is needed to stop the bleeding.

CHAPTER 12

Case Study 1

1. Tests may include barium swallow, upper endoscopy, upper GI series, barium esophagography, esophageal manometry, gastroscopy, breath test, stool antigen test, fluid pH test, biopsy specimen, and radiographic chest films.

2. The symptoms of pain and burning in your throat and chest are caused by the reflux, or upward flow, of fluids from your stomach. These fluids are very acidic and are irritating to your esophagus. The prescribed medication will make this fluid much less acidic so it doesn't further injure your esophageal lining, thus allowing it to heal.

3. Conservative, nonpharmacologic measures include stopping smoking; losing weight; reducing or eliminating alcohol intake; avoiding large meals, high-fat foods, caffeine, and chocolate for 4 hours before bedtime; and elevating the head of the bed 6 inches.

4. Chronic, severe esophagitis may cause tissue cells in your esophageal lining to change to what is considered a precancerous condition. In other words, esophagitis, if left untreated, could eventually lead to cancer.

Case Study 2

1. • "How many loose stools have you had in the last 24 hours?"
   • "Can you describe the appearance of your stools?"
   • "Approximately how much fluid was lost in each stool?"
   • "Can you describe the type and quantity of fluids you've had in the past 24 hours?"
   • "Were you able to keep any of these fluids down?"
   • "Have you had a fever? If so, what was it?"
   • "How often have you been urinating?"
   • "What does your urine look like?"
   • "Do you feel dizzy or light-headed?"

2. Tests mostly likely to be ordered are stool studies, including microscopic examination for parasites and culture for bacterial or fungal infections. Other tests may include serum WBCs, electrolytes, protein, abdominal x-rays, lower endoscopy, and biopsy.

3. While Danielle could be suffering from an intestinal virus, the sudden onset and severity of her symptoms implicate some type of food poisoning caused by the ingestion of food that has spoiled or been contaminated with bacterial or toxic organisms. Other possibilities include ingestion of insecticides, lead, mercury, or other substances.

4. Prevention of dehydration relies on liberal intake of fluids, including water, diluted fruit juice, rehydration solutions such as Pedialyte, diluted electrolyte sports drinks, Jell-O, Popsicles, and broth. Fluids which worsen dehydration should be avoided; these include caffeinated and alcoholic beverages.

Case Study 3

1. Tests may include a barium swallow with abdominal films, but shouldn't if bowel perforation or ischemia exists. Plain radiography or CT scan may be done. Laboratory tests may include complete blood count (CBC) and electrolytes.

2. Adhesions are scar tissue that develops after a previous abdominal surgery. Mrs. Hernandez most likely developed adhesions secondary to her prior abdominal surgeries.

3. Ingesting any food or fluids at this time will simply worsen her symptoms, and she will vomit up whatever she takes in. However, she will likely be given IV fluids to treat her dehydration.

4. She will not be allowed to eat or drink, and a nasogastric tube may be inserted to decompress her stomach and relieve her nausea and vomiting. Medications may be given to control nausea and promote abdominal peristalsis. She will be given IV fluids and may also receive electrolytes and antibiotics as needed. She will be monitored for return of bowel function and may undergo surgery if the obstruction does not resolve spontaneously.

Multiple Choice

1. d. Esophageal varices: varicose veins of the distal end of the esophagus

2. c. Hiatal hernia: part of the diaphragm around the base of the esophagus weakens and allows a portion of the stomach to slide upward into the thoracic cavity

3. b. Peritonitis: potential complication of appendicitis

4. c. Ulcerative colitis: chronic inflammation of the innermost lining of the rectum and colon

5. c. Hepatitis C: the most common reason for liver transplantation

Short Answer

1. Dental caries and gingivitis

2. See Table below.

3. The majority of peptic ulcers are caused by infection with *Helicobacter pylori*, which is responsive to antibiotic therapy.

	Cause and risk factors	Description	Incidence	Treatment
Apthous ulcer	Familial tendency, immunologic factors, vitamin deficiency, stress, smoking cessation, injury to the mouth, food allergies, menstruation, fatigue, some types of toothpaste, and some diseases	Small, acutely painful ulcers with gray-yellow centers and reddened halos, occurring on the inner lips, gums, or floor of the mouth	Peak incidence in young people (school age to young adulthood); slightly more common in women	No specific treatment; mouthwashes, saline rinses, topical anesthetics, lozenges, and analgesics may reduce pain and discomfort
Cold sore	Caused by herpes simplex virus type 1 (HSV-1); triggers for outbreaks include fever, stress, mouth injury, hormones, and exposure to sun and wind	Small hard spot, usually on the lip, that tingles and then develops into a painful vesicle	Very common because it is contagious	Topical anesthetics and oral analgesics; antiviral drugs may shorten the course

CHAPTER 13

Case Study 1

1. Type 1 diabetes is caused by an autoimmune response. This means your body's immune system is attacking some of the specialized cells in your pancreas that are responsible for producing insulin. Insulin helps glucose, a type of sugar, get into the cells of your body so it can be used for energy. Because your pancreas isn't able to produce insulin anymore, your blood glucose level gets too high while your cells go hungry.

2. When your blood sugar gets really low you might feel tired, restless, hungry, dizzy, irritable, and confused. You might also feel shaky, break into a cold sweat, and feel like your heart is beating irregularly or thumping harder than normal. When your blood glucose rises too high you might notice that you are really tired, thirsty, and hungry, and you may pee so much that you become dehydrated. Others around you might notice that your skin is dry and flushed and that you act confused.

3. If you notice symptoms of low blood sugar, you should eat some type of simple sugar right away, like glucose tablets, orange juice, nondiet soda, or hard candy. Then you should eat a snack or meal of complex carbohydrates and protein, like a peanut butter sandwich or a hamburger. If you notice symptoms of high blood sugar, you should check your blood glucose level and take your insulin according to the guidelines your doctor has given you.

4. It can drop too low if you use too much insulin, don't eat enough food, exercise too strenuously, or are ill with vomiting or diarrhea. It can rise too high if you don't use enough insulin or miss insulin doses, eat too much food, are less active than usual, are under extra stress, or have some types of illness or infection.

5. Unfortunately, no. Insulin must be administered by injection because it is destroyed by stomach acid.

6. It is very important that you develop good habits to care for your feet so that you can prevent complications. Here are some things you should get in the habit of doing every day. Some of these you could do first thing in the morning or before going to bed at night.

   • Inspect your feet every day using a mirror, so you can look at the soles.

- Wash your feet with a mild soap and luke-warm water, and then dry them gently and thoroughly.
- Apply lotion to keep skin soft.
- Trim your toenails carefully, clipping straight across to avoid ingrown nails.
- See a podiatrist to treat corns, calluses, and any sores that aren't healing.
- Always wear good-fitting shoes, even in the house, and never go barefoot.
- Break in new shoes very carefully so you don't get blisters.

- Put on fresh, clean socks every day.
- Don't wear sock with tight tops.
- Inspect your shoes before putting them on to make sure there is nothing inside.
- Wear house slippers and keep a night-light on when you get up during the night, to prevent foot injury.
- Tell your doctor right away if you notice redness, soreness, or breaks in the skin of your feet.

Case Study 2

	Hypothyroidism (Martha)	Hyperthyroidism (Ana)
Cause (thyroid level)	Inadequate levels of thyroid hormones	Excessive thyroid hormones
Metabolism	Diminished	Increased, stimulated
Energy level and mental state	Fatigue, mental apathy, physical sluggishness	Anxiety, nervousness, insomnia, depression
Hair changes	Dry, brittle	Thinning
Body weight	Gain	Loss
Temperature sensitivity	Intolerance of cold	Intolerance of heat
Thyroid-gland size	Enlargement (goiter)	Hypertrophy (goiter)
Diagnostic-test results	High plasma TSH and low free thyroxine	Decreased TSH and increased thyroid hormones
Treatment focus	Lifelong administration of synthetic thyroid hormones and addition of iodine to diet	Medications to suppress thyroid function and surgical removal of part or all of the thyroid gland

Case Study 3

1. Addison disease is an illness that involves gradual failure of the adrenal glands, which results in too little production of steroid hormones. Cushing syndrome is a disorder caused by too much production of cortisol.

2. Addison disease is usually caused by gradual autoimmune destruction of the adrenal glands. Cushing syndrome is caused by chronically high levels of cortisol, as happens when patients take glucocorticoids to suppress their immune systems after organ transplantation, their levels of corticotropin-releasing hormone and ACTH are too high (these hormones stimulate cortisol production), or pituitary or adrenal tumors cause increased secretion of ACTH.

3. Patients with Addison disease are often asymptomatic early on and then develop vague complaints of weakness, fatigue, anorexia, weight loss, nausea, vomiting, abdominal pain, dizziness, postural hypotension, and increased skin pigmentation, causing a bronze coloration of the skin. Life-threatening hyponatremia and hyperkalemia can develop.

   Patients with Cushing syndrome develop increased fat distribution on their upper body, face, neck, and torso; their extremities tend to be thin. Their skin becomes thin and fragile, bruising and injuring easily and healing poorly. They also develop pink-purple striae on the thighs, buttocks, arms, breasts, and abdomen. Other signs and symptoms include osteoporosis, fatigue, weakness, anxiety, irritability, depression, hyperglycemia, and hypertension. Women develop hirsutism and irregular menses; men experience decreased libido and fertility. Children with Cushing syndrome tend to be obese and grow slowly.

4. For Addison disease, corticosteroids such as prednisone must be given as a replacement. Treatment of Cushing syndrome, by contrast, is aimed at suppressing cortisol production and secretion.

Multiple Choice

1. d. Hirsutism: male pattern of body-hair development

2. c. Graves disease: diseased retina caused by poorly controlled diabetes

3. a. Increased thirst

4. d. Pancreatopathy

5. b. Vasopressin is a hormone that helps the body concentrate urine and conserve water.

Short Answer

1. Retinopathy is a diseased retina, neuropathy is damage to motor and sensory nerves, and nephropathy is diseased changes of the kidneys that can lead to eventual kidney failure.

2. Pituitary dwarfism is a condition of reduced growth and development due to deficiency of growth hormone in childhood.

3. Gigantism occurs when the pituitary gland secretes excessive amounts of human growth hormone during childhood, resulting in an abnormal increase in height and size. Acromegaly occurs when the pituitary gland becomes overactive after the individual has reached adulthood, and it causes abnormal continued growth of the bones and tissues of the face and extremities.

CHAPTER 14

Case Study 1

1. Osteoporosis develops when bones lose minerals and density faster than new bone material can be made. This can be caused by any of the following:
   - inadequate minerals in the diet
   - postmenopausal decrease in hormones
   - not getting enough weight-bearing exercise
   - problems with the thyroid and parathyroid glands
   - some types of medication
   - alcohol and tobacco use
   - advancing age
   - a family history of osteoporosis

2. Unfortunately, there aren't any good signs of osteoporosis that will warn you it is developing until it has become severe. When that happens, you will see changes like those your mother has had: loss of height, kyphosis (hunchback), and fractures of bones in the spine or the hips.

3. Yes, there is. There are several tests that can be done, including x-rays, CT scan, and dual energy x-ray absorptiometry scan. Blood tests may also be done to check your levels of serum calcium and estrogen.

4. There are several things you can be doing now. They include:
   - getting regular weight-bearing exercise, such as walking (30 to 60 minutes three or four times per week) and modest weight lifting
   - consistently taking in adequate amounts of calcium, magnesium, and vitamin D
   - eliminating or minimizing alcohol consumption
   - eliminating tobacco use
   - chatting with your doctor about whether you have any risk of hyperthyroidism, whether you should consider hormone replacement therapy, and whether you are on any medications that might increase your risk

Case Study 2

1. The more common name for this disorder is shin splints. It is a painful condition involving the anterior tibias (shins) and the muscles and tendons that attach to them.

2. Shin splints is caused by irritation of muscles, tendons, and tissues along the front of the shin bone and periosteum (tissue layer covering the bone). It is caused from overuse and physical trauma, in your case probably from running.

3. Flat feet (having very low arches) causes overpronation (rolling inward) of your feet as you run. This increases stress on the muscle along

the front of the leg and could certainly increase your risk of this disorder.

4. There are several things you can do:
   - Rest and elevate your legs as often as you can.
   - If swelling is a problem, apply compression (like with an elastic bandage).
   - Take NSAIDs to help with the pain.
   - Massage your shins with ice several times each day.
   - Wear properly fitting shoes.
   - Consider being evaluated and fitted with orthotic shoe inserts—this will help with the flat arches.
   - Consider changing to a low-impact sport, like swimming or bicycling.
   - Try taping your lower legs and ankles to provide stability; some people find that this helps.

Case Study 3

1. It is commonly called a bunion.
2. The bones of the big toe are improperly aligned (positioned wrong) and point toward the second toe instead of straight ahead.
3. Experts don't agree about whether wearing shoes like high heels with narrow toes causes the condition, but they do agree that it makes it worse.
4. There are some measures that can help:
   - using padding over the bunion to reduce pain
   - resting your feet and avoiding activities that worsen pain
   - applying cold
   - taking NSAIDs (with your physician's approval)
   - getting corticosteroid injections (from your physician)

   - wearing custom-fitted orthotics (shoe inserts) to help realign your foot and toes

Multiple Choice

1. d. Pronation: movement of the arm so the palm is up
2. c. Rotation: motion that turns a body part about its axis
3. b. Sciatica
4. a. Rheumatoid arthritis
5. d. Kyphosis

Short Answer

1. Scoliosis is a lateral, S-shaped curve, kyphosis is an exaggerated thoracic curve (hunchback), and lordosis is an exaggerated lumbar curve (swayback).
2. Any five of the following:
   - RA is more severe than osteoarthritis and can affect other tissues in the body than joints.
   - RA is autoimmune in nature.
   - RA causes affected joints to lose function and possibly move out of alignment, becoming dislocated.
   - Symptoms of RA affect several joints of the body in a bilateral pattern.
   - Rheumatoid nodules may appear beneath the skin on the patient's arms.
   - Patients with RA frequently experience generalized symptoms of fatigue, fever, and weight loss.
   - Patients with RA experience periods of exacerbation and remission.
3. See Table below.

	Similarities	Differences
Symptoms	Fatigue, malaise, and pain	Acute: Redness, heat, edema, fever, and chills Chronic: Skin ulceration, formation of a sinus tract, and drainage
Diagnosis	Culture and sensitivity, x-ray, MRI, and CT	Acute: Elevated white blood cells Chronic: Elevated erythrocyte sedimentation rate
Treatment	Prolonged antibiotic therapy, possible surgery (probable with chronic osteomyelitis)	Chronic: Possible amputation
Prognosis	N/A	Acute: Good Chronic: Guarded

CHAPTER 15

Case Study 1

1. Conjunctivitis may be caused by allergic reactions or bacterial or viral infection. Other causes include the presence of a foreign object in the eye and the splashing of an irritating substance into the eye. In newborn babies, it may be caused by an incompletely opened tear duct.

2. It is extremely contagious. Melissa should avoid touching her eyes and sharing washcloths, towels, or other items that come into contact with her face. She should wash her hands frequently and cleanse her eyes with a separate warm washcloth for each eye.

3. Eyes are typically red, swollen, teary, sensitive to light, and itchy, with a gritty feeling. Drainage may be clear or thick yellow or green.

4. Treatment of conjunctivitis varies with the cause. Symptoms of allergic and viral conjunctivitis respond to application of cool, moist compresses and artificial tears. Severe cases may be treated with anti-inflammatory medications, antihistamines, decongestants, mast-cell stabilizers, and topical-steroid eyedrops. Conjunctivitis that is thought to have a bacterial cause is treated with broad-spectrum antibiotic eyedrops or ointments.

   If a chemical splash is the cause, the eyes must be immediately and thoroughly irrigated with sterile saline, or water if saline is not available. Depending upon the type of chemical and the severity of the burn, treatment may include the use of topical steroids and referral to an ophthalmologist for further care.

Case Study 2

1. He might describe a shadow in the peripheral vision that progresses across the visual field or toward the center, like a veil or curtain being drawn over the visual field.

2. A tear in the retina develops secondary to eye or head trauma and allows vitreous humor to leak through and collect beneath it. This causes the retina to begin to separate and peel away from the underlying tissue. If a blood vessel is included in the tear, bleeding may occur. As more fluid accumulates, the degree of detachment increases.

3. Cryotherapy (freezing) and laser photocoagulation create scar tissue around the retinal tear that prevents fluid from flowing through the hole and collecting behind the retina. Scleral buckling is a surgical procedure in which tiny bands of silicone, plastic, or sponge are sewn to the outer surface of the eyeball. They act like a belt and pull the eye wall inward against the hole, thereby compressing it and helping the retina to reattach. Some of the fluid that has collected behind the retina is also drained though a small slit in the sclera. Vitrectomy is a procedure in which vitreous humor is removed. It is usually combined with a procedure called pneumatic retinopexy, in which a gas bubble is injected into the eye. Afterward, the patient maintains a specified position (often facing downward) over the next several days or weeks so that the bubble pushes against the retinal tear. The bubble expands initially and then is absorbed over the next several weeks. As this occurs, the eye produces vitreous fluid and refills the posterior chamber.

Case Study 3

1. Vertigo is a sensation of moving around in space and extreme dizziness. Tinnitus is ringing or other abnormal sounds in the ears.

2. Treatment is focused on dietary modification, medications to reduce symptoms, and possible surgery. Recommended dietary changes include limiting salt and sugar intake and eliminating alcohol, caffeine, and possibly aspartame. Smoking cessation is encouraged. Bedrest may be advised for acute attacks. A variety of medications are used to relieve symptoms, including antihistamines, anticholinergics, sedatives, antiemetics, anticonvulsants, and corticosteroids. In extreme cases, surgery may be done to relieve pressure or even to destroy or remove part of the inner ear. A vestibular neurectomy (cutting the nerve) may also be done to relieve vertigo.

3. Ménière disease usually begins in one ear only, but after a number of years, half of all patients have bilateral disease. In most cases, progressive hearing loss develops and can become severe. Tinnitus may also worsen over time. However, in some individuals the attacks lessen in severity and frequency over time or even resolve spontaneously and completely— they may then never recur.

Multiple Choice

1. d. Glaucoma: disorder in which increased intraocular pressure results in loss of peripheral vision and eventual blindness
2. c. It is usually preceded by an upper respiratory infection.
3. b. Labyrinthitis
4. c. Presbyopia: age-related vision loss
5. a. Cholesteatoma

Short Answer

1. Acquired cholesteatoma usually develops secondary to otitis media when the TM has been perforated. The skin of the TM then grows through the hole into the middle ear. As it grows, the cholesteatoma can destroy the ossicles. Chronic swelling of the eustachian tube leads to negative pressure within the middle ear, which pulls the TM in the wrong direction. This creates a cyst that fills with sloughed skill cells and debris. When the cyst becomes inflamed and infected, it may cause degeneration of the ossicles.
2. Patients with foreign bodies in the ears are usually children under 5 years of age.
3. Otitis externa
4. Entropion is a condition in which the edges of the eyelid are turned inward and rub the surface of the eye. It usually affects the lower eyelid. Ectropion is a condition in which the lower eyelid is turned outward and droops more with aging.
5. A hordeolum is an infection of a sebaceous gland at the base of an eyelash. A chalazion is a small cyst in the eyelid. It differs from a hordeolum in that it is usually larger and less painful. Over time it develops into a small, nontender nodule in the center of the eyelid. In contrast, a hordeolum localizes to the edge of the eyelid and remains painful.

CHAPTER 16

Case Study 1

1. Most fetal blood bypasses the lungs, because the placenta provides oxygen and nutrients.
2. Blood returns to the heart from the body by entering the right atrium. Nearly two-thirds of it then flows into the left atrium through an opening called the foramen ovale. From there, blood flows into the left ventricle and out through the aorta. Only about one-third of the blood that enters the right atrium flows down into the right ventricle and then out through the pulmonary artery. Instead of going to the lungs, most of it is shunted through the ductus arteriosus into the aorta.
3. Shortly after birth, the umbilical cord is clamped and the infant is separated from the placenta. This is also when the infant's first breaths are taken. These things bring about a change in circulation. A greater amount of blood flows to the lungs, where it picks up oxygen. The ductus arteriosus no longer serves a purpose, and it begins to constrict and seal shut. As larger amounts of blood flow into the left atrium from the lungs, the increased pressure causes the septum primum, a one-way flap, to close over the foramen ovale. This, in turn, causes all blood returning to the right atrium to flow down to the right ventricle and on to the lungs through the pulmonary artery.
4. An atrial septal defect is a condition in which there is a hole between the right and left atria that allows blood flow between the two chambers. Mostly, oxygenated blood that has just returned to the left atrium from the lungs flows into the right atrium.

    A ventricular septal defect is a condition in which there are one or more holes in the septal wall that separates the right and left ventricles.

    Patent ductus arteriosus is a condition in which the ductus arteriosus, normally present in the fetus, fails to close within 10 days after birth. As a result, blood continues to flow abnormally between the pulmonary artery and the aorta.

    Tetralogy of Fallot is a condition in which an infant is born with a group of four different heart defects: a large ventricular septal defect, an overriding aorta, pulmonic stenosis that causes obstruction of outflow from the right ventricle, and hypertrophy of the right ventricle.

Case Study 2

1. Duchenne muscular dystrophy and Becker muscular dystrophy
2. They cause progressive muscle weakness.
3. DMD

4. Both forms nearly always affect boys. DMD is the most common type in children and affects very young boys, around ages 2 to 6. BMD affects boys in their adolescence or early adulthood.

5. DMD is caused by an absence of dystrophin. Individuals with BMD produce some of this protein, but it is either too little or of poor quality. DMD and BMD are X-linked genetic disorders passed from female carriers to their sons.

6. The symptoms of both are similar. With DMD, symptoms occur as early as age 2. Walking may be delayed and children appear clumsy, fall frequently, and have difficulty rising from lying or sitting. Generalized muscle wasting and weakness first affects voluntary muscles of the shoulders, pelvis, and thighs. The calves may appear enlarged. This can be misleading, because it is caused by fat accumulation rather than muscle development. The child walks with an odd, waddling gait and may walk on his toes or the balls of his feet, with the belly stuck out and shoulders held back. This is an attempt to maintain balance. He may struggle to raise his arms and will lose the ability to walk around age 7 to 12. Eventually, respiratory and cardiac muscles are affected; patients typically enter the final stages of the disorder in their late teens or early 20s. Approximately one-third of individuals with muscular dystrophy also have learning disabilities.

    The course of BMD is similar but slower and less predictable. Consequently, diagnosis may not occur until the patient's late teens or adulthood. The pattern of muscle wasting and loss of functioning is similar to that in DMD, though more variable. These individuals may not lose the ability to walk until their middle or late 30s.

7. The prognosis for patients with muscular dystrophy depends upon the type and severity of the condition and on the patient's access to medical care. Those with DMD often die before the age of 20 and rarely survive past 30. Life expectancy is better for those with BMD; they often survive into their middle or late adult years.

Case Study 3

1. The cause of cryptorchidism is not clearly understood. The testicles develop within the abdomen and usually descend into the scrotum between 28 and 40 weeks' gestation. Possible risk factors for the condition include abnormalities of the abdominal wall, maternal alcohol abuse, maternal diabetes, and maternal exposure to cigarette smoke or pesticides. Maternal caffeine exposure (more than three cups of coffee per day) has also been implicated.

2. Physical examination will confirm an absent testicle. Further examination may reveal the testicle within the inguinal canal. However, in some cases the testicle is nonpalpable, and further diagnostic testing may be necessary to determine its exact location. This may include pelvic ultrasound or MRI, both of which are generally safe, noninvasive procedures. In some cases genetic testing is necessary to identify or rule out other genetic disorders.

3. Yes, although in most cases no treatment is needed, since the condition often corrects itself within several months. However, if the testicle has not properly descended by the time he is 4 to 6 months old, treatment can be done. It may involve hormonal therapy or surgery to correctly place and anchor the testicle within the scrotum and close the inguinal canal.

Multiple Choice

1. d. Y chromosome: one of two chromosomes that determine gender in humans; determines female gender

2. b. Is inherited by a man from his mother

3. c. It can be diagnosed prenatally.

4. b. Cystic fibrosis

5. a. Pyloric stenosis

Short Answer

1. Neural tube defects (spina bifida occulta, meningocele, myelomeningocele, anencephaly, and iniencephaly), cleft lip, and cleft palate

2. They are both chromosomal disorders that involve the sex chromosomes. Both usually cause infertility. Diagnosis is confirmed for both with karyotype testing.

3. Fetal alcohol syndrome causes damage to the central nervous system and affects other organs and tissues in the body as well. Physical defects of FAS include heart defects, growth deficits, malformed facial features, malformed extremities, poor muscle tone, and decreased physical coordination. Learning and

behavioral disorders are common. Children with FAS frequently struggle with impaired attention span, memory deficits, hyperactivity, faulty judgment, poor impulse control, and sensory (hearing, vision) and communication problems. Infants with FAS also struggle with sleep and sucking and feeding.

CHAPTER 17

Case Study 1

1. Basal cell carcinoma is the most common type of skin cancer and therefore the type Arcelia is likely to see the most.
2. Malignant melanoma
3. Malignant melanoma
4. Australia
5. Ultraviolet exposure from sunlight or tanning beds, childhood sunburns, fair skin, red hair, and family history
6. The warning signs of malignant melanoma can be remembered by the ABCDE system:
   - **A**symmetry: The mole is irregular in shape; one half does not match the other half.
   - **B**order: The edges of the mole are irregular, notched, scalloped, or blurred.
   - **C**olor: Varying shades of color appear throughout, including tan, brown, black, blue, red, and white.
   - **D**iameter: The mole is larger than 6 millimeters, or displays new growth.
   - **E**volution: The appearance of the mole changes over time, or symptoms of bleeding or itching develop.

Case Study 2

1. We aren't sure about the specific cause. Risk factors include a history of cryptorchidism (undescended testicle), HIV infection or AIDS, age between 15 and 34, Caucasian race, and a family history of testicular cancer.
2. Patients with testicular cancer often don't have symptoms in the early stages. Signs and symptoms include a lump or enlargement in the testicle, which may or may not be painful; a dull ache within the groin or abdomen; a feeling of heaviness within the scrotum; scrotal edema; breast enlargement; fatigue; and malaise.
3. We might perform testicular ultrasound, which is highly effective. A solid mass is a sign of a malignant tumor, because most other testicular conditions involve the presence of fluid. If findings are suspicious, then tissue biopsy would be done to confirm the diagnosis. Blood tests might also be done. Alpha-fetoprotein and human chorionic gonadotropin, two proteins called tumor markers, in the blood may indicate the presence of a testicular tumor. A CT scan may also be done to help stage the cancer and identify whether it has spread to other organs.
4. No. The prognosis is good when diagnosis is early but declines as the cancer becomes more advanced. Overall, there is a 95% rate of successful treatment.
5. You did the right thing by coming in. In the future, you should perform a testicular self-examination every month. This will help you become familiar with how your testicles normally feel and increases the odds that you will notice changes early. If you notice lumps or bumps that are different from normal and persist for more than 2 weeks, then you should definitely see a doctor so it can be checked out. However, you might find it reassuring to know that many other disorders besides cancer can explain testicular changes.

Case Study 3

1. Yes, nearly 150,000 people are diagnosed with this type of cancer every year in the United States.
2. Unfortunately, we don't completely understand what causes cancer. But we do know that some of the risk factors for this type of cancer are a history of inflammatory bowel disease; family history of colorectal cancer; sedentary lifestyle; low-fiber, high-fat diet; obesity; and alcohol and tobacco use.
3. It is common for patients to have no symptoms in the early stages. When symptoms do occur, they can include a variety of things, like a change in bowel-elimination pattern, blood in the stools, abdominal pain, pallor (pale skin), anemia, and, as in your case, intestinal obstruction.
4. Once in a while people notice this, but quite often any blood that is there is not obvious.
5. Yes. Routine screening tests are the best way to catch it early. They include fecal occult blood tests and lower endoscopy.

6. Among patients whose colorectal cancer is detected early, the survival rate is 90%. However, in 61% of cases, metastasis has occurred by the time of diagnosis. The prognosis then is more guarded and depends on how the patient responds to treatment.

Multiple Choice

1. d. Supportive surgery: surgery done to remove cancerous tissue and cure the patient
2. c. Myeloma: cancer that originates within the eyes
3. b. Presence of the *BRCA1* or *BRCA2* gene
4. c. Wilms tumor: postmenopausal Caucasian women
5. a. Avoid iron-rich foods because they can cause constipation.

Short Answer

1. The seven warning signs of cancer are change in bowel or bladder habits, a sore throat that does not heal, unusual bleeding or discharge, thickening or a lump in the breast or other area, indigestion or difficulty swallowing, obvious change in a mole or wart, and nagging cough or hoarseness.

2. Treatments include various combinations of surgery (lumpectomy, partial mastectomy, total mastectomy, and modified radical mastectomy), radiation, chemotherapy, and hormone therapy.

3. Have regular oral and dental hygiene checkups; minimize your alcohol intake; avoid tobacco products; prevent or treat gastroesophageal reflux disease; eat a diet that is high in fiber, rich in fruits and vegetables, and low in fat; follow measures to avoid contracting hepatitis B; and follow measures to protect and strengthen your immune system.

CHAPTER 18

Case Study 1

1. With both disorders, Marco would have a hard time paying attention for more than a short amount of time and has a hard time prioritizing and getting things done. The main difference with ADHD is that he would also have a very hard time sitting still for long and would prefer to be moving around.

2. We still don't know for sure what causes it, but we think it might be a combination of things. It does seem to run in families, so there might be something about it that is genetic. But that does not mean that you did anything wrong. Some children may have something about their brain and the chemicals in their brain that is different from other people, and there may even be other causes that we still are not sure of.

3. Children with ADD and ADHD have a very hard time getting organized and do tend to lose things. Other common behaviors include difficulty staying on task and finishing what they start, being impulsive and distractible, making careless mistakes, difficulty paying attention, struggling with schoolwork, feeling restless, talking a lot, blurting out comments or answers, interrupting others, and difficulty waiting in lines or taking turns.

4. You are making a good start by learning about the disorder. That will help you to better understand your son's behavior. Some other things you can do are:
   - Communicate frequently with his teacher and be sure to go to conferences.
   - Check with Marco every day about homework or notes from his teacher.
   - Provide an uncluttered area for him to do his homework.
   - Designate a regular homework time but allow him to take frequent breaks.
   - Do not expect perfection; reward him for good behavior.
   - Help Marco develop organizational skills. For example, you might pick out a place for him to put his backpack when he comes home from school each day, and you might want to get him his own calendar for his wall, that he can write on.
   - Arrange a meeting with the school psychologist if you are concerned that Marco's needs are not being met.

Case Study 2

1. If you and Josh's parents are concerned, then they should make an appointment to discuss this with Josh's doctor. I can tell you that many children experience some degree of stuttering during their early years. It usually goes away within several weeks or months. Fewer than 5% of children who stutter experience a more significant and longer-lasting problem.

2. We aren't sure. Children who stutter may process speech and language information in different parts of their brain. Genetics might be a factor, since the problem appears to run in families. Acquired stuttering may occur after a stroke, after administration of certain drugs, or as a reaction to unusually stressful circumstances.

3. Since the problem only started recently and most cases resolve on their own, he probably doesn't need any treatment. When it is performed, treatment is aimed at helping patients speak and communicate more smoothly and effectively. Patients are taught to monitor the pace at which they speak, to pronounce words in a slower, more relaxed manner, and to control their breathing. Other therapies include relaxation techniques, hypnosis, and delayed auditory feedback (a technique that enables speakers to hear their own voices a fraction of a second later, similar to an echo). In some cases, medications such as neuroleptics may also provide some benefit. Should treatment become necessary, you would need to work with Josh's doctor and a speech and language pathologist to figure out the best treatment plan for him.

Case Study 3

1. Munchausen syndrome

2. Munchausen syndrome is a puzzling disorder without a clearly identifiable cause. Efforts to gather statistical data have been complicated by the fact that patients excel in concealing the true cause or nature of their symptoms, sometimes conceal their true identities, and are extremely resistant to psychiatric evaluation. Patients seem not to be motivated by secondary gain, as with many other disorders, but rather seek the illness, hospitalization, and invasive procedures as a primary goal. The disorder also differs from hypochondria in that hypochondriacs truly believe they are ill whereas patients with Munchausen syndrome *desire* to be.

3. Diagnosis of Munchausen syndrome is extremely challenging because of the patient's elaborate efforts to be deceptive. Actual physical disorders must be ruled out or treated as appropriate. When the disorder is suspected, a psychiatric evaluation is necessary. However, patients are generally very resistant to this and may respond angrily by "firing" their physician

and leaving to seek out another physician at another facility to repeat the pattern there. Whenever possible, a psychiatrist performs an evaluation. To make the diagnosis, certain criteria must be met, including evidence that the patient is either faking or self-inducing the disorder and that the patient is motivated to be viewed as ill but is not motivated by financial or legal gain.

4. While patients with Munchausen syndrome are eager to undergo treatment for physical ailments, they are extremely resistant to admit to or accept treatment for their psychiatric disorder. A gentle approach that helps the patient avoid embarrassment is most effective. Psychotherapy is aimed at behavior modification to reduce the use or misuse of medical care. When possible, family members are included in therapy aimed at eliminating any rewarding of the illness behaviors. Medication may be useful in treating related disorders, such as anxiety or depression. However, this must be carefully monitored, since the patient may misuse prescribed medications. In some cases, hospitalization in a psychiatric facility may be necessary.

Multiple Choice

1. b. Avoidant personality disorder: chronic, excessive psychological dependence on others

2. d. Hallucination: false, unfounded belief

3. c. Dysgraphia is a type of learning disorder.

4. c. Delirium is an acute, reversible state of agitated confusion marked by disorientation, hallucinations, or delusions.

5. a. Your mood and energy level should both improve within 7 to 10 days.

Short Answer

1. Strategies that improve quantity and quality of sleep include:
   - going to bed and getting up at the same times each day
   - avoiding stimulants such as caffeine or tobacco in the evening
   - eating a light-fat snack in the evening, if hungry, but avoiding large, high-fat meals
   - exercising during the day, not before bedtime
   - using meditation or relaxation exercises to relax the body and mind

- creating a calm, quiet, dark, soothing environment in which to sleep
- creating a bedtime routine or ritual, such as reading, taking a warm bath, or stretching
- avoiding performing activities in the bedroom that are not related to sleep (working, watching TV, eating, etc.)
- not napping during the day
- masking environmental noise by wearing earplugs or creating white noise with a fan or sound machine
- getting out of bed for a while if you are awake for more than 30 minutes
- getting up, writing yourself a note, and putting it where you are sure to see it in the morning, if you are worried about forgetting to do something
- making an organized, prioritized list of things you need to do the next day and putting it where you are sure to see it in the morning
- giving yourself permission to simply "rest" rather than sleep; this may lower your stress and help you relax, and you might "accidentally" fall asleep without even realizing it

2. The key feature is manipulation of others without any regard for their feelings or for right and wrong. Signs include destructive or negative behaviors such as setting fires, cruelty to animals, theft, aggression toward others, intimidation of others, commission of crimes, abuse of drugs and alcohol, and abuse or neglect of children. Other behaviors are more subtle, but just as destructive, such as lying and manipulating others for selfish gain, usually in a completely charming manner. They are also easily frustrated and prone to irritation and anger.

3. Population most commonly affected: Females
Social norm conformed to: Thinness
Amount of food eaten: Those with anorexia eat too little, while those with bulimia eat large quantities of food during binges.
Body weight: Those with anorexia become dangerously thin, while the body weight of those with bulimia fluctuates but usually remains in the normal range.
Physical signs and symptoms: Those with anorexia display signs and symptoms of very poor nutrition (poor growth, anemia, hypothermia, thinning hair, dizziness, and dry, pale skin). They also display psychological symptoms that include intense fear of weight

gain, perfectionism, memory difficulties, obsessive or compulsive tendencies, low self-esteem, depression, and moodiness. Malnutrition and weight loss may be mild or severe.
Those with bulimia display signs and symptoms of purging, including esophagitis, sore throat, or sore mouth; tooth erosion; bloodshot eyes; sores, calluses, or scars on the hands or knuckles; irregular heartbeat; abnormal bowel function; fatigue; and dehydration.
Shared deadly complication: Heart failure

CHAPTER 19

Case Study 1

1. Any number of approaches could work. One might be to say something like: "I used to think that too, but I was surprised to learn that Biowarfare has been common throughout history.

2.
- 600 BC—Assyrians poisoned their enemies' wells with ergot that contained mycotoxins.
- 184 BC—Hannibal's army launched earthen pots filled with poisonous snakes onto their enemies' ships.
- 1346 (and later)—Plague-infected corpses were launched by military troops over the walls of enemy cities.
- 1767—British soldiers gave smallpox-infested blankets to Indians as "gifts" to intentionally cause an epidemic.
- 1930s—Japan used biological weapons against China, killing tens of thousands.
- 1940s and 1950s—The United States developed sites in Maryland, Mississippi, Utah, and Arkansas to develop and study biological weapons.
- 1960s—The Vietcong placed feces-contaminated spears in pits to trap and kill their enemies.
- 1979—An explosion in a military compound in the USSR resulted in the accidental release of anthrax spores, killing approximately 1,000 people.
- 1984—Members of the Rajneeshee cult in Oregon contaminated salad bars in The Dalles in an effort to influence the outcome of an election, making more than 750 ill and hospitalizing 40.
- 2001—Twenty-two people in the United States developed anthrax after exposure by mail; several of them died.

Case Study 2

- potential for dissemination as an aerosol
- potential for mass casualties
- initially benign presentation of victims
- need for a sophisticated medical and governmental response
- potential for widespread panic
- potential to cause diseases that can be transmitted from person to person

Case Study 3

1. It was virtually eliminated from the human population, and there seemed to be no need for continued vaccinations.

2. The term *pox* is from a Latin word that means "spotted," and it refers to the rash of raised bumps that develops on those who are infected with smallpox.

3. Smallpox is spread through respiratory secretions and secretions from lesions. It may also be spread indirectly through contact with contaminated objects, such as clothing or blankets.

4. A macular rash develops in the mouth and then spreads quickly to the rest of the body. It progresses through papular (bumps), vesicular (clear blisters), and pustular (pus-filled blisters) stages. The pustules subsequently rupture and form scabs that leave disfiguring scars. The acute symptomatic stage typically lasts 14 to 21 days.

   A key way to distinguish smallpox from chickenpox is that smallpox lesions spread over the body very quickly (within 24 hours) and are all in the same stage at the same time. Furthermore, the lesions are most prevalent on the face, hands, and legs. The lesions of chickenpox, by contrast, appear over a much longer period of time (14 days), are in multiple stages of development at the same time, and are most prevalent on the face and trunk.

Multiple Choice

1. d. Botulism: the classic symptoms include nausea, anorexia, bloody diarrhea, fever, and severe stomach pain

2. a. Vaccination is currently available to some members of the armed forces, laboratory workers, and those who need to work in contaminated areas.

3. c. The Aum Shinrikyo group

4. b. The causative organism is usually found in the soil.

5. c. Early symptoms are similar to those of influenza.

Short Answer

1. Any five of the following:
   - creation of a response plan
   - identification and training of response teams to work at local and state levels
   - ensuring the availability of resources to provide accurate testing and appropriate treatment
   - collection and storage of antibiotics
   - creation of a national database to facilitate the identification and tracking of cases
   - coordination of nationwide sharing of information
   - creation of educational programs and resources for the media, the general public, and health-care professionals

2. The CDC maintains a surveillance system for botulism cases based upon reports from health-care providers. Two antitoxins are available and are being stored in a variety of locations across the nation.

   An investigational botulism vaccine has been used for military and high-risk laboratory personnel in the recent past. While this vaccine is no longer in production, another one is currently under development. Efforts are planned to develop a means of rapidly detecting and diagnosing botulism by the year 2013.

3. If *Francisella tularensis* were used as a biological weapon, it would likely be aerosolized. Inhalation of the organism causes severe, life-threatening respiratory illness, and systemic infection without rapid, aggressive treatment. Because the bacteria exist readily in nature, they could be isolated and developed in sizable quantities in the laboratory. However, the manufacture of an efficient and effective aerosol weapon would take significant sophistication.

CHAPTER 20

Case Study 1

1. Ms. McKenna's pain is chronic, because she has had it daily for 20 years.

2. Subjective data would be her verbal statements describing her pain.

3. Nonmalignant—rheumatoid arthritis is not a type of cancer.

4. She may well be depressed, but rheumatoid arthritis is known to be a devastating illness that causes severe pain. Furthermore, chronic pain is much more likely to cause depression, rather than the reverse. The depression, in turn, could cause difficulty coping effectively with the pain. She may need to be treated for both, but it is unfair to her to suggest that her problem is merely one of being depressed.

Case Study 2

1. Age has little impact on an individual's ability to feel pain, but it may affect the expression of pain (very young patients may cry and thrash about, while some teens and adults may refrain from such a response, and elderly patients may be afraid to complain at all).

   Fatigue increases the perception of pain and diminishes coping skills, while being well rested diminishes pain perception and increases tolerance of pain. Neurological impairment can interfere with the perception of pain.

   Experience with severe or unremitting pain increases the fear of its return and increases pain perception.

   Effective coping skills help patients respond to and manage injury, pain, and fear. Dysfunctional coping skills hinder this response.

   Cultural factors affect patients' responses to and interpretations of the meaning of pain.

2. For many years the response was woefully inadequate. This was due in part to an inadequate understanding of pain, inadequate strategies for managing pain, and exaggerated fears about the abuse of medication and about side effects. In an effort to address the problem, some health-care organizations have developed standards and guidelines for the evaluation and management of pain. Pain has been labeled as the fifth vital sign as a reminder that it should be evaluated as frequently as temperature and blood pressure.

3. • All patients have the right to have their pain assessed and managed.
   • Staff are to be competent in the assessment and management of pain.
   • Patients and family members are to be educated about effective pain management.

• Symptom management is to be addressed during discharge planning.
• All care (described above) is to be documented.

Case Study 3

1. This information will help him begin to understand the degree of control that she believes she has over events in her life. It may indicate how motivated she will be to take charge of her health and invest the time and effort needed to get better.

2. Biofeedback could teach her to control her autonomic nervous system. This involves the use of a variety of technologies that provide feedback about physiological functions. These include electromyography, which provides feedback about muscle tension; skin sensors, which provide feedback about skin temperature; electroencephalography, which provides feedback about brain-wave activity; and electrodermal response, which provides feedback about the activity of the sweat glands. Feedback is given by way of sounds through headphones or blinking lights when changes occur in pulse, blood pressure, brain waves, or muscle contractions. This would help her develop an increased awareness of her body, thereby giving her greater control over it. Once the technique is learned, she could reproduce the results without the need for technology. Through this process she could improve circulation and muscle relaxation, which may relieve or reduce her pain. She would probably master the skill after 10 or 12 sessions.

   Hydrotherapy typically occurs is specially designed therapy pools. She could participate in weight-bearing exercises that may be difficult for her on dry land. Water creates buoyancy and supports a large percentage of the body weight. This allows greater participation in therapy without causing damage or excessive discomfort. It also removes the fear of falling, thereby decreasing her fear and anxiety. The water is kept warmer than in a typical swimming pool, which helps to promote relaxation and flexibility. Water provides resistance against body movement, which adds a dimension of strength training that is not possible on dry land. Finally, most patients find therapy in the water to be much more enjoyable than dry-land therapy.

Multiple Choice

1. b. Subjective: observable, measurable, and analyzable
2. c. Endorphin: inactive substance that has no inherent medicinal value
3. d. The cause of chronic pain is often unclear.
4. d. TENS units work by delivering neurotransmitters to the central nervous system.
5. a. Iontophoresis delivers small electrical pulses to specified parts of the body with electrodes placed on the skin.

Short Answer

1. Patients may be left wondering why they are still in pain. When they learn of the deception, the trust relationship between them and their health-care providers is destroyed. Sadly, they tend to mistrust health-care providers thereafter. Patients deserve to be treated with respect, dignity, and honesty. They also are legally and ethically entitled to make informed decisions. This isn't possible when critical information is kept from them.

2. • Identify and address the patient's beliefs and concerns regarding health issues and needed changes.
   • Help patients understand the whys. Most people feel more enthusiastic about making changes once they understand how they will benefit.
   • Start with small, realistic, achievable steps.
   • Invite the patient to identify individual learning goals.
   • Work new behaviors into the existing routine; this makes change feel less drastic and more possible.
   • Ask the patient for a commitment to take specific steps.
   • Connect the patient to a support person or support group.
   • Consult with physicians about appropriate referrals for professional consultation. Examples include registered dietitians, diabetes educators, physical therapists, and psychologists.
   • Identify a plan for follow-up and let the patient know that you will be monitoring progress.
   • Express concern and care. A persuasive statement from a health-care professional can be influential.
   • Express confidence in the patient's ability to succeed.

3. Any three of the following:

Myth: Healthcare providers can determine whether or not the client's pain is real.
The pain experience is completely subjective. Health-care providers have no way to see, feel, or measure a patient's pain. Objective physical changes may or may not be apparent, but their absence should never be taken as proof of the absence of pain. It is important to remember that physical indicators associated with acute pain are rarely seen in those suffering from chronic pain. It is also important to remember that people express pain differently based upon a variety of personal, social, and cultural factors. Finally, health-care providers should remember to treat their patients in the same manner that they themselves would wish to be treated, which means that they choose to believe them or at least give them the benefit of the doubt and then respond in a compassionate manner.

Myth: The very young and the very old have a decreased perception of pain.
There is little evidence that age impacts pain perception. Individuals in these two groups often have a compromised ability to communicate what they are feeling, which may lead others to mistakenly assume that they feel less pain. Health-care professionals must be very careful never to make such assumptions and should always err on the side of providing more rather than fewer comfort measures.

Myth: Men/Women perceive pain more (or less) than those of the opposite gender.
Myth: Men/Women have a greater (or lesser) tolerance for pain than those of the opposite gender.
Such topics always generate a lively discussion with opinions going both ways. However, there is no evidence to support the belief that men and women experience more or less pain or have a higher or lower tolerance for it. Such beliefs generally arise from assumptions based upon differences that may be seen in the expression of pain. However, it is important to remember that pain is subjective and may be expressed in a wide variety of ways by men and women of different cultures.

Myth: Individuals who take opioid analgesics run a high risk for becoming addicted.
According to the American Pain Society, misunderstandings about addiction and unfairly labeling patients as addicts has resulted in unjustified withholding of opioid medications.

Studies show that the risk of addiction from the treatment of acute pain with opioid medication is nearly zero (<1%). Evidence shows that individuals who take opioid analgesics for pain stop taking the medication when the pain ends.

Use of opioid medications by those with chronic pain has not been well studied, so the risk of addiction is not clearly known. However, there is reason to believe that opioid use by patients with chronic pain, who are properly evaluated and well managed, increases their productivity and overall quality of life without producing the feared ramifications.

Addiction is a compulsive disorder in which an individual becomes preoccupied with obtaining and using a substance, the continued use of which results in a decreased quality of life.

Myth: People with chronic pain should never be treated with opiates.
Given the long-standing concerns that healthcare providers have had about the potential for medication abuse among those with chronic pain, it is important to point out the difference between **physical dependence, tolerance,** and **psychological addiction.** Both physical dependence and tolerance are naturally occurring phenomena in those who take opioid medication on a regular basis for an extended period of time. Tolerance refers to the fact that over time, the body loses sensitivity to opioids and their pain relieving effects. As a result, there may be a need for an increased dosage to achieve the same results. Physical dependence is said to have occurred if the individual experiences a withdrawal syndrome when the medication is suddenly discontinued. Neither of these phenomena reflects immoral, unethical, or illegal behavior or intent on the part of the individual. Neither do they indicate anything about the individual's moral character. They simply describe a physiological response to the continued presence of the opioid medication.

Health-care providers should refrain from using the terms "addict" or "addiction" in reference to their patients because of the negative implications associated with such terms. Addiction has been defined in a variety of ways. Descriptors include compulsive, maladaptive, disabling, relapsing, chronic disease, drug-seeking, and dependence. Results of addiction are described in terms of adverse or negative psychological, physical, economic, social, health, and legal consequences.

Drug abuse is a real problem and healthcare providers are sure to encounter some patients who may be drug-seeking. However, they must be very careful about labeling patients as "drug seekers," since such labels can easily promote bias against patients and negatively affect the quality of care provided. Furthermore, it is important to note that healthcare providers are making assumptions which may or may not be true. The behaviors of patients who are drug-seeking might be very similar to patients who are relief-seeking. This is called **pseudoaddiction.** These people seem preoccupied with obtaining opioids because their desire to obtain opioids is directly related to the poor pain relief they have experienced. Once their pain is well managed, the drug-seeking behavior will generally disappear.

In an effort to respond to misconceptions about the risk of addiction when treating patients with chronic pain, the World Health Organization issued this recommendation:
Step 1: Use of NSAIDs and adjuvant medication
Step 2: Use of weak opioids and adjuvants
Step 3: Use of strong opioids and adjuvants
These steps are to be taken in the order listed until the patient has achieved satisfactory relief and management of his pain. However, in the case of patients with cancer pain, the recommended order is reversed. Strong opioids should be used initially if needed to get the patient's pain under control, followed by a reduction to the point that adequate pain management is maintained.

Myth: The risks of side effects of opioid medications outweigh the benefits.
Common side effects of opioid medications include respiratory depression, sedation, and gastrointestinal (GI) problems, including nausea, vomiting, and constipation. Health-care providers often recite the risks of these side effects as reason to discontinue or withhold opioids.

Certainly these side effects are a potential problem for any patient taking opioids. However, they can usually be minimized or managed and are not an acceptable reason to withhold treatment.

Risk of sedation and respiratory depression are greatest when opioid medication is first given to an individual who has little or no experience with them. Therefore, dosage strength and frequency should be conservative until the patient's response has been determined. Medication can then be increased as necessary, as indicated by the physician, to achieve the best result. Over time, people actually develop a tolerance for these side effects and will experience less of a problem with either sedation or respiratory depression.

It is also worth noting that unrelieved pain is exhausting. When individuals finally achieve pain relief, they may, for the first time in a long while, be able to relax and sleep. This is not the same thing as being over-sedated and can be easily distinguished by noting whether the person's respiratory rate is depressed and whether he or she is easily awakened.

GI side effects tend to be more ongoing but in most cases can be minimized or managed through a variety of strategies. Nausea is lessened by taking medication with food and by the administration of antiemetic (anti-nausea) medication. Constipation may be prevented or managed by dietary modification (increase of fluid and fiber) as well as the use of medications such as stool softeners and laxatives. Lastly, it is worth noting that people respond differently to different medications and a certain amount of trial and error may be necessary to find the best medication for any given individual.

Myth: People with a history of chemical dependency should never be treated with opioid medication.
There is no question that these patients present unique challenges. However, to accept this statement as an iron clad rule does a grave disservice to this patient population. Health-care providers should treat each patient individually, taking all factors into consideration. A careful medical history should be gathered along with information about the individual's history of substance abuse. Whenever possible, it is generally considered preferable to avoid prescribing opioid medication if adequate pain control can be achieved by other means. However, there are times when this is not possible, and it is never acceptable to withhold opioid medication as a viable treatment option for those suffering severe, unrelieved pain. The American Pain Society states that those with known addiction have been shown to benefit from judicious use of opioids to manage postoperative pain, cancer pain, and even forms of recurrent pain.

When health-care providers do prescribe medication for such individuals, their tendency is to keep doses low out of fear of worsening their dependency. However, these patients often require more than the typical dose of opioids to achieve adequate pain relief because they may have a tolerance. In addition, such individuals typically are more sensitive to pain than the average person because their body has stopped producing endorphins. When the decision is made to prescribe opioids for such patients, it should be done thoughtfully, and such patients should be monitored carefully by their primary health-care provider.

Myth: People with chronic pain can learn to develop a greater tolerance for it.
The phrase "just learn to live with it" has been recited all too often to patients who endure chronic pain, and it sends with it the message that health-care providers no longer care and are giving up on any efforts to provide help. It also implies that patients should somehow be able to turn down their sensitivity to pain and feel it less. The first message is sad, the second is absurd, and both are unacceptable.

Those with chronic pain sometimes accept the reality of continued pain, but this is not the same thing as developing a tolerance for it. Their suffering continues and, if anything, is worsened by their feelings of abandonment and isolation.

Myth: Those who complain of chronic pain are really just depressed.
Living with chronic pain takes a severe toll. It is physically, emotionally, psychologically, and spiritually exhausting. Add to this feelings of abandonment and isolation, and the result may be feelings of helplessness and hopelessness. Is it any wonder then, that such individuals are prone to depression?

Depression is indeed a problem among those who suffer from chronic pain. However, it is unfair to assume that the depression caused the pain when, in fact, the reverse is more likely true. In any case, one certainly compounds the other. Unrelieved pain contributes to feelings of depression, and depression certainly impairs the individual's ability to cope effectively with pain. Furthermore, it seems to actually increase their pain sensitivity. Caring and compassionate health-care providers should, therefore, address both issues without implying judgment.

Index

Page numbers followed by f indicate figures; t, tables; b, boxes.

H